Theoretical Nursing
Development and Progress

J.B. LIPPINCOTT COMPANY
Philadelphia

New York   *St. Louis*   *London*   *Sydney*   *Tokyo*

Theoretical Nursing
Development and Progress
Second Edition

Afaf Ibrahim Meleis, R.N., Ph.D., F.A.A.N.

Professor, Department of Mental Health,
Community, and Administrative Nursing
School of Nursing
University of California
San Francisco, California

Acquisitions Editor: David Carroll
Coordinating Editorial Assistant: Amy Stonehouse
Project Editor: Virginia Barishek
Indexer: Ann Cassar
Design Coordinator: Kathy Kelley-Luedtke
Production Manager: Caren Erlichman
Production Coordinator: Sharon McCarthy
Compositor: TCSystems
Printer/Binder: R.R. Donnelley & Sons Company

1 3 5 6 4 2

Library of Congress Cataloging-in-Publication Data

Meleis, Afaf Ibrahim.
    Theoretical nursing : development and progress / Afaf Ibrahim
Meleis.—2nd ed.
      p. cm.
    Includes bibliographical references.
    Includes index.
    ISBN 0-397-54823-0 :
    1. Nursing—Philosophy.   I. Title.
    [DNLM: 1. Philosophy, Nursing.   WY 86 M519t]
    RT84.5.M45   1991
    610.73'01—dc20
    DNLM/DLC
    for Library of Congress   90-6504
                                           CIP

To Soad Hussein Hassan, R.N., Ph.D.—a maverick—for exemplifying humanism and commitment, for encouraging feminism and autonomy, for accepting challenge and diversity, for tolerating rebellion, for sponsoring inquisitiveness, and for being my mother.

And
To Mahmoud Meleis, Ph.D.: for caring without knowing; for knowing and challenging without understanding; and then, for understanding and supporting.

PREFACE

The rationale for writing the first and the second editions of *Theoretical Nursing: Development and Progress* parallels some developmental phases in my career. I wrote the first edition because I was inspired by nurses who have dared to conceptualize and theorize in a practice discipline and because I was privileged to have worked with some significant mentors who have, knowingly or unknowingly, supported my evolving ideas and showed me the ropes.

The writing of the second edition, however, was inspired by a completely different group of mentors and supporters: the readers of my writings in general and of the first edition in particular. They are the students who thought the book helped them to demystify theory; the clinicians who shared with me the ways by which they were able to connect their expertise and their practice with theoretical nursing; the colleagues who have taken the time to write or call analyzing, critiquing, and extending the ideas I have presented; the conference audiences who persisted in their attempts to meet with me and to discuss and debate ideas; and others who through serendipitous meetings were ready with comments, examples, and recommendations. One particularly significant comment I have heard repeatedly was that the ideas conveyed in the first edition have *"touched their lives in a meaningful and profound way."* My response to these readers is *"not as much as your comments have touched mine."* All these comments were thoughtful, stimulating, and challenging. In short, the intense interactions with nurses (national and international educators, students, administrators, clinicians, researchers, theoreticians), my international research on women, and my research on immigrants in the United States have all helped in shaping the modifications and changes reflected in this second edition.

For those who understood, those who did not understand, those who challenged me, those who supported my arguments, as well as those who provided counterarguments, I have learned a great deal from you and I have attempted to reflect all that in this edition.

Once again, here is a synthesis that reflects a pride in our discipline, a respect for our heritage, a concern about health care for those who need it the most, a belief in our abilities to develop knowledge, and a belief in the potential of knowledge development in empowering our profession as well as our clients. I share these ideas with you, claiming neither finality nor closure. I only share them to initiate, maintain, and support dialogues about theoretical nursing. If you are moved to discuss, challenge, refute, critique, support, extend, or discard any of the ideas presented here, I will consider that writing the second edition was a worthwhile endeavor.

Many people helped me to accept the challenge of writing the second edition. David Carroll, my editor at J.B. Lippincott Company, proposed the second edition and encouraged and supported my efforts with advice and prompt responses. Barbara Mow, reluctant at first to undertake typing this project, then tackled it with enthusiasm and zeal, demonstrating throughout a commitment to perfection and deadlines.

There is no project of this magnitude that does not attract questions, discussions, and solicited or unsolicited advice from family members and friends. These daily subtle or unsubtle inquiries ("How far along are you in writing the second edition?" "Aren't you finished yet?") from many continents in the world kept me focused and ensured progress. It is much easier to maintain deadlines than to attempt to justify delays to all these interested family members and friends. Therefore, they all have played a significant role in my accepting to do the second edition and in completing it.

The attention given my work by my sons, Waleed and Sherief, and their constant attempts to understand my perspective have been enormously valuable at many more levels than could be given justice here. To them I offer my special appreciation for their intellectual support.

Mahmoud, my friend and husband, continues to give of himself, his time, and his energy, in supporting all aspects of my professional, academic, and personal life, as well as in such tangible ways as reviewing and verifying references, citations, tables, and figures.

Afaf Ibrahim Meleis, R.N., Ph.D., F.A.A.N.

PREFACE TO THE FIRST EDITION

"How long did it take you to write your book?" is perhaps the most frequently asked question of a writer. It is not a question that can be answered with any degree of precision. Thoughts, ideas, and analyses exist long before they ever become written and translated into an articulate whole. If there is an answer to the question above, maybe it could be that it all started in 1969 when Dorothy Johnson asked me to teach her theory classes while she was on sabbatical leave. I owe a great deal to her and I learned a great deal from her. Not only did she leave an indelible impression upon me, but she provided me with the first opportunity to test my ideas about theory; I have been teaching theory ever since.

However, it is possible that I began this book even earlier. When I started my graduate work at UCLA in 1964, the late Burton Meyer challenged me to identify the theoretical underpinnings for my research and practice. His questions—incomprehensible at the beginning—were the impetus for my interest in theory, an interest that was then fostered by many others. Ralph Turner continued to challenge me with his critiques of my research, continued to help me by smoothing the rough edges of my conceptualizations, and continued to provide for me, in his presence, a model of scholarliness. To both of these men I am indebted for their profound influence. I am also grateful to Martha Rogers and Abe Kaplan, who managed to ignite my interest in both philosophy and humanism.

The discussion, analysis, and debates with students over the past years while teaching theory in the United States, Europe, and the Middle East have sharpened my ideas and have challenged me to further develop my thoughts and to refine the focus contained in this book. My students have been among my staunchest supporters and my best critics; I greatly value the impetus to ideas and insights that these ongoing dialogues have provided.

I would like to acknowledge the anonymous reviewers of this manuscript. Their exhaustive and extensive reviews and critiques have been pivotal in the development of the book. I hope I have done justice to their recommendations and that I have matched their seriousness in criticism with equal seriousness in revision. *Vive la* collegial skepticism!

Cheyney Johansen is a true author's companion. She typed and edited the numerous drafts, starting from a prospectus to a completed manuscript. I have appreciated her striving for perfection, her involvement and sense of pride in the book, and, most of all, the energy and dedication with which she approaches her work.

I am grateful to the J.B. Lippincott Company staff for their support from inception to completion. John Connolly's innovative approach and Paul Hill's unwavering support have helped immensely to bring the book to fruition.

It is nearly impossible to express in words the appreciation I feel toward my friend and husband, Mahmoud. He provides joy, insights, wisdom, challenge, and support to my life that is reflected in all of its facets, including this book. He and my sons, Waleed and Sherief, actively participated in the thinking and writing process by asking questions, participating in discussions, and assuming more family responsibilities. What I have learned from them is incalculable, and my debt to them is enormous.

Afaf Ibrahim Meleis, R.N., Ph.D., F.A.A.N.

CONTENTS

Theoretical Nursing
Development and Progress

Part *1*

Our Theoretical Journey

*U*ncovering the role that theory plays in our daily experiences is the first step of the theoretical journey proposed in this book. The two chapters in this part describe the journey and its destinations: Chapter 1 describes the assumptions of the journey, the organizational plan, and the supporting material; Chapter 2 sets the stage for the journey by providing key definitions of theoretical terms.

Chapter 1

Introduction

By unfolding the development of our theoretical past, we gain insights that improve our understanding of our current progress, and we are empowered to achieve our disciplinary goals. By looking at our theoretical present, we see shadows of our past as well as visions of our future. Reconstructing our theoretical heritage is a process that involves reconstructing our present reality. The intent of the journey proposed in this book is to demonstrate the progress of nursing through analyses of the philosophical assumptions, the theoretical methods, and the theoretical threads in the discipline. We will perform these analyses in ways that value our experiences as nurses, in ways that support and enhance our progress, and in ways that allow us to proactively develop theories that represent and guide our nursing actions. Synthesizing insights of the past with visions of the future can enhance creativity in the discipline of nursing, significantly furthering its development and progress.

This book is designed to unfold the thought processes inherent in nursing, to analyze the origins of nursing ideas, and to contribute to the ongoing dialogue about the role of theory in the development of the discipline of nursing. Its intent is to provide the reader with the knowledge base necessary to understand the theoretical present of nursing and to begin to formulate ideas for the future.

The development of the discipline of nursing has progressed by leaps and bounds in the last decade. Few would dispute the notion that theory in general has been responsible for this development, yet many still question its effect. The thesis of this book is that the evolution of the discipline of nursing and its scholarliness is greatly intertwined with its focus on theory and theory development. The discussions go beyond this thesis to delineate boundaries of nursing knowledge, origins of knowledge, theories that guided the development of nursing's scientific base, and criteria of truth that the discipline may or may not employ. While the book intends to provide the reader with a sense of history, the process itself helps to unfold a futuristic course.

The ideas contained in this book are articulated to vehemently compete with any work that denigrates the theoretical history of nursing—past, present, or future. At the same time, the ideas complement and are intended to collaborate with all other writings of colleagues on theory and metatheory. When I provided critique, I attempted to voice it from our perspective and to analyze from within the contextual forces and constraints.

It is not the intent of this book to promote a certain epistemological perspective, a certain theory, or a certain set of ontological propositions over any others. Instead, this book explores, discusses, analyzes, critiques, compares, and contrasts different epistemologies, theories of truth, and nursing theories. It delineates components of theory and criteria for theory critique. It describes different strategies used in the development of nursing theories and the consequences of each strategy. This book is intended to be used by those who want to understand a significant aspect of the nursing discipline that has been dichotomized with practice and shadowed by an emphasis on education of nurses. It attempts to promote understanding, not by dissecting the discipline of nursing into separate compartments, but rather by emphasizing nursing as a discipline that is based on philosophy, theory, practice, and research. Although the focus is on nursing theories, the relationships and interdependence among research, art, philosophy, and practice are highlighted and explicated.

This book is based on several assumptions:

- ○ Understanding theory and its role is enhanced by exploring the origin of ideas and the processes by which ideas develop into theories.
- ○ Pluralism in nursing theories is desirable and inevitable; therefore, an exploration of existing theories is essential for improving the utility of theory and for continuing the development and progress of the discipline.
- ○ A critical assessment of the history of theoretical thought will pave the way for development of theories that further describe and prescribe nursing practice. This understanding will help delineate issues that could be resolved in the future.

Theory is no longer a luxury in nursing. There was a time when using theory was equated with developing a conceptual framework to be used only as a guide to curriculum development. Theory now is part and parcel of the nursing lexicon in education, administration, and practice. We need to understand its role in the discipline, the processes and strategies used to develop it, the most accepted criteria used to analyze and critique it, and how to use it to enhance the discipline.

THE THEORETICAL JOURNEY

Like all journeys, the journey proposed for you, the reader, could be short or long, detached or involved, superficial or profound, simple or complex, preplanned or spontaneous, and structured or discovered. Like all journeys, this one has maps, destinations, lampposts, detours, setbacks, surprises, disappointments, and insights. Like all journeys, you will get out of it what you put into it. It has been my experience in sharing this journey with others through teaching, research, or practice that the insights gained and advancements in knowledge made depend on complete openness to the journey, on true involvement in all its aspects, and on synthesizing this journey with personal experiences.

Therefore, you are invited to embark on a long journey that spans the theoretical past, present, and future of our discipline. You are also encouraged to reflect on your own theoretical journey and to compare and contrast your journey with that of the discipline. Both journeys will take on different meanings—the insights from one journey will enhance the insights from the other.

The following are some questions to guide a reflective approach to your journey:

- ○ How did you come to define theory, nursing, human beings, and health? What values and assumptions do these definitions hold, and what courses of action are dictated by those values?
- ○ What theories guided you in your assessment of your patients, in your research projects, and in your teaching methods? Why did you select these theories? How congruent are the ontological beliefs of these theories with your own? With those of the discipline of nursing?
- ○ What criteria did you use in selecting or rejecting theories to guide your actions? Are these the same as or different from those criteria used in selecting or rejecting nursing theories?
- ○ In what ways do you demonstrate your critical assessment of progress in theoretical and scientific nursing? Are these critiques illuminated by a true understanding of daily experiences of members of the discipline? Are these critiques guided by a nursing perspective?

ORGANIZATION OF THE BOOK

To improve the potential of achieving the goals of understanding the role of theory in the development and progress of the discipline and understanding the role of members of the discipline in developing and constructing theory, this book is organized in parts and chapters according to potential illuminations throughout the journey. It is divided into seven major parts.

Part One describes terms of the journey into the past and the future; it includes this introduction, assumptions to guide the journey, and the lampposts that define key elements of the journey.

Part Two presents a historical analysis of the discipline's progress toward its present theoretical perspective. Stages of development and milestones leading to the next phase are discussed. A proposed pattern of progress unique to the discipline of nursing is explored. Forces and barriers are discussed that may have affected theory development and therefore indirectly affected the scholarly evolution of the discipline of nursing. Different theories of progress are explored, and the course of development of nursing knowledge is traced, compared, and contrasted with the development of other sciences.

Part Three focuses on an analysis of the discipline as it is perceived by its members at the beginning of the 1990s. It is devoted to a description of the domain of nursing, its central problems, and its scholarliness and includes discussion of the tools that have contributed to nursing's scholarly standing and the criteria by which a scholarly discipline is assessed. Part Three also proposes models to be considered in developing theories.

Part Four evolves from the analysis provided in Parts One, Two, and Three. In this part, the relationship between the theoretical past and theoretical present and the structure, processes, and meaning of effective theories are delineated and discussed. Nursing metatheorists have debated about the nature of nursing and its underpinnings: whether nursing is basic or applied science, whether its theories are unique or borrowed, and whether its theories are conceptual models or applied theories. The first chapter of this part provides a discussion of the major sources and resources for theory development and the major historical issues related to nursing theory. The second chapter focuses on strategies, processes, and tools essential to the development of theories. Several major strategies are considered and exemplars are included. Part Four concludes with a model for the description, analysis, critique, and testing of theory.

Part Five focuses on our theoretical present. It begins with a classification of nursing theories according to their paradigmatic origins and then presents a discussion of domain concepts as they have emerged from these existing theories. The balance of this part is devoted to the utilization of the model for theory description, analysis, critique, and testing that was proposed in the previous part for analyzing selected theories in nursing. The selections, based on the theories' central questions, are matched with the domain concepts.

Part Six discusses conclusions and future directions. A future course is charted, and means for achieving that course are proposed.

Part Seven is divided into two chapters. The first contains an abstracted analysis of selected central writings on metatheory and nursing theory. It is not intended as a comprehensive compilation of abstracts of everything that has been written about metatheory and theory; rather, it is intended as a beginning—but central—collection that you are encouraged to use as a model for your own collection of analytical abstracts. The analyses are intended to provide a beginning point for discussion and debate. The last chapter in this part, the final chapter of the book, contains an extensive and considerable bibliography on metatheory, on paradigms that have been used in nursing, and on nursing theory.

Sections 1 through 12 of that chapter, containing the metatheory literature, are organized around common themes in nursing and theory, such as philosophy and methods, theory development in nursing, forces and constraints in theory development, theory and science, theory and research, theory and practice, theory and education, and theory analysis and critique. Section 13 contains writings about nursing theories by theorists or by others who have used the theories for research practice, education, or administration. You can find all the writings related to a theory—to the best of my knowledge—by looking under the theorist's last name in this section. Asterisked citations in this entire chapter indicate citations that have been abstracted and analyzed in the previous chapter under metatheory or theory.

Sections 14 through 24 contain writings on several central paradigms that have influenced the discipline of nursing, including psychoanalytical theory, symbolic interaction, developmental systems, adaptation, and role theories. Section 25 provides a descriptive list of audio and video tapes that have been created to explicate theorists' ideas.

This book is designed to be used sequentially as well as nonsequentially. This free use of each chapter and each part necessitates a slight repetitiveness of ideas. The repetitions are intended to emphasize and expand on significant themes and to present the same or similar ideas with a different analytical posture. This book ideally should be employed in five teaching/learning units: the first focusing on Parts One and Two; the second on Part Three; the third on Part Four; the fourth on Part Five; the fifth on Part Six. Part Seven provides the necessary supportive material for each of the parts.

ON A PERSONAL NOTE

Writing and reading books are both existential experiences and ongoing, evolving processes. Neither the reader nor the writer is the same person after reading or writing a book, nor are their ideas and viewpoints the same. A book is never complete because ideas are never complete. Yet at some point a project needs to be abandoned so that others can explore its ideas in order to modify, extend, affirm, refine, or refute their own—all of which, if shared with the author, will allow her to do the same.

I urge you to consider this book complete as well as incomplete, a temporarily abandoned project that represents my own thinking and analysis. It incorporates my past, present, and future, intermingled with the past, present, and future of nursing and of nurse theorists. It is from all of this that my present interpretation of theoretical nursing has evolved, but this continuous, evolving process is presented here with temporal boundaries. Therefore, if I misinterpreted any theorists' or metatheorists' admonitions, it was unintentional, and my critique should be viewed as an honest epistemological interpretation bounded by cognitive, historical, and sociocultural meanings of the time.

I firmly believe that without the theorists and metatheorists and their writings, this book would not have been written, nor would it have been necessary. Interpretations and selections of theorists and metatheorists and their ideas were not guided by desire for omission but rather by limitations imposed by time and space. The conceptualizations of all theorists and all the analyses of the metatheorists, whether included in this text or not, provide the tapestry that depicts the future of theoretical nursing.

Finally, I have tried to avoid language that suggests stereotypical views of the nurse, patient, and physician, but there were times when comprehension, clarity, and simplicity took precedence. Because the majority of nurses are women, I have used "she" to encompass both "she" and "he." I have done the same elsewhere with "he."

Chapter 2

Theory: Who Needs It . . . What Is It?

THE DESTINATION: THEORY AND THEORETICAL THINKING

The destination of our theoretical journey is to achieve a useful level of theoretical thinking and to further the development of theoretical nursing.

Theory is the goal of all scientific work; theorizing is a central process in all scientific endeavors; and theoretical thinking is essential to all professional undertakings. This book is about theory, theorizing, and theoretical thinking. It is about theoretical activities that have occupied·clinicians, theoreticians, and researchers. It is about how we have been theorizing and using theory, perhaps without attaching the label of theory to these activities. It is also about how we can continue to advance the discipline of nursing through knowledge development, how we can enhance professional nursing through the process of nurses conceptualizing their actions, and how we can facilitate better care for clients through theory-based policies. This book does not provide recipes for achieving these goals; instead, it provides ideas intended to enable you, the reader, to pursue your own goals, to develop your own recipes, and to share your insights and wisdom with your colleagues.

Despite the tremendous progress made in the theoretical development of the discipline of nursing, as demonstrated in the explosion of theoretical writing, there remains confusion about the role of theory in the development of knowledge and about the role of researchers and clinicians as theorists. As is true in all other disciplines, it is natural and expected for some nurses to declare themselves only clinicians, only theoreticians, or only researchers. Yet it is cause for concern when theorization, theory development, and theory utilization are seen as ivory tower activities, removed from other scientific and professional processes because they are activities that clinicians and researchers perform in some form or other, with varying degrees of intensity, throughout their careers.

Increasingly, nurses are demonstrating more commitment to the activities associated with theory. This commitment is manifested in the language that nurses use to describe the activities that occupy them, for example, when they refrain from using non-criteria-based adjectives to describe theory utilization in nursing. Skepticism and non-criteria-based critiques that are founded on limited knowledge and a paucity of criteria are not helpful in making changes or in developing knowledge. Healthy skepticism and criteria-based critiques that are based on knowledge are, however, essential to the development of knowledge.

Theory and theoretical thinking are not limited to theoreticians in the discipline. Theoretical thinking is integral to all the roles played by nurses, including those of researcher, clinician, consultant, and administrator. In research, for example, theoretical thinking could be demonstrated in all aspects of the research process. First, it is demonstrated in identifying the phenomenon within the domain of nursing, in differentiating between relevant and irrelevant phenomenon, and in deciding how the research questions are related to the theoretical domain of nursing and to the focus of nursing practice. In a human science, theoretical thinking is also demonstrated when and if the researcher attempts to determine the importance of the research questions and answers to humanity, as well as the significance of the research topic or focus to the researcher. Theoretical thinking helps in raising questions about the meaning of the researcher's personal commitment to the research process. When these questions are raised, discussed, and answered, a process of theoretical thinking has already occurred.

Second, after defining a phenomenon, theoretical thinking continues to guide the process of research (Quinn, 1986). The researcher seeks theories that can help explain this phenomenon or that can prescribe a nursing action for it. If theories are available, then the researcher evaluates them to decide on the most useful theory for the research process—one that will help to expand knowledge. Evaluation of theories is as much the business of the theoretician as it is the business of the researcher and the clinician. The researcher evaluates whether a theory should be tested as well as whether and in which ways the findings of the research can help refine and extend the theory. The clinician evaluates theories for utilization in practice. This evaluation of a theory, for research or practice, is integral to the whole process of theorizing and demonstrates another aspect of theoretical thinking.

Third, after evaluation, propositions are developed to guide the research process or to test the theory. Fourth, after testing a theory or propositions of a theory, the researcher may complete the task by simply describing the findings or by interpreting those findings in relationship to the original theory, perhaps choosing to refine, extend, or modify the original theory. Each of these activities is theoretical in nature and represents theoretical thinking and theory- building, and each of these activities should be acknowledged as an aspect of engaging in the work needed to develop theoretical nursing.

The professional clinician goes through a similar process in deciding what to assess in her clients, the timing of assessment, how she defines the needed actions, and what interventions are best for the situation. Some of these decisions are based on theory, others could be the impetus for theoretical development. These processes predicate processes of analysis and development described in this book. To enhance an understanding of these processes, definitions of some key concepts are proposed as a baseline.

DEFINITIONS

There are many ways to define each concept employed in developing, evaluating, and using theories. I encourage you to become knowledgeable about the different definitions and to select the options that are most congruent with your own philosophical values. The following definitions are limited in depth and scope, and are provided only as guidelines for your refinements and extensions.

Philosophy

Philosophy is a distinct discipline in its own right, and all disciplines can claim their own philosophical bases that form guidelines for their goals. Philosophy is concerned with the values and beliefs of a discipline and with the values and beliefs held by members of the discipline. Individuals' values and beliefs may or may not be congruent with those of the discipline. Philosophy focuses on providing the framework for asking both ontological and epistemological questions about central concepts of the discipline. It also provides the assumptions that guide theories.

The philosophy of a science deals with the values that govern the scientific development and the justification of the discipline. It helps in defining or questioning priorities and goals. Philosophical inquiries help members of the discipline to uncover issues surrounding priorities and to analyze these priorities against societal and humanistic priorities.

Science

Science is a unified body of knowledge about phenomena that is supported by agreed-upon evidence. Science includes disciplinary questions and it provides answers to questions that are central to the discipline. These answers represent wisdom based on the results of data that have been obtained through the different designs and methodological approaches. These answers are also the seeds from which science evolves and develops. There are different approaches to evaluating and judging scientific findings: support of truth through repeated findings; tentative consensus among a community of scholars supporting aspects of evidence; tentative consensus among other subcommunities attesting to descriptions of reality; and the use of objective criteria by members of the community (Brown, 1977; Popper, 1962; Kuhn, 1962).

Domain

Domain is the perspective and the territory of the discipline. It contains the subject matter of a discipline, the main agreed-upon values and beliefs, the central concepts, the phenomenon of interest, its central problems, and the methods that are used to provide some answers in the discipline. A domain includes the players and the actors who help ask and answer the questions. The actors for the domain of nursing are the clinicians, the researchers, the theorists, the metatheorists, the philosophers, the teachers, the consultants, and the ethicists.

Phenomenon

Phenomenon is all aspects of reality that can be consciously sensed or experienced. Phenomena within a discipline are those aspects that fall within the domain or the territory of the discipline. A phenomenon is the term, description, or label given to describe an idea about an event, a situation, a process, a group of events, or a group of situations. A phenomenon may be temporally and geographically bound. Phenomena can be described from evidence that is sense-based (*e.g.*, something seen, heard, smelled, or felt) or from evidence that is grouped together through thought connections (*e.g.*, the observation that more children die in pediatric intensive care units on the 3:00 to 11:00 p.m. shift than on other shifts). In the latter example, simply observing the deaths does not make the phenomenon; it is the connection between the deaths and the specific shift that makes it a phenomenon. As another example, taking a certain amount of time to adjust to new time zones, having trouble remembering, experiencing foggy thinking, and being indecisive may all be part of the phenomenon related to flying across time zones.

Concept

Concept is a term or label used to describe a phenomenon or a group of phenomena. Concept denotes some degree of classification or categorization. A concept provides us with a concise summary of thoughts related to a phenomenon; without such concise labeling, we would have to go into great detail to describe the phenomenon. Notice the difference between describing the phenomenon of what happens to individuals who travel from one time zone to another through detailing their sleep disturbances, the changes in their moods and eating habits, and so forth, and summarizing all those details through the concept of "jet lag." The latter is a more concise and efficient way of communicating.

Theory

Theory is an organized, coherent, and systematic articulation of a set of statements related to significant questions in a discipline that are communicated in a meaningful whole. It is a symbolic depiction of aspects of reality that are discovered or invented for the purpose of describing, explaining, predicting, or prescribing responses, events, situations, conditions, or relationships. Theories have concepts that are related to the discipline's phenomenon. These concepts relate to each other to form theoretical statements.

Paradigm

The definition of paradigm is closely associated with Kuhn (1970), who introduced the concept to those members of the scientific community interested in philosophical discourses. Critics and supporters of Kuhn's work have created a multitude of meanings for paradigm, which was further confused by the many usages of the term that Kuhn demonstrated in his own writings. Kuhn himself reported a critic's finding of "twenty-two different" usages of paradigm in his writings (Kuhn, 1977, p. 294). Paradigm is defined as those aspects in a discipline that are shared by its scientific community. To dispose of the confusion created by his multiple use of paradigm, Kuhn (1977, p. 297) proposed to replace it with "disciplinary matrix." A *disciplinary matrix* includes the shared commitments of the community of scholars, the shared symbolic generalizations, and the exemplars, which are the shared problems and solutions in the discipline. The varied and at times conflicting definitions of paradigm within and among disciplines makes its use in nursing problematic.

Assumptions

Assumptions are statements that describe concepts or connect two concepts that are factual, accepted as truths, and represent values, beliefs, or goals. These statements represent the thread that holds different aspects of knowledge together. Assumptions are the taken-for-granted statements of the theory, the concept, or the research that preceded. When assumptions are challenged, they become propositions. Assumptions emanate from philosophy; they may or may not represent the shared beliefs of the discipline.

Nursing Theory

Nursing theories are reservoirs in which findings related to nursing concepts, such as comfort, healing, recovering, mobility, rest, caring, enabling, fatigue, and family care, are stored. They are also reservoirs for answers related to significant nursing phenomena, such as post-stroke levels of cognition, refusing a rehabilitation regimen for myocardial infarction patients, and revolving admissions.

The definition of nursing theory has been most problematic, as demonstrated by many exchanges in the nursing literature. Many concepts have been used interchangeably with theory, such as conceptual framework, conceptual model, paradigm, metaparadigm, theorem, and perspective. The multiple use of concepts to describe the same set of relationships has resulted in more confusion and perhaps in less use of nursing theory.

There are several types of theory definitions, the first four of which were identified by Chinn and Jacobs (1987):

1. The first type of definition focuses on the structure of theory, as exemplified by McKay (1969), who defined theory as "logically interrelated sets of confirmed hypotheses" (p. 394). This definition incorporates research as a significant step in theory development and discounts conceptualizations that are based only on mental processes. Therefore, using this definition would not allow for consideration of any of the current nursing theories as theories.

2. The second type of definition focuses on the goals upon which the theory is based. Different theorists, such as Dickoff and James (1968), define nursing theory as "a conceptual system or framework invented for some purpose" (p. 198). Not only do they focus on outcomes and consequences because of their premise that prescriptive theory should be the ultimate goal for all theory activities in nursing, but they also do not distinguish in their definition between conceptual framework and theory. Indeed, theory is defined in terms of a conceptual framework. This definition also brings to our attention the potential for inventing nursing reality (Chinn and Jacobs, 1987, p. 65); and mental images are therefore not restricted to the discovery of reality but to the construction of reality.

3. The third type of definition alludes to the tentative nature of theory, as exemplified by Barnum (1990). Barnum defines theory as "a statement that purports to account for or characterize some phenomenon" (p. 1). Barnum goes on to emphasize that the source of nursing theory is not "what is" but what "ought to be" and that existing conceptualizations are indeed nursing theories because, she asserts, quibbling over labels of theory, concept, framework, and so forth only "leads one to worry over labels rather than to look at the substance of the given thesis" (p. xi). Barnum's definition is significant in a number of ways. It acknowledges that theories are always in the process of development (Chinn and Jacobs, 1987), that existing conceptualizations are theories, and that invention is as much an arena for theory development in nursing as discovery is.

4. The fourth type of definition focuses on research and is exemplified by Ellis (1968). Ellis defines theory as "a coherent set of hypothetical, conceptual, and pragmatic principles forming a general frame of reference for a field of inquiry" (p. 217). Ellis' definition reminds us that theory is developed for the purpose of guiding research. This definition assumes that practice guides theory development, theory guides research, and research guides theory.

5. A fifth definition emerged from the first four and was articulated by Chinn and Jacobs (1987). They define theory as:

A set of concepts, definitions, and propositions that projects a systematic view of phenomena by designating specific interrelationships among concepts for purposes of describing, explaining, predicting, and/or controlling phenomena (p. 70).

According to this definition, when concepts are defined and interrelated in some coherent whole for some purpose, we have a theory. The definition leaves the door wide open for using theory in practice and research and does not restrict theory to research-verified propositions. This definition exemplifies the multiple usages of theory.

6. A sixth type of definition focuses on nursing phenomena and is exemplified by Fawcett (1989). Nursing theories "are made up of concepts and propositions," they address "phenomena with much greater specificity than do conceptual models," (p. 17) and they address "the metaparadigm phenomenon of person, environment, health, and nursing by specifying relationships among variables derived from these phenomena" (p. 22). This type of description adds a new dimension to the definition of nursing theory: the specific, agreed-upon nursing concepts. (See Table 2-1 for a summary of these different types of definitions for nursing theory.)

The definition of nursing theory adopted in this text was based on the following:

○ The work and the definitions of previous theorists, particularly their common themes, was taken into account.
○ Theorists and utilizers have used different labels interchangeably to describe their conceptualizations, and criteria for selection of

Table 2–1
Types of Theory Definitions

Chinn and Jacobs (1987) identify four types:
1. Definitions focusing on structure
2. Definitions focusing on practice goals
3. Definitions focusing on tentativeness
4. Definitions focusing on research

From these, Chinn and Jacobs (1987) present a fifth type:
5. Definitions focusing on concepts and the use of theory in practice as well as research

Fawcett (1989) provides a sixth type:
6. Definitions focusing on nursing phenomena

---

the different labels (model, paradigm, science, theory, framework) are not always entirely clear and are sometimes used to describe similar structures. For example, the utilizers of theory have used "models" and "theories" interchangeably; although some usage differentiated between models and theories, such differentiation was not completely clear. Models are considered structures of concepts preexisting theory, or as structures of concepts evolving from theory. (Refer to Chapter 19, where a cursory review of article titles will document this multiple usage).

A deliberate decision was made to avoid the fine-line debates about what to call existing conceptualizations. These differences are tentative at best and hair-splitting, unclear, and confusing at worst. Some theorists who differentiate between theory, metaparadigm, conceptual framework, and model have provided analyses that tend to overlap the properties of each of these concepts. If, indeed, conceptual models are more abstract, less specific, and contain fewer defined concepts and testable propositions, then their linkages with research and practice should not be expected. Because the utility of these models in practice and research have in fact been evaluated, and the linkages between theory and practice, research, education, and administration have been addressed by the utilizers, the properties of the existing conceptualizations do not lend themselves to the label "conceptual models." (See Chapter 9 for specific examples.) Therefore, the differences between the different labels (theory, metaparadigm, conceptual frameworks, and so forth) are differences in emphasis rather than substance and are not worth the debate or the creation of new esoteric entities to describe the mental images of nurse theorists. The usefulness of one label over another has not helped the differentiation and has only managed to create more ambiguity for the novice and the experienced alike.

When comparing nursing theories with theories in other fields, such as role theory in sociology or psychoanalytical theory in psychology, we often find that some of our nursing theories may be as specific or as unspecific as those theories, or as abstract or as concrete—so why do we continue to unwittingly downgrade nursing theory by relegating it to a conceptual framework status when other conceptualizations have been called theory?

Theories are always in the process of development. Therefore, a theory in process should not be considered a conceptual framework; it is simply in an expected stage in the process of development.

Even if some theorists and utilizers prefer to continue to use one particular label over another, multiple theory usage may be the rationale. Theories could be used as conceptual frameworks when

concepts from different theories are linked together to form a new whole, as theoretical frameworks when concepts from some theory are given new meanings or new linkages, or as conceptual models when a theory is used as a prototype or is modeled in form or structure.
To consider the existing conceptualizations as models and frameworks for nursing as a whole is to convey the idea that nursing is conceptualized in one way and according to one model. Therefore, other conceptualizations may be excluded prematurely by the one-particular-model advocate. Proponents may ask: How can we see the world through different pairs of glasses simultaneously? (Further development of these ideas can be found in Chapter 9.)

The position taken in this book is that existing nursing conceptualizations are theories that could be used to describe and prescribe different aspects of nursing care. They are not competing models; they are complementing theories that may provide a conceptualization of different aspects, components, or concepts of the domain. They also address a specific aspect of nursing. Nursing theory is then defined as an articulated and communicated conceptualization of invented or discovered reality (central phenomena and relationships) in or pertaining to nursing for the purpose of describing, explaining, predicting, or prescribing nursing care. Therefore, not only is nursing theory an articulation of phenomena and their relationships that depicts existing or imagined reality, but such articulation has to be communicated.

Nursing theories evolve from extant nursing reality as seen through the mind of a theorist who is influenced by certain historical and philosophical processes or events. They also may evolve from a perception of ideal nursing practice, tinted by one's history (personal, professional, and disciplinary) and philosophy. Theory here is a tool for the development of research propositions (see the left side of Fig. 2-1). Theory is also a goal, a reservoir in which findings (both quantitative and qualitative) become more coherent and meaningful. The cyclical nature of theory, practice, philosophy, history, research, and science is depicted in Figure 2-1. Taken together, all these domains constitute the knowledge base for nursing theory.

Examples of phenomena and relationships depicted in nursing theories are:

A nursing client is conceptualized as a self-care agent.
A nursing client is a biopsychosocial and cultural being.
A nursing client is a system with a number of behavioral subsystems.
A nursing client is conceptualized as a conglomerate of needs.
A nursing client is a system of such modes as interdependence,
    self-concept, roles, and psyche, among others.
Person–environment interactions are the focus of nursing care.
Health and illness behavior is a product of person–environment
    interactions.

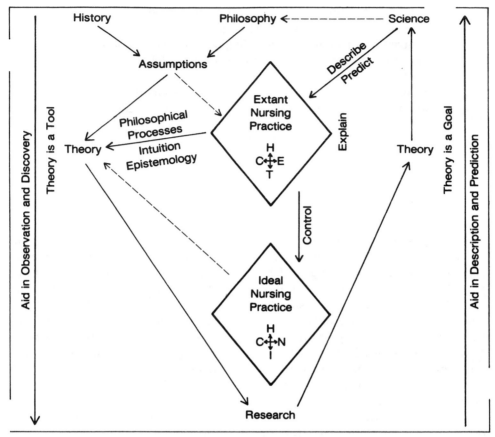

Figure 2–1. Knowledge base for nursing theory (H, health; C, client; T, transitions; E, environment; ⟺, interactions and process).

Communication is a tool for diagnosis and intervention in nursing.

An efficient, functional, productive interaction has several components: sensing, perceiving, conceiving.

A goal of interaction is to develop rapport, which in turn enhances patient care.

The focus of intervention is the client's environment.

Environment is a composite of energy fields.

Nursing care deals with manipulation of environment.

Nursing provides self-care needs only until the client or a significant other is capable of providing self-care.

A nurse is conceptualized as performing a number of functions designed to meet the patient's needs.

TYPES OF THEORIES

Nursing needs theories based on discovery of phenomena and relationships depicting realities from patients' and nurses' perspectives. To accomplish its goals of optimum health and well-being, nursing needs theories based on effective and efficient clinical therapeutics. An operational method of theory development is incongruent with its process of assessing, diagnosing, and intervening (Kritek, 1978). Therefore, the types of theories that nursing needs could be conceptualized on a grid, with process, assessment, diagnosis, intervention, and consequences as columns and description and prescription as rows. The following theories result from this grid.

Descriptive Theories

Descriptive theories are theories that describe a phenomenon, an event, a situation, or a relationship; identify its properties and its components; and identify some of the circumstances under which it occurs. Although descriptive theories have an element of prediction (for example, when a phenomenon occurs and when it does not occur), their contribution to knowledge is mainly to help sort out observations and meanings regarding the phenomenon. Descriptive theories describe a phenomenon, speculate on why a phenomenon occurs, and describe the consequences of that phenomenon; therefore, they have explanatory, relating, and predicting utility. Descriptive theories are complete theories and have the potential for guiding research.

There are two types of descriptive theories. The first type is the *factor-isolating, category-formulating,* or *labeling theory.* This theory describes the properties and dimensions of phenomena. The second type is the *explanatory theory,* which describes and explains the nature of relationships of certain phenomena to other phenomena. Examples of descriptive theories are the descriptions of the life processes of a nursing client, person–environment interactions in health and illness, health status, ways of assessment, types of diagnosing, disruptions of life processes, and interventions. Descriptive nursing theories are those theories that help describe, explain, and predict nursing phenomena and relationships between nursing phenomena. Descriptive theories are not action-oriented and do not attempt to produce a situation.

Types of descriptive theories in nursing include:

Life processes;
Person–environment interactions;
Assessment;
Diagnosis;
Descriptions of alterations in life processes; and
Clinical therapeutics.

Prescriptive Theories

Prescriptive theories are those theories addressing nursing therapeutics and the consequences of interventions. A prescriptive theory includes propositions that call for change and predict the consequences of a certain strategy of nursing intervention. A prescriptive theory should designate the prescription and its components, the type of client to receive the prescription, the conditions under which the prescription should occur, and the consequences. It articulates the conditions in the life process, person–environment interactions, and health status that need the prescription and the effect on the client's life process, health status, and interaction with his environment. Prescriptions may also be focused on the environment.

In summary, all theories used in nursing to understand, explain, predict, or change nursing phenomena are nursing theories, whether or not they evolved out of other theories, other paradigms, other disciplines, nursing experiences, diagnoses, nursing processes, or nursing practices, and whether or not they were developed by nurses. If we must differentiate between different types of theory, then such differentiation is meaningful only in terms of the goals and not the source of the theory. Theories that are developed to understand and explain human processes in health and illness are pure or basic theories. In other words, they are theories with a descriptive focus. Theories that are developed to control, promote, and change are nursing practice theories, or prescriptive theories (Crowley, 1968).

Theory Components

Theories are made up of assumptions, concepts, propositions, and exemplars. The structural components of descriptive and prescriptive theories differ somewhat.

Structural components of descriptive theories include:

Clients' state or condition; and
Patterns of responses to conditions, situations, or events, analyses of contexts of conditions and responses, and analyses of promoting and inhibiting contexts.

Structural components of prescriptive theories include:

Definition of clients' situation;
Nursing therapeutics;
Process by which therapeutics is implemented;
Patterns of desired status or consequences; and
Context for desired/undesired status and for therapeutics.

USES OF THEORY

Theory and Research

The objective of theory is to formulate a minimum set of generalizations that allow one to explain a maximum number of observable relationships among the variables of a given field of inquiry. The theory sets limits on what questions to ask and what methods to use to pursue answers to the questions. The relationship is cyclical in nature; the results of the research can then be used to verify, modify, or falsify a theoretical proposition. Nursing theories have provided a limited impetus for nursing research. Nursing research has depended more on educational, sociological, and psychological theory than on nursing theories. Nursing theories provide the boundaries within which scientists conducting research in nursing can explore significant problems of the field. In doing so, the potential for development of nursing knowledge increases.

Theory and Practice

The primary use of theory is to guide research. Through interaction with practice, guidelines for practice will evolve. Research validates and modifies theory. Theory then guides practice. Until empirical validation or modification is completed, theory can be given practical validation and can therefore be allowed to give direction to practice.

Theory provides the nurse with goals for assessment, diagnosis, and intervention. A nurse working as part of a health care team focuses on those aspects of care that are delineated in theory for a more effective assessment of a health care client. If the goals are health maintenance, promotion of self-care, and enhancement of stability during the illness episode, then the nurse has an intellectual checklist by which the levels of health, self-care needs and abilities, and stability are assessed. Diagnosis is related to those areas in which the nurse plans an intervention.

Theory is a tool that renders practice more efficient and more effective. Just by being goal-directed, our energies in assessing extraneous areas are minimized. If no nursing goals exist, the nurse might use energy and time inefficiently by considering areas of assessment or intervention that may be handled more efficiently and expertly by other members of the health care team.

There are other uses for theory. Language of theory provides us with common grounds for communication and with labels and definitions for phenomena; therefore, nursing practice could be described and explained by common concepts. These common concepts allow us to communicate succinctly with each other. More effective and efficient communication can eventually lead to further theory development as concepts are refined, sharpened, extended, and validated. Well-defined concepts with conceptual and construct validity enhance the cyclical communication between practitioners, theorists, clinicians, and educators. The world of nursing can become more coherent, more goal-oriented, and more efficient.

Professional autonomy and accountability are enhanced by theory use in practice. Being able to practice by scientific principles allows nurses the opportunity to accurately predict consequences of care and the range of patient responses. Articulation of our actions, goals, and consequences of actions enhances our accountability. If we can clearly talk about our purpose and what we hope to accomplish, perhaps other professionals and patients can do that too. Defining the focus and the means to achieving that focus and being able to predict consequences increase our control of our practice and therefore increase our autonomy. As stated by Fuller (1978),

> The autonomy of a profession rests more firmly on the uniqueness of its knowledge, knowledge gathered ever so slowly through the questioning of scientific inquiry. Nursing defined by power does not necessarily beget knowledge. But knowledge most often results in the ascription of power and is accompanied by autonomy (p. 701).

In summary, theory helps to identify the focus, the means, and the goals of practice. Using common theories enhances communication, increasing autonomy and accountability to care. Theory helps the user gain control over subject matter (Barnum, 1990). All these in turn help bring about further refinements of theory and better relationships between theory, research, and practice. Figure 2-1 identifies the relationships between theory, research, practice, and philosophy.

REFERENCES

Barnum, B.J. (1990) *Nursing theory: Analysis, application, and evaluation* (3rd ed.). Boston: Little, Brown & Co.

Brown, N.H. (1977) *Perception, theory and commitment: The new philosophy of science.* Chicago: University of Chicago Press.

Chinn, P.L. and Jacobs, M.K. (1987) *Theory and nursing: A systematic approach.* St. Louis: C.V. Mosby.

Crowley, D.M. (1968) Perspectives of pure science. *Nursing Research,* 17(6), 497–501.

Dickoff, J. and James, P. (1968) A theory of theories: A position paper. *Nursing Research,* 17(3), 197–203.

Ellis, R. (1968) Characteristics of significant theories. *Nursing Research,* 17(3), 217–222.

Fawcett, J. (1989) *Analysis and evaluation of conceptual models of nursing* (2nd ed.). Philadelphia: F.A. Davis.

Fuller, S. (1978) Holistic man and the science and practice of nursing. *Nursing Outlook,* 26, 700–704.

Kritek, P. (1978) The generation and classification of nursing diagnosis: Toward a theory of nursing. *Image,* 10(2), 33–40.

Kuhn, T.S. (1962) *The structure of scientific revolutions.* Chicago, IL: University of Chicago Press.

Kuhn, T.S. (1970) *The structure of scientific revolutions* (2nd ed.). Chicago, IL: University of Chicago Press.

Kuhn, T.S. (1977) *The essential tension.* Chicago, IL: University of Chicago Press.

McKay, R. (1969) Theories, models and systems for nursing. *Nursing Research,* 18(5), 393–399.

Popper, K. (1962) *Conjecture and refutations.* New York: Basic Books.

Quinn, J.F. (1986) Quantitative methods: Descriptive and experimental. In P. Moccia (Ed.), *New approaches to theory development.* New York: National League for Nursing.

Part 2

Our Theoretical Heritage

*T*he discipline of nursing is beginning to establish itself as a theoretical field. The process of its evolution follows a unique path, a path that is not clearly understood by those who measure nursing progress and development against the scientific revolutions of the physical and natural sciences. The origins of the nursing development path can be traced through a study of its research tradition or theory tradition, or both. This part, which includes Chapters 3, 4, and 5, traces the historical development of nursing theory and theoretical nursing. The course of the evolution of nursing as a theoretical discipline is mapped and discussed. Forces and constraints that nurses confronted in their quest to establish theoretical nursing are analyzed.

The development of the discipline of nursing is conceptualized as evolving in stages. The premise upon which the discussion proceeds is that all stages preceding the philosophy stage contribute to the development of theoretical nursing. Milestones in every stage are delineated, and the influence of each milestone on nursing theory is explored. The relationships between theory, science, practice, and philosophy are also explored.

Forces and barriers in the development of theory in nursing are identified. The roles of nurses—as nurses, as predominantly women, and as nurse theorists in the development of nursing theory against many odds—are explored and discussed. Different theories of the development and progress of nursing knowledge and of meaning, understanding, and truth are discussed, and the impact of these theories on nursing is analyzed. Part Two concludes with propositions that reject the idea that the development of the discipline of nursing follows either a revolutionary or an evolutionary path. An integrative process is proposed to describe the unique nature of progress in nursing.

Chapter 3

On the Way to Theoretical Nursing: Stages and Milestones

Ever since nurses started to care for human beings in an orderly and organized way, they have been involved in some form of theorizing. Concepts of care, comfort, communication, protection, healing, and health, among others, were utilized to guide clinical practice before they were labeled as the beginnings of nursing theories. They were not communicated in articulated wholes to describe nursing and nursing care actions. Serious labeling and communication of theories in nursing took place between 1950 and 1980.

First attempts in theoretical nursing were made by Florence Nightingale in the late 19th and early 20th centuries to describe nursing focus and action in the Crimean War. Nightingale was prompted to articulate her ideas in numerous publications for different goals. Among these goals were gaining support for a national need for nurses, achieving the education of nurses, and exposing the unhealthy conditions and environment endured by English soldiers during war situations.

Subsequent attempts in theorizing were published by American nurse educators in the mid-1950s, prompted by the need to justify different levels of nursing and the need to develop curricula for the different levels of nursing educators. To improve curricula, a handful of pioneer nurses combined their clinical expertise with educational goals and a forward vision to describe a mixture of "what are nursing goals" and "what ought to be the aims of nursing." These early theorists were aware that by developing programs that represented a nursing perspective, they would help nursing students, that is, future clinicians, to focus on nursing concepts and problems rather than on medical concepts and problems. Groups were formed and committees were constructed to answer such questions as: What is nursing? What do nurses do? and How unique is nursing from other health science disciplines? Others went further to ask: What is nursing knowledge?

Perhaps the best way to consider the history of nursing theory and to put nurses' interest in theory during the 1980s and 1990s in perspective is to consider dominant themes in the different stages of the development of nursing knowledge.

There is an implicit assumption here that those themes discussed in the literature are indicative and representative of what the discipline was interested in at different times. In addition to delineating these themes, an analysis of the theory literature itself provides us with specific milestones that may have helped the development of theoretical nursing. Both approaches provide insights into how nursing evolved into its current status.

In this chapter, then, the stages that have influenced knowledge development are traced and defined. The central themes in this chapter are:

Stages that mark the development of theoretical nursing; and
Milestones in the development and use of theoretical nursing.

STAGES IN NURSING PROGRESS

Since the time of the Crimean War, nursing has gone through many stages in its search for a professional identity and domain. It is interesting to note that our analysis and evaluation of nursing's theoretical thought, the patriarchal societies we live in, and the view and status accorded nurses and nursing may make it appear as if each of these stages was a deviation from the goal of establishing the discipline of nursing. However, each of these stages has indeed sharpened and clarified the dimensions needed for the establishment of the scientific aspects of the discipline, promoting or leading to a scholarly evolution of the nursing discipline. Each stage has helped nurses come closer to identifying the domain of nursing, defining its mission, and defining its theoretical base. Progress in the development of theoretical nursing is definable in terms of five stages: practice, education and administration, research, theory, and philosophy.

Stage of Practice

The Western version of nursing as an occupation dates from the late 19th century and the early 20th century, a product of the Crimean War. Out of the need to care for the wounded warriors, Florence Nightingale organized a group of women to deliver care under her supervision and that of the war surgeons. Nightingale focused on hygiene as her goal and environmental changes as the means to achieve that goal.

The Eastern version of the beginning of nursing gives credit to Rofaida Al-Islamiah, who accompanied the prophet Mohammed in his Islamic wars. She, too, organized a group of women and she, too, focused on hygiene and environment in caring for the wounded. In both Eastern and Western versions of the beginnings of nursing, a woman saw the need for organizing other women to care for the wounded in wars.

During this stage, the mission of nursing was defined as providing care and comfort to enhance healing and a sense of well-being and to create a healthy environment that helps in decreasing suffering and deterioration. Nurses defined their domain to include the patient and the environment in which the care is offered.

Both Nightingale and Al-Islamiah created and monitored the environment in which the caring was taking place. The stage of practice gave nursing its *raison d'etre*, its focus, and its mission. Theoretical writings by Nightingale (1946) describing the care goals and process are testimony to the potential for nurses to articulate practice activities theoretically. These writings also point to the potential for nursing as a field of practice to be articulated theoretically.

Stage of Education and Administration

From that early focus on practice and the concomitant traditions of apprenticeship and servitude, there was a shift to questions related to the constitution of the nursing curriculum. The "how to" of practice eventually was translated into what curriculum to develop and how to teach it. Almost three decades were spent experimenting with different curricula, ways of preparing teachers, modes of educating administrators for schools of nursing and for service, and ways of preparing nurse practitioners. During this stage there was a focus on the development of functional roles for nurses. The dominant themes of this stage evolved out of education and administration roles.

The significance of this stage in the theoretical development of the discipline lies in the impetus it provided nurses to ask questions related to the domain of nursing. In developing curricula that are geared toward preparing nurses for different educational levels, nurses asked such questions as: What is nursing? How different is nursing care as provided by a diploma graduate, an associate degree graduate, a bachelor of science graduate, or a master's degree graduate? These questions prompted nurses to articulate the core of nursing theory (Henderson, 1966). In a curious way, it is during this stage that the theoretical ideas of the pioneering American nurse theorists were born. A focus on teaching and education, therefore, may have paved the way for the further development of theoretical nursing.

Stage of Research

The focus on education, curriculum, teaching, learning strategies, and administration led educators to an interest in research. Experts in nursing curricula recognized that without research and a systematic inquiry into, for example, the aims of teaching/learning modalities and the teaching/learning milieu, education of nurses could not be improved. Therefore, the research interest focused on questions related to curricula.

How to teach, how to administer, how to lead, and which strategies would be more effective in teaching and administering were the questions that led to the development and expansion of nursing research (Gortner and Nahm, 1977). The first nursing research journal—titled *Nursing Research*—in the United States (and in the world) was established in 1952, and both the Southern Regional Educational Board (SREB) and the Western Council for Higher Education in Nursing (WCHEN) were developed in the mid-1950s and mid-1960s, respectively. Their objectives called for improving nursing education, enhancing nursing research productivity, and raising the quality of research. The journal, the standards, and the meetings of the SREB and WCHEN helped nursing develop its scientific norms—that "set of cultural values and mores governing the activities termed scientific" (Merton, 1973).

Criteria for reviewing scientific papers were established, based on the assumption that scientific inquiry must be judged by peers. Thus, nurse researchers began to abide by Merton's norm of universalism, the impersonal evaluation of a research product by some objective criteria (Merton, 1973, p. 270). Universities also held the same expectations for nursing faculty that they held for other faculty; specifically, members of faculty in schools of nursing were required to develop their ideas and communicate them in the scientific arena through publications in refereed journals and scholarly presentations in meetings. Therefore, when seen in the context of science, the "publish or perish" dogma was not unrealistic but was rather another norm governing nursing science. Nurses were now involved in that communality—the sharing of ideas—and their research was subjected to the scrutiny of their peers and anonymous critics (Gortner, 1980; Merton, 1973).

Nursing's initial attempts at introducing ideas and sharing research results were met with severe and, at times, devastating criticism by other nursing colleagues. (Those who participated in the early research conferences may remember the lengthy and severe research critiques that may not have considered the stage of nursing research development and that traumatized researchers and audience alike.) As a result, and in addition to universality and communality, two other norms evolved: objectivity and detached scrutiny. Objective criteria for research evaluation, which were identified and shared, provided a turning point—a scholarly medium for research refinement and further development (Leininger, 1968).

The stage of research development made major contributions to contemporary scholarly nursing. It was also the stage in which tools of science left a major mark on curricula through the new offering of research classes and statistics courses and through the several publications in which major research tools and instruments were compiled and combined.

These, then, were the beginnings of nursing inquiry and science. During this stage, as in other sciences, researchers emphasized scientific syntax—the process rather than the content of research (Kuhn, 1970). The binding frameworks or depositories of collected facts were still lacking. Nevertheless, the syntax of the discipline had been formulated.

Stage of Theory

Eventually, the fundamental questions about the essence of nursing—its mission and its goals—began to surface in a more organized way. An incisive group of leaders, nurses who believed that theory should guide the practice of nursing, wrote about the need for theory, the nature of nursing theory, how philosophers viewed theory, and how nursing theory ought to be shaped. Although nurse theorists' conceptual schemata for the discipline of nursing appeared during the education and administration stages of the discipline, it was not until the stage of theory emerged that they were taken seriously.

During this stage there were arguments about whether nursing was merely a chapter of medicine or whether it was part of the biological, natural, or physical sciences (analogous to the earlier Cartesian concept that biology is simply a chapter of physics). The Cartesian concept was rejected (biology is indeed a distinct and autonomous science), and nursing continued to resist the implication that it was a part of medicine. It became clear to a new breed of nurse leaders—the philosophers and the theorists (or conceptualists, as some referred to them)—that nursing could not be reduced to a single science that inquires into just one aspect of man, just as biology is not reducible to physics. Nursing is complex, necessitating its intrinsic autonomy in content and methods.

The search for conceptual coherence evolved from a preoccupation with syntax to the disciplined and imaginative study of the realities of nursing and the meaning and truths that guide its actions (Table 3-1). The development from preoccupation with scientific method to speculation and conceptualization in nursing is reminiscent of the development of philosophical thought in the 18th and 19th centuries. The 18th century was greatly influenced by Newton and by Bacon, who was in turn influenced by Descartes. The 19th century was dominated by Kant, whose hypothetical, deductive, and metaphysical approach encouraged the speculative nature of science. The speculators in nursing began to construct realities as they themselves saw them, and their imaginative constructs evolved from their philosophical backgrounds and from their educational inclinations.

It was natural for theory development to be influenced by the paradigms of other disciplines, by the educational background of nurse theorists, and by the philosophical underpinnings of the time. Therefore, we find premises stemming from existentialism, analytical philosophy, and pragmatism guiding the development of those theories, sometimes explicitly and very often implicitly. Nurses also adopted concepts and propositions from other paradigms, such as psychoanalysis, development, adaptation, and interaction, as well as from humanism, to guide its assessment and its action. Theories were developed in response to dissatisfaction with isolated findings in research. The emerging theories addressed the nature of the human being in interactions and transactions with the health care system as

Table 3–1
Characteristics of the Beginning of the Stage
of Theory Development

- ○ Use of external paradigms to guide theory
- ○ Uncertainty about discipline phenomena
- ○ Discrete and independent theories
- ○ Separation between research, practice, and theory
- ○ Search for conceptual coherence
- ○ Theories used for curricula
- ○ The goal of a single paradigm prevails

well as the processes of problem solving and decision making for assessment and intervention.

Although certain theoretical concepts were synthesized from diverse paradigms, most nursing theories, such as subsystems of behavior, role supplementation, therapeutic touch, and self-help, were definable and analyzable only from the nursing perspective. Theories offered a beginning agreement on the broad intellectual endeavors and the fundamental explanatory tasks of nursing. This stage offered knowledge of relevant phenomena, but there was continued uncertainty about the discipline of nursing and its intellectual goals. Just as in nuclear physics, when the first achievement was not one of observation or mathematical calculation but one of intellectual imagination, conceptual schemata evolved before there was any clear recognition of nursing's empirical scope. In nursing, the theories helped the discipline to focus on its concepts and problems.

Rogers (1970) offered a conception of nursing that focused on the constant human interaction with the environment. Johnson (1980) developed the notion that a human being—a biological system—is also an abstract system of behavior centered on innate needs. Levine (1967) and Orem (1971) proposed guidelines for nursing therapeutics that preserve the integrity of the human being, the psychology, the community affiliation; in short, the entire person. Orem reminded us that the human being is perfectly capable of self-care and should progress toward that goal (Orem, 1985).

Because of the earlier focus on education and professional identity, because the National League for Nursing stipulated a conceptual framework for curricula, and because the truth of a theory had not yet been established using the empirical positivists' criteria of corroboration, emergent theories were not used to guide practice or research but were instead used to guide teaching; consequently, scientific energies were dissipated in developing curricula that corresponded to these theories.

Although theories may have influenced practice through students, such influence was not documented in the literature that focused more on theory in educational programs. As an educator who was a member of a school that used nursing theory (also called a model) as a framework for the curriculum, I experienced the conflicts that graduates of the program encountered when they wanted to use the nursing framework that they learned in their education program in practice and were unable to do so because of its novelty and its esoteric concepts. Whether the use of nursing models in education rendered nursing care more effective and efficient is a matter left to speculation and was evidenced only in isolated incidents. The graduates of programs that were based on nursing theories in the early and mid-1960s should be encouraged to write analytical descriptions of how upon graduation they used their different theoretical programs in practice.

The nagging questions continued. What fundamental process does nursing represent? Which are its units of analysis? These questions continued to be answered because of the need for a guiding paradigm and the search for a universal theory, culminating in the search for a universal theory with explanatory power for all dimensions of nursing. One is reminded that Galileo and Descartes liked to talk of the scientist's task as that of being able to decipher once and for all the secrets of nature and to arrive at the "one true structure" of the nature of the world. However, that was a Platonic ideal rather than a plain description of the task of scientific research. Later, scientists began to discard this line of pursuit. Physicists and physiologists "now believe that . . . we shall do better in these fields by working our way toward more general concepts progressively, as we go along, rather than insisting on complete generality from the outset" (Toulmin, 1977, p. 387). Toulmin proposed that "human behavior in general represents too broad a domain to be encompassed within a single body of theory" (p. 387). When scientists accept the need for multiple theories, and when they accept the process nature of science, it will be a "sign of maturity rather than defeatism" (p. 387) within the discipline.

Because nurse scientists searched for one theory for the entire discipline, the task was either overwhelming and too highly abstract (Rogers, 1970) or too simplistic and reductionist (Orem, 1971). The sentiment of practitioners was to question the possibility and usefulness of an encompassing theory, as evidenced by the meager literature throughout the 1960s and 1970s on nursing practice utilizing nursing theory. The desire for a single conceptual framework to guide the nursing curriculum was carried to nursing practice. Nurse practitioners believed that there was also a movement toward making a choice between theories and adhering to that one particular theory. Because none of the theories addressed all aspects of nursing, nurse practitioners avoided nursing theory, ignored it, or refused to use it. A myth was being formed. However, many nurses were beginning to abandon the notion of a universal theory to describe and explain nursing phenomenon and units of analysis and to guide nursing practice, just as physicists did when they abandoned the 17th-century hope that a universal science of nature could be developed within the framework of fundamental ideas of classical mechanics.

Three themes in nursing that evolved during this stage were: acceptance of the complexity of nursing and the inevitability of multiple theories; acceptance of the need to test and corroborate major propositions of differing theories before dismissing any of them; and the idea that concepts or theories remaining in the field, through a cumulative effect, become the basis for the development of a specific perspective. Dualism and pluralism were the norms of the stage of theory. It was also during this stage that nursing developed the boundaries necessary to focus its inquiry and the flexibility necessary to allow expansion through creative endeavor.

Stage of Philosophy

As nurses began reflecting on the conceptual aspects of nursing practice, on defining the domain of nursing, and on the most appropriate methods for knowledge development, they turned to philosophical inquiries. The focus during this stage was on raising and answering questions about the nature of nursing knowledge (Silva, 1977; Carper, 1978), the nature of inquiry (Ellis, 1983), and the congruency between the essence of nursing knowledge and research methodologies (Allen, Benner, and Diekelman, 1986). During this stage, philosophy was considered an attempt to understand philosophical premises underlying nursing theory and research (Sarter,

1987), and an attempt to develop philosophical inquiry as a legitimate approach to knowledge development in nursing (Fry, 1989).

This stage influenced profoundly the intellectual discourse in nursing literature. It was during this stage that epistemological diversity was accepted and the need for ethical, logical, and epistemological inquiries was legitimized—as evidenced in the numerous philosophically based manuscripts accepted for publication (Ellis, 1983).

This stage was also marked by a scholarly maturity in the discipline, as its members acknowledged the limitation of appropriate tools to investigate fundamental and practical issues. Assumptions about wholeness of human beings, contextual variables, and holism of care called for congruent investigative tools, and nurse scholars acknowledged the complexity of capturing nursing phenomenon using existing tools (Stevenson and Woods, 1986). Accepting limitations while maintaining the reality of the contextuality and complexity of the phenomenon represents a marked scholarly maturity and the potential to focus on the development of appropriate tools.

MILESTONES IN THEORY DEVELOPMENT

The progress and development of theoretical nursing is marked by several milestones. Milestones are identified through an analysis of theoretical literature that appeared in selected nursing journals between 1950 and 1990. These milestones substantially changed the position of theory in nursing and profoundly influenced the further development of theoretical nursing. Each milestone is defined and briefly described here (Table 3-2). Identifying and defining these milestones challenges others to explore the impact each milestone may have had on the progress and development of nursing knowledge.

Table 3–2
Theory Development in Nursing: Milestones

Prior to 1955	From Florence Nightingale to nursing research
1955–1960	Birth of nursing theory
1961–1965	Theory: A national goal for nursing
1966–1970	Theory development: A tangible goal for academics
1971–1975	Theory syntax
1976–1980	A time to reflect
1981–1985	Nursing theories' revival: Emergence of the domain concepts
1986–1990	From metatheory to single domain theory

Prior to 1955—From Florence Nightingale to Nursing Research

The significant milestone of the period before 1955, which has influenced the subsequent development of all nursing science, was the establishment of the journal, *Nursing Research*, with the goal of reporting on scientific investigations for nursing by nurses and others (Fig. 3-1). The journal's most significant goal was to encourage scientific productivity. The establishment of the journal was a confirmation that nursing is indeed a scientific discipline and that its progress will depend on whether or not nurses pursue truth through an avenue that respectable disciplines take, namely research. Although Nightingale may have provided the beginning impetus for research and theory, her impact was most keenly felt in nursing education. Education of nurses had predominantly taken place in diploma programs, but there was a beginning unrest regarding a different route for nurses' education.

This period was otherwise uneventful for nursing theory, except in that the establishment of nursing research publications provided the framework for a questioning attitude that may have set the stage for inquiries into theoretical nursing.

1955–1960—The Birth of Nursing Theory: The Columbia University Teachers College Approach

Although Florence Nightingale's ideas about nursing, focusing on the relationship between health and environment, were developed in the early 1900s, it was not until the mid-1950s that nurses began to articulate a theoretical view of nursing. Questions grew out of an interest in changes in educational preparation of nurses from diploma to baccalaureate programs and out of concerns about what to include or exclude in curricula and about what nurses needed to learn in order to function as nurses.

Columbia University's Teachers College, in response to this concern, offered graduate programs that focused on education and administration. The theories taught were mainly educational and administration theories, and graduates were prepared to be competent educators and administrators. Although the focus was not on nursing science or on nursing theory, it is significant to note that most theorists who offered a conception of nursing during that decade were educated at Teachers College; these were Peplau, Henderson, Hall, Abdellah, King, Wiedenbach, and Rogers (Table 3-3).

Being prepared in the functional roles and experiencing a sense of competency in preparing syllabi, staffing patterns, and so on may have freed the creative abilities of these scholars for other aspects of the scholarly process, such as theory development or conceptual model development. Therefore, it may have been other experiences and programs that directly influenced these scholars in their theoretical pursuits (*e.g.*, Rogers' doctoral preparation at Johns Hopkins). However, whatever the other experiences were, it appears that the philosophy of Teachers College indirectly left an impact, not only on psychiatric theory and research, but also on theoretical thinking in all of nursing (Sills, 1977).

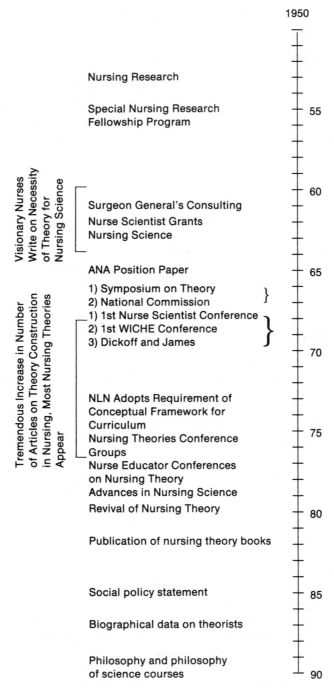

Figure 3–1. Chronology of the development of theoretical nursing.

Table 3–3
Nursing Theorists: 1950–1980

1952	Hildegarde Peplau. *Interpersonal relations in nursing*. Also published 1962, 1963, 1969.
1955	Virginia Henderson. *Textbook of the principles and practice of nursing* (with B. Harmer). Also 1966, 1972, 1978.
1959	Dorothy Johnson. *A philosophy of nursing*. Also 1961, 1966, 1974.
1959	Lydia Hall. *A philosophy of nursing*. Also 1964 (and by others, 1975).
1960	Faye Abdellah. *Patient-centered approaches to nursing*. Also 1965, 1973.
1961	Ida Jean Orlando. *The dynamic nurse-patient relationship*.
1963	D. Howland and E. McDowell. A hospital system model.
1964	D. Howland and E. McDowell. The measurement of patient care: A conceptual framework.
1964	Joyce Travelbee. *Interpersonal aspects of nursing*. Also 1969, 1971, 1979.
1964	E. Wiedenbach. *Clinical nursing: A helping art*. Also 1967, 1969, 1970, 1977.
1966	Myra Levine. Adaptation and assessment.
1966	M. Harms and F. McDonald. A new curriculum design.
1967	Myra Levine. *Introduction to clinical nursing*. Also 1969, 1971, 1973.
1968	Imogene King. A conceptual framework of reference for nursing. Also 1971, 1975.
1969	Joyce Travelbee. *Interventions in psychiatric nursing*. Also 1971 (1979).
1970	Martha Rogers. *An introduction to the theoretical basis of nursing*. Also 1980.
1970	Sister Callista Roy. Adaptation: A conceptual framework for nursing. Also 1974, 1976, 1980, 1984.
1971	Imogene King. *Toward a theory for nursing: General concepts of human behavior*.
1971	Dorothea Orem. *Nursing: Concepts of practice*. Also 1981, 1982, 1985, 1991.
1972	Betty Neuman. The Betty Neuman health-care systems model. Also 1989.
1976	Josephine Patterson and L. Zderad. *Humanistic nursing*. Also 1988.

For complete citations, see Chapter 19 under appropriate authors.

Peplau (1952), using Harry Stack Sullivan's theory title and concepts to develop her own, produced the first articulated concept of nursing as an interpersonal relationship with components of interpersonal processes central to nursing needing to be elucidated and analyzed. The field of psychiatric nursing subsequently was based on Peplau's ideas. Other theories that evolved in the 1960s were based on those early conceptions of nursing. For example, Virginia Henderson, with Bershan Harmer, developed the early seeds of a nursing theory that was then published in the mid-1950s in a textbook on the principles and practice of nursing.

The request from the International Council of Nursing to define nursing and its mission led to the subsequent International Council of Nursing statement in 1958 that appeared in a publication with wide distribution and that was adapted internationally (Henderson, 1966, p. 15). The message given by both Peplau and Henderson was that nursing has a specific and unique mission and that this mission has some order and organization that can be communicated. These articulated wholes represented the beginnings of theories in nursing.

Abdellah's nursing theory, evolving from her work at Columbia University, is another example of the influence of that school on theoretical nursing (Abdellah, Beland, Martin, and Matheney, 1961). Abdellah's doctoral dissertation in 1953 at Teachers College, under the leadership of Hildegard Peplau, focused on determining covert aspects of nursing problems. The results of her research were subsequently published in *Nursing Research*, marking the beginning of her attempts at theorizing the nursing care process. Her conceptualization of nursing care evolved out of the dissertation research and out of another study that was completed in 1955 on the needs of patients for nursing care. The latter was based on data collected from patients, nurses, and doctors. Abdellah developed her conception of what nursing is by focusing attention on patients rather than on techniques (Abdellah, Beland, Martin, and Matheney, 1961).

Other theorists' ideas were formulated around the need for a binding framework to guide curricula, but their writing and publications did not have the instant impact that Peplau's, Henderson's, and Abdellah's had on theoretical nursing. Their conceptions were slow to have an impact on nursing. Orem's ideas were first published in a guide for developing a curriculum for practical nursing in 1959. Patient needs were also the focus. Hall developed, in 1959, and implemented, in 1963, a concept of nursing based on needs and interpersonal relations at the Loeb Center for Nursing and Rehabilitation. One can see the influence of both Peplau and Henderson in her writing (Hall, 1963).

Independent of the Teacher's College group of theorists, Johnson was beginning to play a central role in conceptualizing nursing. Johnson's (1959) analysis of the nature of science in nursing was undoubtedly a milestone in drawing attention to the potential of nursing as a scientific discipline and in advocating the development of its unique knowledge base. At that time Johnson tentatively suggested that nursing knowledge is based on a theory of nursing diagnosis that is distinct and different from medical diagnosis. The substantive matter for such diagnosis, the beginning of Johnson's theory, was starting to be formulated at this time. (See Chapter 19 for appropriate citations for each theorist.)

Another milestone in nursing progress was the establishment of the special nursing research fellowship program to facilitate, support, and encourage nurses' education for research careers.

1961–1965—Theory: A National Goal in Nursing

From a reduced conception of a human being as "an illness" or "a surgery," with signs and symptoms, nursing theory, in the late 1950s, refocused nursing attention on the individual as a set of needs and nursing as a set of unique functions. Still, a reductionist approach to nursing existed. The 1960s, with its turbulent society, the Camelot goals of harmony and coexistence, and the influence of Peplau may have prompted the refocusing of nursing from its stated mission of meeting patients' needs to the goal of establishing a relationship between the nurse and client. If relationships are effectively established through interpersonal relationships (as previously articulated by Peplau, 1952, and as advocated by a new group of theorists), then nursing care can meet the needs of the patient—not as defined by nurses but as perceived by the patient.

During this period, the Yale School of Nursing's position, influenced by the Columbia Teacher's College graduates who became faculty members at Yale, was beginning to be formulated. Nursing, to them, was considered a process rather than an end, an interaction rather than content, and a relationship between two human beings rather than an interaction between unrelated nurse and patient. Social forces that helped the Yale group to develop their ideas into concepts of nursing were multifold. Federal grant money was available for preparation ranging from psychiatric nursing to teaching positions, for identifying psychiatric concepts in nursing, and for the development of an integrated curriculum. The availability of time and resources, therefore, was significant in providing the necessary push as well as the appropriate environment in which to reflect on nursing's mission and goals.

Although the work of the faculty of the Yale School of Nursing may have profoundly influenced nursing research in the United States in the 1960s, its influence on theory was not quite as marked at the time. There was a revival of that impact in the 1980s as nurses acknowledged Yale's strategies for theory development; this is evidenced by the reconsideration of Orlando's work (Schmieding, 1983; 1987; 1988) and by the paradigmatic shift in nursing research to phenomenology (Oiler, 1982; Omery, 1983; Silva and Rothbart, 1984). These writers' conceptualization of nursing therefore was not the milestone that prompted the evolution of the next stage of theory. Rather, it was the American Nurses' Association's (ANA) position paper in which nursing was defined as care, cure, and coordination and in which theory development was identified as a most significant goal for the profession of nursing, that may have been influential in the further development of theoretical nursing (ANA, 1965).

Two other significant developments occurred during this period. Federal support was provided to nurses wishing to pursue doctoral education in one of the basic sciences. It is important to note that the graduates of these programs are those who, in the mid-1970s, further developed metatheoretical ideas. The second development was inauguration of the journal, *Nursing Science.* Although short-lived, it was a medium for exchange of ideas on theory and science in nursing and a confirmation that nursing is an evolving science with theoretical principles and underpinnings.

1966–1970—Theory Development: A Tangible Goal for Academics

With the ANA's recommendation that theory development was of highest priority in the profession, and with the availability of federal support, a symposium sponsored by Case Western Reserve University was held as part of the nursing science program. This symposium was divided into three parts. The part focusing on theory took place on October 7, 1967 and was considered a milestone during this period (Table 3-4). The papers were published in *Nursing Research* one year later. These publications lent support to what were previously considered simply perceptions and conceptions of theoretical nursing from an isolated number of theorists. Not only did a group of significant people in nursing get together to discuss theory in nursing, but the official scientific journal of the field recognized the significance of these proceedings by publishing them.

Nurses also received confirmation from two philosophers and a nurse theorist who had been involved in teaching nurses at Yale for five years that theories are significant for the practice of nursing, that the practice of nursing is amenable to theoretical development, and that nurses are capable of developing theories (Dickoff, James, and Wiedenbach, 1968). The presentations and the subsequent publications influenced the discipline of nursing quite profoundly, as evidenced by the classic nature of those publications and by the acceleration in publications related to theory. Nursing theory was defined, goals for theory development were set, and the confirmation of outsiders (people outside the field of nursing, non-nursing philosophers) was productive.

Although the insiders (the nurse theorists) may have charted the course of action for theory development, the doubts and skepticism about theory (from the critics who viewed theory as scientific and as evolving from an empirical, positivistic model) that dominated nursing until then were somewhat squelched by the presentations and discussions that went on during that significant meeting in which Dickoff and colleagues presented their metatheory of nursing. (The evidence for skepticism is derived from omission rather than commission. When theories were used during this period, they were used in conjunction with education and not in practice or, except for the New York and Yale students, in research. Refer to the theory literature in Chapter 19 for documentation of the omission.)

The metatheorists in nursing started their questioning during this period. Questions of this era were related to what types of theories nurses should develop rather than to the nature of the substantive content of those theories. The first metatheorists were Ellis (1968) and Wiedenbach (Dickoff, James, and Wiedenbach, 1968). Dickoff and James (1968), philosophers by training, addressed metatheoretical concerns that focused on types of theories and content of theories. Debates occurred about whether the theories should be basic or borrowed, pure or applied, descriptive or prescriptive.

Accomplishments at this stage can be summarized as:

Nursing is a field amenable to theorizing.
Nurses can develop theories.
Practice is a rich area for theory.
Practice theory should be the goal for theory development in nursing.
Nurses' highest theory goal should be prescriptive theory, but it is
    acceptable to develop descriptive and explanatory theories.

Table 3–4
Theory Development in Nursing: A Historical Perspective

1860	Florence Nightingale addresses the need for research and the educational preparation of nurses.
1900–1950	Diploma schools served as major source of nurses—the Flexner Report for Medicine.
1952	*Nursing Research* first published.
1955	Establishment of the Special Nurse Research Fellowship Program in the National Institute of Health, Division of Nursing
1959	D.E. Johnson. The nature of a science of nursing. *Nursing Outlook, 7,* 292–294.
1960	R.N. Schlotfeldt. Reflections on nursing research. *American Journal of Nursing.* 60(4), 492–494. (The primary task of nursing research is to develop theories that serve as a guide to practice.)
1961	Surgeon General's Consultant Group on Nursing appointed to advise the Surgeon General on nursing needs and to identify the appropriate role of the federal government in assuring adequate nursing services in the nation. This group strongly supported nursing research and recommended a substantial increase in funds.
1961	D.E. Johnson. Patterns in professional nursing education. *Nursing Outlook,* 9, 608. (Nursing science may evolve more easily through the identification of common but major problems of patients that are of direct concern to nursing.)
1962	Nurse Scientist Graduate Training Grants Program
1963	*Nursing Science* first published
1963	M.E. Rogers. Some comments on the theoretical basis of nursing practice. *Nursing Science,* 1, 11–13. (The theoretical base of nursing practice is nursing science . . . a body of scientific knowledge characterized by descriptive, explanatory, and predictive principles . . . developed through synthesis and resynthesis of selected knowledges from the humanities and the biological, physical, and social sciences. . . . It assumes its own "unique scientific" mix through selection and patterning of these knowledges.)
1963	M.E. Rogers. Building a strong educational foundation. *American Journal of Nursing,* 63(6), 941. (The explanatory and predictive principles of nursing make possible nursing diagnosis and knowledgeable intervention toward predictable goals . . . nursing science is not additive, but creative.)
1964	D.E. Johnson. Nursing and health education. *International Journal of Nursing Studies,* 1, 219. (Nurses must be socialized as scholars and must develop commitment to inquiry and skill in the use of scientific knowledge.)
	J.S. Berthold. Theoretical and empirical clarification of concepts. *Nursing Science,* 406–422.
	M.I. Brown. (Spring) Research in the development of nursing theory. *Nursing Research,* 13, 109–112. (Assesses progress of theory development in nursing and emphasizes need for explicit relationship of research to theory.)
	F.S. Wald and R.C. Leonard. (1964) Toward development of nursing practice theory. *Nursing Research,* 13(4), 309–313.

(*continued*)

Table 3–4 (Continued)

1965	American Nurses' Association. Educational preparation for nurse practitioners and assistants to nurses: A position paper.
	P. Putnam. A conceptual approach to nursing theory. *Nursing Science*. 430–442.
1967	V.S. Cleland. The use of existing theories. *Nursing Research*, 16(2), 118–121.
1967	L.H. Conant. (Spring) A search for resolution of existing problems in nursing. *Nursing Research*, 16, 115.
	Symposium on Theory Development in Nursing. (Reported in *Nursing Research*, 1968, 17(3).)
1967–1970	National Commission for the Study of Nursing and Nursing Education, Jerome F. Lysaught, director.
1968	First Nurse Scientist Conference on The Nature of Science in Nursing. Sponsored by University of Colorado School of Nursing, Dr. Madeleine Leininger, chair. (Reported in *Nursing Research*, 1969, 18(5).)
	First Annual WCHEN Communicating Research Conference
1968	J. Dickoff and P. James. A theory of theories: A position paper. *Nursing Research*, 17(3), 197–206. (Professional disciplines are obligated to go a step further than explanation and prediction in theory construction, to the development of prescriptive theory.)
	J. Dickoff, P. James, and E. Wiedenbach. Theory in a practice discipline: Part I. Practice oriented theory. *Nursing Research*, 17(5), 415-435.
	Idem. Theory in a practice discipline: Part II. Practice oriented theory. *Nursing Research*, 17(6), 545-554.
	R. Ellis. (1968) Characteristics of significant theories. *Nursing Research*, 17(3), 217–222.
	D. E. Johnson. Theory in nursing: Borrowed and unique. *Nursing Research*, 17(3), 206-209.
	M. Moore. Nursing: A scientific discipline. Forum, 7(4), 340–347.
	J. L. Sasmor. Toward developing theory in nursing. *Nursing Forum*, 7(2), 191–200.
1969	G. Mathwig. Nursing science: The theoretical core of nursing knowledge. *Image*, 3, 9–14, 20–23.
	R. McKay. Theories, models, and systems for nursing. *Nursing Research*, 18(5), 393–399.
	C. M. Norris (Ed.). Proceedings: First, second, and third nursing theory conference. University of Kansas, 1969 and 1970.
1971	F. Cleary. A theoretical model: Its potential for adaptation to nursing. *Image*, 4(1), 14–20.
	I. M. Harris. Theory building in nursing: A review of the literature. *Image*, 4(1), 6–10.
	M. Jacobson. Qualitative data as a potential source of theory in nursing. *Image*, 4(1), 10–14.
	J. F. Murphy (Ed.). *Theoretical issues in professional nursing*. New York: Appleton-Century-Crofts.
	I. Walker. Toward a clearer understanding of the concept of nursing theory. *Nursing Research*, 20(5), 428–435.

Table 3–4 (Continued)

1972	M. Newman. Nursing's theoretical evolution. *Nursing Outlook*, 20(7), 449–453.
	NLN Council of Baccalaureate and Higher Degree Programs approved its "Criteria for the Appraisal of Baccalaureate and Higher Degree Programs in Nursing," including criterion stating that curricula should be based on a conceptual framework.
1973	M. E. Hardy. The nature of theories. In M. Hardy (Ed.), *Theoretical foundations for nursing*. New York: MSS Information Corporation.
	The Nursing Development Conference Group. (1973) *Concept formulation in nursing: Process and product*. Boston: Little, Brown & Co.
1974	M. E. Hardy. Theories: Components, development, evaluation. *Nursing Research*, 18, 100–107.
	A. Jacox. Theory construction in nursing: An overview. *Nursing Research*, 23, 4–13.
	D. E. Johnson. Development of theory: Requisite for nursing as a primary health profession. *Nursing Research*, 18, 372–377.
1975	Nursing Theories Conference Group. (Formed out of a concern for the need for materials to help students of nursing understand and use nursing theories in nursing practice.)
1978	Advances in Nursing Science. S. K. Donaldson and D. Crowley. The Discipline of Nursing. *Nursing Outlook* 26(2), 113–120.
1979	M. A. Newman. *Theory Development in Nursing*. Philadelphia: F. A. Davis.
1982	M. J. Kim and D. A. Moritz. *Classifications of Nursing Diagnosis*. New York: McGraw-Hill.
1983	L. O. Walker and K. C. Avant. *Strategies for Theory Construction in Nursing*. New York: Appleton-Century-Crofts
	J. Fitzpatrick and A. Whall. *Conceptual Models of Nursing: Analysis and Application*. R. J. Brady Co.
	P. L. Chinn and M. K. Jacobs. *Theory and Nursing: A Systematic Approach*. St. Louis: C. V. Mosby.
	H. S. Kim. *The Nature of Theoretical Thinking in Nursing*. New York: Appleton-Century-Crofts.
	I. W. Clements and F. B. Roberts. *Family Health: A Theoretical Approach to Nursing Care*. New York: John Wiley & Sons.
	P. L. Chinn. *Advances in Nursing Theory Development*. Rockville: Aspen Systems.
1984	J. Fawcett. *Analysis and Evaluation of Conceptual Models*. Philadelphia: F. A. Davis.

1971–1975—Theory Syntax

There was a period, just before the research enterprise in nursing focused on answering significant questions in the field, when nurse researchers focused on discussing and writing about research methodology. A parallel exists in the area of theory. The period from 1966 to 1970 resulted in a beginning focus on theory development, which was followed by attempts at identifying the structural components of theory (refer to Table 3-4). Metatheorists dominated this period. The emphasis was on articulating, defining, and explicating theory components and on the processes inherent in theory analysis and critique. Nurse theorists were no longer questioning whether nursing needed a theory or whether or not theory could be developed in nursing; questions of this period focused on what is meant by theory (Ellis, 1968, 1971; Walker, 1971), on what are the major components of theory (Hardy, 1974; Jacox, 1974), and on ways to analyze and critique theories (Duffey and Muhlenkamp, 1974). Education of nurses in basic, natural, and social sciences through the federally supported nurse–scientist programs produced a cadre of nurses who shared a common goal: the establishment of the unique knowledge base of nursing. Discussions of what constituted theory and the identification of theory syntax seemed to be the means to achieve that goal.

Just before the close of this period, a milestone was achieved. Just as the ANA acknowledged the significance of theory development during the previous period, the National League for Nursing not only acknowledged theory but also made theory-based curriculum a requirement for accreditation. Schools of nursing were expected to select, develop, and implement a conceptual framework for their curricula. This requirement for accreditation was both a moving force and a major barrier to theory development. To use theory for curriculum development further heightened awareness of academic nursing to the significance of theory and to the available nursing theories. However, this requirement diverted the goal of developing theories for practice (those theories that would answer significant questions related to practice) to the goal of utilizing theory for education. Nevertheless, this milestone increased the use of theory and discussions about theory and prompted more writing about the syntax of theory to help academicians and students understand and use theories in curriculum and teaching. The limited number of journals that acknowledge and promote theoretical nursing, the focus on promoting the publication of empirical research findings, and the growing financial difficulties of some journals were barriers to written exchanges on theory and theorizing.

1976–1980—A Time to Reflect

Nurse theorists were invited to participate in presentations, discussions, and debates in conferences sponsored by nurse educators, marking a significant milestone in the progress of theoretical nursing. A national conference devoted to nursing theory and the formation of the Nursing Theory Think Tank in 1978 further supported the direction of the profession toward the utilization of existing theory and the development of further theory to describe and explain nursing phenomena, to predict relationships, and to guide nursing care (Preview, 1978). This was the time for nurse academicians, who had utilized nursing theories as guiding frameworks for curricula, to consider putting theory to other uses, particularly in practice.

The inauguration of the journal, *Advances in Nursing Science*, with its focus on "the full range of activities involved in the development of science," including "theory construction, concept, and analysis" and the application of theory, was another significant milestone during this period (Chinn, 1978) (refer to Table 3-4). The focus of the journal on theory and theory development added more support to the significance of theoretical nursing and simultaneously gave nurses who were interested in theory the necessary medium in which to present and discuss their ideas. It allowed for the questioning and debate that is necessary for the development of theoretical bases in any discipline.

This period is characterized by questioning if nursing's progress would benefit from the adoption of a single paradigm and a single theory of truth (Carper, 1978; Silva, 1977). More sophisticated debates about what types of theory nursing needs (Beckstrand, 1978a, 1978b, 1980) and about issues in theory (Crawford, Dufault, and Rudy, 1979) appeared in nursing literature. A more solid commitment to the development of theory emerged, combined with a specific direction to nurses' efforts in theory development (Donaldson and Crowley, 1978; Hardy, 1978). The links between theory and research were considered and discussed (Batey, 1977; Fawcett and Downs, 1986), the path was charted for bridging the theory–research gaps between theory and practice (Barnum, 1990), theory and philosophy were examined (Silva, 1977), and the role of each in the development of nursing knowledge was clarified (refer back to Fig. 2-1). Domain concepts were beginning to be identified, and their acceptance was demonstrated in the next period.

1981–1985—Nursing Theories' Revival: Emergence of the Domain Concepts

In this period, theory began to be questioned less and pluralism debated less. This period was characterized by an acceptance of the significance of theory for nursing and, furthermore, by the inevitability of the need for the development of nursing theory. Doctoral programs in nursing incorporated theory into their curricula and considered it a core content area, ranking it at the top of all other core content (Beare, Gray, and Ptak, 1981).

A review of theory literature during this period reveals the lack of debate on whether or not to use theory—practice versus basic theory, or borrowed versus nursing theory. Instead, there appeared to be more writing on the examination of nursing theories in relation to different research and practice problems and on comparisons between the different conceptualizations (Jacobson, 1984; Spangler and Spangler, 1983). Questions of this period included: What have we learned from theory? and How can we use theory? The latter was a question that clinicians began to ask.

Knowledge of the syntax emerging from the previous period was used to analyze existing theories (Fawcett, 1984; Fitzpatrick and Whall, 1983). In addition, existing theories came to be thought of as the means to develop unique nursing knowledge. Concepts central to nursing were identified, and existing theory, the source of the identified concepts, was in turn re-examined in terms of further development and refinement (Crawford, 1982; Reeder, 1984).

This period was characterized by the nursing *theory advocates* who pleaded for the use of a nursing perspective in general or for the specific utilization of nursing theory (Adam, 1983; Dickson and Lee-Villasenor, 1982). (See *Advances in Nursing Science, Journal of Nursing Administration*, and *American Journal of Nursing* for examples of the American advocates and *Journal of Advanced Nursing* for examples of international advocates.) Another group also emerged during this period: the *theory synthesizers*. The differences between the advocates and the synthesizers was in the level of the scope of analysis. The advocates promoted nursing theory and demonstrated its use in research projects or in a limited practice arena. The synthesizers, on the other hand, went beyond that limited use to describe and analyze how nursing theory had influenced nursing practice, education, research, and administration. The synthesizers are exemplified by, but not limited to, Fitzpatrick and Whall (1983) and Fawcett (1984). The Rogerian First National Conference (1983), in which theoreticians, practitioners, and researchers discussed the utility of Rogers' theory from different perspectives, is a different example of an effective synthesis of different uses of a theory. The planners of this conference belong to the group of theory synthesizers.

A few of the synthesizers graduated from New York University in the mid-1970s. It is too early to determine a pattern among the synthesizers as a school of thought. One thing that cannot be ignored is made evident by a review of the titles of doctoral dissertations in nursing from New York University from 1941 to 1983, which affirm the significance of that school in nursing research and nursing theory. Most of the titles indicate a nursing perspective, and there appears to have been an attempt at cumulative knowledge development. How and in what ways such a pattern may have influenced and may continue to influence theory development is an area worth further investigation and analysis.

This period was characterized by an acceptance of theory as a tool that emanates from significant practice problems and can be used for practice and research. This period was also characterized by a greater clarity in the relationship between theory and research than between theory and practice.

The only remaining confusion during this period was related to semantics. Conceptual models were referred to as conceptual frameworks, theories, metatheories, paradigms, and metaparadigms and, when differentiated, boundaries were not totally clear and properties not entirely distinct.

1986–1990—From Metatheory to Single Domain Theory

Three characteristics of this period were epistemological debates, ontological analyses, and an increase in concept development and analyses. The epistemological debates included questions related to describing alternative approaches to knowledge development, such as the use of phenomenology, critical theory, and feminist or empiricist methodologies (*e.g.*, Allen, 1985; Allen, Benner, and Diekelman, 1986; Hagell, 1989; Leonard, 1989). Although the debates were focused on knowledge development in general rather than on theoretical development of the discipline, these debates were related as well to the development of theoretical nursing.

Effective analyses were those that focused on ontological beliefs related to central nursing concepts, for example, environment (Chopoorian, 1986; Stevens, 1989), and health (Allen, 1985 and 1986; Benner, 1984). These analyses added substantially to a more contextual approach to understanding each concept. These analyses also raised the awareness and the consciousness of nurses to the necessity of using frameworks that allow for an integrative, holistic, and contextual description of nursing phenomena, phenomena that go beyond the individual clients. Such frameworks, these authors demonstrated, maintained the integrity of the basic ontological beliefs that have historically guided nursing practice, for example, holism, integrated responses, and relationship with environment.

The third milestone of this period was an increase in writings related to concept development. These developments were different from earlier theory developments that included answers to such general questions as, What is nursing? These analyses were more practice-oriented, were integrative, and represented early attempts in the development of single domain theories. This was also the period in which a plea for substance was made (Meleis, 1987; Woods, 1987; Chinn, 1987; Downs, 1988). These authors echoed the sentiment of other discipline members by urging discourse that was more focused on substantive issues that were confronting health care recipients.

Process debates became more a potential force for theory development when and if they were grounded in substantive disciplinary content. Therefore, instead of debating whether critical theory or feminist theories were more appropriate as a philosophical base for the discipline, one may argue whether it was more effective to view environment or comfort from either or both perspectives. Such substantive debates then would add to or revise parameters and dimensions of that area of knowledge.

CONCLUSION

This chapter presented significant historical themes that are related to an interest in theoretical nursing. Progress and development in theoretical nursing was defined in terms of stages and milestones. A view of historical development offers a significant perspective upon which current and future theoretical thinking can be built. Analysis of present development is deficient without tracing these historical themes.

ACKNOWLEDGMENTS

The first part of this chapter is based on: A.I. Meleis (1983) The evolving nursing scholarliness. In P.L. Chinn (Ed.), *Advances in nursing theory development*, pp. 19–34. Reprinted with permission of Aspen Publishers, Inc., © 1983.

REFERENCES

Abdellah, F.G., Beland, I.L., Martin, A., and Matheney, R.V. (1961) *Patient-centered approaches to nursing.* New York: Macmillan.

Adam, E. (1983) Frontiers of nursing in the 21st century: Development of models and theories on the concept of nursing. *Journal of Advanced Nursing*, 8, 41–45.

Allen, D. (1985) Nursing research and social control: Alternative models of science that emphasize understanding and emancipation. *Image*, XVII(2), 58–64.

Allen, D.G. (1986) Using philosophical and historical methodologies to understand the concept of health. In P.L. Chinn (Ed.), *Nursing research methodology: Issues and implementation.* Rockville, MD: Aspen Systems.

Allen, D., Benner, P., and Diekelman, N.K. (1986). Three paradigms for nursing research: Methodological implications. In P.C. Chinn (Ed.), *Nursing research methodology: Issues and implementations.* Rockville, MD: Aspen Systems.

American Nurses' Association. (1965) Educational preparation for nurse practitioners and assistants of nurses. *American Journal of Nursing*, 65(12), 106–111.

Barnum, B.S. (1990). *Nursing theory: Analysis, application and evaluation* (3rd ed.). Boston, MA: Little, Brown & Co.

Batey, M.V. (1977) Conceptualization: Knowledge and logic guiding empirical research. *Nursing Research*, 26(5), 324–329.

Beare, P.G., Gray, C.J., and Ptak, H.F. (1981) Doctoral curricula in nursing. *Nursing Outlook*, May, 311–316.

Beckstrand, J. (1978a) The notion of a practice theory and the relationship of scientific and ethical knowledge to practice. *Research in Nursing and Health*, 1(3), 131–136.

Beckstrand, J. (1978b) The need for a practice theory as indicated by the knowledge used in conduct of practice. *Research in Nursing and Health*, 1(4), 175–179.

Beckstrand, J. (1980) A critique of several conceptions of practice theory in nursing. *Research in Nursing and Health*, 3(2), 69–80.

Benner, P. (1984) *From novice to expert: Excellence and power in clinical nursing practice.* Menlo Park, CA: Addison-Wesley.

Carper, B.A. (1978) Practice oriented theory: Part 1. Fundamental patterns of knowing in nursing. *Advances in Nursing Science*, 1(1), 13–23.

Chinn, P.L. (1978) A model for theory development in nursing. *Advances in Nursing Science*, 1(1), 1–11.

Chinn, P.L. (1987) Response: Revision and passion. *Scholarly Inquiry for Nursing Practice: An International Journal*, 1(1), 21–24.

Chopoorian, T.J. (1986) Reconceptualizing the environment. In P. Moccia (Ed.), *New approaches to theory development.* New York: National League for Nursing.

Crawford, G. (1982) The concept of pattern in nursing: Conceptual development and measurement. *Advances in Nursing Science*, 5(1), 1–6.

Crawford, G., Dufault, K., and Rudy, E. (1979) Evolving issues in theory development. *Nursing Outlook*, 27(5), 346–351.

Dickoff, J. and James, P. (1968) A theory of theories: A position paper. *Nursing Research*, 17(3), 197–203.

Dickoff, J., James, P., and Wiedenbach, E. (1968) Theory in practice discipline: Part 1. Practice oriented theory. *Nursing Research*, 17(5), 415–435.

Dickson, G. and Lee-Villasenor, H. (1982) Nursing theory and practice: A self-care approach. *Advances in Nursing Science*, 5(1), 29–40.

Donaldson, S.K. and Crowley, D. (1978) The discipline of nursing. *Nursing Outlook*, 26(2), 113–120.

Downs, F. (1988) Doctoral education: Our claim to the future. *Nursing Outlook*, 36(1), 18–20.

Duffey, M. and Muhlenkamp, A.F. (1974) A framework for theory analysis. *Nursing Outlook*, 22(9), 570–574.

Ellis, R. (1968) Characteristics of significant theories. *Nursing Research*, 17(3), 217–222.

Ellis, R. (1971) Commentary on Walker's "Toward a clearer understanding of the concept of nursing theory." *Nursing Research*, 20(6), 493–494.

Ellis, R. (1983) Philosophic inquiry. In H. Werley and J. Fitzpatrick (Eds.), *Annual review of nursing research*. New York: Springer.

Fawcett, J. (1984) *Analysis and evaluation of conceptual models of nursing*. Philadelphia: F.A. Davis.

Fawcett, J. and Downs, F.S. (1986). *The relationship of theory and research*. Norwalk, CT: Appleton-Century-Crofts.

Fitzpatrick, J. and Whall, A. (1983) *Conceptual models of nursing: Analysis and application*. Bowie, MD: Robert J. Brady Company.

Fry, S.T. (1989) Toward a theory of nursing ethics. *Advances in Nursing Science*, 11, 9–22.

Gortner, S.R. (1980) Nursing science in transition. *Nursing Research*, 29(3), 180–183.

Gortner, S.R. and Nahm, H. (1977) An overview of nursing research in the United States. *Nursing Research*, 26(1), 10–33.

Hagell, R.I. (1989) Nursing knowledge: Women's knowledge. A sociological perspective. *Journal of Advanced Nursing*, 14, 226–233.

Hall, L.E. (1963) Center for nursing. *Nursing Outlook*, 11, 805–806.

Hardy, M.E. (1974) The nature of theories. In M.E. Hardy (Ed.), *Theoretical foundations for nursing*. New York: MSS Information Corporation.

Hardy, M.E. (1978) Practice oriented theory: Part 1. Perspectives on nursing theory. *Advances in Nursing Science*, 1(1), 37–48.

Henderson, V. (1966) *Nature of nursing*. New York: Macmillan.

Jacobson, S.F. (1984) A semantic differential for external comparison of conceptual nursing models. *Advances in Nursing Science*, 6(2), 58–70.

Jacox, A. (1974) Theory construction in nursing: An overview. *Nursing Research*, 23(1), 4–13.

Johnson, D.E. (1959). A philosophy of nursing. *Nursing Outlook*, 7(4), 198–200.

Johnson, D.E. (1980) The behavioral system model for nursing. In J.P. Riehl and C. Roy (Eds.), *Conceptual models for nursing practice* (2nd ed.). New York: Appleton-Century-Crofts.

Kuhn, T.S. (1970) The structure of scientific revolutions. In Neurath, O. (Ed.), *International encyclopedia of unified science* (2nd ed.). (Vol. 2) Chicago: University of Chicago Press.

Leininger, M. (1968) The research critique: Nature, function, and art. *Nursing Research*, 17, 444–449.

Leonard, V.W. (1989). A Heideggerian phenomenologic perspective on the concept of the person. *Advances in Nursing Science* 11(4), 40–55.

Levine, M.E. (1967) The four conservation principles of nursing. *Nursing Forum*, 6(1), 45–59.

Meleis, A.I. (1987) ReVisions in knowledge development: Being vs. becoming or being and becoming. *Health Care for Women International*, 8, 199–217.

Merton, R.K. (1973) *The sociology of science: Theoretical and empirical investigations*. Chicago: University of Chicago Press.

Nursing Theory Think Tank. (1979) *Advances in Nursing Science*, 1(3), 105.

Nightingale, F. (1946) *Notes on nursing: What it is and what it is not.* Philadelphia: J.B. Lippincott Company.

Oiler, C. (1982) The phenomenological approach in nursing research. *Nursing Research*, 31(3), 178–181.

Omery, A. (1983) Phenomenology: A method for nursing research. *Advances in Nursing Science*, 5, 49–63.

Orem, D.E. (1971) *Nursing: Concepts of practice.* New York: McGraw-Hill.

Orem, D.E. (1985) *Nursing: Concepts of practice* (3rd ed.). New York: McGraw-Hill.

Peplau, H.E. (1952) *Interpersonal relations in nursing.* New York: G.P. Putnam's Sons.

Preview: The Second Annual Nurse Educator Conference. (1978) *Nurse Educator*, 3(6), 37–39.

Reeder, F. (1984) Philosophical issues in the Rogerian science of unitary human beings. *Advances in Nursing Science*, 6(2), 14–23.

Rogerian First National Conference. (1983, June) New York University, New York.

Rogers, M. (1970) *An introduction to the theoretical basis of nursing.* Philadelphia: F.A. Davis.

Sarter, B. (1987) Evolutionary idealism: A philosophical foundation for holistic nursing theory. *Advances in Nursing Science*, 9(2), 1–9.

Schmieding, N.J. (1983) An analysis of Orlando's nursing theory based on Kuhn's theory of science. In P.L. Chinn (Ed.), *Advances in nursing theory development.* Rockville, MD: Aspen Systems.

Schmieding, N.J. (1987) Problematic situations in nursing: Analysis of Orlando's theory based on Dewey's theory of inquiry. *Journal of Advanced Nursing*, 12, 431–440.

Schmieding, N.J. (1988) Action process of nurse administrators to problematic situations based on Orlando's theory. *Journal of Advanced Nursing*, 13, 99–107.

Sills, G.M. (1977) Research in the field of psychiatric nursing 1952–1977. *Nursing Research*, 26(3), 281–287.

Silva, M.C. (1977) Philosophy, science, theory: Interrelationships and implications for nursing research. *Image*, 9(3), 59–63.

Silva, M.C. and Rothbart, D. (1984) An analysis of changing trends in philosophies of science on nursing theory development and testing. *Advances in Nursing Science*, 6(2), 1–13.

Spangler, Z.S. and Spangler, W.D. (1983) Self-care: A testable model. In P.L. Chinn (Ed.), *Advances in nursing theory development.* Rockville, MD: Aspen Systems.

Stevens, P. (1989) A critical social reconceptualization of environment in nursing: Implications for methodology. *Advances in Nursing Science*, 11(4), 56–68.

Stevenson, J.S. and Woods, N.F. (1986) Nursing science and contemporary science: Emerging paradigms. In G.E. Sorensen (Ed.), *Setting the agenda for the year 2000: Knowledge development in nursing.* (Publication No. G-a170, 3M, 5/86.) Kansas City, MO: ANA.

Toulmin, S. (1977) *Human understanding: The collective use and evolution of concepts.* Princeton, NJ: Princeton University Press.

Walker, L.O. (1971) Toward a clearer understanding of the concept of nursing theory. *Nursing Research*, 20(5), 428–435.

Woods, N.F. (1987) Response: Early morning musings on the passion for substance. *Scholarly Inquiry for Nursing Practice: An International Journal*, 1(1), 25–28.

Chapter 4

From Can't to Kant: The Fantastic Voyage

The journey from the days of Florence Nightingale to modern nursing has been long, hard, and bumpy. Nightingale's attempts to establish professional nursing based on nursing's unique concern with the environment for promotion of health were pre-empted by an illness-oriented training that was dependent on other professions for existence and on hospitals for training and sustenance. Nursing has travelled from apprenticeship to education, from hospital service and training to the university, from mere implementation of doctors' orders to accountability and autonomy, from practical to theoretical applications.

The journey has included a major detour through the land of "Can't": a land of perceived inability to conceptualize or generalize; a land that espoused practice, concreteness, and practical relevance as antithetical to generalizations, universal propositions, and theories. The decades of the 1970s and 1980s mark our emergence from this land and our going back on course, back to where Nightingale began. Upon our return, however, we are more experienced, more assured, and more trusting in our perceptions; we are more accepting of the varied meanings of experience and of its roles in the theoretical development of nursing.

We are reminded in this journey of Immanuel Kant, a dominant 19th-century philosopher, who maintained that reality is not only a thing in and of itself but is also constructed by those who experience it. Reality in nursing history has been a synthesis of conditions that predisposed nurses to a nontheoretical existence and an *a priori* perception that helped to structure a lack of acceptance of theoretical generalizations.

Kant aptly distinguished between perception of experience and sensation of experience. Sensation of experience is confounded by temporal and spatial limitations. Experience, the basis of knowledge, has, in nursing, been dependent on this or that procedure as performed at a certain moment, or on the knowledge of this or that patient occupying a certain space and existing at a certain moment. Although knowledge begins with experience, Kant maintained that this does not mean that all knowledge evolves from experience. To him, our experiences have two components: an *a priori* impression of what may be experienced and impressions as they are actually received. Understanding is a synthesis of both. Therefore, a human being—a knowing, active, and experiencing subject, not a passive recipient— interprets and analyzes impression data in a certain way. That certain way—the *a priori* form by which experiences are shaped—is a synthesis of something that is out there and something that is constructed by the person experiencing it (Copleston, 1964).

Increasingly, during the journey of nurses from early to modern times, experience took on different meanings with more profound explanations. Experience provided the impetus for describing and explaining phenomena central to nursing and perhaps was responsible for the invention of new therapeutics for the change or control of unwanted events related to health care. Some nurses are better prepared than others to consider cosmic connections between people, events, and procedures and to incorporate the relationships of seemingly discrete variables to help them better understand events crucial to health care. The journey, still in progress, brings us closer to more efficient and effective theorizing in nursing to help us define more functional and useful descriptions, explanations, predictions, and prescriptions of nursing care.

Why was the journey long and complex? Why did nursing go through such detours of seemingly nontheoretical periods and, more important, why did nurses appear to reject theory and theorizing during the journey, practically forcing the detour into the nontheoretical existence? Even when a small handful of nurses attempted to return, to put nursing on course by providing a theoretical view of what nursing is, it was almost two decades after the development of these conceptions that their notions and their stance began to be accepted. And why is it that some skeptics in nursing were still saying, in the latter part of the 20th century, that theory or theorizing in nursing is antithetical to the practice of nursing, that nursing practice is either a practically or theoretically oriented situation and therefore choosing one standpoint leaves no room and no need for the other? What conditions have prompted the beginning acceptance of theoretical nursing?

This chapter considers the forces that have both hindered and fostered the development of nursing theory. Kant's writing on the synthesis between reality as a separate entity and reality as constructed by the subject who is experiencing it helps us understand the two meanings of these forces. Human and knowledge barriers and human and knowledge forces are two sides of the same coin. We can analyze these forces as both negative and positive in the development of nursing theory. The content may be the same (the sensation in Kant's analysis), but the form distinguishes between forces as barriers and forces as resources. Together, content and form (provided by sensation and mind) enhance knowledge and understanding of the dynamics of the journey from no theory to theory. As we begin to perceive constraints in a new light and through a new lens, we can shift the negative power of constraint to a positive force, and we can reconstruct new realities and develop new blueprints that are more congruent with the mission of nursing and health care needs nationally and internationally.

BARRIERS TO THEORY DEVELOPMENT

Human Barriers: Nurses as Nurses

The type of student who is selecting nursing, the kind of education nursing students receive, and the nature of nursing may all have been related to the paucity of developments in nursing theory or to the rejection of the theoretical nature of nursing, particularly when education of nurses was confined to hospitals and before baccalaureate programs became the norm. Evidence of these relationships varies from speculative to more empirical and verified. Prior to the 1970s, women who chose to enter nursing may have done so because of its service orientation rather than its professional potential. Nursing may have attracted non-career-oriented individuals who were looking for an occupation that allowed them to get in and out conveniently as their families demanded. A decision to become a nurse may have depended on an image of nursing that was glamorized in the media but that was also paradoxically servile.

Whether nursing still attracts a unique group of individuals who are substantially different from students entering other fields is becoming increasingly debatable. Students are becoming attracted to nursing for its financial potential, its career possibilities, and its potential impact on society. There are no reported data to substantiate that shift; however, it is apparent to educators that attitudes of nursing students are changing drastically as changes occur in other spheres of life, in other professions, and in economic status. Several nursing programs now attract graduates from other disciplines, more nurses are seeking graduate degrees, and fewer nurses are enrolling in diploma programs.

One example of this shift in attitude is the influx of graduate students (graduates from other fields) into community college nursing or baccalaureate nursing programs. These students are often women who are older and therefore more developmentally mature and more intellectually sophisticated. They have already experienced academic life, and they knowingly and deliberately selected a different educational path that has the potential for leading to financial independence and a career. These differences between nursing students of the past and students of the present may suggest a difference in attitudes toward nursing and its professional status as well as its theoretical underpinnings.

Although differences between students who select nursing and those who select other professions are inconclusive due to the sparseness of research, there are indications that nursing education itself has created differences between nursing students and other students. Education plays a major role in training the mind to think beyond immediate action, to question situations, to link events, to generalize and, in short, to conceptualize.

Nursing education has a long history of squelching curiosity and replacing it with conformity and a nonquestioning attitude. Nursing education in the past prepared nurses to think of themselves as the handmaidens of physicians, the executors of doctors orders, and the implementers of hospital policy. It managed to socialize students to roles that are not congruent with scholarship and discovery.

Any independent thinking or critical attitude was the antithesis of what was expected of a nurse. Because nursing education was based more on apprenticeship, training, and experience than on ideas, knowledge, and learning, the nurse graduated only to find herself far more dependent on the medical and hospital systems than on her own problem-solving abilities. The educational system in nursing did not help nurses come to see themselves as sources of knowledge.

Theory creation is an active process, but early research characterized nurses as passive (Cleland, 1971; Edwards, 1969). The social climate in which nurses practiced did not encourage debate or freedom to experiment.

> [T]he subculture of nursing has encouraged the perpetuation of a feminine world that emphasizes routine and repetition, intuition and magical thinking, respectful obedience for authority, and covert rather than overt methods of control. Such a subculture does not provide a fertile field for the growth and development of curiosity and challenge of the status quo, both so necessary to scientific inquiry and scholarship. As a result, a number of nurses . . . have chosen to move to other disciplines for the substantive background and the mental stimulation so necessary to scholarly development. (Benoliel, 1975, p. 25)

Functional orientation—the act of performing procedures rather than thinking, reflecting, and problem solving—is a theme apparent in the discipline of nursing (Loomis, 1974). The concept originated in the early inclusion of nursing training programs in hospital settings that socialized nurses to become intellectually subordinate.

The hospital's role was to provide service within its means; its role in education was minimal. Therefore, when hospitals agreed to take on the education of nurses, they did so to improve patient care and to save money. It was acceptable to have nurses work very long hours and to allow them to attend lectures only when education did not interfere with the service they were providing. Nursing students were the lowest on the totem pole; they were taught how to respect physicians, how to believe in physicians, and how to totally submit to the hospital routine. Essentially, nurses were taught "intellectual subordination" (Bullough, 1975, p. 229).

Nursing students worked 12-hour shifts and were even further exhausted by being sent on home visits to bring in more revenue that was direly needed by the hospital. Decisions about home care were not predicated on goals of nursing nor on the outcome of nursing care but rather on the need for an economic boost through the use of students as cheap labor. As a result, nurses developed an attitude of task-orientation and, for the most part, did not take time to think or reflect, which maintained nursing at a practical rather than a theoretical level. Doing and thinking are not mutually exclusive. Unfortunately, however, the education nurses received fostered an unquestioning acceptance of authority and a subservient attitude.

> The weight of past tradition, the subordination of nurses, the sex segregation, and the apprenticeship model in nursing education have left a mark on the attitudes of present-day nurses. (Bullough, 1975, pp. 229–230)

The qualities necessary for theory development are thinking, reflecting, questioning, and perceiving the self as being capable of developing knowledge. The education nurses received did not develop these qualities, nor did it reinforce these qualities in those who had them.

Nursing has also suffered from the paternalism of hospital administration and medical staff (Ashley, 1977). This paternalism has been internalized as the rules and regulations created by others have been replaced in recent years with rules and regulations created by nurses for nurses. Questioning is still discouraged, rebelliousness is unthinkable, and disobedience is punished, but attrition is a personal option and many, indeed, resort to it.

Early on, the nurse's role was equated with a woman's or mother's role in the family, and the physician's role was equated with that of the father, the head of the family. Therefore, just as wives and mothers were relegated certain prescribed roles, the nurse was also plagued by the image of the sacrificing, altruistic, submissive placater, the fixer-of-all—a role detrimental to the creativity essential for theoretical thinking. Thinking, creating, and questioning were reserved for the head of the family. It is perhaps that same image that has helped perpetuate the duality of science and practice. Compassion (a characteristic of nurses in practice) cannot be replaced by the rigor, calculation, objectivity, and coolness of the scientist or the theoretician, though perhaps it could be complemented by such characteristics.

Academic nurses, on the other hand, suffered from this concept of nursing just as greatly but in a different way. Because they were far removed from patient care, they were more interested in theorizing about student learning or curricula than about patient environment. Being new themselves to the halls of academia, they dissipated their energies in the struggle to prove they belonged there. They competed with others in more established disciplines and shied away from those in practice who pointed their finger at these ivory-tower colleagues and said, "Your theories are too theoretical and your research is too esoteric; what do you know about practice anyhow?" or "Stick to teaching and leave practice to us."

The attitude of nurses toward theory development, shaped by personal attributes upon entry into nursing or by educational and practice environments that are antithetical to theorizing and scientific endeavors, was also greatly influenced by the reward structure in the profession. Recognition of nurses was based on immediate actions, and rewards were based on expedient doing. Even today, rewards are more easily bestowed on nurses in clinical roles or nurses in teaching roles than on those engaged in research or theory development. Rewards for scholarliness are not as tangible as rewards for these other roles, they are slow to come by, and the rationale for the rewards is not as well-defined, especially when the discipline is still developing and has no agreed-upon standards for reward (Gaston, 1975). In addition, the subculture of nursing has not promoted competition, not even constructive competition, which is essential in the development of theoretical ideals. What Benoliel said about competition in research applies to theory development:

> If scientific inquiry and production of knowledge are dependent on
> individuals who thrive on open competition, then perhaps the slow
> development of research in nursing is tied to a lack of competitive spirit

among nurses in idea development. Reflecting on nursing's origins as a form of women's work, I find this slow development not too surprising. Compliance with the rules rather than challenge of authority has been an organizing theme in much of nursing's history, and a subculture that places high value on conforming behavior is not fertile soil for the development of practitioners who are comfortable with the aggressive rivalry of scientific endeavors.

The subservient and self-effacing posture that nurses have traditionally held in their working relationships with physicians is not an effective stance for nurses engaged in scientific study. Rather, those who seek to be purveyors of new nursing knowledge can only do so when they carry a sense of self-confidence that permits them to see and experience the positive values of open competition in the world of ideas. (Benoliel, 1973, p. 8)

Finally, collaboration, a hallmark of success in nursing practice and an activity about which nurses are most familiar, has not been attached to the scholarly development of disciplines. So, even this, which nurses can do well, was not acknowledged as a significant characteristic of development and progress in scientific disciplines until the late 1980s when Gilligan (1984) and others described and explained the differences in development between men and women. Women's development was described in terms of connection and collaboration. A tolerance for these differences was beginning to appear in the late 1980s, and with it came a slow acceptance of alternate indicators to progress and development.

Human Barriers: Nurses as Women

Slowness in the development or acceptance of nursing theory can also be attributed to sex-role stereotyping. Theory development is a laborious process that requires flexibility in time, access to leisure time, access to resources, and freedom from apprehensions, none of which women possess or obtain as readily as men have in the past (Keller, 1979). The Western view pictures a woman as a hard-working, home-bound person whose energies should be confined to rearing children and caring for a family. Many women have internalized this role ascribed to them by society. Even when women tried to break away from societal stereotypes, they were beset by the need to both fulfill the new employment roles and maintain their function in the old roles. The result has been overload—hardly conducive to reflecting, questioning, and cumulatively developing theory. As Cole (1981) noted, "It is in the domain of informal activities in science that the biggest gaps between men and women remain" (p. 388).

About 95% of nurses are women; therefore, the sex-role identity of nurses cannot be ignored when we discuss theory development and the potential for theoretical thinking. Nursing has always been an occupation with predominantly feminine characteristics, and it is still stereotyped with nurturing roles such as those of wife and mother. Whether the image of nursing as a feminine role evolved out of recruitment of women into nursing or whether women were recruited into nursing because of its feminine image is a moot question. Ever since Nightingale recruited only women to accompany her to the Crimean War area to care for the wounded, the image of nurse was fused with the ministering, sacrificing, and altruistic image of women. The same pattern also was demonstrated in the Eastern image of a nurse, Rofaida Al-Islamiah, who is considered the mother of nursing in the Middle East. There is little doubt that many of the issues facing nursing emanated from the feminine image of nursing and the idea of nursing as a profession for women, particularly in societies in which women are relegated to secondary status (Dachelet, 1978; Heide, 1973; Wren, 1971).

Many characteristics of women have been considered antithetical to creativity and scientific productivity. There is ample evidence indicating that women are reared and socialized differently than men from the minute they utter their first cry of life, which may lead to some differences between their cognitive structures. Women are considered more affective, more subordinate, more emotional, less aggressive, and less achievement-oriented, and they are generally expected to apply rather than to create. Because ours is a patriarchal society, these differences, which could have been considered simply as differences without any value judgments, have been judged as negative toward women. In addition to this attitude, which has been more than devastating to women, women are also beset with many roles to juggle and many struggles to survive in career-oriented jobs (May, Meleis, and Winstead-Fry, 1982). Generally, women are conditioned to consider a professional career as secondary to family and home, which has not allowed them to reserve their energies for more creative endeavors such as theory development and theory testing.

Creativity and scholarly productivity embody curiosity, intellectual objectivity, the ability to be engaged in decision making, and independent judgment. These are socially desirable attributes so long as they are not adopted by women. Because nursing did not insist on independence or active striving for success, it has generally been perceived as a profession congruent with what is expected of women. Furthermore, nursing embodies subjectivity in care-giving, dependence on others for decision making, and expressiveness in relationships—all considered female traits.

Even when women broke away from the mold, they suffered ambivalences. Horner (1972) demonstrated that anxiety in many women is created by achievement-related conflicts. Those qualities that are essential for "intellectual mastery," such as independence and active striving, are not female qualities. Therefore, women who defy the conventions of sex-appropriate behavior usually pay the price in anxiety.

Until very recently, the message was, women are different, are less than men, and nursing is also different. The attributes that women should strive for and maintain are epitomized in nursing. Therefore, women believed the congruence between societal expectations of women and nurses. The self-fulfilling prophecy of what education women should have and how they should act as women and nurses lingered on. As a result, women who entered nursing, at least until the 1970s, had identified strongly with the roles of wife and mother and either believed that nursing would prepare them for the natural roles of women or that the nursing role was a way to earn a living until a knight came along and rescued them from the drudgery of full-time work. For most women, a career was not supposed to coexist with marriage and motherhood, so a woman had to choose between the two. Men, however, could easily combine career, fatherhood, and being a husband.

The self-identity of nursing students lay in their womanhood rather than in their profession. Women in nursing were different from women studying other professions in other ways as well. The self-concept of women who selected nursing, teaching, and dental hygiene included a perception of low autonomy, less chance for advancement, and less need for intellectual stimulus. They also asserted, by selecting nursing, that they had more favorable attitudes toward marriage and family. Students in nursing in the late 1960s and early 1970s ranked home and family roles as number one and career roles as number two, with their own identity being attached more to the former and less to the latter roles (Cleland, 1971; Olesen and Davis, 1966).

On the job, nurses' productivity was demonstrated by their constantly doing, by their sense of urgency, and by their appearing busy. However, their identity remained first and foremost ascribed to simply being women. Their type of productivity was devalued because women were socialized to believe that what they do is of little worth and below the level of what men do. Their identity also suffered because they were allowed to receive validation mainly through the capacity to bear children and rear children, not through intellectual achievement, career advancement, or financial gain. Male productivity, on the other hand, was valued, and men's identities were attached to doing, not being.

There were other perceived differences between men and women that might have retarded the development of nursing theory. For one thing, women in science were, in general, engaged in less scholarly production than men (Cole, 1981). Also, because nursing was fairly new to the scholarly arena, it was apparent that

> New scholars in the field have more obstacles and ambivalences to overcome
> in their attempt to integrate the scholarly role with the repertoire of other
> roles that constitute the self-concept. (May, Meleis, and Winstead-Fry, 1982,
> p. 23)

Sex-role stereotyping has also impeded nursing in one more way. Many women have come to believe the stereotypes that they are unintellectual, subjective, and emotional (Keller, 1979). Women have become prejudiced against each other, have reinforced the myths against each other, and have perpetuated the myth about their inability to think theoretically and to develop theories (Goldberg, 1968).

Two patterns that have existed in nursing for some time may thus be questioned. These are the rejection of nursing theories for some two decades and the predominance of theories, utilized by nurses, that have been developed by men who are not nurses. Is it possible that the slow adaptation and utilization of nursing theories may have occurred because they were theories developed by women and nurses as compared with other theories that were developed by men who were not nurses? These are questions worthy of further exploration by those interested in sex-role identity and perceptions and knowledge development in nursing.

Human Barriers: Nurses as Theorists

Nurse theorists themselves have sometimes acted unwittingly as barriers to the further development of theory. In the minds of practitioners, theorists who were associated with educational institutions were castigated for being far removed from practice. The language that theorists used separated them from their colleagues in practice and other nursing arenas. The language of theories appeared to be esoteric to the rest of the nursing world, to say nothing of the outside world. A nursing client as an energy field, a system of behavior, or a self-care agent were all new and ill-defined concepts. To complicate matters, educators translated nursing theory to curricula rather than to propositions for testing. This intensified the schism between theory and practice and supported the perceived lack of relationship between theory and practice.

Nurse theorists, easily accessible to their immediate colleagues, appeared to practitioners to be remote and inaccessible. Academics in general are perceived to represent the ivory tower and are perceived far less to represent the real world. The lack of intertheory discussions and debates added a new dimension to the many intradisciplinary schisms. Schisms also appeared between disciples of the various theories.

All theorists agree that the discipline of nursing needs to concur on the phenomena, perspectives, and problems that are central to the field and to the mission of nursing. But to select adaptation, homeostasis, self-care, need fulfillment, or effective nurse–patient interactions as the mission of nursing may mean concentrating exclusively on one mission to the exclusion of others. This may have been misinterpreted and the theorists may have been perceived as preaching one binding philosophy, one theory, or one conceptual model to guide nursing's research and practice. To accept one theory (argued the practitioners, the educators, and the researchers) that has not been subjected to practice application, research validation, or the test of time (to the exclusion of others) was unacceptable. Misconceptions, such as believing it was necessary to have only one theory, drew the few believers further away from theoretical nursing.

Though there is no published documentation for this analytical posture, the lack of debate about and among nursing theories in the 1960s and 1970s may in itself be an indication of such a misconception. There were numerous debates, though, among and between faculty members and clinicians regarding which theory to utilize and the inadvisability of such a choice. These debates were more ideological than substantive. Therefore, we can propose that nurses have been harsh in critiquing nursing theories, perhaps because (1) the theories did not appear to evolve from an empirical base, (2) these theories were developed by women, and (3) each theory in itself was not able to describe, explain, and predict all nursing phenomena. Harshness was also apparent in criticism of the nurse theorists for taking risks, which is another manifestation of what Ryan (1971) called "blaming the victim."

> Nurses have been admonished for contributing to their own oppression and inhibiting nursing from achieving the status of a profession (Stein, 1972). Much energy and time has been wasted, through intradisciplinary battles

between nursing service and nursing education and over types of educational programs and levels of entry into practice. Nurses invalidate other nurses by bringing in "experts" from other disciplines to tell nurses how to do things that are already being done by nursing "experts." This blaming, self-flagellation, and infighting must be recognized by nurses as deriving from the more general social problems of women. And, like women generally, nurses must understand that they alone are not to blame for these problems. (Yeaworth, 1978, p. 75)

Knowledge Barriers

Knowledge barriers also inhibit development in theoretical nursing. Knowledge barriers are manifested in the use of knowledge developed by other disciplines, the reluctance to use nursing theory that has been developed within the discipline by members of the discipline, and the further development of knowledge that is more pertinent to the fields of preparation of nurses (*i.e.*, disciplines from which nurses received their doctorates before the development of doctoral programs in nursing).

An interesting phenomenon persists in nursing—the *what is imported is superior* phenomenon, in which the imported is far more meaningful than that which is domestic and developed by nurses. By imported we mean theories developed by individuals other than nurses and those developed in a field other than nursing. Sometimes this importing of theories was done for legitimate reasons, but many times it was done with no rationale other than the obvious: someone who was not a nurse developed it, and it emerged from a non-nursing paradigm, therefore, it must be good. This is apparent in the unquestioning use of theories from other disciplines, the lack of reluctance to attribute the label of theory to conceptualizations that evolve from a non-nursing discipline (*e.g.*, role theory, when sociologists are still debating whether role is a concept, a construct, or a theory), and the concomitant reluctance to attribute the label of theory to nursing conceptual schemes.

Nursing has been shadowed first by the biomedical model and then by numerous other paradigms; therefore, the notion of knowledge development was left up to those in the different fields that are related to nursing. Few in those related fields saw fit to push nurses to look for their own individualized umbrella, their own perspective, their own paradigm. As expected, disciplines prefer to prepare their own students for research careers that include research in nursing rather than to prepare nurses for such careers.

> Sociologists, psychologists, and physiologists are much more comfortable with the idea of providing members of their discipline to do the research for nursing than with the idea of providing doctoral preparation for nurses who then return to nursing to apply their knowledge. (Yeaworth, 1978, p. 75)

Because they had few role models who combined nursing and another field in their graduate programs and because they were away from nursing practice while studying theory and research, nurses with doctorates in non-nursing fields tended to explore phenomena using their new field's binoculars and neglected to synthesize the findings into theoretical nursing. The result has been to explore propositions from sociology, psychology, education, or physiology. These explorations often have implications for nursing practice but not for nursing theory. Many of these nurses educated in other disciplines may have believed that nursing had nothing unique to offer and therefore maintained that the quest for a unique domain is a quest for separation and noncollaboration. To some, to condone nursing theories and nursing's need to develop theories was to support a separationist notion.

Theory itself was a barrier. First, nurses said they needed theories to prove that nursing is a profession, not simply an occupation. The one thing nursing lacked in its quest for professionalism was a systematic, coherent body of knowledge with boundaries. Theories fulfilled this requirement but, as a result, were suspected of being developed for professionally selfish reasons. This turned off the practitioners, and theorists found themselves spending a great deal of energy trying to justify their theories rather than developing them any further or making them more useful.

Another misguided goal evolved. Educators began to believe that theory—which was then called "conceptual framework"—was needed to develop conceptually based curricula. In fact, the National League for Nursing required that a curriculum should have a well-articulated conceptual framework as a requirement for accreditation. The rationale was that if students were prepared in these programs, they would go out and be agents of change in practice. Thus, from 1965 to 1975 faculty everywhere began to rush around trying to fit square pegs into round holes. The result were curricula that overwhelmed students with esoteric content rarely used in practice after graduation. In fact, the schism that existed between the languages of clinicians and educators had convinced students of the uselessness of the esoteric content even before their own graduation and initiation into the work force.

Many graduate students have commented on trying to revive the knowledge of nursing theory they gained in their baccalaureate years, knowledge that to them had not been useful in practice. Upon returning to school, however, they were grateful their baccalaureate program had been based on one of the nursing theories. The academic need for those theories has been established. Many of us had been lulled into thinking that using conceptual frameworks was the way to develop theories and theoretical thinking. Therefore, focusing on conceptualizing curricula caused us to lose sight of the reason for it in the first place: *nursing practice* and *patient care*.

Another goal was for nursing to have a disciplinary status based on scientific foundations; this required the existence of theories. Theories, then, appeared to be a means to establish nursing as an academic discipline, one that is distinct from medicine and deserving of professional status. All these are worthy goals for nursing. They will not be achieved, however, by developing theories to guide curricula; theories must be developed through asking and answering the significant questions of the field. The central goal is the provision of effective nursing care of clients in any society. Significant questions arise from this goal, and theories help us understand, explain, predict, and prescribe the care. Secondary gains, then, comprise a professional and disciplinary status for nursing. During the 1980s and 1990s, nurses have realized the primacy of the goal of providing care to clients and have restructured their goals.

Conceptual Barriers

All these barriers—history, culture, and environment—contribute to the lack of conscious use of nursing theories, inhibit the potential for developing theories, and may have created conceptual barriers for nurses. Conceptual blocks are those closed gates that prevent nurses from perceiving or developing nursing phenomena beyond the immediate problem-solving need. Conceptual blocks, according to Adams (1974), are caused by perceptual, cultural, and environmental obstacles. Cultural and environmental blocks were discussed previously; the following section discusses perceptual blocks.

> Perceptual blocks are obstacles that prevent the problem solver from clearly
> perceiving either the problem itself or the information that is necessary to
> solve the problem. (Adams, 1974, p. 13)

When used as a framework to describe the nursing situation, perceptual blocks may appear in the following six forms, as described by Adams (1974). First, a nurse may have difficulty delineating a phenomenon that is worthy of pursuance theoretically. She may be unable to perceive meaningful clues, she may focus on tangential issues, use *a priori* paradigms that do not permit a nursing perspective, or fail to see a phenomenon because of the lack of a defining framework.

Second, some nurses may put closer boundaries on a phenomenon—more acceptable boundaries in terms of societal expectations—to the detriment of understanding the phenomenon. For example, suppose an immigrant was admitted to the emergency room three times in the six weeks following his successful triple by-pass surgery. Each time there was a question of another myocardial infarction, and each time the infarction was unsubstantiated. The causes of the unwarranted emergency room appearances were recorded as noncompliance, or diagnostic problems in the emergency room, or inability to communicate signs and symptoms. In this case, a premature closure on the phenomenon of repeated appearance prevented a careful exploration of the phenomenon within the context of the immigrant's experience and the cultural meanings attached to heart problems.

Similarly, a third perceptual block is lack of experience in considering a phenomenon from different perspectives.

Nurses also fall prey to a fourth type of perceptual block that is related to paradigms that have guided us for many generations and make us see what we expect to see. If we see the world through the biomedical model, we tend to see signs, symptoms, and biomedical antecedents. Our stereotypes of cultures and social classes and our likes and dislikes in values limit our perceptions and create blocks.

Immersion and experience are two-edged swords in theoretical development. While both are essential in describing theoretically clinical practice, they also tend to prevent us from seeing a phenomenon from fresh perspectives. Anthropologists and sociologists have discussed this fifth perceptual block and advise distancing to allow a return to a fresh start. Another strategy is to consciously keep a journal of events related to the phenomenon. Putting the journal aside and picking it up again later permits the distancing and diffuses what Adams calls the problems of "saturation" (1974, p. 25).

The final perceptual block to be aware of is the nurse's potential inability to permit and accept all senses and intuitive inputs in delineating and developing a phenomenon theoretically.

FORCES AS RESOURCES

Human Resources: Nurses as Nurses

Theory is a mental image and conception of reality. Tools for theory development are similar to tools that nurses use in their clinical practice and with which they are most experienced. One of the most significant tools for theorizing is the ability to observe. Nurses have ample opportunity to learn how to observe, to sharpen their observations, and to use all their senses in collecting data. Observation is central to nursing practice; observation comes easily to the experienced clinician.

Another significant tool for theorizing is the ability to record what actually is happening in a nursing care situation. Nursing records offer a wealth of information and are patient-specific, temporally limited, and have space boundaries that do not allow for generalization. With other tools—thinking and reflecting—providing legitimation for developing theories, the observation and recording of data could become the impetus for more general descriptions. Each one of these nursing care situations could become an exemplar for further generalization.

Examples from our theoretical history substantiate these abilities and their relationship to theory development. Nightingale reflected on the many functions and activities that nurses performed during the Crimean War. While in bed (Nightingale spent the last 30 years of her life in bed), she had uninterrupted time and resources to collate observations, critique actions, analyze perceptions of nursing, and arrive at the first systematic, comprehensive concept of nursing.

The field of nursing itself, a source for theory development, is a gold mine for those who wish to articulate its many components and incorporate them into theory. Nurses are dealing with many phenomena that need describing and explaining, and they are responsible for helping clients achieve their health goals through a wide range of activities, ranging from assessing to evaluating, from the technical to the highly abstract. A world of information exists in nursing that needs to be described and put into order.

Unlike other disciplines that have doubtful social significance, nursing is needed as a human service and is sanctioned for its significance to health care. Nurses in practice settings spend a good deal of time with patients, and because practice is one of the most significant sources of theory, the central ingredient for theory development is therefore available.

In the 1960s, in the wake of nursing education and its attempt at integration, the Yale school of thought evolved to represent developing theories by observing patients, cajoling nurses to articulate what they had accomplished in patient care, and composing a view of nursing—its mission, its goals, and its prescription. These nurse educators used observation and recording skills they had mastered as nurses, and they utilized nursing clinicians' abilities to do the same. The result was an early conceptualization of nursing as an interpersonal process, which is useful to this day. One must consider, however, that federal funding at the time allowed those nurses the free time and flexible schedules to think, reflect, and develop theories.

Whereas earlier nursing education had been a deterrent to theory development, nursing education since the beginning of the 1980s has been a force headed toward its enhancement. When faculty of doctoral nursing programs in the United States were asked what they considered the core content in their respective programs, highest in rank order were nursing theory, theory development, and conceptual formulation (Beare, Gray, and Ptak, 1981). Students and recent graduates from doctoral programs in nursing, beginning in the 1980s, were practically the first purebreds in the science of nursing. The generation immediately preceding them had experienced a true hybrid of a multitude of programs. Therefore, it is natural that these purebred individuals address the central questions in the field by engaging in the much needed processes of theory development and organization of nursing knowledge. Many master's programs in the United States also offer nursing theory, and a few undergraduate programs are beginning to orient their students to the need for theorizing and for utilizing nursing theory in practice.

Other quests make the nature of nursing a moving force in theory development. Theoretical knowledge is viewed as a "basis for power" (Chinn and Jacobs, 1987). Therefore, as nurses attempt to achieve their professional autonomy, theory becomes a most significant mechanism. As the novices recognize that they can defend ideas better when they approach the argument or debate from a theoretical basis, they will tend to use theory more. As the experienced push to have their services acknowledge nursing care outcomes as distinguishable from outcomes of other kinds of care, they will use theory to articulate their mission, their goals, and their focus. A move toward autonomy is indeed a moving force toward theory development and utilization.

Autonomy is linked to communication about patient care among nurses and between nursing and other health care professions. Communication is enhanced when it is in an understandable language that is common, if not to all health care professionals, then at least among nurses themselves. Communication is enhanced when it evolves from some guiding framework. As nurses value and respect each other's observations and diagnoses, and as they search for a common language with which to communicate, a language that represents nursing's goals and missions more than immediate patient care, then theory becomes a means to achieve better communication. Therefore, the quest for better communication about patient care and about patient care outcomes is a quest for theory development. Nursing practice and nursing education are present-day forces toward theorizing in nursing.

Finally, experiences of nurses as experts in nursing practice were formally acknowledged in the 1980s as a most significant source for nursing knowledge (Benner, 1984). Describing expert nursing practice as seen and practiced by nurses was considered a valued source if not the most significant source for articulating in a meaningful and coherent whole the fundamental and practice aspects of nursing.

Human Resources: Nurses as Women

Theorists and researchers are beginning to produce evidence to refute some of the myths surrounding female identity. Recent empirical investigations and theories do not show sex-role differentiation in sensitivity to social cues, in affiliative behavior, or in nurturing behavior. Women are neither more empathetic nor more altruistic than men. Although the myth surrounding these differences still lingers, data are increasingly refuting them (Meeker and Weitzel-O'Neill, 1977). Therefore, some of the attributes of women that have been linked to lower productivity and paucity in theoretical thinking are questioned by more contemporary researchers. These new findings, though, are still limited in distribution and in their power to refute earlier findings presented in this chapter. More research and more widespread distribution of knowledge about productivity-oriented female attributes is occurring in the current decade.

In the meantime, the feminist movement has done a great deal of consciousness-raising of women in general and nurses in particular. It has attempted to dissipate some of the myths that have been true barriers to the development of women for a long time. Nurses are beginning to identify more with feminist movement ideals and with a view of nursing as a career rather than merely as a stepping stone toward motherhood (Moore, Decker, and Dowd, 1978; Stein, 1972). Research supports the presence of that shift. Graduate, baccalaureate, and associate degree program students were found to have self-images more in harmony with the image of professional nursing (Stromborg, 1976). The shift is toward an image of independence, competence, and intellectual achievement, characteristics more congruent with a person who engages in idea development.

New research findings demonstrate that nursing students are not qualitatively different from other female college students in their sex-role identity and personality constructs (Meleis and Dagenais, 1981). These new studies are either dispelling the earlier myths that nursing students manifest more feminine characteristics than other women in college or are demonstrating that drastic changes have occurred for women, and particularly for nurses.

When feminine characteristics of nursing students in programs at the three educational levels (diploma, associate, and baccalaureate) were compared with normative data of women in general, results demonstrated that nurses are generally similar to female college and university students in a number of personality constructs. When there were differences, they were congruent with what is expected in practice professions; that is, they did not differ in autonomy but rather in practical aspects (Meleis and Dagenais, 1981). Education plays a more significant role in perception of self than in sex-role identity. Changing sex-role identities through dispelling some of the myths surrounding women's abilities makes the environment more receptive to women's creativity in knowledge development.

Changing society's expectations of women and science are other forces in theory development in nursing. There are some attributes that women possess that may have been perceived in the past as inappropriate and incongruent with creativity but that are becoming more accepted in today's society. Women have been described as intuitive. Increasingly, as Eastern and Western modes of knowledge development merge, intuition is seen in a more positive light and, indeed, as essential in idea development, as a component in different patterns of understanding reality, and as an accepted method for scientific inquiry (Carper, 1978; Silva, 1977). Intuition is part of the philosophical process, the mental labor that is central to the process of developing theories. Intuition played a significant role in Einstein's discovery and in Darwin's articulation of the evolutionary theory. Intuition, the "curse" of women's abilities, is a force in the 1990s for women's potential. Intuitive awareness of personal and social phenomena is a resource for women in nursing (Adams, 1972).

Although women may have been caught in a "compassion trap" of always being available as helpers in the past, Adams (1972) suggests that, as a result, women possess an attribute that is significant in today's world: flexibility. Women, as an oppressed minority, learned to deal with difficult situations when others controlled access to resources. In the process, they learned how to be flexible and how to be innovative in finding alternative resources essential for their development and for accomplishing their goals.

> Persons with these sensitive capacities undoubtedly perceive reality
> differently than those who occupy positions of social power and dominance,
> yet their perceptions have much to contribute to knowledge about nurturing
> and the care-taking process. (Benoliel, 1975, p. 26)

Women's contextual cognitive style has been learned in a life of socialization. Juggling roles is more congruent with the contemporary need to consider sociocultural variables in scientific questions. Changes in sex-role identity, changes in the image of women, and a growing respect for intuition as a pattern of knowing, flexibility, and resourcefulness are all significant forces in theory development.

Women in nursing have an added advantage over women in other disciplines. Women scientists—in physics, chemistry, and social and behavioral sciences, among others—are a minority in their own fields. They have experienced prejudices, less support, and outright discrimination in resource allocation, among other social ills that result from the competition with a dominant group by an oppressed group. In such unfair competition, men tend to win to the detriment of women's progress in these disciplines (Cole, 1981).

The overwhelming majority of nurses are women; therefore, conflicts resulting from intradisciplinary sex-role competition are nonexistent. Female nurses have full citizenship within their own discipline. Moreover, we hope that the lessons we have learned from other disciplines will not permit prejudices against male nurses.

Creative energy can be freed from the sex-role struggle for the benefit of theory development.

Women and nurses have exhibited a sense of humility as a corollary to humanity, which may have previously prevented them from generalizing beyond the immediate situation (Dickoff, James, and Wiedenbach, 1968). This sense of humility is now being replaced by self-assurance as nurses articulate their conceptualization of reality.

Knowledge as a Force and a Resource

Knowledge breeds knowledge; the more knowledge we need, the more we are stimulated and challenged to further develop an understanding of phenomena. Theory development in nursing is enhanced by the wealth of theoretical knowledge we already have. The theories developed by nurse scholars provide an impetus for further refinement and development. They lead to an agreed-upon set of concepts that are central to nursing and point to phenomena of interest to nursing. They have set the stage for the next steps.

Debates surrounding which theories to develop, how to develop them, and whether or not to develop them have helped to further clarify the mission of nursing. With a preliminary identification of content and a beginning articulation of methodology, the course is now clear for smoother sailing. All this has set the stage for shaping skills in analytical and critical thinking and has stimulated more nurse scholars to pursue further development in theoretical nursing. Nursing has the potential for developing a feminist approach to science, or even a nonsexist science, by converting "value-free technology" to a "humane technology" that incorporates self-care (Ardetti, 1980).

Old paradigms of knowledge are being challenged by new paradigms, prompted by two significant social movements: the feminist movement and the women's health movement (McPherson, 1983). Essential components of the new paradigm represent a shift to include humanitarianism, holism, the incorporation of sociocultural content, perceptions of subjects of research, subjects and researchers collaborating in the research process, and a qualitative approach. The "new paradigm" is not new to nursing. Its newness stems more from social acceptance as the public is becoming more aware of ways to develop knowledge and demanding participation in the process. The newness is in the congruence rather than in a shift in thinking. There is wider acceptance of components of the "new paradigm" by consumers who care. That is a force that will help nurses further develop knowledge. The energy that used to be expended by those defending components of a paradigm that was incongruent with a prevailing scientific perspective can now be channeled from the creativity of reaction to the creativity of action.

A new world view is emerging, a view that has even changed physics from the mechanistic conceptions advanced by Descartes and Newton to a more holistic and ecological view (Capra, 1983). The new world view is congruent with women's views of science and nurses' views of health. It is a view that has shifted focus from a causative view to a more interpretive view. It is heightened by phenomenology and qualitative research.

Conceptual Resources

To use all senses, experiences, and intuition requires involvement and immersion in situations as a whole, and to describe patterns of responses theoretically requires longer periods of engagement in situations where nursing phenomena occur. The nature of nursing, the process of nursing care, the history of the profession, and the predominant gender orientation of the profession enhance the conceptual resources for nurses. Nurses are trained to observe, to record, to analyze, and to solve problems. Whether we admit it or not, we tend to use our own and others' experiences in providing care, and in doing so we rely on all our senses and intuitions, just as we rely on science principles to guide our action.

Nurses spend long hours with patients, families, and communities; this time allows an understanding of patterns of behaviors rather than isolated incidents. Diversity in nurses and in their cultural, educational, and socioeconomic backgrounds can be a resource to allow for diverse views, a safeguard against premature closure on a phenomenon and against narrow perspectives. Diversity in care-givers, in some instances considered problematic, could become a useful resource for theoretical development. This resource could help remove perceptual blocks.

Nurses have effective interviewing skills for which they have been meticulously trained. They have mastered questioning, they know how to prioritize, and they know how to participate in dialogue. They have opportunities to confirm observations and hunches during clinical rounds at the end or beginning of shift reports, during impromptu meetings at the nurses' stations, in meetings with other members of the family, and during their many regular daily roles and activities that involve talking, listening, questioning, answering, and writing. Each one of these tasks enhances perception, and each is a resource and an asset for conceptualization.

Other Forces for Theory Use and Development

The journey to theoretical thinking has been a progression through self-effacing stops, self-doubt detours, humility delays, collisions with opposing and dominating paradigms, and near-misses due to embarking on unfamiliar territory or unpaved terrain. Nursing and nurses are emerging theoretically stronger and far better prepared to embark on a task of theoretical clarification. The quality of the journey could be enhanced by coaching, mentorship, and sponsorship toward the development of the scholarly role.

Nurses are no longer resistant to the use of nursing theory in their practice or to their potential involvement in theory development. Rather, they are asking how they can use theory and looking for those they can emulate in the process. One example of nurses' interest in theory was a national conference held in 1983 by clinical specialists, in which the topic of theory development and utilization dominated a full half day of the two-day conference (Clinical Nurse Specialists, 1983).

Planners of the conference were concerned about the responses of the attendants to what might appear as highly abstract ideas not directly related to everyday care issues. The results were astonishing, the evaluations were heartening, and the request came for another session the following year, focusing on how to bring acceptance to theory utilization and development in clinical areas (Clinical Nurse Specialists, 1984). In short, nurses were asking for role modeling, role clarification, and role rehearsal—all properties of mentorship (May, Meleis, and Winstead-Fry, 1982).

> Mentorship is an intense relationship calling for a high degree of involvement between a novice in a discipline and a person who is knowledgeable and wise in that area. . . . In the process of helping the beginning scholar to fit resources to her needs and capabilities, the mentor provides options, opens up new opportunities, and helps to make corrections. This means that, on cognitive and affective levels, the mentor is involved with the novice as a whole person and feels a sense of responsibility for her (May, Meleis, and Winstead-Fry, 1982, p. 23).

Role modeling, which is teaching by example and emulation, then fosters the learning of these behaviors (Bandura, 1962; Meleis, 1975). Role clarification provides an opportunity to understand the subtle intricacies of the role to be emulated. What does it mean to have a role in the theoretical development of nursing? What cues are needed to perform that role? Role clarification in theory use and development may include spelling out the differences between the various theories, the different strategies in theory development, the different barriers to use of theory, and some strategies for handling all of these. Mentorship also includes opportunities for role rehearsal. Use of theory in theoretical patient care studies and use of different strategies in theory development are examples of staged situations to practice behaviors central to the use and development of theory (May, Meleis, and Winstead-Fry, 1982; Meleis and May, 1981).

Time and sociocultural conditions are right for the development of theoretical nursing, which in turn is significant for patient care, and nurses are "going for it." If, indeed, there is a woman's way to understand the world, and if there are areas of knowledge that are better understood when seen through the eyes of women and through the use of feminine logic, then nursing is ready on all of these accounts, and nurses are well-prepared to pursue that knowledge.

Nursing education can provide supportive conditions through programs that focus on scholarly productivity (Meleis and May, 1981; Meleis, Wilson, and Chater, 1980). Theory and theory development should not be limited to graduate programs. Theoretical thinking should be the *modus operandi* for conscientious patient care from day one in nursing education. Nursing practice has an equal commitment to provide avenues by which nurses can communicate their findings in theoretical terms and can have the opportunity to translate their hunches into theoretical terms. Nurses in the appropriate atmosphere should be able to try using different theories in practice for the purpose of refining and extending them.

Similar supportive environments could be provided by nurse administrators to help in the development of a theoretical culture that allows dialogues, debates, and discussions that go beyond the immediate day-by-day problem solving and decision making. Strategies to be used by nurse administrators and educators for the enhancement of theory development include creating a theoretical culture, supporting critical thinking, refocusing dialogues and discussions on concepts, defining nursing territory, exploring ambiguous ideas, allowing uncertainty about phenomena to linger, avoiding premature closure on ideas, facing views of phenomena from different perspectives, and providing such resources as library time, observation time, and writing time (Jennings and Meleis, 1988; Meleis and Jennings, 1989; Meleis and Price, 1988).

CONCLUSION

Nurses are now in the land of Kant rather than the land of "Can't." Kant maintained that knowledge depends on experience and experience on observation, but observations by themselves do not form experience nor give meaning to experience. Observations have to be organized *a priori* by the mind in order to develop into knowledge. In so organizing our observations, we tend to reconstruct reality.

Nurses may have reconstructed the meaning of theoretical constraints into forces that foster the further development of theoretical nurses. They can use the tools of practice for theory development, relying on the same abilities they have used for practice, research, teaching, administering, and translating these skills to theorize and to use theory, perhaps thereby becoming convinced that their experiences comprise the appropriate impetus for theory development.

The synthesis between continental rationalism and British empiricism espoused by Kant may be helpful in increasing our knowledge of nursing realities.

REFERENCES

Adams, J. (1974) *Conceptual block busting: A guide to better ideas.* San Francisco: W.H. Freeman and Co.

Adams, M. (1972) The compassion trap. In V. Goernick and B.K. Moran (Eds.), *Women in sexist society.* New York: Signet Books.

Ardetti, R. (1980) Feminism and science. In R. Ardetti, P. Brennan, and S. Cavrak (Eds.), *Science and liberation.* Boston: South End Press.

Ashley, J.A. (1977) *Hospitals, paternalism, and the role of the nurse.* New York: Teachers College, Columbia University.

Bandura, A. (1962) Social learning through imitation. In M.R. Jones (Ed.), *Nebraska symposium on motivation.* Lincoln: University of Nebraska Press.

Beare, P.G., Gray, C.J., and Ptak, H.F. (1981) Doctoral curricula in nursing. *Nursing Outlook,* 29(5), 311–316.

Benner, P. (1984) *From novice to expert: Excellence and power in clinical nursing practice.* Menlo Park, CA: Addison-Wesley.

Benoliel, J.Q. (1973) Collaboration and competition in nursing research. In *Communicating nursing research: Collaboration and competition.* Boulder, CO: Western Interstate Commission for Higher Education.

Benoliel, J.Q. (1975) Scholarship: A woman's perspective. *Image,* 7(2), 22–27.

Bullough, B. (1975) Barriers to the nurse practitioner movement: Problems of women in a woman's field. *International Journal of Health Services*, 5(2), 225–233.

Capra, F. (1983) *The turning point: Science, society, and the rising culture.* New York: Bantam.

Carper, B.A. (1978) Practice oriented theory: Part 1. Fundamental patterns of knowing in nursing. *Advances in Nursing Science*, 1(1), 13–23.

Chinn, P.L. and Jacobs, M.K. (1987) *Theory and nursing: A systematic approach* (2nd ed.). St. Louis: C.V. Mosby.

Cleland, V. (1971) Sex discrimination: Nursing's most pervasive problem. *American Journal of Nursing*, 71(8), 1542–1547.

Clinical Nurse Specialists Annual Conference (1983, February 17–18) San Francisco, CA.

Clinical Nurse Specialists Annual Conference (1984, February 16–17) San Francisco, CA.

Cole, J.R. (1981, July/August) Women in science. *American Scientist*, 69, 385–391.

Copleston, F. (1964) *A history of philosophy. Modern philosophy: Kant.* (Vol. 6, Part II). Garden City: Image Books.

Dachelet, C.Z. (1978) Nursing's bid for increased status. *Nursing Forum*, 17(1), 18–45.

Dickoff, J., James, P., and Wiedenbach, E. (1968) Theory in practice discipline: Part 1. Practice oriented theory. *Nursing Research*, 17(5), 415–435.

Edwards, C.N. (1969) The student nurse: A study in sex-role transition. *Psychology Report*, 25(3), 975–990.

Gaston, J. (1975) Social organization, codification of knowledge, and the reward structure in science. *Journal of Social Psychology*, 18, 285–303. (Koln, Germany)

Gilligan, C. (1984) *In a different voice: Psychological theory and women's development.* Cambridge, MA: Harvard University Press.

Goldberg, P. (1968, April) Are women prejudiced against women? *Trans-Action*, 5, 28–30.

Heide, W.S. (1973) Nursing and women's liberation—A parallel. *American Journal of Nursing*, 73(5), 824–827.

Horner, M. (1972) Toward an understanding of achievement-related conflicts in women. *Journal of Social Issues*, 28(2), 157–175.

Jennings, B. and Meleis, A.I. (1988) Nursing theory and administrative practice: Agenda for the 1990s. *Advances in Nursing Science*, 10(3), 56–69.

Keller, M. (1979) The effect of sexual stereotyping on the development of nursing theory. *American Journal of Nursing*, 79(9), 1585–1586.

Loomis, M.E. (1974) Collegiate nursing education: An ambivalent professionalism. *The Journal of Nursing Education*, November, 39–48.

May, K.M., Meleis, A.I., and Winstead-Fry, P. (1982) Mentorship for scholarliness: Opportunities and dilemmas. *Nursing Outlook*, 30(11), 22–28.

McPherson, K.I. (1983) Feminist methods: A new paradigm for nursing research. *Advances in Nursing Science*, 5(2), 17–36.

Meeker, B.F. and Weitzel-O'Neill. (1977, February) Sex roles and interpersonal behavior in task-oriented groups. *American Sociological Review*, 42, 91–105.

Meleis, A.I. (1975) Role insufficiency and role supplementation: A conceptual framework. *Nursing Research*, 24(4), 264–271.

Meleis, A.I. and Dagenais, F. (1981) Sex-role identity and perception of professional self in graduates of three nursing programs. *Nursing Research*, 30(3), 162–167.

Meleis, A.I. and Jennings, B. (1989). Theoretical nursing administration: Today's challenges, tomorrow's bridges. In B. Henry, C. Arndt, M. DiVincenti, and A. Marriner (Eds.). *Dimensions and issues in nursing administration.* Boston: Blackwell Scientific Publications.

Meleis, A.I. and May, K.M. (1981) Nursing theory and scholarliness in the doctoral program. *Advances in Nursing Science*, 4(1), 31–41.

Meleis, A.I. and Price, M. (1988) Strategies and conditions for nursing: An international perspective. *Journal of Advanced Nursing*, 13, 592–604.

Meleis, A.I., Wilson, H.S., and Chater, S. (1980) Toward scholarliness in doctoral dissertations: An analytical model. *Journal of Research in Nursing and Health*, 3, 115–124.

Moore, D.S., Decker, S.D., and Dowd, M.W. (1978) Baccalaureate nursing students' identification with the women's movement. *Nursing Research*, 27(5), 291–295.

Olesen, V.L. and Davis, F. (1966, Spring) Baccalaureate students' images of nursing: A follow-up report. *Nursing Research*, 15(2), 151–158.

Ryan, W. (1971) *Blaming the victim*. New York: Random House.

Silva, M.C. (1977) Philosophy, science, theory: Interrelationships and implications for nursing research. *Image*, 9(3), 59–63.

Stein, L.I. (1972, April) Liberation movement: Impact on nursing. *AORN Journal*, 15(4), 67–85.

Stromborg, M.F. (1976) Relationship of sex-role identity to occupational image of female nursing students. *Nursing Research*, 25(5), 363–369.

Wren, G.R. (1971, March/April) Some characteristics of freshman students in baccalaureate, diploma, and associate degree nursing programs. *Nursing Research*, 20(2), 167–172.

Yeaworth, R. (1978) Feminism and the nursing profession. In N. Chaska (Ed.), *The nursing profession: Views through the mist*. New York: McGraw-Hill.

Chapter 5

Toward the Development of the Discipline of Nursing: Epistemological Issues

Epistemology is the branch of philosophy that considers the history of knowledge. It raises and answers questions related to the origin, the nature, the methods, and the limitations in knowledge development and outlines the various criteria by which knowledge is accepted. This chapter will discuss several issues that have preoccupied the discipline of nursing in the past. These are:

Theoretical growth: Revolution, evolution, or integration;
From the received view to the perceived view; and
From correspondence to Weltanschauung.

Understanding how knowledge evolves, how science is accumulated, and how knowledge is accepted is essential for development and progress in any field. Such understanding helps to further define goals to be pursued, either for the individual scientist or for the discipline as a whole (Andreoli and Thompson, 1977; Baer, 1979; Carper, 1978; Silva, 1977). Therefore, a study of epistemological issues helps us to accomplish the following:

○ Increase our awareness of the complexity and diversity of perspectives, views, and theories (sometimes conflicting) of scientific progress, truth, and the methodology of truth;
○ Distinguish between different kinds of problems in knowledge and development and therefore deliberately pursue those that seem most germane to the theoretical progress of the nursing discipline; and
○ Deal with potential epistemological constraints, however inappropriate, that evolve from *de facto* acceptance of one view, one theory, or one perspective without careful study of alternatives.

During the past two or three decades, we have accumulated a good deal of nursing knowledge about caring, interacting, promoting healthy environments, supplementing roles, enhancing recovery, and supporting healing. If we allow our knowledge to continue to develop haphazardly, disconnectedly, or aimlessly, it may not progress as expediently as we wish, or in the direction we choose. A period of reflection on the course of the development of nursing's knowledge base, particularly its theoretical progress, allows us to appreciate our progress and, at the same time, gives us the pause necessary for a more organized future development.

The concern in this book is the role of theory in the development of nursing knowledge, although it is understood that knowledge encompasses far more than theory—it includes research, common sense, and philosophy as well as extant and ought-to-be nursing practice. The following discussion is about, but not limited to, the evolution of theory in nursing.

THEORETICAL GROWTH: REVOLUTION, EVOLUTION, OR INTEGRATION

Scientific growth has been studied by many philosophers and scientists. Several theories have been advanced to describe patterns of scientific progress based on retrospective analysis of physical and social science progress. The question of how sciences develop, which has occupied philosophers of science, has also become one of nursing's significant questions. What processes did nursing go through leading to its current stage of development? To answer these questions, nurses have resorted to patterns that have been previously identified. Utilizing patterns that are more congruent with scientific progress in the physical sciences may have impeded the theoretical growth of the discipline of nursing.

A Theory of Revolution

Kuhn (1970, 1977), a physicist by training, is credited with developing the revolutionary theory of scientific development. *Revolution* is defined by *Webster's Third New International Dictionary* as "a sudden, radical, or complete change" characterized by "overthrowing" fundamental changes.* Kuhn's theory is based on this definition and is congruent with its sentiment. Sciences, to Kuhn, develop by leaps and bounds only through periods of crisis in which theories compete, anomalies are identified, and inadequacies are highlighted—leading to predominance of one theory over all others.

This period of scientific unrest is followed by a tranquil period that Kuhn calls normal science. This period marks the acceptability of one theory over all others. Normal science is a period when members of the field accept in a unified way a common paradigm. The transition from a crisis to normal science marks a scientific revolution. Kuhn asserts that scientific revolutions are inevitable for the development of a science and that scientific development is noncumulative, meaning an

---

* By permission. From *Webster's Third New International Dictionary* ©1986 by Merriam-Webster Inc., publisher of the Merriam-Webster® dictionaries.

aspect of one theory that is useful is not added to another competing theory to render it more useful. The competition between paradigms does not evolve into collaborative paradigms; rather, only one prevails to the destruction of others. In other words, older paradigms, whether or not useful on the whole or in part, are incompatible with newly conceived paradigms (Kuhn, 1970).

Kuhn is a prolific writer and speaker who should be amply credited for giving credence to the philosophy of science as a field worthy of exploration and investigation. His central ideas are:

1. A paradigm is defined as an entire repertoire of beliefs, values, laws, principles, theory methodologies, ways of application, and instrumentation.
2. A paradigm encompasses substantive theoretical assumptions about the subject matter of the discipline and methodological strategies as well as a degree of consensus about theory methods and techniques.
3. A paradigm includes the questionable areas in the field and some puzzle solutions that could act as examples to help members of that scientific community solve the remainder of the normal science problems in the discipline.
4. A discipline matures when it has such a paradigm. Prior to its paradigmatic stage, however, there is haphazard and variable fact-finding in the processes used to answer the discipline questions. This period is characterized as a preparadigmatic stage of the discipline. The movement toward a paradigmatic stage occurs only when one of the paradigms becomes dominant and is accepted by the community of scholars. It is then and only then that the period of normal science is achieved.

The process is a revolutionary one characterized by sudden changes, and its cornerstone is competition. Development is not possible without competition, the result of which is the predominance of one paradigm over all others. The revolution occurs because none of the earlier paradigms work any more. A paradigm may be thrown away and replaced by another competing paradigm because the exemplar attached to it is more successful and others in the field are in agreement with it. Rejection of all other paradigms occurs at this time.

Once a paradigm dominates, competition is halted because one paradigm clearly prevails. This is the period of normal science. Collaboration, then, replaces competition, and the scientific community prevents any alternative paradigms from emerging during this period. Even when theoretical or methodological issues evolve, the scientific community avoids and ignores them, permitting the continuing dominance of the prevailing paradigm.

Kuhn's ideas led to a belief that disciplines develop by convergence. Converging on one paradigm is then accepted as the goal of disciplines to lead them to progress. A *convergent process* is a closed rather than an open process—a process that is antithetical to the nature of science, which is characterized as being open to new development and tolerant of competition.

The term *paradigm* was substituted in Kuhn's later writing with *disciplinary matrix*, denoting the same definition of paradigm but with the addition of *shared exemplars* (Kuhn, 1970, pp. 181–210). Because content boundaries of paradigms are not entirely explicit but rather implicit, exemplars are provided to identify the problems and the solutions in the discipline. They are models for problems and solutions that are accepted by scientists during the period of normal science.

Kuhn's ideas have been both revered and criticized. Many writers have taken issue with his admonitions and questioned the capability of his theory to describe and predict the developmental process in the progress of science. More specifically, Kuhn's notion of the development of scientific disciplines through crises and through scientific revolutions has fostered numerous debates in the field of philosophy of science. There are those who have pointed to historical inconsistencies between Kuhn's analysis of several of the established scientific disciplines and his generalization about such developments; these inconsistencies point to the harmonious coexistence between numerous competing paradigms.

In the view of those who have pointed out such inconsistencies, coexistence between competing paradigms leads to appropriate debates within a given field. Critics pointed out disciplines that were established in spite of having no single guiding framework. Why, Dudley Shapere asks, should we only have the extremes, the absolute differences in competing paradigms (thus a crisis) or the absolute identity within one paradigm (thus a revolution) followed by normal science? (Shapere, 1981, p. 58) Is it not possible to have, at any one point in time, both similarities and differences, both competition and collaboration?

Laudan also challenged Kuhn's assertion and proposed that competition is continuous and that scientific disciplines include a variety of coexisting research traditions (1981, p. 153). Laudan identified five major flaws in Kuhn's philosophical view of the development of scientific discipline (1977, pp. 74–76). These have implications for nursing.

1. "Kuhn's failure to see the role of conceptual problems in scientific debates and in paradigm evaluation." Kuhn appears to be using only a positivistic view of science by comparing the number of facts a theory is able to address and the congruence between these facts in theory and in real life. An empirical view addresses elements in verification and falsification of theories; but no conceptual coherence, logic, social congruence, or other significant components of usefulness.
2. "Kuhn never really resolves the crucial question of the relationship between a paradigm and its constituent theories." Does a paradigm encompass all theories? Do theories explain and describe the paradigm or vice versa? Which gives evidence to the other?
3. The notion of a prevailing paradigm does not allow for the changes and discoveries that characterize our present science, where misconceptions are corrected, parts of theories are justified,

and others are changed. Scientific discovery is a continuous process; present-day tools allow for a fast pace. Kuhn's theory of scientific development appears to provide a rigid structure that limits the continuous development of theories and the continuous correction of the paradigm's weaknesses, which may become apparent over time.

4. Kuhn does not advocate explicit articulation of paradigms or disciplinary matrices. Therefore, such implicitness does not account for nursing's attempt to make the boundaries of the discipline explicit or the assumptions debatable, nor does such implicitness promote the many controversies that Kuhn considers essential to the development of science. Scientists can debate explicit matrices but can avoid implicit ones.

5. "Because paradigms are so implicit and can only be identified by pointing to their *exemplars* (basically an archetypal application of a mathematical formulation to an experimental problem), it follows that whenever two scientists utilize the same exemplars they are, for Kuhn, *ipso facto* committed to the same paradigm" (Laudan, 1981, p. 85). If more scientists work in this way, we come closer to a revolution. Some exemplars have been used in nursing by nurses who hold divergent views about the most basic conceptual and methodological questions. Helping people cope with transitions is an area providing exemplars in health/illness transitions, developmental transitions, or situational transitions. These exemplars have been treated effectively by those who adhere to psychoanalytical views and just as effectively by those adhering to sociocultural views in nursing. Therefore, the exemplars themselves would not mean commitment to some paradigm. Commitment to one paradigm over another is apparent only by making paradigms explicit and not by maintaining implicitness.

Finally, a sixth flaw apparent in Kuhn's philosophy has been identified by Toulmin (1972):

6. How the transitions from competing paradigms to revolution to normal science take place is not clear in Kuhn's writing. Does a community of scholars hold a mass meeting to denounce one competing paradigm and adopt another? Considering that, according to Kuhn, followers of each paradigm are supposedly entrenched in the paradigm they use and do not always seem to communicate, nor do they always share a common language or world view, how could they agree on one rather than another paradigm? Contrary to Kuhn's ideas regarding the lack of communication during the crisis period, Toulmin offers many

historical examples of careful communication, debate, discussion, or proposed modification in physics before any minute change was made or any modification was incorporated into the established body of the discipline (Toulmin, 1972, p. 10).

Some nursing scholars seem to have accepted Kuhn's theory of progress and have adhered to the position that nursing is following the same patterns of revolutionary development as the other physical sciences analyzed by Kuhn. Nursing progress has thus been measured against the canons proposed by him (Hardy, 1978). The result has been a negatively critical assessment of nursing progress and anticipation of a nursing scientific revolution in which one paradigm prevails and is accepted by the nursing community. According to these scholars, nursing is in its preparadigmatic stage. It is possible that the nursing scientific revolution may never come, not because nursing is not progressing but because there may never be periods of normal science. Other natural and behavioral science disciplines continue to progress and continue to have competing paradigms to describe and predict the phenomena of their disciplines. In addition, the notion of one paradigm is not acceptable to sciences, particularly to nursing, which deals with human beings and complex health/illness situations.

Some nurses have presented a view of nursing as something that has arrived at the beginnings of a paradigm (Munhall, 1982; Newman, 1983). However, the process depicted does not demonstrate competition, rejection, and dominance as much as an evolutionary process. Therefore, the appropriateness of using the revolutionary theory to describe progress and development of nursing knowledge is questioned, and other theories are discussed.

A Theory of Evolution

Evolution denotes change in a certain direction, unfolding from lower to higher and from simpler to more complex and headed in the direction of greater coherence. Evolution denotes a sense of continuity and gives the impression of long-term cumulative changes. An evolutionary view of a scientific discipline combines instances of intellectual innovation that are complemented by a continuing process of critical assessment and selection. An evolutionary stand acknowledges competition but accepts the inevitability of cumulation in knowledge development. An evolutionary stand also acknowledges the significance of the genealogy of ideas in the progress of knowledge.

Toulmin (1972) used the evolutionary theory of Darwin as the basis upon which he formulated the evolution of knowledge development. He identified four basic principles for Darwinian theory. These four principles have their counterparts in the evolution of scientific disciplines. *First,* each discipline contains its own body of concepts, areas of concern, methodologies, and goals, all of which can change drastically but slowly through a mutable process. Nevertheless, there is a definite continuity that can be detected in the major ideas of the discipline. Conceptual thoughts in each of the disciplines, while having coherence and continuity, also manifest slow, long-term changes, with each new conceptual thought based on previous ideas, and with the more developed concepts superseding older ones.

Second, all ideas, concepts, and methodologies are given a chance to compete, to be discussed, to be weeded out. Only the discoveries and innovations that fit will flourish and survive from one generation to the next. This process of retention of some conceptual thoughts, mutation of others, and rejection of still others explains the stability of intellectual thought in disciplines and accounts for transformations into new theories.

Third, marked substantive changes in the field are possible when a number of conditions exist. One important condition is the existence of qualified people in the discipline who are capable of inventing new ideas, exploring new problems, and developing new theories. An evolutionary position presupposes the presence of an arena for debate, critique, and competition of ideas and concepts. Another necessary condition is that there be enough openness in the discipline to allow for new ideas to develop and survive long enough to prove their suitability or to be refuted.

Fourth, the selection of the more useful ideas, concepts, and theories is based on which of them helps to meet the demands of the local intellectual environment within the discipline. The selection process is also based on the congruence between the demands, the issues, the current problem areas of the issues, and the innovative ideas that are being offered (Toulmin, 1972, pp. 139–143). Other competing ideas continue to be adhered to, refined, and further developed.

An evolutionary process of knowledge development contains such units of analysis as merits, competitions, demands, and successes. When contrasting the Darwinian zoological evolutionary process of the species with the Toulmin intellectual evolutionary process of disciplines, one finds a pattern of development based on innovation, the comparison of ideas, survival of the fittest, and selection. One theory, one set of ideas that may have more explanatory power to resolve some significant conceptual problem, is generally selected over another previous theory. It may incorporate parts of the previous theory and reject other parts. Progress in the physical sciences is not revolutionary, according to Toulmin, but evolutionary. It has taken a cumulative pattern.

The evolutionary theory of knowledge presupposes that the problem areas of the field and the criteria for truth and explanation are agreed upon. In addition, certain conditions should exist as indicators that a discipline has developed cumulatively. These conditions, the first four of which have been identified by Freese (1972), are:

1. Modification of truth value: generalizations are cumulative when one generalization modifies a previous generalization; that is, one generalization causes change to or from truth, falsity, or indetermination. An empirical confirmation of the second generalization modifies the truth inherent in the first.
2. Modification of antecedent value: generalizations are cumulative if the empirical verification or falsification of a second subsequent generalization modifies the antecedent in the first generalization.

Change of one to the other of the following would fulfill this condition: necessary but not sufficient, sufficient but not necessary, necessary and sufficient, sufficient with necessity indeterminate, and necessary with sufficiency indeterminate.

3. Premise or derivation in a deductive chain: this applies to cases in which a confirmed proposition in one theory becomes a premise preceding another proposition in another theory. Theory is cumulative when the propositions of one theory are based on or help modify the premises of another theory.

4. Space–time independence: theories are cumulative when their propositions transcend geography and time.

5. Practice–research–practice dependent link: this link presupposes modification of practice based on theory or research, or vice versa. Cumulation occurs when a direct ripple effect occurs between practice and research.

If we accept these premises for cumulative knowledge, then physical sciences (using revolutionary criteria) are based on paradigms and (using the evolutionary process) are established disciplines. Social and behavioral sciences, on the other hand, are classified as being in a preparadigmatic stage or are, in Toulmin's terms, "would-be disciplines." One can readily detect conditions of cumulation in the physical sciences, very little of which exists in the social and behavioral sciences or, indeed, in nursing.

Propositions emanating from theoretical nursing do not fit in a deductively tight, logically interrelated cumulative model. Systematic cumulative development that begins from a common point and expands upward to become another canon cannot be detected in nursing knowledge. If cumulation is the unit of analysis for the evolution of disciplines, then nursing scientific development is not closely congruent with either a revolutionary or an evolutionary concept. Rather, it has followed a course that may be considered unsystematic, haphazard, and lacking direction—if we impose on it the two theories discussed previously.

A Theory of Integration

It is possible that the development of the discipline of nursing did not follow a strictly revolutionary or evolutionary path. The revolutionary one would deny nursing's scientific status and the evolutionary one presumes systematic development with research based on theory and theory evolving out of research. The discipline of nursing evolved through peaks, valleys, detours, circular paths, retracing of steps, and series of crises as well as through an evolutionary process. Features that are unique to the discipline of nursing are:

○ The development of nursing theory was not based on the research of the discipline, nor does nursing's research add up to a theory (Batey, 1977; Fawcett, 1978).

○ Competing ideas exist simultaneously and have existed for decades (different research methodologies, conceptual approaches to care, comfort, and pain). Competing theories are being used even within the same institution. To be sure, there are areas of agreement: significance of environment, focus on health and coping, interest in transitions, fascination with human responses to health and illness. Although each of these concepts may be viewed from a different theoretical background, there is an initial agreement.

There is an initial agreement on major concepts that are central to the discipline of nursing; different theories explain, describe, and predict the different concepts. In some instances there are different theories that best explain different situations related to the same concept. Human conditions dictate the appropriateness of different uses of theories.

There is an agreement that the discipline of nursing incorporates professional practice, research, education, and teaching. One could argue, too, that the discipline has been in continuous crisis over the origins of its knowledge base for many years (practice, teaching, or administration) and that the agreement now is that knowledge develops, for the most part, from clinical practice, but other ideas coexist. There are also areas of disagreement, such as the nature of the nursing client and the methodology most congruent with the subject matter of nursing and its philosophical stand.

○ In a discipline that deals with human beings, it is perhaps not feasible that only one theory should explain, describe, predict, and change all the discipline's phenomena. For example, medicine utilizes the biomedical model based on the structure and function of biological systems; however, it also utilizes a variety of means for auscultation, palpitation, and laboratory tests by computer or mechanical means, all of which are accompanied by different theories that compete but coexist (Frank, 1957, pp. 356–358).

A case for paradigmatic pluralism has to be made in nursing because there is a need for theories about people, interactions, illness, health, and nursing interventions. In fact, currently there are many different theories that, although seen by some as competing with each other, address different relationships and focus on different phenomena, thereby actually complementing each other. These theories evolved from a variety of paradigms (adaptation, system, and interactionist, among others). Nursing deals with human behavior, and

> human behavior in all its aspects whatever does not lend itself to explanation by a single, completely general and comprehensive theory; instead, the desire for a single, all-embracing "scientific psychology" may itself prove to be a will-o'-the-wisp. Certainly, a

similar will-o'-the-wisp had to be disregarded before modern physics
could become the discipline it now is; and the reasons why this was
so throw some light on the contemporary state of behavioral science
(Toulmin, 1972, p. 386).

○ Nursing acts in an open system and has to be influenced by and be
  responsive to society at all times. How can we afford convergence
  only? Nurses' and clients' actions are shaped by each other and by
  their social environment. In this there is an analogy between
  nursing and sociology (Urry, 1973).
○ There are many communities in nursing, but there is not one
  community that could act as a unit to support one competing
  theory over another, nor are there unified communities in any of
  the other disciplines. If we decide to wait for that total agreement,
  perhaps we will not be able to work diligently on the much needed
  conceptual clarity and the further development of existing
  competing thoughts.
○ A compromise between the old and the new concepts exists in
  nursing. Researchers focus on the family and on the individual, on
  parts of individuals and on wholes, they use quantitative and
  qualitative techniques, and they explore administrative and clinical
  questions.
○ In instances in which there are changes, old paradigms are
  redefined rather than totally rejected. For example, even as there is
  a revival of Nightingale's concept of nursing, new paradigms, such
  as Rogers', are redefining her ideas.
○ It is the presence of competing theories, competing schools of
  thought, and debatable ideas that makes a discipline a scholarly
  one. The right to question, critique, and challenge have
  characterized all advanced disciplines (Toulmin, 1972, p. 110). If
  nursing were to adopt a revolutionary philosophy for its growth, it
  could put an end to this significant property of scholarliness
  (Laudan, 1977, pp. 73–76). Competition, creativity, and innovation
  are the hallmarks of scientific growth.

The discussion thus far has attempted to address the unique features of
nursing that may make an evolutionary or revolutionary development unsuitable for
describing nursing development (at best) and that may distort such developments
(at worst) (Table 5-1).

Nursing progress seems to have charted its own path; ideas that were rejected in one stage of development have been accepted at a different stage. Examples of this are the early rejection of nursing theories, the more recent revival of
Nightingale's concept of nursing and her focus on health and environment, the
preoccupation with quantitative research methodology in the 1960s, the more
recent revival of meaning of experience, and the greater acceptance of alternate
designs for research such as phenomenology. Ideas have been cumulative at times

Table 5–1
Comparison Among Three Processes of Progress in the Discipline: Revolution, Evolution, and Integration

Revolution	Evolution	Integration
Sentiment		
Aggression: Crises	Adaptation	Change
Interaction		
Competition	Cumulation	Collaboration
Goals		
Conquering	Building	Progressing
Overthrowing	Developing	Understanding
Process		
Substitution	Lower to higher	Openness
Elimination	Selection	Flexibility
	Simple to complex	Contemporary and traditional
Discontinuity	Continuity	Innovation
Pattern of Development		
Convergence	Mutation	Diversion
	Slow, long range	
Reasoning		
Adversary	Logical	Dialectic
Mode		
Rejection	Acceptance	Understanding
Evaluation		
Criticize to destroy	Analyses to construct	Dialogue to develop
Environment		
Critical	Restrictive	Supportive
Challenge		
Options		
No option during normal science	Limited options	Open/unlimited options
Units of Analysis		
Paradigms	Merits	History
Changes	Competitions	Patterns
	Demand	Development of members

(*continued*)

Table 5–1 (Continued)

Revolution	Evolution	Integration
	Success	Number of unique phenomena identified
		Quality of questions answered
		Actualizing relationships between research, theory, and practice
Nursing		
Preparadigmatic	Would-be discipline	Discipline

and unrelated to previous stages at others. Toulmin (1972), in spite of his interest in cumulation, observed that

> [t]he leading ideas current at any stage in the development of 20th-century social science have tended to resemble those current two or three generations before, more than they have resembled those of the immediately previous generation (p. 385).

Popular theories of knowledge development call for a pattern of progress that is not manifested in its entirety in nursing. Therefore, nursing progress has been minimized, and its delays and limitations have been highlighted. An integrative process of development allows for an explanation of competitions and collaborations, acceptances and rejections, cumulations and innovations, peaks and valleys, reconsideration, development, evolution, and convolution. *Webster's Third New International Dictionary* defines a *convolution* as a complex, twisting, winding form or design.*

Integration is neither a nonpattern nor a negative pattern, rather it allows for pendulum swings and is explained as a pattern in progress. It is not a pattern toward the conventional idea of progress, toward a paradigm; it is a pattern of progress depicting nursing's accomplishments and its solid theoretical present through accommodation, refinement, and collaboration between thoughts, ideas, and individuals. This pattern of progress does not underestimate the further need for progress that is inherent in all scientific disciplines. It allows for careful critique of what has been accomplished and what is yet to be accomplished.

Table 5-1 illustrates the differences and similarities between the three processes of knowledge progress discussed here. When the progress of nursing is analyzed through each of the three philosophical views, different conclusions can be drawn. To a revolutionist, nursing is in a preparadigmatic stage; to an evolutionist, nursing is a would-be discipline; to an integrationist, nursing has achieved a disciplinary status. A careful assessment of patterns of growth and development in

* By permission. From *Webster's Third New International Dictionary* ©1986 by Merriam-Webster Inc., publisher of the Merriam-Webster® dictionaries.

nursing, milestones, stages, and phenomena identified demonstrate the quality and significance of questions asked and answers provided. These units of analyses represent a synthesis between research, theory, and practice. When nursing is analyzed in terms of these, then it has achieved a disciplinary status.

FROM THE RECEIVED VIEW
TO THE PERCEIVED VIEW

A number of philosophers in nursing are concerned that nurses have adopted a limited view of science that is in direct contradiction to nursing's philosophy, its heritage, and its goals. The view perceived by these writers could be summarized under the rubric of "the received view," which others may call the scientific method (Suppe, 1977). The received view is philosophically old and outdated, but its effects lingered longer in nursing than in the field of philosophy of science (Suppe and Jacox, 1985).

The *received view* in any discipline usually denotes a set of ideas that are not to be challenged, the philosophical equivalent of being engraved in stone. It is the same premise that declares that holy books were received and therefore should not be challenged. Received view is also a label given to the "empirical positivism" movement or to "logical positivism," a 19th-century philosophical movement closely aligned with Rudolf Carnap and rooted in the celebrated Vienna circle of philosophers. This circle, which met regularly during the 1880s in a seminar led by Moritz Schlick, a professor of philosophy at the University of Vienna, advocated an amalgamation of logic with the goals of empiricism in the development of scientific theories (Runggaldier, 1984). Eventually, the concept of "positivism" was dropped and replaced with "empiricism" to avoid the connection with Auguste Comte, whose ideas were coming into disfavor at that time. When Carnap joined the University of Chicago in 1936, logical empiricism was introduced to the United States (White, 1955, pp. 203–225).

The following are the tenets of logical empiricism:

1. Statements that cannot be confirmed by sensory data and through sensory experiences are not considered theoretical statements worthy of pursuing. As a result, they are disqualified as common sense statements and are therefore nonsense. Predictive statements that have no sensory data corroboration are not scientific. A direct relationship has to exist between experience and a meaningful theory.

2. True statements are only considered to be those that are *a posteriori*. That is, they are based on experience and known from experience.

3. Positivists regard most traditional metaphysics and ethical considerations as meaningless. Positivists regard such questions as possessing "emotive" meaning and as being "cognitively meaningless" (White, 1955).

4. Analyses of theories are based on analyses of completed theories, and completed theories are based on empirical data (Suppe, 1977, p. 125). The context of justification—that is, the verification and falsification of completed theory propositions—is the only significant context for consideration by scientists and philosophers alike. On the other hand, the contexts of discovery, such as conceptual issues, contexts within which theories are developed, logic in theory development, and usefulness, should be within the province of the sociologists of knowledge: the psychologist and historian (Reichenback, 1968).

5. Because the received view considers theories to reflect *a posteriori* depictions of reality, documented by sensory experiences, it therefore follows that propositions of theories are presented in a symbolic, formal, and axiomatic manner. There is room for *a priori* analysis, although it is only mathematical in nature.

6. Science is value-free, and there is only one method for science, which is the scientific method.

The "ghost of the received view" loomed over nursing in its quest for a scientific base, according to Webster, Jacox, and Baldwin (1981). Others, such as Watson (1981) and Winstead-Fry (1980), also joined in blaming nursing's slow scientific progress on the insistence of its leaders to use the outdated scientific method as its model and to strive for one scientific method. The scientific method that they were speaking of is one that is based on the received view, one that espouses "reductionism, quantifiability, objectivity, and operationalization" (Watson, 1981, p. 414).

As a result, significant holistic problems in nursing have been ignored because they are neither reducible, quantifiable, nor objective. The scientific method adapted by nursing reduced a problem to its smallest unit or its most insignificant form and stripped it of the rich context from whence it emanated (Newman, 1981). The scientific method, oriented toward quantitative methods and highly accepted and respected, could not address theory and developing theory; therefore, it has not helped nursing to develop meaningful theories or advanced nursing to its projected goal of a scientific discipline.

There is some justification in blaming the received view for the slow progress and development of nursing. Many examples exist that support the view that nurses have been somewhat disillusioned by a philosophical view of science that is outmoded and ineffective. One example is the many theoretically disconnected but methodologically immaculate research projects that nurses have produced, a view that is shared by Batey (1977). However, there is more evidence than we have been led to believe supporting the view that nursing has, in fact, considered and followed a scientific path that is broader in scope and more integrative in approach than the received view.

Nursing theorists who have worked diligently to give us their conception of the discipline of nursing have not followed a received view approach. They have offered a number of conceptualizations that encompass the whole of nursing—a perceived view—based on their experiences and incorporating ideas that are subjective, intuitive, humanistic, integrative and, in many instances, not based on sense-oriented data.

Discovery of field concepts, theory development, and processes of theorizing in nursing has not been based on the received view or on a structured and strict scientific approach. The context of discovery of these ideas has been traditional: case studies, personal anecdotes, and group insights. Acceptance of those visions that emanated from our nurse theorists has been slow because the theories have been branded by some as unscientific. Therein lies the problem.

To generalize, saying that nursing has followed a positivistic path is akin to saying that physics has followed an intuitive one. The theoreticians in nursing, those who have developed conceptualizations encompassing the field as a whole, have used the *perceived view*, which is a combination of phenomenological and philosophical approaches, as alternate methods of theory development. (See Chapters 7–10 for support of this view.) Perhaps the scholars in the field who believe that knowledge emanates from the context of justification have helped to orient nursing toward considering concepts such as sensory data, verification, and falsification as ways to accept or reject nursing conceptualizations. These scholars have therefore precipitated the early mass rejection of nursing theory as well as the continuous rejection by many in the field who are skeptical about the use or the effectiveness of nursing theories.

What we see in nursing today is a shift from the insistence of a few to adhere to the scientific method. Instead of ignoring nursing theoretical perspective until all propositions are tested and verified, there is a move toward analysis of theories that are in process, as evidenced by the outpouring of books and articles that focus on and encourage the further development of nursing theory. There is a belief that analyses of these theories does not begin when theories are accomplished facts or when they are accepted or rejected. Rather, proposed analyses take into account other epistemic factors related to the context of discovery. This context calls for explorations to discover which questions are more significant and which answers will be more acceptable. It is a view of science that accepts values, subjectivity, intuition, history, tradition, and multiple realities; a view that is more congruent with nursing and its commitment to human beings (Munhall, 1982; Oiler, 1982; Winstead-Fry, 1979).

To summarize, perhaps the dominant evaluative criteria for nursing research by our funding agencies has been a received view approach. In the meantime, the guiding paradigm for nursing practice, nursing theory, and, for that matter, nursing education has been more open, more variable, more relativistic, and more subject to experiences and personal interpretations. It has used a holistic approach, a view based on perceptions of both the clients and the theoreticians of their experiences; therefore, a perceived view.

Table 5–2
Comparison of the Received and Perceived
Views of Science*

Received View	Perceived View
Objectivity	Subjectivity
Deduction	Induction
One truth	Multiple truths
Validation and replication	Trends and patterns
Justification	Discovery
Prediction and control	Description and understanding
Particulars	Patterns
Reductionism	Holism
Generalization	Individuation
Empirical positivism	Historicism

* *Based on Meleis, A.I. (1985)* Theoretical nursing, *Philadelphia: Lippincott; and Stevenson, J.S. and Woods, N.F. (1985)* Nursing science and contemporary science: Emerging paradigms. *In G. Sorenson (Ed.),* Setting the agenda for the year 2000: Knowledge development in nursing. *Kansas City, MO: American Academy of Nursing.*

It was perhaps the incongruence between the perceptions of the few (who evaluated research for publishing and for funding) and the perceptions of the majority of nurses (scientists, theoreticians, and clinicians) regarding knowledge development that delayed the acceptance of the perceived view. The research evaluators were slow in accepting the perceptions of the nursing majority. The views of the former, although leaders in nursing, did not seem to reflect the viewpoint of the majority in nursing. Table 5-2 demonstrates some of the similarities and differences between the received and perceived views.

TRUTH: FROM CORRESPONDENCE TO WELTANSCHAUUNG

There is another subject of concern to those who are inquisitive about nursing's progress toward the development of its knowledge. What criteria have been used by nursing to accept or reject its theoretical notions? What concepts of truth should be used in the future? When do experiences become knowledge, and when does knowledge become truth? Does reality exist or appear?

Philosophers since Plato have addressed these epistemological questions. Over the centuries, three views have emerged: correspondence, coherence, and pragmatism (Armour, 1969; Kaplan, 1964).

The first view is that of *correspondence*, which, with its careful rules, calls for sensory data, very small variables, and operational definitions. For generations, this view has dominated science, research, and theory construction in the physical and natural sciences. It is the method of truth upon which the received or scientific view is based. Indeed, there are many philosophers of science who consider truth by correspondence and the received view one and the same. However, the received view and truth represent two different processes. The former addresses the process of research, the methodology by which data are collected and theories are developed; the latter attends to examining realities, the results of the findings. While the former asks what to do to know, the latter asks how to know.

The empiricists, such as Bertrand Russell, and rationalists, such as J.E. McTaggart, preferring to view truth through correspondence, have designed a set of rules and norms against which theory development and research are expected to be analyzed. The most significant norm is that of truism of facts and their correspondence with the theories that encompass them. One of the most significant correspondence norms is total objectivity, a separation of the observer from the observed world. Validation is based on congruence between propositions and reality; that reality being one reality, an existing reality, and not reality as it may appear to different viewers. The theorist's role is to match the world with assertions and match the facts with concepts.

The positivists assert that correspondence truth is achieved through corroboration by verification. Popper (1959) modified the positivist view and developed the argument for falsification. He asserted that the central concept in scientific discovery is "demarcation." *Demarcation criteria* require that we consider a proposition scientific only if it has the potential for being falsified. Verification of the opposite statement occurs with multiple incidents of falsification of the statement through experience. Once a proposition is countered by a single falsifying instance, it should be rejected. On the other hand, it is not scientific if it does not have the potential for falsification. Continuous attempts to falsify statements make the scientific process rigorous. Truth is achieved when we have exhausted all attempts at falsifying propositions.

Although Popper warns against the potential for any entirely conclusive statement due to problems of reliability in testing, we nevertheless come closer to the truth by testing and retesting with the objective of attempting to nullify and to falsify the proposition under exploration. To the correspondence theorists, whether verification or falsification is the focus, truth is achieved through sensory data and controlled experiments. The correspondence of existing reality, of facts and propositions, is the goal. No room exists for metaphysics, for conceptual truths, for multiple realities, or for perceptions of reality. There are other problems when viewing truth in mainly correspondence terms. If facts exist, are not facts already affected by the concepts introduced to explain the facts?

Truth through *coherence* differs considerably from truth through correspondence. The truth through coherence is manifested in the logical way in which relationships and judgments relate. While the norms for correspondence are verification and falsification with sensory data, the norms for coherence are an integration of relationships, simplicity of presentation, and a certain beauty of propositions. When separate components of a phenomenon "suddenly fall into a pattern of relatedness, when they click into position," then truth has been achieved (Kaplan, 1964 p. 314). Truth according to this theory endures, but perhaps in a more transitory fashion, in ways that may not be reproducible but are no less recognizable. If the proposition is sufficient for today, then there is truth in it.

The coherence norms of logic, simplicity, and aesthetic presentation appear to be norms to be utilized for both the context of discovery and the context of justification. They are most suitable, however, for the discovery of apparent realities. They lend themselves more to the evaluation of concepts that are in the process of development than those in the process of testing. Though norms of correspondence and coherence may appear to contradict each other, it is nonetheless possible to consider them as complementary. While using the coherence norms to judge and evaluate theories, we can also use correspondence norms to judge propositions that evolve out of research.

In the 1930s, a third type of theory about truth was advanced by a group of American philosophers called pragmatists. In fact, according to Leslie Armour (1969), there are two types of *pragmatic* theories of truth. *First*, an assertion is true if it produces the right type of influence on its followers. In other words, a proposition is declared to be true when its usefulness is determined by its users. Experience and the ability to solve problems are two of the norms considered in this view of truth. *Second*, a proposition or any theorized relationship is true if it receives confirmation from a person or persons who may have conducted the right investigations or who are designated as significant by the community of scholars. Pierce (cited in Kaplan, 1964) suggests that, according to this theory, a consensus between significant theoreticians or investigators is what constitutes truth.

Pragmatic truth is not as dependent upon evidence as it is upon observation—upon a declaration of effectiveness by whatever methods the significant members of a community of scholars use. These measures of effectiveness may be subjective, political, social, or objective. To the proponents of this view, "a theory is validated, not by showing it to be invulnerable to criticism, but by putting it to good use, in one's own problems or in those problems of co-workers" (Kaplan, 1964).

A pragmatic theory of truth allows for validation of theories through restructuring, use of new techniques, or even better awareness and realizations of the meaning of old relationships. The value of these new relationships lies not in the answers they may provide as much as in the new questions they may ask and the consequences that result from their use (Kaplan, 1964). Humanity, tentativeness, subjectivity, collectivity, and usefulness are all qualities attached to this concept of pragmatic truth, which evolved out of the Chicago school of thought. (See Table 5-3.)

Table 5–3
Comparison of Different Theories of Truth

Correspondence	Coherence	Pragmatic
Norms		
Corroboration	Logic	Experience
Contexts		
Context of justification	Context of experience	Context of discovery and justification
Goals		
Acceptance/rejection	Support	Understanding
Reality		
One		Multiple
Role of Theorist		
Match world with assertions	Match with world of assertions	Match with users
Distance		Humanness
Evaluation		
Verification	Simplicity	Utility
Falsification	Beauty	Problem solving
Process		
End	Process	Process
Validation		
Congruence between propositions and reality	Endurance of ideas	Consensus of users

There are some conceptual problems that are not as well-addressed by any one of the theories of truth in isolation. Laudan identified three (1977, p. 54). The first of these problems is an intrascientific problem, which results from two theories representing two domains that are inconsistent. An example may be Rogers' (1970) view of a unitary human being as an energy field and behavior as the manifestation of the pattern and organization of the energy field, which presupposes a methodological approach to the study of a human being and his energy field as a whole. Johnson (1974), on the other hand, views a social behavioral system with seven subsystems revolving around subsystem goals and manifested in observable behavior. Johnson presupposes a study of man by reducing man to behaviors.

Because of the theoretical incompatibility between the two fundamental views of the nursing client, the nursing community may attempt (perhaps prematurely) to accept one in favor of the other. The theorist's commitment to adequacy and effectiveness may also prompt one to concede to the other. Either of those alternatives to resolving the problem may not do so because of the level of conceptual and methodological knowledge. To reject Rogers' conception of a unitary human being as an energy field and behavior as a manifestation of pattern and organization of the energy field will either create a reductionist scientific school of thought in nursing or will prompt Rogers, a committed theorist, to continue to work on developing a more adequate theory of the unitary human being. The latter is an acceptable option for scientific development, but the former may impede development because of its prematurity.

It is also possible that the newness of nursing as a discipline makes it easier to reject both competing views in favor of another, more established view of a human being (such as a person as a biological system) to the detriment of solving the central problem. Neither correspondence nor coherence criteria could solve this issue; it is best addressed through a pragmatic approach to truth.

Nursing has also been beset by other philosophical inconsistencies (Munhall, 1982). Existential and pragmatic philosophies have dominated clinical nursing, and positivistic, empirical philosophies have attempted to dominate the academic discipline. This theoretical confusion has only managed to impede nursing's theoretical development. Laudan refers to such conflict between emerging conflicting theoretical and methodological paradigms as normative difficulties. Those who believe that nursing has been dominated by the correspondence norm would attribute the early rejection of nursing theories to this paradox.

There was a belief that the only credible theories in nursing were those that were inferred from observable data. Others asserted that a nursing philosophy that espoused holism, integration, and health was in direct conflict with its methodology of reductionism, objectivity, logic, measurement, verification, and falsification. Where does the truth lie? Which of the two options should nursing follow—the methodological view or the philosophical premise? Who determines the truth—the methodologists or the theoreticians? None of the norms in isolation would provide us with the truth. A combination of all may bring us closer.

The third difficulty that confronts theorists and cannot be resolved by any one of the theories, Laudan calls "prevalent world view difficulties" (Laudan, 1977, p. 61). This phenomenon is observed when the myths, the beliefs, the history, and the practice are in opposition with the developing theories. The prevalent nursing view ascribed to by clinicians is that nursing is practical and skill-oriented and that its principles as well as its skills are derived from other disciplines. Nursing is not theoretical, says this world view, or academic.

Tension also exists between the researchers, who hold the world belief that theories develop only from research, and the theoreticians, who believe that theories are culminations of experience, history, and intuition as well as research findings. There have been many "world views" in nursing, with very few ascribing to a theoretical world view. Weltanschauung attempts to address the many problems that none of the truth theories are able to address in isolation.

Weltanschauung: The Multiple Truths in Nursing

Weltanschauung is defined as "a comprehensive world view, especially from a specified standpoint." Suppe (1977), in offering alternatives to correspondence norms and to the received view, suggested that what is needed is a different way by which theories are analyzed. According to Suppe, Weltanschauung is:

> [an] analysis of theories which concerns itself with the epistemic factors governing the discovery, development, and acceptance or rejecting of theories; such an analysis must give serious attention to the idea that science is done from within a conceptual perspective which determines in large part which questions are worth investigating and what sorts of answers are acceptable; the perspective provides a way of thinking about a class of phenomena which define[s] the class of legitimate problems and delimits the standards for their acceptable solution. Such a perspective is intimately tied to one's language which conceptually shapes the way one experiences the world. (p. 126)

There is a Weltanschauung, or world view, of truth in theoretical nursing that includes an integration of norms emanating from different theories of truth. It combines rigor and intuition, sensory data as they exist and as they appear, perceptions of the subject and of the theoretician, and logic with observable clinical data. What have been advocated by different theorists and researchers merely as norms for acceptance of propositions are not contradictory norms because in some situations, events, and experiences, one set of norms is more appropriate than another. Some research in nursing has been guided by the positivists' views and by correspondence. Some theory development has been guided by these norms as well; for example, Orlando and Johnson focused on observable, verifiable behavior in developing theories (Johnson, 1974; Orlando, 1961). Rogers spoke of experiences beyond the five senses (1970).

Nursing theoreticians, however, would not have developed their theories if they adhered to correspondence norms. There are numerous examples that nursing has utilized a pragmatic theory of truth. Johnson, in 1974, spoke about criteria for acceptance of knowledge as based on social responsibility and about how knowledge and nursing action should make a valuable difference in the people's lives. Whether the model guiding nursing is right or wrong is a social decision and not a theorist's or researcher's decision exclusively.

Rogers (1970), in conceptualizing a unitary man as an energy field, spoke of experiences beyond the five senses and therefore could not use correspondence norms to verify her conceptualization, but instead used coherence norms. Many others supported the necessity of considering coherence norms in conceptualizing nursing and suggested that truth emanated from logic (Batey, 1977; Beckstrand, 1978a, 1978b; Dickoff, James, and Wiedenbach, 1968).

The Weltanschauung of truth in nursing theory uses validation, verification, simplicity, logic, consequences, clients, theorists, and actual or potential experiences as norms against which truth of the theory is compared. It accepts multiple realities and "a composite of realities" (Oiler, 1982). It accepts different expressions, different sources, and criteria such as a number of solved problems within a discipline (Laudan, 1977).

CONCLUSION

Three epistemological issues may have influenced the course of theory development in nursing and, indeed, all knowledge in nursing. The first addressed the
course that nursing has taken to achieve a disciplinary status. Two prevailing
theories of progress were discussed and analyzed: revolution and evolution. Neither
could adequately describe the unique path that nursing has taken, and both cast a
dark shadow on nursing progress because accomplishments in nursing could not be
entirely credited under either of them. A third approach of integration was proposed
as being more congruent with nursing progress. It takes into account the nature of
nursing and its detours.

The second issue is related to the pull between the received view of science
and the perceived view. The former provided the canons for acceptance and rejection of the road that nurses have taken in theory development, but perhaps is a more
acceptable approach to analysis and evaluation of work within the context of
justification. The perceived view, the guiding paradigm for nursing practice, nursing
theory, and, for that matter, nursing education, has been more open, more variable,
relativistic, and subject to experience and personal interpretations. It is a view that
is holistic in approach, a view that is based on the perceptions of both the client and
the theoretician. The perceived view is more appropriate for the context of discovery.

The third subject that has created issues of acceptance and rejection of
nursing knowledge comprises questions such as: What counts as truth? How do we
go about finding it? What criteria do we have for acceptance of nursing's major
questions, assumptions, and answers? Three theories of truth were discussed and
related to the view of truth that has emerged in nursing.

Progress in nursing has been unique and phenomenal in acceleration in the
past decade. Theorists and researchers in nursing began in the late 1980s to accept
the differences between nursing and other sciences, the uniqueness of nursing, and
the capabilities of its scholars to develop knowledge. Nursing deals with wholeness,
perceptions, experiences, multiple realities, appearances of phenomena, and the
existence of phenomena. Whether it needs to or should use any of the theories of
truth discussed in this chapter is up to you, the reader, and the future theoreticians
in nursing. This chapter intended to bring you present-day discussions and to
encourage you to go beyond this limited discussion to explore theories of probabili-
ties and theories that espouse the use of the criteria of a number of solved problems
within a discipline rather than truth theories.

REFERENCES

Andreoli, K.G. and Thompson, C.E. (1977) The nature of science in nursing. *Image*, 9(2),
   32–37.
Armour, L. (1969) *The concept of truth.* Assen: Van Gorcum and Co.

Baer, E.D. (1979) Philosophy provides the rationale for nursing's multiple research directions. *Image*, 11(3), 72–74.

Batey, M.V. (1977) Conceptualization: Knowledge and logic guiding empirical research. *Nursing Research*, 26(5), 324–329.

Beckstrand, J. (1978a) The notion of practice theory and the relationship of scientific and ethical knowledge to practice. *Research in Nursing and Health*, 1(3), 131–136.

Beckstrand, J. (1978b) The need for a practice theory as indicated by the knowledge used in conduct of practice. *Research in Nursing and Health*, 1(4), 175–179.

Carper, B.A. (1978) Practice oriented theory: Part 1. Fundamental patterns of knowing in nursing. *Advances in Nursing Science*, 1(1), 13–23.

Dickoff, J., James, P., and Wiedenbach, E. (1968) Theory in a practice discipline: Part 1. Practice oriented theory. *Nursing Research*, 17(5), 415–435.

Fawcett, J. (1978) The relationship between theory and research: A double helix. *Advances in Nursing Science*, 1(1), 49–62.

Frank, P. (1957) *Philosophy of science.* Englewood Cliffs, NJ: Prentice-Hall.

Freese, L. (1972) Cumulative sociological knowledge. *American Sociological Review*, 37(4), 472–482.

Hardy, M.E. (1978) Practice oriented theory: Part 1. Perspectives on nursing theory. *Advances in Nursing Science*, 1(1), 37–48.

Johnson, D.E. (1974) Development of theory: A requisite for nursing as a primary health profession. *Nursing Research*, 23(5), 372–377.

Kaplan, A. (1964) *The conduct of inquiry: Methodology of behavioral science.* San Francisco: Chandler Publishing Company.

Kuhn, T.S. (1970) The structure of scientific revolutions. In Neurath, O. (Ed.), *International encyclopedia of unified science*, 2nd ed. (Vol. 2). Chicago: University of Chicago Press.

Kuhn, T.S. (1977) *The essential tension: Selected studies in scientific tradition and change.* Chicago: University of Chicago Press.

Laudan, L. (1977) *Progress and its problems: Toward a theory of scientific growth.* Berkeley: University of California Press.

Laudan, L. (1981) A problem-solving approach to scientific progress. In I. Hacking (Ed.), *Scientific revolutions.* New York: Oxford University Press.

Munhall, P.L. (1982) In opposition or apposition. *Nursing Research*, 31(3), 175–177.

Newman, M. (1981, October) Methodology of pattern. Paper presented at the Nursing Theory Think Tank, Denver, CO.

Newman, M.A. (1983) The continuing revolution: A history of nursing science. In N.L. Chaska (Ed.), *The nursing profession: A time to speak.* New York: McGraw-Hill.

Oiler, C. (1982) The phenomenological approach in nursing research. *Nursing Research*, 31(3), 178–181.

Orlando, I.J. (1961) *The dynamic nurse-patient relationship.* New York: G.P. Putman's Sons.

Popper, K. (1959) *The logic of scientific discovery.* London: Hutchinson.

Reichenback, H. (1968) *The rise of scientific philosophy.* Berkeley: University of California Press.

Rogers, M. (1970) *An introduction to the theoretical basis of nursing.* Philadelphia: F.A. Davis.

Runggaldier, E. (1984) *Carnap's early conventionalism: An inquiry into the historical background of the Vienna circle.* Amsterdam: Rodopi.

Shapere, D. (1981) Meaning and scientific change. In I. Hacking (Ed.), *Scientific revolutions.* New York: Oxford University Press.

Silva, M.C. (1977) Philosophy, science, theory: Interrelationships and implications for nursing research. *Image,* 9(3), 59–63.

Stevenson, J.S. and Woods, N.F. (1986) Nursing science and contemporary science: Emerging paradigms. In G. Sorenson (Ed.), *Setting the agenda for the year 2000: Knowledge development in nursing.* Kansas City, MO: American Academy of Nursing.

Suppe, F. (Ed.). (1977) *The structure of scientific theories* (2nd ed.). Champaigne: University of Illinois Press.

Suppe, F. and Jacox, A.K. (1985) Philosophy of science and the development of nursing theory. In *Annual Review of Nursing Research,* 3, 241–267.

Toulmin, S. (1972) *Human understanding: The collective use and evolution of concepts.* Princeton, NJ: Princeton University Press.

Urry, J. (1973) Thomas S. Kuhn as sociologist of knowledge. *British Journal of Sociology,* 24(4), 462–473.

Watson, J. (1981, July) Nursing's scientific quest. *Nursing Outlook,* 29(7), 413–416.

Webster, G., Jacox, A., and Baldwin, B. (1981) Nursing theory and the ghost of the received view. In J.C. McClosky and H.K. Grace (Eds.), *Current issues in nursing.* Oxford: Blackwell Scientific Publications.

White, M. (1955) *The age of analysis: 20th century philosophers.* Boston: Houghton Mifflin.

Winstead-Fry, P. (1979, June) Defining clinical content of nursing. In *Proceedings of the 1979 forum on doctoral education in nursing.* San Francisco: University of California.

Winstead-Fry, P. (1980) The scientific method and its impact on holistic health. *Advances in Nursing Science,* 2(6), 1–7.

Part 3

Our Discipline

*A*s members of the discipline prepare for the last decade of the 1900s, they can pause and reap the benefits of the early struggles. Our discipline claims a domain of study, scholarly progress, and philosophical debates and discourses that are indicative of a sophisticated reflective stand. The discipline of nursing is always progressing and developing, and its members are caring and involved, yet they are able to take stock of the need to participate in activities that may help in organizing and structuring nursing's knowledge base.

This part of our journey focuses on contemporary analyses of the discipline. In Chapter 6, the domain of nursing is described, and the central concepts are defined. Properties and indications of the scholarliness of nursing are analyzed in Chapter 7 within the context of the history of theoretical development of the discipline. In Chapter 8, several perspectives that emerged to guide the development of theoretical nursing are briefly presented and related to the nature of nursing and its mission.

Chapter 6

The Discipline of Nursing and Its Domain of Knowledge

A *discipline* has been defined as "a unique perspective, a distinct way of viewing all phenomenon, which ultimately defines the limits and nature of its inquiry" (Donaldson and Crowley, 1978, p. 113). Webster defines a discipline as "a particular field of academic study," as well as the "training expected to produce a specific type or pattern of behavior" (Webster's II, 1984). A discipline includes a specified branch of knowledge, the rules that govern this knowledge, and ways by which an order and rules are applied to knowledge (Webster's II, 1984).

The discipline of nursing, therefore, includes the content and processes related to all roles that nurses play, including administrator, teacher, politician, clinician, and consultant. A discipline also includes the theories developed to describe, explain, and prescribe as well as the research findings related to the discipline's central phenomenon and the knowledge from related disciplines that is essential for informing members of a particular discipline (Fig. 6-1). All disciplines are formed around a domain of knowledge.

A domain of knowledge is the crux of a discipline. A *domain* is a territory that has both theoretical and practical boundaries. The practical boundaries represent the current state of investigative interests that emerge from questions that are significant to members of the domain. The theoretical boundaries are formulated by visionary questions of members. These visionary questions are not bound by, or limited to, current concerns of the members of the discipline.

Current questions that may determine the territory of nursing include whether nursing should involve caring for people who are not able to care for themselves in the face of illness or anticipated known illness. Theoretical boundaries may necessitate considering questions about caring for individuals who are in hemispheric transition or who may reside in a space shuttle for an extended period of time. Some elements of the theoretical boundaries are similar to practical boundaries, for example, a focus on human beings; others require some modification, for example,

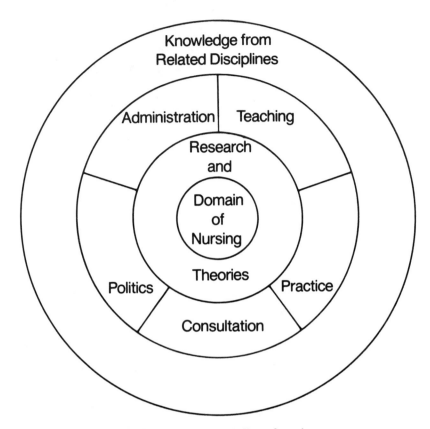

Figure 6–1. The discipline of nursing.

the content of the environment—that the earth environment may have similar as well as different characteristics from other planet environments.

THE DOMAIN OF NURSING

Domains are defined differently by different philosophers of science. The following definitions of a domain synthesize some aspects of Kuhn (1970), Merton (1973), Parsons (1968), and Toulmin (1972).

- A domain has some broad basic concepts.
- It contains the major problem areas of the field that make up the canons for significant statements.
- Some units of analysis used in its investigations are identified.
- There is evidence of beginning agreement and genealogy of ideas.
- Its members allow for a synthesis of a number of paradigms.
- Its members are knowledgeable about the different schools of

thought, and they acknowledge and accept the use of different paradigms.

○ There are accumulated experiences of its members. These experiences are respected, critically assessed, and accepted. The grounds for analysis and critique are clear and subject to debate.

○ The norms and the tools for knowledge development are defined within the domain. These norms and tools emerge from the domain goals and are congruent with its shared assumptions.

○ A domain informs and is informed by all outer circles of the discipline (see Fig. 6-1). That is, a domain is revised and developed through the wisdom and expertise of members of the discipline, through accumulated research and theory, and through knowledge developed in other disciplines. Therefore, a domain has certain focal elements of stability, but the nature of its content is dynamic and responsible to changes occurring in other spheres.

When we consider nursing analytically, we find that there are numerous indications that nursing is indeed a discipline with a particular perspective. That perspective is defined by and within its domain. The central problems of the domain of nursing may be examined by other sciences; however, the centrality of these problems to the domain is what determines primary domain affiliation. Comforting patients during intrusive procedures may be of concern to a number of health science disciplines, but comfort of clients during all life processes related to health and illness situations as well as ways by which comfort is enhanced are central concerns of nurses and nursing.

Some interests of some disciplines overlap others. An example of another discipline that may encounter such overlap is engineering. Premises upon which the discipline of engineering is built may come from physics, chemistry, economics, and behavioral sciences, but the synthesis is uniquely engineering for the purpose of describing, explaining, and predicting phenomena central to engineering, for example, the shielding of nuclear power plants. The problem of shielding is central to the field of nuclear engineering but only peripheral to physics, chemistry, and other sciences.

The nursing domain does not simply encompass results of research (*i.e.*, nursing science), nursing theories, or nursing practice, rather it encompasses knowledge of nursing practice (also used by Newman, 1983), which is based on philosophy, history, former practice, common sense, research findings, theory, and genealogy of ideas (Fig. 6-2). The nursing domain encompasses units of analysis, congruent methodology, nursing processes, holistic approaches to assessment, and other practice and methodological procedures that are essential to knowledge development. Central components of the nursing domain are:

Major concepts and problems of the field;
Processes for assessment, diagnosis, and intervention;
Tools to assess, diagnose, and intervene; and

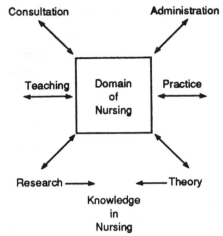

Figure 6–2. The domain of nursing.

Research designs and methodologies that are most congruent with
nursing knowledge.

Theoretical boundaries of the nursing domain result from an explication of the
first three components listed. Research designs and methodologies evolve from
acceptable philosophical principles in nursing and complement knowledge development related to its central concepts, problems, and goals of the discipline.
Research designs and methodologies also help identify and develop components of
the domain of nursing. Nursing theories are a component of the domain of nursing,
and they provide nurses with different perspectives on nursing and nursing phenomenon.

In 1975, Yura and Torres delineated and described the major concepts used in
baccalaureate programs that were central to the different conceptual models and
frameworks used for nursing curricula. Four focal concepts emerged: person,
society, health, and nursing (Yura and Torres, 1975). The centrality of these concepts in the discipline of nursing continued to be supported through the 1980s. For
example, Newman (1983) asserted that the "domain of nursing has always included
the nurse, the patient, the situation in which they find themselves, and the purpose
of their being together, or the health of the patient" (p. 388). Therefore, she agreed
that the major components of concern to nursing are "nursing (as an action), client
(human being), environment (of the client and of the nurse-client), and health."
Others modified the list to exclude environment (Barnum, 1990), or they expanded
the meaning of "person" to encompass both human being and patient (Barnum,
1990), or they redefined "client" to mean "pluralities of persons and internal units,
such as families, groups, and communities" (Schultz, 1987, p. 71). Nursing theory, it
was argued by some, could include one or more of these concepts (Fawcett, 1989),
for example, client, society, health, or nursing, or, others argued, nursing theories

should include the concept of nursing as an activity in addition to any one of the other concepts (Flaskerud and Halloran, 1980), such as any set of "commonplaces" (nursing act, patient, health, nurse–patient relationships, nursing acts and health, and patient and health), as long as "any given nursing theory—directly or by implication—differentiates nursing from other disciplines and activities" (Barnum, 1990, pp. 7 and 8). Still others emphasized that nursing theories should include health and direction for nursing action in order to facilitate the process of health (Newman, 1983, p. 390). None of the positions objected to inclusion of all domain concepts, if indeed a theory is able to address them all.

As indicated, there were variations in the recommendations of metatheorists in what, how many, and which central concepts should be included in nursing theories. The position adopted in this text has its own unique features also, but it falls within general patterns of agreement within the discipline. Concepts identified as central to the domain of nursing are nursing client, transitions, interaction, nursing process, environment, nursing therapeutics, and health. It is proposed that the nurse interacts (*interaction*) with a human being in a health/illness situation (*nursing client*) who is in an integral part of his sociocultural context (*environment*) and who is in some sort of transition or is anticipating a transition (*transition*); the nurse–patient interactions are organized around some purpose (*nursing process, problem solving, or holistic assessment*), and the nurse uses some actions (*nursing therapeutics*) to enhance, bring about, or facilitate health (*health*).

It is argued here that theories developed to describe any of the concepts listed above are nursing theories when the ultimate goal is related to the maintenance, promotion, or facilitation of health and well-being, even though the theory may not specify the nursing actions. It is also argued that nursing is an encompassing concept that includes all the concepts listed previously and is therefore defined by them. It would be an instance of tautological conceptualizing to define nursing by all the concepts and then include nursing as one of the concepts. Other disciplines may use nursing theories for different goals, and nursing theories therefore lose the original goal, become adapted, and become "shared" theories (Barnum, 1990).

A conceptual definition is provided for each of the central concepts in nursing. These definitions, evolving from contemporary shared knowledge in nursing and from a current world view, are provided as working definitions. The reader should use them as a springboard for further development and refinement.

The Nursing Client

The most central concept within the domain of nursing is the recipient of care or the potential recipient of care—the nursing client. Although a client is also central to a number of other disciplines, the perspective from which that client is considered is invariably different and evolves from the domain of the discipline. Nurses have claimed that individuals are the focus of their actions ever since nurses began caring for patients and ever since they attempted to describe the care they provide. For example, Nightingale described nursing as having to "put the patient in the best condition for nature to act upon him" (Nightingale, 1946, p. 74). Others spoke of nursing in terms of helping individuals develop their self-care activities (Orem, 1988) and doing what needs to be done to help individuals adapt to their illness or environment (Roy, 1984).

To illustrate, when a physician thinks of a person, the image that is conjured up is an image of biological systems with structure and function. That image may include a person's occupation, family, socioeconomic class, or other variable; however, the central image is of a biological system. When a sociologist thinks of a person, on the other hand, she thinks of roles, status, interaction, and significant others, of individuals as part of a society. When a psychologist thinks of a human being, she thinks in terms of intrapsychic processes. A human being to a cell biologist is made up of groups of cells.

Nursing theories claim that nursing focuses on the person whose needs are not met because of illness or the person who needs help in maintaining or enhancing wellness. Nurse theorists provide us with several views of our clients. A nursing client probably is a composite of all of the conceptions provided by these nurses theorists, and perhaps the context determines which image is more central at the time. Some of these conceptions are complementary, while others are based on conflicting value systems. The following are some examples of nurse theorist's conceptions of the nursing client:

○ The nursing client has a set of basic human needs (Abdellah (1969)—21 problems; Henderson (1966)—14 daily activities; Orem (1988)—the deficit between self-care capabilities and self-care demands). The focus of nursing is on assisting with activities to fulfill the client's needs.
○ The nursing client is an open system, an adaptive being who changes to accommodate outside changes.
○ A nursing client is conceptualized as a person in disequilibrium or at risk of disequilibrium due to insufficiency or incompatibility between one or more of the subsystems.
○ A nursing client is a person who is unable, or is at risk of being unable, to be a self-care agent.

These theories provided us with varied conceptions described in the social policy statement (ANA, 1980). These conceptions should be used as guidelines for analyses to determine which conceptions are more congruent with the values and the mission of the discipline (Allen, 1987). A *nursing client* is defined here as a human being with needs who is in constant interaction with the environment and has an ability to adapt to that environment but, due to illness, risk, or vulnerability to potential illness, is experiencing disequilibrium or is at risk of experiencing disequilibrium. *Disequilibrium* is manifested in unmet needs, inability to take care of oneself, and nonadaptive responses.

Theoretical developments of phenomena related to nursing clients encompass but are not limited to six areas.

1. Research and theories to describe philosophical principles governing views of human beings in nursing, including analyses of values and norms related to human beings and their relationships;
2. Research and theories that relate to the fundamental process of responses to human and environmental conditions that are considered within normal ranges;
3. Research and theories to describe, explain, and predict responses of human beings to health and illness situations;
4. Research and theories to describe human responses to nursing therapeutics;
5. Research and theories to describe groups, communities, and organizational responses to health and illness and nursing therapeutics; and
6. Theoretical development of person models that are congruent with the disciplinary values.

One of the discipline's immediate goals is to discover and develop techniques and methodologies to capture the holistic nature of human beings and the nature of integrated responses to the environment that are considered central to the domain of nursing. Until this goal is realized, nurses may have to continue to resort to a more reductionist approach to the study of clients.

Examples of the types of theories that need to be developed are (1) descriptive theories (*e.g.*, patterns of normal responses); (2) explanatory theories (*e.g.*, how and why different groups of clients respond in certain ways to noxious stimuli); and (3) prescriptive theories (*e.g.*, how and in what ways nurses enhance a sense of comfort or well-being in clients).

Transitions

Nurses deal with people who are experiencing transition, anticipating transition, or completing the act of transition. Transition denotes a change in health status, in role relationships, expectations, or abilities. It denotes changes in needs of all human systems. Transition requires the person to incorporate new knowledge, to alter behavior, and therefore to change the definition of self in social context. Transitions are developmental, situational, or health/illness events. Two significant developmental transitions may be associated with health problems (both psychosocial and biophysiological): the transition from childhood to adolescence, which has the potential of being associated with ensuing problems such as substance abuse and teen pregnancies; and the transition from adulthood to mature adulthood, a period accompanied by gerontologic problems relating to identity, retirement, and chronic illness.

Another transition falling within the domain of nursing is the situational transition, which includes the addition or loss of a member of the family through birth or death. Each situation requires a definition or redefinition of the roles that the client (a person or a family) is involved in. The transition from a nonparental role to a parental one, the change from double parenting to single parenting, and the attempts of women to move from the battered role to the nonbattered role are three examples of situational transitions that affect a human being in totality, though we are concerned with them in terms of health. Nurses are also concerned with the transition from institutional care to community care.

The last, but not least important, transition category is the health/illness transition. This category includes such transitions as sudden role changes that result from moving from a well state to an acute illness, from wellness to chronic illness, or from chronicity to a new wellness that encompasses the chronicity. (Tornberg, McGrath, and Benoliel, 1984). Transitions are therefore one component of the nursing domain.

The sociologist, the psychologist, the biologist, and the physiologist are all interested in transitions at the micro and macro levels, and the objective of their interest is to know. Because domains are not only identified by the types of objects with which they deal but also by the questions they ask, differentiating between different domain interests can be done by considering types of questions that nurses ask. Only the nurse is interested in articulating transitions that are bio-psycho-socio-cultural; not only to know but ultimately to have knowledge of the utility of what we know and, in particular, to have ways to effectively use that knowledge. Unlike other academic disciplines, nursing is accountable to the public; it is expected to meet the public's needs.

An example of a multidimensional transitional interest is my own interest in the health care of Arab-Americans, which arose from the needs of health care systems dealing with that population. It concerns immigrants in sociocultural transition and considers the effect of transition on clients' biological, psychological, sociological, and cultural needs and the effect of transitions on health behavior, illness behavior, illness episodes, and coping styles of any group of immigrants to the United States. The interest evolved from a nursing perspective, utilizes a sociological model, and will add to the domain of nursing.

Nursing does not deal with transition of an individual, a family, or a community in isolation from an environment. How human beings cope with transition and how the environment affects that coping are fundamental questions for nursing. Nursing seeks to maximize clients' strengths, assets, and potentials or to contribute to restoration of the client to optimal levels of health, function, comfort, and self-fulfillment. Coping and adapting are multidisciplinary and interdisciplinary concepts. The menopausal experience, for example, is a developmental transition and a multidomain concept. Although research in nursing considers menopause from a bio-psycho-socio-cultural perspective, the sociologist looks at it in terms of societal expectations, with the roles and status normatively accorded the menopausal person. The psychologist views menopause from an intrapsychic perspective; the physician views it in terms of changes in cells in the endocrine system. The nurse researcher considers the subjective meaning of the entire experience, what bio-psycho-socio-cultural variables influence that meaning, what the consequences are for the person as well as for that person's significant others, how the person is adapting to changes, and, finally, how the nurse can help the menopausal person cope with the experience, if indeed there is a need to do so.

Clients in transition share some commonalities. These were defined by Chick and Meleis (1986) and Meleis (1986) as a perception of "disconnectedness from usual social network and social support systems," "temporary loss of familiar reference points or significant objects or subjects," "new needs that may arise," or old needs that remain unmet," and "old sets of expectations no longer congruent with changing situations" (Meleis, 1986, p. 19).

Although each nurse researcher considers the nursing phenomenon according to the basic premises of the field and according to a total view of the human being, the goals of research will dictate the dominant model. For example, one nurse researcher conceptualizes phenomena predominantly from a physiological model, whereas another will use a sociological model. Both explicate nursing phenomena and work toward the goals of enhancing healthful living, an adaptive stance, and a higher sense of well-being. Both are adding to the nursing conceptualization of an experience.

Theories are needed to describe the nature of transitions and normal patterns of responses to transitions, to explain relationships between transitions and health, and to provide guidelines for enhancing a perception of well-being.

Interaction

Some theorists focused on the process and tools of assessment and therefore viewed nursing as an interaction process. Together they provided us with the genesis of one or more interaction theories. They all spoke of properties of the nurse–patient dialogue, of therapeutic interaction, and of the components of interacting as being the sensing, perceiving, and validating of the patient's need for help and the sharing of information. They explicated properties of perception, thought, and feelings during health and illness situations. Together they provided us with a framework that contains major concepts central to nursing. Theories relating these concepts could come from inside or outside nursing. They could evolve from studying the work of the different theories in conjunction with patient care situations or in conjunction with other interaction theories, such as those of Sullivan (1953) and Mead (1937).

Interaction is one of the central concepts in nursing for the following reasons:

- ○ A nursing client is in constant interaction with his environment (Rogers, 1970; King, 1981; Nightingale, 1946). Therefore, nursing focuses not only on individuals but also on monitoring, regulating, maintaining, and changing environments.
- ○ Interaction is the major tool by which nurses assess client's needs and resources, and it is also a central tool in providing nursing therapeutics (Orlando (1961), Wiedenbach (1963), King (1981), Travelbee (1971), Paterson and Zderad (1976).

There is some agreement that interaction is a domain concept and that there are interactions as person–environment interactions (Flaskerud and Halloran, 1980) and nurse–patient interactions (Barnum, 1990). Interaction is considered here in its broadest sense to incorporate both of these types of interactions.

Several kinds of theories related to interactions need to be developed, including the following:

1. Theories that describe normal patterns of interactions of human beings with significant aspects of their environments.
2. Theories that describe normal patterns of interactions between clients and their environments within a context of health and illness, which should account for developmental, sociocultural, and cognitive variations
3. Theories that describe and explain interactions and consequences of interactions that are related to assessment, diagnosis, and interventions

(Kim (1987) identified four sets of variables that are related to client–nurse contacts for providing nursing care: client and nurse, a social context for the contact, a process of interaction, and outcomes. The conceptual linkages between each of these sets of variables are then amenable to theory development (Kim, 1986, p. 105)).

Nurses have claimed nurse–patient interactions as central to the nursing diagnosis; however, Kim (1987) reminded us:

> While there has been a great deal of rhetorical emphasis on the importance of client–nurse interaction in the delivery of nursing care, very little has been done either in theory development or in empirical testing of the theories. There is a rich array of theoretical and empirical work accomplished in sociology and social psychology that is transferable to this nursing domain. There is a need to have an understanding of how the special nature of client–nurse interactions modifies sociological, social, psychological, and communication theories. Much work, therefore, needs to be done to revise and reformulate existing knowledge to explain and predict phenomena in the client–nurse domain. (Kim, 1987, p. 107)

Nursing Process

Another concept that is central to many of the nursing theories is that of the nursing process, although it is not always easy to consider the distinct properties of the nursing process as they differ from interactions. In spite of some overlap, it is proposed here that propositions about the nursing process, about approaches that are more effective in the process of assessing, diagnosing, or providing nursing therapeutics, and about the goals of the nursing process can be derived from the work of several theorists: Abdellah, Henderson, Orem, Orlando, Travelbee, and Wiedenbach. Together they provided nursing with a perspective on assessment, diagnosis, plan for intervention, and evaluation (Abdellah, 1969; Henderson, 1966; Orem, 1988), on the process of defining and attaining goals (King, 1981), and with emphasis on the patient's perception of his own condition (Wiedenbach, 1963). In proposing the nursing process as a concept with the potential for development of middle-range theory, Hall* (1982) makes the following comments:

> Nurses and teachers of nursing find it useful to organize their knowledge in a way that depicts nursing as orderly and sequential. It is also useful because it structures reality and acts as a focus for the nurse's attention. It limits the duration of the nurse's interaction and it spells out clearly the phases or the steps that should occur and in what order. It thus confines the nurse and the patient to a relationship with each other that has a specific function, is temporary, and has signposts that indicate progress.
>
> Therefore nursing needs a process theory because concern with patients inevitably involves a relationship that has temporal elements. Different knowledge and actions are called for as the relationship proceeds through stages from the beginning to the end. The theories, however, need to pay attention to the details of the model itself rather than focus on content. The significant process variables connected with the beginning, the middle, and the end cannot be given short shrift.
>
> One cannot find any theoretical approach in the literature that claims to teach us how to develop a process theory, or even what one is, specifically. There are some examples of this approach, though, and these will be cited in this paper so we can arrive at the elements of a process theory inductively.
>
> From the field of sociology there are no better examples of process theory than those developed by the symbolic interactionists, Becker, Strauss, and Glaser (Becker, 1963; Becker, Geer, Hughes, and Strauss, 1961; Glaser and Strauss, 1964, 1967). These process theories are called, variously, career sequence, commitment, and status passage. They all rest on the assumption that behavior occurs in an orderly sequence that can be observed, recorded, and then generalized as a process. Essentially, the process metaphor presents identity as a series of movements or steps in a sequence. Passage from one sequence to another is a study of the orderly steps or changes over time. Becker says that, when viewed as a process, the variables in this sequence model are a description of the steps in the process accompanied by an explanation of each step.
>
> Becker's (1963) conception of sequential models was developed from Hughes' (1956) work on occupational careers. Becker used Hughes' idea of career as a "moving perspective" to develop his own thoughts on career contingencies and career flow. Becker reasoned that at various stages of the career process, factors come into play such as recruitment, replacement, crucial contingencies, timing, sequencing, and sponsorship. These factors then become the dimensions of the process. Each one serves to further the career, socialize the recruit, foster identity with the occupation, and ensure that critical choices are made with appropriate help. From the point of view of the occupation, the process ensures that the members entering the occupation will have sufficient socialization to develop appropriate attitudes, values, and skills necessary to good functioning.

---

* Reprinted with permission from Beverly A. Hall.

Thus, instead of the simplistic stages depicted by the nursing process, we have a process comprised of stages that presents a moving picture of the significant career variables in each stage and culminates in the achievement of a new identity for the occupational recruit. Becker depicts occupational identity as career process because the two, from his perspective, are inseparable.

Further study of Becker's work, though, reveals that Becker did not use the above theory to establish a middle-range substantive theory of occupational careers. Rather, he went on to develop from this process a formal theory of career process. The variables of recruitment, replacement, crucial contingencies, timing, and sponsorship are the "form" of a career, whether the career is occupational or some other kind. Career is literally a moving perspective, to go back to Hughes, and we can use that "form" to study other processes such as dying and the study of social deviance.

In the case of the deviant, the first step in a deviant career is the commission of a nonconforming act. This is a necessary condition but not a sufficient condition because acts are committed by persons who do not go on to a deviant career. Individuals who are to become deviant learn their careers in the same way people learn any career, by having crucial experiences along the career process that enforce a deviant identity, such as sponsorship, public labeling, and recruitment into the inner circle of a subgroup. Eventually, as the person goes through these stages of a career, the growing commitment strengthens identification as a deviant.

Becker used this same sequence model to study professional careers, marijuana users, and dance musicians. The notion of career sequence was further developed by Glaser and Strauss in their study of status passage in which the sequence model was applied to the dying patient. This latter example is well known in nursing. Glaser and Strauss developed a "low level" theory of dying in hospitals. They then began to apply this to many areas. This step developed the theory of dying into a theory of status passage which has been applied to many areas of status and role change—retirement, career mobility, deviant behavior, and adjustment to the sick role. It is at this stage that Denzin (1970) says we have a multifocused formal theory, that is, one that describes a form that can be applied to a number of substantive areas.

Although Becker, Strauss, and Glaser do not discuss patterns per se, I believe that if a process is developed and studied in its complex detail, it would take on the characteristics of a pattern. A pattern in process theory would appear to be simply a stage or a step in the process that is normative or at least modal, along with the clustered variables in each stage.

Furthermore, these patterns could be developed along the lines of formal sociological theory. That is, we could discover formal patterns that would cut across substantive areas. These would include both process and content. In the so-called nursing process there is virtually no content, although it is implied by the process and could be developed. A good process would lead to the development of content that is inseparable from the form. Form and content can be isolated from each other, just as they are in grammar, so that the form can have life without the content. However, it would seem to me that the content cannot have life without the form. That is the purpose of form; it allows the content to be interpreted.

In summary, nursing could probably benefit by attention to its process in which basic forms would be developed. Formal theory may begin in its development by focusing on a single process. It then becomes multifocused as it is extended to explain phenomena other than that for which it was originally developed.

The nursing process, a tool for nursing practice, was introduced to nursing first by Orlando (1961) and became central to many publications in nursing and has even been considered a framework for nursing practice and nursing education (Yura and Walsh, 1978a, 1978b). Most of the theorists described and discussed the nursing process. Though some components of the process of clinical judgments are an integral part of all professional–client relationships, the process in nursing differs in that the goals of each profession are different. It is proposed here that the nursing process is a central concept in the domain of nursing.

Many nurse metatheorists agree with this position (*e.g.*, Torres, 1986; Walker and Avant, 1989), as demonstrated by the extensive literature on and use of the nursing process, and by those who maintain that emerging theories and models in nursing must consider the nursing process (Thibodeau, 1983). Others question the compatibility of the holistic mission of nursing and the reductionist approach dictated by the use of the nursing process (Barnum, 1987). Barnum (1987) pointed out the potential for other processes in decision making to be more compatible with the holistic principles of nursing, such as the problematic method described by Dewey in 1966. These debates in the nursing literature demonstrate the need for further theoretical development of different processes for assessment and diagnoses and for providing nursing therapeutics.

One significant component of the nursing process that has received the attention of the discipline throughout the 1980s is a taxonomy of nursing diagnoses. The movement toward the development of the taxonomy began in the early 1970s by Christine Gebbie (a graduate of University of California, Los Angeles, a faculty member at UCLA, and a collaborative author with Betty Neuman). The nursing diagnoses described by participants in annual nursing diagnoses conferences were without a binding theoretical framework to guide their development. While these taxonomies appear to be a unifying diagnostic language for communication between nurses, they

> cannot contribute to the development of scientific solutions (*i.e.*, nursing therapeutics), [because] nursing diagnoses that are not developed within an explanatory framework have to be accepted only as descriptive "averages" to be used for the purpose of communication and documentation only. (Kim, 1987, p. 102)

Several types of theories related to the nursing process need to be developed. Examples of these are: theories to describe the actual processes that nurses utilize in assessing, diagnosing, and providing nursing therapeutics to different types and categories of clients; theories to describe nursing diagnoses and those that can "give order to the nomenclature" (Kim, 1987, p. 103); theories to explain diagnostic categories within the different contexts; and theories that explain nurse–patient contacts within the contexts of client variables and diagnostic categories. Processes for assessment, diagnosis, and intervention have emerged as central to nursing and its mission.

Finally, a dialogue about the congruency between a reductionist approach to viewing nursing phenomenon, as assumed through using the nursing process, and the assumptions of holism, needs to go forward. This dialogue began with effective arguments supporting the incongruousness between assumptions inherent in theories of nursing process and the nature of holism in nursing (Barnum, 1987).

Environment

Ever since Florence Nightingale (1946) identified nursing in relation to a focus on optimizing an environment to promote healing and optimal health, environment has been a concept central to the nursing domain. Nightingale considered both the discomfort and suffering that patients experience as results of inadequacies in the environment and nurses' actions as focusing on that environment. We lost track of this concept during the years when the biological systems dominated nursing and when nursing focused on illness, medical treatment, and assistance with a medical regimen. As central as the concept may be, nursing theorists have not addressed it in the same depth and with the same conviction about its centrality as did Nightingale—nor as they did when considering the individual. Clinicians appear to pay lip service to it.

There are those more contemporary theorists who see the environment as central to nursing, particularly human being–environment interaction (*e.g.*, Rogers, 1970; Paterson and Zderad; 1976). To these theorists, environment encompasses energy fields, social systems, family, society, culture, the patient's room, the nurse, and all that surrounds the client. Rogers' theory focuses on a description of person and environment energy fields as inseparable. There is constant interaction between a human being and the environment; the process inherent in such interactions can only be understood through a careful consideration of the environment. This view considers the person and the environment as being in constant interaction and recognizes changes in one as integral and simultaneous to changes in the other. Therefore, the aim of nursing intervention is to promote, maintain, regulate, or change the environment or life processes of people to affect changes in both.

Chopoorian (1986) argued for considering the environment as the central focus for nursing interventions and against the centrality of clients. She developed her thesis by demonstrating the limited roles of nurses in instituting changes if clients are considered the central focus for nursing. In reconceptualizing environment for the discipline of nursing, she suggested that, "nurses develop a consciousness of environment as social, economic, and political structures; . . . as human social relations, . . . as everyday life" (Chopoorian, 1986, p. 47). In reconceptualizing environment for nursing, Chopoorian proposes that this approach has the potential for opening up new opportunities for nurses to make contributions to resolving society's problems (p. 53).

Environment, as a central domain concept, includes immediate client settings, family, significant others, health care professionals, and the socioeconomic and political contexts of the client's families and communities (Hedin, 1986). Stevens (1989) proposes the use of critical theory to illuminate oppressive environmental factors that influence health, hinder human potential and life possibilities, and "restrict their equal and fully conscious participation in society" (p. 63).

Several types of theories related to environment need to be developed. Theories centering on environment are expected to describe properties, components, and dimensions of environment that are healthy or that help in maintaining or in changing health care outcomes, that describe the nursing client's environment, and that promote self-care, adaptation, and effective interventions. In addition, they are expected to guide changes in systems that constrain development, access and equality. Examples are theories to describe healthy environments; theories to describe societal mechanisms in constraining the development and provision of healthy environments; theories that describe and explain access to politics regarding health care; and theories that guide actions for environmental change.

Nursing Therapeutics

Nursing therapeutics is defined as all nursing activities and actions deliberately designed to care for nursing clients (Barnard, 1980). While the nursing process addresses patterns in assessing, diagnosing, and intervening, nursing therapeutics considers the content of nursing interventions and the goals of intervention. The ultimate goal of theory development in nursing is to develop theories that guide the care that nurses give to patients. The existing nursing theories, as categories, provide nursing with the beginnings of nursing therapeutics. For example, interaction theorists suggest that because we define nursing as a process and as an interaction, the problems are in that area; therefore, to these theorists nursing therapeutics are related to making the interaction process more effective. They recommend the use of empathy, validation, and deliberative nursing process.

Examples of other therapeutics are:

Touch (stimulation and repatterning of human fields) (Krieger, Johnson, Weiss, Rogers, Neuman);
Care (Orem, Henderson, Leininger);
Role supplementation (Meleis, Swendsen, Dracup);
Protection (Johnson, Norris);
Manipulation of focal, residual, and contextual stimuli (Roy);
Comfort (Arruda, Larson, and Meleis; Morse); and
Use of self as a nursing therapeutic.

Each of these concepts related to nursing therapeutics could become the nucleus of a single-domain theory in therapeutics.

Health

Health, a goal shared by a number of health professions, emerged as a central goal in nursing in the writings of Florence Nightingale in the mid-1800s. Since then, theorists have considered health with different degrees of specificity, reductionism, and centrality. Health has been accepted as more than the absence of disease, and that concept is becoming more emphasized in nursing (Newman, 1983, 1986; Smith, 1983; Neuman, 1989).

Several different models of health were identified from the nursing literature (Meleis, 1990): health as an absence of disease (Smith, 1983), health as an internal homeostasis (Johnson, 1980), health as adaptation (Roy, 1984; Smith, 1982), health as performing roles and functions (Orem, 1988; Smith, 1982), and an existential view of health that focuses on symbolism and the place of the self in an intricate web of relations among objects and subjects (Paterson and Zderad, 1976; Travelbee, 1971). A sixth model relies on space/time/energy and consciousness expansion; health in this model is viewed in terms of awareness, personal control, personal empowerment, and mastery over body (Newman, 1986; Rogers, 1970). The last model considers the cultural/social/political aspects of health (Allen, 1986; Tripp-Reimer, 1984). For further theoretical development of health as a central concept, the unity and diversity among these models need to be addressed, compared, and contrasted. Several conditions were identified as needing to be included in further theoretical development of health. These are

> the need for focusing on an understanding of the health care needs of
> underserved populations, the potential advantage in using a feminist
> framework, the integration between a static conception of being healthy and
> a process/dynamic/becoming conception of health. (Meleis, 1990, p. 1)

CONCLUSION

The domain of nursing deals with clients who are assumed to be in constant interaction with their environments, human beings who have unmet needs related to their health or illness status, who are not able to care for themselves or are not adapting to their environments due to interruptions or potential interruptions in health. The domain of nursing incorporates a central focus on environments that includes sociopolitical and economic contexts for nursing clients and their significant others. The domain of nursing includes a focus on nursing therapeutics to help in meeting the needs of human beings for health and health care, to enhance adaptation capability, to develop self-care abilities, and to maintain or promote health and well-being. Theory and research are the processes by which the domain concepts and problems are developed, validated, and communicated. Practice, education, and administration are the means by which the domain goals are implemented. All these are part of the discipline of nursing.

REFERENCES

Abdellah, F.G. (1969). The nature of nursing science. *Nursing Research*, 18, 390–393.

Allen, D.G. (1986) Using philosophical and historical methodologies to understand the concept of health. In P.L. Chinn (Ed.), *Nursing research methodology: Issues and implementation*. Rockville, MD: Aspen Systems.

Allen, D.G. (1987). The social policy statement: A reappraisal. *Advances in Nursing Science*, 10(1), 39–48.

American Nurses' Association (1980). Nursing: A social policy statement. Kansas City, MO: ANA.

Barnard, K. (1980). Knowledge for practice: Directions for the future. *Nursing Research*, 29, 208–212.

Barnum, B. (1990) *Nursing theory: Analysis, application, evaluation* (2nd ed.). Boston: Little, Brown & Co.

Barnum, B.J. (1987) Holistic nursing and nursing process. *Holistic Nursing Practice*, 1(3), 27–35.

Becker, H.S. (1963) *Outsiders: Studies in the sociology of deviance*. New York: Free Press.

Becker, H.S., Geer, B., Hughes, E.C., and Strauss, A.L. (1961) *Boys in white*. Chicago: University of Chicago Press.

Chick, N. and Meleis, A.I. (1986) Transitions: A nursing concern. In P.L. Chinn (Ed.), *Nursing research methodology*. Boulder, CO: Aspen.

Chopoorian, T.J. (1986) Reconceptualizing the environment. In P. Moccia (Ed.), *New approaches to theory development*. New York: National League for Nursing.

Dewey, J. (1966) *Democracy and education*. New York: Macmillan.

Donaldson, S.K. and Crowley, D. (1978). The discipline of nursing. *Nursing Outlook*, 26(2), 113–120.

Fawcett, J. (1989). *Conceptual models of nursing* (2nd ed.). Philadelphia: F.A. Davis.

Flaskerud, J.H. and Halloran, E.J. (1980) Areas of agreement in nursing theory development. *Advances in Nursing Science*, 3(1), 1–7.

Glaser, B.G. and Strauss, A.L. (1964) *Awareness of dying*. Chicago: Aldine.

Glaser, B.G. and Strauss, A.L. (1967) *The discovery of grounded theory*. Chicago: Aldine.

Hall, B. (1982, September) The nursing process as a middle-range theory. Paper presented at Nursing Theory Think Tank, Dallas, Texas.

Hedin, B.A. (1986) Nursing, education, and emancipation: Applying the critical theoretical approach to nursing research. In P.L. Chinn (Ed.), *Nursing research methodology: Issues and implementation*. Rockville, MD: Aspen Systems.

Henderson, V. (1966) *The nature of nursing*. New York: Macmillan.

Hughes, E.C. (1956) *Men and their work*. Glencoe, IL: Free Press.

Johnson, D.E. (1980) The behavioral system model for nursing. In J.P. Riehl and C. Roy (Eds.), *Conceptual models for nursing practice* (2nd ed.). New York: Appleton-Century-Crofts.

Kim, H.S. (1987) Structuring the nursing knowledge system: A typology of four domains. *Scholarly Inquiry for Nursing Practice*, 1(2), 99–110.

King, I.M. (1981). *A theory for nursing: Systems, concepts, process*. New York: John Wiley & Sons.

Kuhn, T.S. (1970) *The structure of scientific revolutions*. In Neurath, O. (Ed.), International encyclopedia of unified science (2nd ed., Vols. 1 and 2). Chicago: University of Chicago Press.

Mead, G.H. (1937) *Mind, self, and society*. Introduction by C.W. Morris. Chicago: University of Chicago Press.

Meleis, A.I. (1986) Theory development and domain concepts. In P. Moccia (Ed.), *New approaches to theory development*. New York: National League for Nursing.

Meleis, A.I. (1990) Being and becoming healthy: The core of nursing knowledge. *Nursing Science Quarterly*. (In press.)

Merton, R.K. (1973) *The sociology of science: Theoretical and empirical investigation*. Chicago: University of Chicago Press.

Neuman, B. (1989). *The Neuman systems model* (2nd ed.). Norwalk, CT: Appleton and Lange.

Newman, M. (1983) The continuing revolution: A history of nursing science. In N. Chaska (Ed.), *The nursing profession: A time to speak.* New York: McGraw-Hill.

Newman, M. (1986) *Health as expanding consciousness.* St. Louis: C.V. Mosby.

Nightingale, F. (1946) *Notes on nursing.* Philadelphia: J.B. Lippincott.

Orem, D.E. (1988) *Nursing: Concepts of practice* (3rd ed.). New York: McGraw-Hill.

Orlando, I.J. (1961) *The dynamic nurse–patient relationship.* New York: G.P. Putnam's Sons.

Parsons, T. (1968) *Sociological theory and modern society* (2nd ed.). New York: Free Press.

Paterson, J.G. and Zderad, L.T. (1976) *Humanistic nursing.* New York: John Wiley & Sons.

Rogers, M.E. (1970) *An introduction to the theoretical basis of nursing.* Philadelphia: F.A. Davis.

Roy, C. (1984) *Introduction to nursing: An adaptation model* (2nd ed.). Englewood Cliffs, NJ: Prentice-Hall.

Schultz, P. (1987) When client means more than one: Extending the foundational concept of person. *Advances in Nursing Science,* 10(1), 71–86.

Smith, J.A. (1982) Letters to the editor. *Advances in Nursing Science,* 4(3), xi.

Smith, J.A. (1983) *The idea of health: Implications for the nursing professional.* New York: Teachers College, Columbia University.

Stevens, B. (1989) A critical social reconceptualization of environment in nursing: Implications and methodology. *Advances in Nursing Science,* 11(4), 56–68.

Sullivan, H. (1953) *The interpersonal theory of psychiatry.* New York: W.W. Norton.

Thibodeau, J.A. (1983) *Nursing models: Analysis and evaluation.* Monterey, CA: Wadsworth.

Tornberg, M.J., McGrath, B.B., and Benoliel, J.Q. (1984, April). Oncology transition services: Partnerships of nurses and families. *Cancer Nursing,* 7(2), 131–137.

Torres, G. (1986). *Theoretical foundations of nursing.* Norwalk, CT.: Appleton-Century-Crofts.

Toulmin, S. (1972) *Human understanding: The collective use and evolution of concepts* (2nd ed.). Princeton, NJ: Princeton University Press.

Travelbee, J. (1971) *Interpersonal aspects of nursing* (2nd ed.). Philadelphia: F.A. Davis.

Tripp-Reimer, T. (1984) Reconceptualizing the construct of health: Integrating emic and etic perspectives. *Research in Nursing and Health,* 7, 101–109.

Walker, L.O. and Avant, K.C. (1989) *Strategies for theory construction in nursing* (2nd ed.). Norwalk, CT: Appleton & Lange.

Webster's II. (1984) *New Riverside University Dictionary.* Boston: Houghton Mifflin.

Wiedenbach, E. (1963). The helping art of nursing. *American Journal of Nursing,* 63(11) 54–57.

Yura, H. and Torres, G. (1975) *Today's conceptual frameworks with the baccalaureate nursing programs* (NLN Pub. No. 15-1558, 17–75). New York: National League for Nursing.

Yura, H. and Walsh, M.B. (1978a) *The nursing process: Assessing, planning, implementing, evaluating.* New York: Appleton-Century-Crofts.

Yura, H. and Walsh, M.B. (1978b). *Human needs and the nursing process.* New York: Appleton-Century-Crofts.

Chapter 7

Hypatia, Hatshepsut, and Nursing Scholars: Scholars in Disguise

Hypatia was a renowned Greek philosopher and scholar during the fourth century A.D. (Osen, 1974), and Hatshepsut was the only ruling queen among the pharaohs of Egypt in 2500 B.C. (Wells, 1969). Both demonstrated commitment, persistence, innovation, leadership, and intelligence. Both were true scholars. Both followed similar paths in their lives—different from the universal and mainstream paths that existed at their respective times. Both met death violently, and may have been tortured because they charted different paths for their people, were forceful in expressing their views, and succeeded in making changes.

Hypatia left her mark on the world in the form of innovative devices to study astronomy and to determine the specific gravity of liquids—devices that were praised highly by Socrates. Hatshepsut left her mark in the form of architecturally beautiful temples for her people, peace within her country and between her country and the neighboring countries, and new artifacts in her land. Both women demonstrated a unique brand of scholarship; however, scientists had to dig hard to learn about their work and their stories. Was that because they were women? Can they be judged by the same criteria used to evaluate and judge male mathematicians and male pharaohs?

Is nursing scholarliness different from scholarliness in other disciplines? In this chapter, this question will be raised and discussed. Answers, however, will await the test of time and the test of those philosophers and investigators who may wish to pursue analyses related to this question.

There are many indications now that the nature of disciplines that are oriented to human responses and the nature of disciplines that focus on clinical matters may differ considerably from other disciplines that focus on physical phenomena or are only theoretical in nature. There are also historical indications that the nature of women may provide them with different voices, different stages of development (Gilligan, 1984), and different ways of knowing (Belenky, Clinchy, Goldberger, and Tarule, 1986). Nursing is a combination of the nature of its domain, its historical association with women, and the propensities of all societies to assign caring to its female constituency. Therefore, it is expected that these characteristics may be reflected in nursing's philosophical perspectives, ways of approaching scientific inquiries, educational strategies, curricular content, and in the ethics that govern knowledge development and knowledge utilization.

It is also expected that the scholarliness in disciplines oriented to human responses may require a different set of criteria to judge its progress and development. These criteria would evolve from the people-oriented nature of the clinical and human sciences, and from the struggles that women have endured to achieve equity and receive acknowledgement for their work and respect for their credibility. Scholarliness for such groups will follow, by necessity, different routes headed for different destinations. Nursing falls into this category of disciplines, and nurses, women and men, may represent scholarliness that is more congruent with the nature of nursing and less with the nature of other disciplines.

SCHOLARLINESS IN NURSING

A scholarly discipline has a focus that is evident and significant. Scholarship in a discipline refers to the degree to which its mission is well-articulated and based on excellent research and theory. Scholarship is evident in disciplines in which knowledge and its progress are easily articulated and in which inquiry answers some significant domain questions. Theory provides disciplines with the means to articulate their focuses. Scholarliness combines theory, research, philosophy, and, in disciplines such as nursing, practice, and it is reflected in the synthesis between a discipline's different components. A characteristic of the stage of scholarliness in a discipline is that the relationships between theory, research, philosophy, and practice become more apparent. Nursing is in a stage of scholarliness. It would not have been able to reach this current stage without having gone through the many previous stages discussed throughout this book.

In the early 1960s, nursing theorists developed theories in isolation, researchers pursued questions of interest only to educators or administrators, and practitioners pursued their practices while remaining oblivious to what the other two groups were doing. Yet significant changes have occurred in the relationships between educators, researchers, theoreticians, and practitioners. They are now talking to each other, writing for each other, and working with each other. They are crossing the boundaries to work together and, more important, most of them believe that practice is the *raison d'etre* of nursing. Therefore, theories are being developed to answer clinical questions. These may include broad questions such as: Who are our nursing clients? When does a client need nursing care in addition to or instead of medical care? When do we discharge a client from our care? Or they may include more specific questions pertaining to ways in which we make our patients comfortable, strategies for pain relief, and care of wounds.

These questions should be compared with questions about strategies of teaching, such as modular or individualized instruction, or with questions about styles of leadership, such as maintenance or developmental, both of which were asked in the past and which led to knowledge that was significant but not central to nursing care. The latter questions could be considered practice-oriented if the reason for asking them was to discover the effects of teaching strategies and leadership styles on practice. Nurses are asking questions central to practice and exploring phenomena emanating from and impacting on practice.

Nursing theories to describe, explain, and predict have been developed during the decades of the 1960s to the 1980s to attempt to answer broad questions that were central to the field of nursing. Although they evolved out of interest in the curriculum, they nevertheless addressed practice in its broadest sense. These questions concerned what knowledge is essential for students, how to organize curricula, and what to include and what not to include in a nursing curriculum. Answers came back in the form of theories that addressed the nursing client, environment, transitions, health, nursing process, nursing therapeutics, and strategies for nursing care. The theories attempted to describe the phenomenon of nursing and attempted to chart a theoretical course for nursing actions. So, the beginnings of a scholarly discipline were created.

There are more indications that nursing scholarliness characterizes the 1980s and 1990s (see Table 7-1). Theory and practice were beginning to be interrelated. In clinically oriented meetings, there was an outgrowth of presentations that were theory-based, there were discussions of questions that lent themselves to theory and theory development. A review of nursing practice literature demonstrated a growing awareness of a stronger relationship between theory and practice. We moved away from "how to" to "why," "what if," and "when" in an attempt to generalize, document, and verify phenomena in nursing practice.

The existing nursing theories tended to address imaginative and ideal nursing practice. These theories were visions of what nursing ought to be and what care should be; they were necessary visions of how nursing should move forward to establish its identity and its boundaries. Once the ideal goals were established, modifications of these theories began to be made as nurses described and documented what exists and what goals are attainable. Nurses became more comfortable with looking at their own practice, describing it, and allowing theoretical formulations to emanate from it (Benner, 1984).

Table 7–1
Characteristics of the Stage of Scholarliness

- ○ Relationships between theory, research, practice, and philosophy become more apparent
- ○ Pluralism in paradigms is encouraged
- ○ Boundaries of domain become more identified
- ○ Domain guides nursing practice, research, and theory

There are indications that professional organizations speak a language congruent with that spoken by theorists and clinicians. One example is the social policy statement issued by the American Nurses' Association (ANA) (1980). The statement provided nursing with a national definition of nursing and a direction for practice and was another indication of agreement on nursing concepts and issues. Nursing is defined as "the diagnosis and treatment of human responses to actual or potential health problems," which is congruent with the focus that emerged on human beings' responses (versus nurses' functions, interactions, or relationships) (ANA, 1980, p. 9).

The definition of human responses to actual or potential health problems includes need, condition, concern, event, dilemma, difficulty, occurrence, or fact that can be described within the target area of nursing. It takes into consideration the diversity of human responses in the health/illness situation. One can see the influence of the different theories on the concepts selected in the social policy statement (ANA, 1980). These responses provide us with phenomena on which to base further research and theory development.

A positive relationship between theory and research is not as foreign and unattainable as it was in previous stages. More specifically, research went through a stage of very limited relationship with theory (Batey, 1977). The links between theory and research preceded links between theory and practice and are becoming more apparent. The literature is replete with suggestions of ways in which nurses can use theory to guide research and of ways in which they can use research to build theories (Fawcett and Downs, 1986).

Different philosophical premises infiltrated nursing from the 1960s to the 1990s. Questions about truth drew on the writings of such diverse philosophers as Popper and Kaplan and spanned the gamut of empiricists, rationalists, pragmatists, existentialists, feminists, and critical theorists. Some questioned the received view as a guiding framework; others proposed to incorporate intuitive thinking and combine it with the more traditional Baconian approach to nursing science. Silva (1977) and Benoliel (1977) supported the idea that nursing should not lose sight of the significant notion that truths gained from intuition are as important as truths gained through more traditional research methods.

In the late 1980s, writing in nursing demonstrated a passion for knowledge, a search for the meaning of truth, and an exploration of values guiding practice as well as knowledge; it also indicated that there changes occurred in the outlooks of nursing's pacesetters. As a result, areas of nursing that during a prior generation were not deemed worthy of investigation enticed a new generation of scholars. An examples of this is comfort as an area worthy of investigation (Arruda-Neves, Larson, Meleis, in review; Morse, 1983).

Norms of Scholarliness

An analytical view of the normative structure of nursing supports the notion of scholarliness in nursing. Education and practice came back together during the 1970s and 1980s. Some institutions tried, and succeeded, in having their faculty maintain joint appointments. Theory infiltrated practice, and, from practice, theories evolved. Instead of taking place within the curriculum, tests of theories were done in practice. Research findings demonstrated significant consequences for nursing care through changes in morbidities, mortalities, and quality of life (Fagin, 1981). There was not only tolerance for multiple theories in nursing but there was in addition an evolving view that pluralism in nursing theory is essential (Newman, 1983).

The use of many theories and the acceptability of pluralism was accompanied by an attempt to derive meaning from their relationship to nursing. Representative examples of excellent theoretical frameworks of nursing phenomena appeared increasingly in the nursing literature (Mercer, 1981; Millor, 1981; Norbeck, 1981; Tilden, 1980; Weiss, 1979). These conceptualizations represented openness to multiple approaches (Armiger, 1974; Schlotfeldt, 1981); they comprised a pluralism that was neither addressed nor advocated during the previous stages.

In spite of having developed these conceptualizations at a time when the dominant trend of the philosophy of science was logical empiricism, authors of these new conceptualizations combined the traditional view that concepts were not accessible to empirical testing with the view that concepts generated variables that are testable. Other nursing concepts, such as maternal role attainment, touch, and temperament in battered children, were based on research and premises from interactionist and developmental models and were drawn from natural and physical science. The new propositions allowed for the divergences that were essential for the development of further testable propositions and, eventually, the development of theories.

This process was analogous to other processes in the history of science. Johannes Kepler, for example, developed the four laws of planetary motion by using careful observations painstakingly collected by Tycho Brahe (Bernstein, 1978). By doing so, Kepler opened up new avenues and brought up new questions. Therefore, he used a convergence of Brahe's data and his own ideas to evolve the laws and to allow for more questions and propositions to develop. Extensions and refinements of early data produced refined and usable laws.

Another property of scholarliness in nursing is that of collaboration. The essence of collaboration is that each member of the team has a major contribution to make and that without that contribution the collaborative act has no meaning (Gortner, 1980). All established disciplines require collaboration within and between disciplines. Our discipline demonstrated increased collaboration by leaps and bounds during the 1980s in both research and publications.

Just as the nature and premises guiding the intellectual discipline of nursing are interdisciplinary, there is also synthesis of truth in nursing. Existing notions of truth in nursing are truth as corroboration by falsification, in the Popperian sense, and as logical coherence of arguments in the Aristotelian sense. It is also the prestige and power that prompt members of the discipline to agree on its main concepts, parameters, and units of analysis that are the focal features of the discipline in the sense that Kuhn advanced. It is introspection, conception, and derivation of meaning in the Kantian sense.

Nurses used all these meanings to constitute multiple truths, combining sub-jectivity and objectivity. Because nurses deal with complex phenomena, with hu-man beings, with behaviors, cognitions, and perceptions, the discipline cannot use one meaning of truth to the exclusion of others. Because of the consideration of the relationship between science and humanity during the 1980s, and because of the close relationships between philosophy and science and science and ethics, nursing realized that a singular theory of truth was inadequate and would defy the essence and purpose of nursing. Theories and research in nursing took into consideration the problems that have motivated the construction of the intellectual systems of nursing, such as the use of self in caring and the need for the total involvement of clients in their care.

As we increasingly accepted the shifts from the received to the perceived view, and as we began to acknowledge the uniqueness of our progress (the integra-tive processes discussed in Chapter 5), we looked at questions of truth as archaic, traditional, and useless. Questions of truth were beginning to be replaced by theo-retical questions—to the degree to which theories are able to solve scientific problems. The basic unit of analysis for progress became "the solved problems" in nursing (Laudan, 1981; Silva and Rothbart, 1984).

Tools of Scholarliness

Scholarliness, by definition, requires creativity. Creativity in nursing is manifested in many ways. Rogers, in the late 1960s and early 1970s, used electromagnetic concepts to explain human beings' reactions to health and illness and to give philosophical guidelines to nurses' interventions. She talked about holism before holism became part of our health care language (Rogers, 1970). Orem (1971) spoke of self-care before the initiation of the self-care movement. Travelbee (1966) spoke of spirituality before it infiltrated the rest of the health care disciplines. The human-ists in the discipline articulated the meaning of the experience of loss and death before it became part of our media lexicon.

Creativity is the ability to link seemingly unrelated concepts and to link seemingly unrelated variables (Bronowski, 1956), just as Einstein linked time with space and mass with energy. To Newton, gravity was the concept he created to describe his data. Creativity is the discovery of hidden likenesses. Bronowski (1956) said that the act of creation is original but does not stop with the originator. Kepler's laws that describe the movements of the planets were not arrived at by mounds of corresponding facts that he collected himself or by corresponding readings, al-though both are significant. He speculated, dreamed, used metaphors, and made analogies (*e.g.*, with music), all of which helped to give conceptual order to the data. In the same fashion, Rogers (1970) used the analogy of symphonic harmony to describe a human being's relations with his environment. Creativity is a leap of imagination.

Scholarliness is a process and state that encompasses the norms and tools of science and the norms and tools of theorizing and philosophizing. It includes not only creativity but also the communication of ideas through teaching to enhance the scholarly socialization of its members. Over the decades, nursing added the necessary pieces to the puzzle of scholarliness. Nursing continues to have a high commitment to improve its curricula, its teaching and learning strategies, its methods of evaluation, and its administrative styles. It is one of very few disciplines that isolates the components of research design and methodology and helps students to develop necessary skills to undertake a research career.

Scholarliness is a hallmark of the 1990s because research and theory help explicate major agreed-upon nursing phenomena; because nursing is able to articulate its mission in theoretical terms and with scientific data (Fagin, 1981); because nursing has well-established organizations, scientific journals, and scientific arenas in which to express its views using both scientific and philosophical methods; because it has authoritative reference groups—all of which helped in establishing agreed-upon, well-defined intellectual goals; because it believes in the autonomy of its clients; because it has a pluralistic view of truth that encompasses internal coherence of premises and propositions, external correspondence of truth through sense, and pragmatic truth through metaphysical processes; because it deals with significant problems; because it deals with humanity and is therefore a stage for humanity; because its constituents have both a passion for knowledge and a flair for practice; and finally, because it offers cumulative wisdom. Nursing goals are generally congruent with those of the recipients of its care; nursing operates from a health and holistic approach and purports to enhance coping and harmony with one's environment.

Indicators of Scholarliness in Nursing

Several indicators serve as examples of the scholarly maturity of nursing. *First*, scholarliness is demonstrated through continuity. Continuity is manifested by the important and fundamental questions in the field that are addressed within a conceptual or theoretical scheme to refine and modify ideas over generations of scholars (Gortner, 1980). Answers are not the isolated incidents nursing deals with. The relationship of mechanostimulation on primary or secondary pain; therapeutic touch as a modality for communication, assessment, and intervention; or the consequences of reality-testing on the elderly are linked to other answers to form a whole that belongs to a theory of stimulation or person–environment interaction.

Scholarliness is the ability to delineate the premises upon which one's decisions and questions are based, the ability to do the research that has the potential for replication, the ability to isolate objective and subjective avenues of inquiry, and the ability to put the results within the context of theories. Our scholarly efforts are concentrated on sharpening and refining our knowledge of the central process of the discipline and of transitional situations that are focal to the nursing perspective: the salient features of person–environment interactions, the nature of coping and adapting, the process of development and prevention, and the mechanisms to maintain or change any of these processes.

Through quantitative and qualitative analyses, dimensions of nursing phenomena are being sharpened, subconcepts are being validated, and basic propositions are being tested, all adding to the substantive knowledge. We must not forget, however, that a significant mission of the discipline is not only better care of the patients but the emergence of our clients from the transition situation equipped with the tools to cope with similar or different transitions in life, equipped with ways to promote their health, equipped with means to prevent further illness episodes, and equipped with techniques to deal with stress in life. Thus, we would be helping to merge research, theory, and practice—the concatenation realized as we handle clinical problems more and more with the same ease we handle theoretical and research problems (Barnard, 1980).

The *second* indicator therefore is demonstrated through nursing theories that evolve from practice and are used in education. As practice is joining with education (Schlotfeldt, 1981), the distance between creation of knowledge, corroboration, and use of knowledge in practice is diminishing. This process I shall call concatenation. Concatenation is the condition under which that shortening of distances is occurring. Concatenation also involves joining with the public media to inform the public of nursing's mission and to modify its goals based on public needs. Our local and national media are cooperating in modifying the negative image the public had of nursing experts, and more important, nurses are speaking up, their messages are loud and clear, and they are being heard (Reemtsma, 1981).

The *third* indicator of scholarliness is the development of the National Center for Nursing Research, which was authorized under the Health Research Act of 1985 and was established in 1986. The Center represented a significant milestone in nursing scholarliness, and it affirmed two significant aspects about the discipline of nursing. First, quality nursing care was dependent on a careful and systematic program of investigation; and second, nursing had defined its domain and its thematic characteristics. It made us all very hopeful that there will be increased support and commitment to knowledge development.

The *fourth* indicator of nursing's growing scholarly maturity is the cumulative work through research and theory that is being done on the central concepts in nursing. For example, health of environment is considered as the patients' environment, as the sociopolitical environment, as the administrative environment, and as the environment for students. Studies were developed to explain different components of environment that add to our understanding of environment. The concept may be the same; the different settings help in the development of all components and all properties of the concept. In an innovative study related to environment, Holzemer and Chambers (1986) found that there was a significant relationship between faculty perceptions of the environment's scholarly excellence, available resources, student commitment, and motivation and faculty productivity. Holzemer and Chambers helped us in conceptualizing properties of health environments for students in the same way we conceptualize healthy environments for patients.

The *fifth* indicator is that the nursing domain became more recognizable by nurses in many of their special clinical and functional fields and is utilized as the organizing framework for education, clinical practice, and research.

SCHOLARLINESS REDEFINED

Scholarliness has been described by many writers, with some slight variations in the definition. The common themes are that a scholar is a person who has a high intellectual ability, is an independent thinker and an independent actor, has ideas that stand apart from others, is persistent in her quest for developing knowledge, is systematic, has unconditional integrity, has intellectual honesty, has some convictions, and stands alone to support these convictions. A scholar is a person who is flexible and who respects all divergent opinions (Roe, 1951; Armiger, 1974; Meleis, Wilson, and Chater, 1980, p. 117). In addition, of course, a scholar is a person who is deeply engaged in the development of knowledge in the field. Not all scientists are scholars, nor are all scholars scientists. Scholarliness concerns having a sense of history about a discipline and knowing how one's work fits within the larger framework and goals of the discipline.

Scholarship in nursing may be slightly different from the way it has been described for other disciplines. Our discipline is scholarly if it engages in the development of knowledge that has some significance to humanity and to human beings, if it has a conviction, if it opens doors for those who have the most difficulty in accessing the health care system, and if it encompasses and includes the underserved population. Nursing scholars deal with human beings, and they not only pursue explanation and prediction, they also address understanding of clinical phenomena that may result from clinical knowledge as well as theoretical knowledge.

Unlike other disciplines that may have promoted competition and distancing as hallmarks of their scientific development, the nature of nursing, with its gender orientation and awareness of feminist approaches (see Chapter 8), would necessitate the promotion of cooperation and collaboration over competition and separation. Scholarliness in the discipline means flexibility regarding its theoretical base. Finally, a scholarly discipline is predicated on the soundness of its theoretical base.

Scholarliness in nursing includes the collaborative efforts of all the resources within nursing to work together to develop critical and reflective thinking in students, academicians, and clinicians. *Critical thinking*, according to Dewey (1922), is defined as the ability to suspend judgment on matters of interest. Critical thinking should be fostered by cognitive and affective approaches in the educational and the clinical arenas. The cognitive approach is enhanced by the provision of frameworks for teaching, for discussion, and for clinical practice.

There should be a balance between providing a framework that enhances critical thinking and one that may lead to other frameworks—or it could be a stifling act that prevents a person from seeing other potential avenues in understanding the situation. Critical thinking lies in the balance between framework thinking and flexible viewing of a situation. Critical thinking can also be enhanced by using effective approaches, for example, through the creation of dialogues about patient care situations that are open to debates and critiques. Critiquing existing theories or research is also appropriate for the attempt to develop critical thinking. Scholarship includes the creativity needed to consider ways to develop knowledge in a human science, ways that do not stifle the richness of its phenomena.

Scholarliness necessitated the use of local models of excellence and the promotion of sponsorship as essential. To preach scholarship without demonstrating it in a close working relationship between mentor and mentoree leaves a lot to the imagination of the mentoree that may not be tangible and attainable. Participation in a mentorship relationship with a person who is pursuing scholarship in practice, theory, or research tends to promote the potential of the development of the same characteristics in the mentorees. Scholarliness in a discipline not only depends on the definition of the discipline by those who are inside it; it also depends on how the discipline is viewed by those outside it. We need to make our discipline more public, demonstrate its significance to the health and care of the public. We also need to become involved in the political and policy-making processes and to make a point of speaking to the public directly.

CONCLUSION

One does not develop knowledge to gain the status of scholarliness. Being a scholar is a means toward an end and not an end in itself; it is a means toward empowerment of individuals and empowerment of nursing as a profession. The end goal is patient care that is based on seriously developed knowledge. It is to provide, to enable, and to empower nurses to make the changes they want to make in the quality of patient care. It is to participate in the development of policies that affect the care that is given. That influence is possible only if it comes from a knowledge base. A knowledge base could be developed if we give attention to patterns of knowing in nursing and to the subject matter of nursing.

ACKNOWLEDGEMENTS

This section, dealing with scholarliness, norms of scholarliness and tools of scholarliness, was adapted, with extensive revisions, from the Helen Nahm Lecture I delivered at the University of California, San Francisco, in 1981; and from (by permission) Meleis, A.I. (1983) The evolving nursing scholarliness. In Chinn, P.L., *Advances in nursing*. Rockville, MD: Aspen Systems.

REFERENCES

American Nurses' Association. (1980) Nursing: A social policy statement. Kansas City, MO: American Nurses' Association. Publication Code NP-63 35M 12/80.
Armiger, B. (1974) Scholarship in nursing. *Nursing Outlook*, 22(3), 162–163.
Arruda-Neves, E., Larson, P., and Meleis, A.I. (In review) Comfort of Hispanic Patients: A concept analysis.

Barnard, K. (1980) Knowledge for practice: Directions for the future. *Nursing Research,* 29(4), 208–212.

Batey, M.V. (1977) Conceptualization: Knowledge and logic guiding empirical research. *Nursing Research,* 26(5), 324–329.

Belenky, M.F., Clinchy, B.M., Goldberger, N.R., and Tarule, J.M. (1986). *Women's ways of knowing: The development of self, voice, and mind.* New York: Basic Books.

Benner, P. (1984) *From novice to expert: An excellence and power in clinical nursing practice.* Menlo Park, CA: Addison-Wesley.

Benoliel, J.Q. (1977) The interaction between theory and research. *Nursing Outlook,* 25(2), 108–113.

Bernstein, J. (1978) *Experiencing science.* New York: Basic Books.

Bronowski, J. (1956) *Science and human values.* New York: Harper Colophon Books.

Dewey, J. (1922) *Human nature and human conduct.* New York: Henery Holt.

Fagin, C. (1981, September) Nursing's pivotal role in achieving competition in health care. Paper presented at American Academy of Nursing meeting, Washington, D.C.

Fawcett, J. and Downs, F.S. (1986). *The relationship of theory and research.* Norwalk, CT: Appleton-Century-Crofts.

Gilligan, C. (1984) *In a different voice: Psychological theory and women's development.* Cambridge, MA: Harvard University Press.

Gortner, S.R. (1980) Nursing science in transition. *Nursing Research,* 29(3), 180–183.

Holzemer, W. and Chambers, D. (1986) Healthy nursing doctoral programs: Relationship between perceptions of the academic environment and productivity of faculty and alumni (research). *Research in Nursing and Health,* 9(4), 299–307.

Laudan, L. (1981) A problem solving approach to scientific growth. In I. Hacking (Ed.), *Scientific revolutions.* Oxford, UK: Oxford University Press.

Meleis, A.I., Wilson, H.S., and Chater, S. (1980) Toward scholarliness in doctoral dissertations: An analytical model. *Research in Nursing and Health,* 3, 115–124.

Mercer, R. (1981) A theoretical framework for studying factors that impact on the maternal role. *Nursing Research,* 30(2), 73–77.

Millor, G.K. (1981) A theoretical framework for nursing research in child abuse and neglect. *Nursing Research,* 30(2), 78–83.

Morse, J.M. (1983) An ethnoscientific analysis of comfort: A preliminary investigation. *Nursing Papers,* 15(3), 6–19.

Newman, M. (1983) The continuing revolution: A history of nursing science. In N. Chaska (Ed.), *The nursing profession: A time to speak.* New York: McGraw-Hill.

Norbeck, J. (1981) Social support: A model for clinical research and application. *Advances in Nursing Science,* 3, 43–59.

Orem, D. (1971) *Nursing concepts of practice.* New York: McGraw-Hill.

Osen, L.M. (1974). *Women in mathematics.* Cambridge, MA: MIT Press.

Reemtsma, J. (1981, May) Nurse, where are you? Television news documentary, CBS.

Roe, L. (1951). A psychological study of eminent biologists. *Psychological Monographs,* 65, 1–67.

Rogers, M.E. (1970) *An introduction to the theoretical basis of nursing.* Philadelphia: F.A. Davis.

Schlotfeldt, R.M. (1981,) Nursing in the future. *Nursing Outlook,* 29, 295–301.

Silva, M.C. (1977) Philosophy, science, theory: Interrelationships and implications for nursing research. *Image,* 9(3), 59–63.

Silva, M.C. and Rothbart, D. (1984) An analysis of changing trends in philosophies of science on nursing theory development and testing. *Advances in Nursing Science,* 6(2), 1–13.

Tilden, V. (1980) A developmental conceptual framework for the maturational crises of pregnancy. *Western Journal of Nursing Research*, 2, 667–677.

Travelbee, J. (1966) *Interpersonal aspects of nursing*. Philadelphia: F.A. Davis.

Weiss, S. (1979) The language of touch. *Nursing Research*, 28(2), 76–80.

Wells, E. (1969). *Hatshepsut*. Garden City, NY: Doubleday.

Chapter 8

On Knowing and Understanding: Nurses as Knowers

An epistemology characterized by a perceived perspective as discussed in Chapter 5 of this book does not fully represent the kind of knowledge that needs to be developed and structured in nursing. In the late 1980s and early 1990s, nurse theorists, researchers, and philosophers realized that a sociopolitical and cultural perspective that considers such variables as gender and class is an imperative for the further development of nursing knowledge. This perspective, argued the philosophers and the theorists in nursing, is more congruent with the nature of the discipline of nursing, the historical development of the discipline, and the nature of nurses as developers and utilizers of theory.

The discipline of nursing combines academic and professional approaches to knowledge development, a history of second-class citizenship, a history of devaluation of its mission of caring, and a history of oppression of its members that reflects worldwide oppression of women and subordination of nurses to other bureaucratic and professional structures. Therefore, by necessity, its members may be more in tune to examining and analyzing similar processes that may be encountered by nursing clients. By necessity, too, these experiences shed different lights on analyses and interpretations of the progress and development of the discipline.

This chapter offers a discussion of the nature of the discipline of nursing and proposes congruent ways of knowing. Three perspectives believed to be essential in influencing the development of nursing theories are presented, discussed, and compared. The intent of this chapter is not to provide a comprehensive account of all perspectives that could be used as frameworks for the development of nursing theory; rather it is to present a selective array of perspectives that nurse theorists, scientists, and philosophers have discussed extensively in the literature during the late 1980s and beginning 1990s. The perspectives selected for the brief presentation that follows are reflective of these dialogues and are the ones I believe will influence substantially the process and the content of nursing theories during the last decade of the 20th century.

This chapter has three other purposes. Types of nurses as proactive agents for the creation of theory are proposed and presented to stimulate the reader to consider potential diverse ways by which nurses may discover knowledge and create theories. A presentation of types of knowledge for which theories could be developed, knowledge that is congruent with the nature of the discipline and its members, is provided. The final purpose of this chapter is to propose for your critical consideration two contrasting models for the development of theories. These models are not inclusive of all other potential models; they are to be considered only as prototypes allowing for many variations. They are intended to guide the development of more specific approaches to theory and to complement existing theory development methodologies.

NURSING: A HUMAN SCIENCE

The science underlying the discipline of nursing has been described as a human science. A human science has several properties, each of which is significant in selecting appropriate strategies for knowledge development. McWhinney (1989) identified some of these properties.

1. A human science focuses on human beings as wholes and advocates understanding the particulars in terms of the whole.
2. A human science has at its core an understanding of experiences as lived by its members.
3. A human science deals with meanings as seen and perceived by its members. Meanings include those attached to responses, symbols, events, and situations.
4. To be able to understand meanings and experiences, a scientist needs to enter into a meaningful dialogue with participants. Interaction is the prime source of meanings and perceptions of experiences. Participants in the activities of knowledge development are those who are developing and structuring knowledge and those about whom knowledge is developed. All participants have to verify the meanings of these experiences.
5. "The scope for generalization for a human science is limited" (p. 298). A generalization has to be made within a context, therefore generalization may be presented in terms of patterns.
6. Some conditions, situations, behaviors, and events are reducible for purposes of description.

Nursing as a human science is concerned with the experiences of human beings and with health and illness matters. Because these experiences are shaped by history, significant others, politics, social structures, gender, and culture, nurses also are concerned with how these perspectives shape actions and reactions of human beings. It is precisely that concern that makes nursing a practice discipline.

NURSING: A PRACTICE-ORIENTED DISCIPLINE

What do we mean when we say that nursing is a practice-oriented discipline? Although nursing may use basic and applied knowledge to achieve its goals, it is still a practice-oriented discipline. The reason it is a practice-oriented discipline is that its members seek knowledge of human beings' responses to health and illness in order to help in monitoring and promoting health, to help in caring for them, to help in assisting them to care for themselves, and to help in empowering them to develop and use resources.

Nurses need basic knowledge to understand the basic phenomena related to the goals and the mission of nursing, for example, how certain groups of people tend to seek help, how certain connections tend to maintain their balance and health, and different patterns of responses to such events as pain, intrusive interventions, hospitalization, and discharge. Basic understanding of such phenomena as comfort, touch, confusion, ambiguity, sleeplessness, and restlessness is essential for the subsequent development of applied knowledge. Applied knowledge is that which provides guidelines to maintain, ameliorate, develop, inhibit, support, change, advocate, clarify, or suppress some of these basic phenomena. Both basic and applied knowledge are the cornerstones of nursing as a practice-oriented discipline.

The goal of knowledge development, then, is to learn how to better care for clients; therefore, caring activities may be congruent with activities involved in knowledge structuring, particularly since the focus of and participants in both activities are human beings. There is knowledge for the sake of knowledge and there is knowledge to provide better nursing care to people of the world. Neither nursing as a discipline nor nurses as scientists whose mission is to develop knowledge related to caring for human beings can afford to have the bulk of their time spent in developing knowledge for the sake of knowledge.

Thus, the purposes of knowledge development and the structuring and organizing of nursing as a human science and a practical discipline (by that I mean engaging in research and/or theory development) are:

Empowerment of the discipline of nursing;
Empowerment of the nurses; and
Empowerment of clients to care for themselves, to take advantage of resources available to them.

If these are the main purposes for developing knowledge in nursing, then we have to consider approaches to knowledge development that make these purposes possible. To empower the discipline and its members, nurses should look for and identify the same skills that made them effective and caring clinicians and build on these skills as well as other skills that could enhance knowledge development. These skills are related to the goals of knowing and understanding.

On Knowing

Knowing includes knowledge based on observations, research findings, clinical manifestations, and scientific approaches. Knowing is more dependent on sense data, but it includes other types of data too. To understand is to connect bits of knowledge in a relational form to other broader statements. For example, we know that women who work outside the household tend to work a double shift at home. We also know that women who work outside the house tend to have better mental health than women who work inside the house. An inference about what types of support and health care these women need is based on this knowledge.

Housework, on the other hand, is an activity that was not acknowledged as work or leisure, an activity with no set hours, wages, or rewards, an activity with no retirement benefits (Harding, 1988, p. 87). Considering the findings within this context of meanings may prompt a consideration of the forces and constraints in utilizing resources that are developed especially for promotion of health of women who are primarily engaged in housework. That involves understanding. Understanding, therefore, includes putting the experience and situation of women within a historical context, looking at gender and social issues. It includes a consideration of values and the meanings of housework constraints.

Knowing results from careful systematic research or from repeated experiences in clinical practice. Reflecting on that knowledge and interpreting the meanings of relationships, as seen and experienced by all parties concerned, and putting that which is known within a context of feelings, values, and different perspectives is what brings us closer to understanding.

On Understanding

Understanding includes interpretation, a total comprehension of other human beings' responses based on their "feelings, ideas, choices, and purposes" as they experience the situation, and as they express their own meanings and understanding of the situation through their own words and through their own responses (Schwartz and Wiggins, 1988, p. 143). The degree to which we need to develop that understanding depends on the extent to which we want to and the how significant our attempt to achieve that level of understanding is. It also depends on the degree to which the other person is willing to be understood, because true understanding not only illuminates the situation, it also uncovers weaknesses and flaws as well as strengths and abilities.

Health and illness situations require a level of understanding that is not required from other situations in which two strangers might come in contact with each other. However, a true understanding of how individuals experience and respond to health and illness mandates an understanding of what a group of people value in life, what priorities they have, how they usually respond to disruptions in their lives, how they prefer to express their discomfort, and what are the most comfortable ways by which they usually prefer to express their feelings.

Knowing about specific groups' perceptions of health and illness, patterns of help-seeking behaviors, and patterns of responses to uncomfortable situations is essential for the level of understanding required to develop an intervention plan, whether that intervention plan is as specific as postoperative deep breathing or maintaining prenatal appointments. Knowing about the extent to which an immigrant is connected to individuals and events in his country of origin may help a nurse clinician understand the out-of-pattern expressions of pain and discomfort to a seemingly less painful experience. Knowing about normal patterns of touch between members of the opposite sex in different social classes may help a health care provider understand when (and when not) to communicate this way.

Understanding includes making connections and achieving syntheses that may go beyond the perception and knowledge of the client or the provider (Schutz, 1967; Habermas, 1971). Understanding has been advocated by interpretive scientists (Allen, 1988, p. 98) as the hallmark for knowledge development in nursing. This understanding includes yet goes beyond specific research findings; it includes yet goes beyond the experience that evolves from the practice arena; it includes yet transcends knowledge awareness from primary theoretical formulations.

Understanding is predicated on knowing about phenomena, knowing about the contexts in which certain phenomena occur, and knowing about patterns of presentation of these phenomena. Knowing about the different roles women enact, knowing about the stresses, strains, and satisfactions in these roles, knowing role theory, knowing the relationships between levels of role involvement and number of roles and health status are all important and significant for developing an understanding of why and when women tend to seek care for themselves or for their children and how they choose to maintain or enhance their health. That level of understanding is also achieved through a deliberate effort to reflect theoretically on some of these concepts and put them together in an organized way to describe and explain some central problems in nursing. Examples of central problems are patterns of maintaining and developing health and patterns of seeking health care.

Jaspers, a physician and a philosopher, addressed the laws of understanding as follows (Jaspers, 1963; Schwartz and Wiggins, 1988, pp. 153–155):

1. Empirical understanding is an interpretation. The data provide the impetus for interpretation and therefore interpretation is not absolute but is subject to other interpretations—and therefore may be theoretical.

2. Understanding opens up unlimited interpretations. To have understanding as a goal frees the researcher to consider many different interpretations. These different interpretations should be subjected to more data to gain support or refutation.

3. Understanding moves in deepening spirals. Starting from parts to understand a certain behavior, one goes to the whole to put the behavior in context and then comes back to the part for better understanding. The process increases understanding.

4. Opposites are equally meaningful. The same evidence could be interpreted in two opposite ways. In doing that, we are attempting not to settle for preconceived notions and we are attempting to understand the synthesis between the opposites. Schwartz and Wiggins (1988, p. 154) give an example:

   We can understand the stoicism of a patient as stemming from bravery and nobility. But we can also understand this same stoicism as motivated by profound fears and a complete inability to face up to a difficult predicament.

5. Understanding is inconclusive. Not all feelings, meanings, and values can be expressed in understandable ways, and not all interpretations are willingly shared.

6. To understand is to illustrate and expose. To really comprehend, both positive and negative aspects of any group or person have to be exposed. Ethical considerations of the balance between exposure and illumination need to be considered.

Should nursing knowledge help us to know, to understand, or to care? Do each require different approaches to knowledge development? Can these approaches substitute for each other, or do they complement each other to enhance knowledge development? I believe that the predominant goals for research are to know and that the predominant goals for theoretical development of the discipline are to understand. I am not saying that one leads exclusively to knowing and one leads exclusively to understanding. I am using the concept "predominant" to differentiate between goals. Imagine knowing and understanding on two continuums. Imagine each going from none to high. Research findings and theorizing could be plotted on the two continuums. Research findings tend to be toward the higher end of the continuum of knowing and may be the middle of the understanding pole, while theorizing tends to be on the higher pole of understanding and may be the middle of the knowing pole.

PERSPECTIVES FOR THEORY DEVELOPMENT

Approaches to knowledge development—including theory development—should be analyzed against the properties of human science, the mission of a practice-oriented discipline, and the balance among knowing, understanding, and caring.

Three perspectives for research have been identified in nursing literature. These perspectives are addressed here in relationship to theory development.

Empiricism is presented here, once again, as a point of departure in comparing it with other perspectives. The rationale for the choice of empiricism as a perspective for the development of theories is obvious in its universality, its vast followers and supporters, and its appeal as the perspective *sine qua non* with scientific developments. Empiricism is then compared with two other perspectives: the feminist perspective and critical theory perspective (see Table 8-1 for a comparison of these three perspectives.)

Empiricist Perspective

A theory for empiricists is a product of research findings that is used as a framework for further research. The empiricists' observations are not contextual and usually focus on single behaviors, events, or situations. Theorizing for empiricists is based on sense data supported by a set of value-free assumptions. Empiricists develop theories by providing precise, well-defined, operationalized concepts—measurable variables. Empiricists are objective, separated, distanced from their theories, they treat the theories as objects and are reluctant to share insights related to findings or evolving ideas with their clients or research subjects. The language they use is research-specific and their approach is inductive. Statistical model building is a significant tool for theory development by the empiricists.

Empirical theories are based on careful and impeccable research studies that are geared to finding relationships between different variables and finding support for a multitude of statements—all geared to answering a set of well-defined questions. Empiricists' theories are well-understood by colleagues from other disciplines, and when theory development is discussed, it is more likely to be understood in relationship to the development of empirical theories.

Table 8–1
Perspectives for the Development of Nursing Theory

Empiricist	Feminist	Critical Theory
Units of Observation		
Acontextual	Human beings	Social structure
Behavior	Gender	Power
Event	Experience	Political structure
Situation	Totality	
	Uniqueness	
	Perception of meanings	
		History
		Relationship with structure
Strategies for Theory Development		
Multiple research findings	Experience of participants	Experience of participants and nonparticipants
	Analysis of situation and context	Analysis of context
	Advocacy	Action

(*continued*)

Table 8–1 (Continued)

Empiricist	Feminist	Critical Theory
Assumptions		
Axiomatic facts	Personal	Societal values critiqued and selected
Value-free	Disciplinary	
	Societal values critiqued	
Concepts		
Precise	Considered within gender orientation	Not essential
Operationalized		
Not acontextual	Analytical statements	
Provide a framework	Patterns	
Unit of analysis		
Goals/Uses		
Theory development	Theory development	Emancipation
Truth-finding for discipline	Consciousness-raising	Structural
	Awareness of participants	Awareness structure
	Illumination	Understanding
Theorist		
Objective	Engaged	Observer of social structure and proactive participant
Separated	Connected	
Distanced		
Secretive		
Approach		
Inductive	Inductive	Creation of new structures
	Deductive	
	Retroductive	
	Philosophical analysis	
Use		
Know	Understand	Change
Starting Point		
Research question	Experience	Structure
	Response	Organization
		Political
Language		
Research-specific	Gender-specific	Philosophical
		Political

Gender Orientation and Feminist Perspectives

The history of nursing attests to how the concept of gender permeates and pervades every aspect of the discipline. Nursing has been predominantly a female profession and continues to be in the 1990s, as female nurses claim about 97% membership in the profession. That is, despite some studies' efforts to open the profession more to men and despite the many contributions men have made to nursing, nursing remains a woman's profession and thus continues to be saddled with all the accompanying issues related to the values of women's work, women's contributions, and the relationship between nursing and other predominantly male professions.

This history could be used to the advantage of the discipline and its clients by attempting to use it as a perspective for the development of gender-sensitive theories. Understanding the constraints inherent in these experiences and the lack of participation in shaping the structure and the goals of inquiry may sensitize nurses to similar experiences of clients.

Gender-sensitive theories are theories that are based on connections between the theorist and the subject matter and the involvement of the theorist with the subjects of the theory in the development and the interpretation of the theory (McPherson, 1983; Sherwin, 1987; Stacy and Thorne, 1985). The goal of gender-sensitive theories is understanding rather than just knowing; the goal is based on uncovering and including personal experiences of the nurse and client and evolves from considering the totality of the experiences, responses, and events described theoretically as well as from giving similar consideration to the experience and the context of the theorist (Hagell, 1989).

A feminist perspective could be utilized not only in understanding issues related to women as clients or women as providers, but as a perspective for developing an understanding of all nursing clients, regardless of sex, gender, race, or culture. It could be utilized to understand, to explain, to raise consciousness, and to develop theories to bring about needed changes for nursing clients (Duffy and Hedin, 1988; Jagger, 1988).

While the assumptions of the empiricists may lean toward value-free axioms and facts and truths derived from previous research findings, assumptions evolving from feminist perspectives are acknowledged as value-laden and include personal, disciplinary, and societal values (Harding, 1986).

Gender-sensitive theories could be based on similar principles that have been discussed in conjunction with gender-sensitive research. Cook and Fonow (1986) defined some guidelines for conducting gender-sensitive research. These guidelines are modified and offered for guiding the development of theories related to recipients of care in nursing. Thus, gender-sensitive theories are theories that

- ○ Consider gender as a basic feature and a central agenda in the theory;
- ○ Provide guidelines for raising consciousness about the experiences described within the theory, heighten understanding of the role of a social system or organization in relationship to these experiences;

- ○ Challenge any norms of objectivity that create distances between participants or between theory subject matter and participants in the theory development;
- ○ Provide a critique of situations and circumstances that may interfere in healthful living;
- ○ Enhance empowerment for options, for understanding, for decision making, or for self-care;
- ○ Decrease any potential of exploitation;
- ○ Enhance advocacy and provide guidelines for advocacy; and
- ○ Provide guidelines for changes, including institutional and organizational changes.

In caring for patients or clients, nurses knowingly or unknowingly have adhered to some of these principles. In fact, some nurse theorists have described nursing using the very principles in the 1960s and 1970s (Travelbee, 1963; Paterson and Zderad, 1976). However, these principles may have been overshadowed by a quest for empiricalization of theories to render the nursing discipline theoretical and scientific. By considering their caring mission, nurses, whether theoreticians or researchers, may be able to synthesize their goals for caring and knowing and thus develop theories that enhance understanding of the situation, the daily experience, and responses of clients.

Gender-sensitive perspective is not to be construed as a substitute for nursing theories. It is a framework that guides the kind of phenomena that nursing theorists may select for development, the approach by which such theories are developed, and the interpretation of findings related to this phenomenon. A gender-sensitive perspective is a framework that guides nurses to study phenomena that represent and emanate from the lives of their clients, phenomena that are important to these clients, phenomena that reflect and are related to the quality of their lives or their health care and that may be seen as problematic from their perspective (Harding, 1987).

Feminist theorizing "seeks to bring together subjective and objective ways of knowing the world" (Rose, 1983, p. 87). A nursing theory that is developed using a feminist perspective is one that values the experiences of the developer, values her intuitions and analyses, values the client's world, and values the client's sociocultural and political perceptions. It is one that includes a sensitive understanding of the conditions that impinge on clients' responses and one that is representative of clients from different sociocultural backgrounds. Nursing theories, whether they are guided by a feminist perspective or an empirical perspective, should continue to inform members of the discipline. Therefore, these theories remain closely connected to the domain of nursing with its focus on responses of human beings and their environments to health and illness situation.

Critical Theory Perspective

Critical theory is a philosophical perspective that emanates from the Frankfurt school of thought and was further developed in West Germany by Habermas (1971) and Gadamer (1979).

> Critical social theory begins with a premise . . . [that] a fully rational social
> decision must be made in a context in which participation is not distorted by
> internal or external constraints (Allen, 1988, p. 93).

To Habermas (1971), there are three distinct but connected approaches to scientific inquiry. These approaches are empirical/analytical, historical hermeneutic, and critical-oriented. The three approaches include the technical, practical, and emancipatory interests. All three types of knowledge and approaches to knowledge development are essential for the development of knowledge for human sciences. Habermas (1971) further proposed that technical problems are best understood through an empirical/analytical approach, practical problems through a historical hermeneutic approach, and problems that include issues that are critical to human beings through emancipatory approaches. The latter incorporates both the empirical/analytical and the historical hermeneutic approaches in a higher-order synthesis. The goal of the critical-oriented inquiry is an active reflective stand that includes changes that are emancipatory (Holter, 1987; Allen, 1985; Habermas, 1974).

The feminist theorists focus on gender inasmuch as the critical theorists focus on power and emancipation through reflection and action. Theories developed through this perspective provide ways of understanding the sociopolitical structure and patterns of oppression of clients within such a structure and also provide guidelines for a reflective approach to the situation and ways by which the subjects of theory are transformed and emancipated from unequal power structures (Bernstein, 1978; Habermas, 1979). The goal of a theorist here is to develop some means by which the participants can be put on the road toward emancipation from oppressive social structures. The goal is not only to understand, but to change and to do so drastically. Reflection, understanding, and action are the hallmarks of a nursing theory developed within this perspective.

A nursing theory developed within this perspective offers a focus on social structure, power, and political structure as units of analyses, a "critique of power and ideology" in existing societal structures in which the nursing client interacts (Allen, Benner, and Diekelmann, 1986). It is a theory that incorporates an understanding of a phenomenon or a situation by all involved parties; it provides insights about the health/illness situation and a framework of what is to be done about it. Therefore, an equal partnership between the subject matter of a theory and the developer of the theory has to be maintained.

Critical theory is not a substitute for nursing theory; rather, it is a framework or a perspective that informs the phenomena to be considered theoretically, guides the approaches for developing them, provides ways by which the phenomena are to be interpreted, and suggests approaches for handling these phenomena.

NURSES AS KNOWERS

Although nursing is a field of study open for men and women, the predominance of women in nursing must not be ignored when considering women as knowers. Women are agents of knowledge whose characteristic activities provide a grounding that is different from and in some respects (in some disciplines based on human science) preferable to men's grounding (Harding, 1988, p. 83). Harding makes this argument:

> What it means to be scientific is to be dispassionate, disinterested, impartial, concerned without abstract principles and rules, but what it means to be a woman is to be emotional (passionate), interested in and partial to the welfare of family and friends, concerned with concrete practices and contextual relations. (Harding, 1988, p. 83)

The question that forms the basis for this section is: Are nurses' approaches to knowing, understanding, and formulating conceptualizations unique? The rationale for this question is described in Part Two of this book. There are indications in the literature of the 1980s and 1990s of the uniqueness of women's developmental processes and women's ways of describing their experiences. The unique ways by which experts in general analyze, judge, and make decisions about situations were discussed and defined by Dreyfus and Dreyfus (1985).

In using this framework, Benner and Tanner (1987) demonstrated how nurses use intuition in expert clinical judgment. Six key aspects of intuitive judgment were identified and discussed in a study that included 21 nurses who were defined by their colleagues as experts. Nurses demonstrated their ability to make judgments by using their intuitive expertise to recognizing patterns of relationships in situations that are not readily recognizable by others, by detecting similarities between situations through common-sense understanding, by "knowing how" in a way that is not definable in common scientific terms, by having a "sense of salience" (that is, recognizing priorities), and by using "deliberative rationality" (shifting perspectives for better understanding) (Benner and Tanner, 1987). These processes involved a level of intuition that has been devalued by nurses for its lack of scientific bases. Are any of these characteristics for caring congruent with those needed for knowing and understanding? The uniqueness of nurses' capacity to know and the unique ways by which they demonstrate that knowing and understanding are proposals that should be seriously considered.

That there are different processes of knowing is a proposal that has been supported by a number of key publications in the 1980s. For example, Belenky, Clinchy, Goldberger, and Tarule (1986) identified five different types of knowers. Schultz and Meleis (1988) theorized that these types could be found in nursing. Types of theories and levels of development of theories may be influenced by the ability of nursing theorists to uncover knowledge of the different types, to be able to hear and reflect the voices of the different knowers in theoretical development.

If the five types of knowers identified by Belenky and colleagues (1986) are defined from a nursing perspective, the following is what we might find:

1. **Silent knowers** are those nurses who tend to accept the voices of authority and thus learn to be silent. These nurses know their practice, their teaching, or their administrative practice, but may not be able to articulate what they know through abstract thought

for theoretical development and may not have the language to express their analysis or interpretation of the phenomenon. Their work, insights, and wisdom are invisible because they are not represented or because theorists have not been able to retrieve them for further theoretical development. Could these silent knowers conceptualize their understanding of phenomenon in ways that are more congruent with their propensity to develop theories?

2. **Received knowers** believe others are capable of producing knowledge that they can follow and reproduce. They believe in external authorities' abilities to generate knowledge, but not in their own or their peers' abilities to do the same. These people depend on and value the expertise of others. Many nurses have contented themselves in using the works of others, believing those works to be far superior to anything they themselves could create. Examples are the different theories and paradigms that we have bought into and used for years without questioning.

3. **Subjective knowers** depend on their personal experiences. These knowers believe and depend on their own inner voices and inner feelings. Knowledge to them is "personal, private, and subjectively known and intuited," and truth "is an intuitive reaction—something experienced, not thought out, something felt rather than actively pursued or constructed" (Belenky, Clinchy, Goldberger, and Tarule, 1986, p. 69). Although these knowers find it difficult to articulate the processes used to arrive at the knowledge, they have the wisdom that holistically looks and explains complete situations. Knowledge from nursing practice as articulated by subjective knowers could inform the discipline of nursing in ways that no other knowledge could. This is the knowledge that Carper (1978) referred to as personal knowledge and Benner (1984) as expert knowledge.

4. **Procedural knowers** depend on careful observations and procedures. They are the rationalists among us. These are the people who communicate procedures, rules, and regulations, and thus may be best suited for developing empirical or procedural theories.

5. **Constructed knowers** view all "knowledge as contextual, they experience themselves as creators of knowledge and value both subjective and objective strategies of knowing." These knowers integrate the different ways of knowing and the different voices (including the silent voice). To them, "all knowledge is constructed, and the knower is an intimate part of the known" (Belenky, Clinchy, Goldberger, and Tarule, 1986). To subscribe to this view is to accept the never-ending process of knowledge development, to accept that theories are always in process, to

accept that frames of reference are constructed and reconstructed, and to accept that situations as well as knowledge are contextual and subject to different interpretations (Schultz and Meleis, 1988).

Are there different types of knowers in nursing? In considering the major theoretical and research literature from the 1970s through the 1990s, patterns of knowing emerge. These patterns are tentative and are in the process of development; nevertheless, I think they represent patterns of theorizing in nursing:

The synthesizers are those conceptualizers who are able to connect already developed ideas, analyze them, and arrive at new wholes. These new wholes make for a more effective explanation and interpretation of already existing knowledge.

The leap theorizers are those who amass research or clinical data and reduce these data to abstract ideas. They are the conceptualizers who are able to make leaps to generalizations to create challenging theoretical questions and answers.

The bush describers are those who know how to describe relationships that have been empirically identified and verified. They usually are reluctant to go beyond these specific findings.

The out-of-discipline theorizers are those who see the world of nursing through the glasses tinted by other disciplines. Therefore, when engaging in conceptualizing and answering questions, they select those that are more accepted and more central to other disciplines. At the same time, however, their findings and conceptualizations shed some light on nursing problems, however minor those problems are to the core of nursing.

The conceptualizers are those who are discovering, identifying, and exploring the discipline's concepts. These concepts may be central or tangential.

The integrated theorizers are those who are as comfortable with theorizing as with researching or practicing. More importantly, these are individuals who have synthesized the different aspects of their problem of interest and have been able to develop conceptualizations in which clinical, research, and theoretical insights are contained.

ON THEORIZING IN NURSING

Each of these agents of knowledge is important to the development, structuring, and organizing of the knowledge base of the discipline, particularly when one considers that practice-oriented disciplines such as nursing may have different patterns of knowing. Four patterns of knowing have been identified in nursing, empirical (the science of nursing); aesthetic (the art of nursing); personal knowledge, which is concerned with the quality of interpersonal contacts, promoting therapeutic relationships, and individualized care; and ethics, which includes the moral component of nursing (Carper, 1978). Fry (1988) reminded us that these patterns are neither complete nor static.

Jacobs-Kramer and Chinn (1988) uncovered patterns of expressions related to each pattern of knowing by which credibility of knowledge within each pattern is assessed. Three related patterns of theoretical formulations were also proposed by Schultz and Meleis (1988) who maintained that the development of theory could not be, and in reality is not, dependent on any particular source. Practice, theory, and empirical findings could all be theory sources (see Chapter 9 for sources of theory and Chapter 10 for strategies of theory development from each source). Therefore, they identified clinical, conceptual, and empirical theories as the types of theories to develop in nursing. The three types of theories are not totally distinct or mutually exclusive; they should only be treated as prototypes. The emphasis on the differences does not preclude hybrid theories that are developed from knowledge emanating from any or all sources (see Table 8-2 for a comparison of these three types of theories).

Table 8–2
On Theorizing in Nursing: Types of Theories

Clinical	Conceptual	Empirical
Phenomena		
Discovered	Discovered	Created
Concepts		
Emerge from phenomenon	Used as per theory or redefined	Used as is redefined Modified due to research
Propositions		
Linkages evolve from experience	Theoretical properties evolve from theory	Deduced from theory
Theory		
Descriptive/explanatory	Descriptive	Descriptive
Prescriptive	Explanatory	Predictive
Purpose		
Explain	Explain	Explain
Prescribe	Development of theory	Development of theory
Development of theory		Researcher
Clinical practice		
Approach		
Clinical experience	Conceptualization	Measurement testing
Evaluation		
Guided by practice situation	Guided by theory	Guided by research

Thus, theorizing in nursing evolves from extending other theories, abstracting from practice, or synthesizing research findings, or any combination of these types. The differences are in how the phenomena are identified, the nature of concepts, and the origins of the propositions. Although all theory may be developed to describe, explain, prescribe, or predict, there are differences in the purposes of each type as well as in the approaches to the development of each type. Evaluation and testing of each theory type would be expected to correspond with its nature and use. The challenge for members of the discipline is in the development of patterns of establishing credibility for each type. Each type of theory is briefly described next.

Clinical Theories

Clinical knowledge results from engaging in the gestalt of doing and caring. Florence Nightingale developed her ideas from her work with the wounded soldiers in the Crimean War; her theory of environment evolved from clinical work. Clinical knowledge could be the result of personal and subjective knowing. There are numerous examples in the literature, particularly in the clinical literature, that provide descriptions of clinical examples that are the sum total of the wisdom of clinicians. The question is, How we can enhance that knowledge and how we can establish its credibility? This credibility may have been based in the past on the fact that it worked! However, because we are trying to establish a case for the significance of this knowledge, perhaps we need to think of some established ways that will render some of this knowledge acceptable.

Clinical theories use what feminist psychologists call "connected knowing," that is, developing theories collaboratively through interpersonal relations with clients and through being connected with what another person may be experiencing. These theories have been described in different ways by different authors. They have been defined as narrative, naturalistic, or clinical concepts. Theories that evolve from a clinical setting have richer clinical context and a longer span; their credibility may be enhanced for other clinicians, and they are developed from concrete experiences.

Conceptual Theories

The second type of theory is one that is abstracted and generalized from other theories and goes beyond personal experiences. Nursing theorists have provided us with many examples of this type of theorizing. Their work is a product of their reflecting about phenomena they consider central to the discipline of nursing; their theories are products of theoretical reflections based on other prototype theories. The criteria for accepting theories have been described by a number of metatheorists as falling within the norms of coherence and corroboration. The criteria for accepting theories that are developed from conceptual knowledge involve the extent to which members of the discipline find them useful in illuminating the discipline of nursing. Therefore, a set of criteria for evaluating these theories are expected to evolve from their origins and objectives.

Empirical Theories

The third type of theory is knowledge that results from research, whether that research is historical, phenomenological, interpretive, or empiricist. Criteria for establishing the credibility of theories that evolve from each of these research traditions have yet to be developed. Theories that are empirical are amongst the most accepted types and are usually the better established.

MODELS FOR METATHEORY

The combination of philosophical perspectives discussed in this chapter, ways of knowing, and types of themes suggest the evolving of two central complementary models for the development of nursing theories. These models evolved from our history, our mission, our propensity to knowing, and our gender orientation. These models are not inclusive of all approaches to theory development; rather they appear to represent evolving disciplinary approaches. They do not correspond to any particular philosophy in its totality; for example, Model 1 is not to be equated with an empirical, neopositivist philosophical stance nor should Model 2 be exclusively equated with phenomenological approaches. These models are modified to represent the nature of knowing and understanding in nursing. I propose that we think of these models as intrinsic to the discipline of nursing and as emerging from its needs and goals. The use of these models could provide support for the kind of knowing and understanding needed in the discipline of nursing. Both models can be analyzed against the social policy statement defining nursing, the nature of nursing as a human science, and the phenomenon that represents the nursing focus.

The premise upon which these two models are developed is that both are equally essential for the development of the discipline of nursing. To avoid labeling that may cast shadows on either model, I prefer to call them Model 1 and Model 2 (see Table 8-3 for a summary comparison of the two models).

Model 1

The unit of observation for Model 1 is more definable than the Model 2 unit of observation; it is more concise, operational, and amenable to being reduced to variables. An example is support. Support is further defined and operationalized into tangible or intangible support, which is further operationalized into tangible daily support for family members. Each of these concepts is carefully defined. The assumptions upon which the theory is developed are carefully delineated and support for each is provided.

Model 1 theory development evolves from a research tradition, whatever that tradition may be; therefore, theories are carefully and immediately connected with existing or evolving research. A theorist using Model 1 will not venture sharing her theory until completed and supported and, when it is shared, it is provided to the scholarly community. Its theory development derives its support through documen-

Table 8–3
Models for Metatheory

Model 1	Model 2
Unit of Observation	
Defined, concise, operational	Behaviors, events, or situations embedded in a context
Predefined	
A particular aspect	Human being and environment
Assumptions	
Axioms	Context
Value-free	Value-laden, beliefs, action
Concepts	
Defined, operationalized *a priori*	Emerge from clinical, research, or theory
Propositions	
Operationalized	Descriptive, explanatory statements
Relationship between concepts	
Theory Development	
Theory evolves from a research tradition	Theory evolves from theory, practice, research
Conditions	
Conciseness, source, facts	Perceptions, meanings, patterns, context
Tools for Development	
Observation	Collaboration
Research designs	Dialogue
Research findings	Intuition
	Experiences
	Diaries
	Self
Reasoning	
Logical development	Connective
Context	
Documentation of justification	Documentation of discovery
Theorist	
Distanced, objectified, not active participant	Engaged, attached, acting, developing
Purpose	
Explain, predict	Describe, explain, understand

(continued)

Table 8–3 (Continued)

Model 1	Model 2
Theory Use	
Congruency with evidence	Congruency with human values
Focus	
Knowing	Understanding
	Caring
Criteria for Evaluation of Phenomena	
Centrality and closeness to cutting edge in discipline	Significance to discipline, to theorist, to humanity
Validity, reliability	
Evaluation	
Critique	Description
Testing	Analysis
	Testing
Criteria for Analysis	
Validity and reliability of concepts	Theorist experiences
Operationalizability	Social structure
Research	Values
Criteria for Testing	
Empirical evidence	Understanding
Statistical methods	Usefulness
Corroboration	Intuition
	Coherence
	Comprehensiveness
	Support from experience
Validity	
Universality	Diversity of exemplars
Replicability	
Stands the test of time	
Norms	
Universal	Contextual
Observation	Reflection
Ordered	
Time	
Defined time period	Time and historically embedded
Transcends time	

(continued)

Table 8–3 (Continued)

Model 1	Model 2
Approach	
Analysis of findings	Reflection
Not contextual	Analysis
	Forward leaps
	Historical and structural context
Language	
Evidence	Understanding
Generalizability	Intersubjectivity
Replicability	Consistency
	Consensus
Goals	
Probability	Pattern
Prescription	Identification
	Liberation
	Change
	Consciousness-raising
Dissemination	
Professional audience	Subjects
	Policy makers

tation of its central questions and answers. The criteria used for evaluating it are its ability to explain and predict phenomena, the centrality of the questions and answers to the discipline's cutting edge, and its potential for more universal use.

Model 1 is still based on some shared assumptions that nursing is a human science and that its mission as a practice-oriented discipline is to care for people. Therefore, theories developed as a result of Model 1's approach are not the same type of theories that may evolve from empiricist, neopositivist, phenomenologist, or any other traditions that may be more appropriate for other disciplines. Model 1 represents the nature of nursing phenomena, nurses' ways of knowing, and the mission of nursing. It may represent a synthesis of other disciplines, or it may represent a new whole, tailored for nursing. It is a model awaiting discovery, created from our history and created for our future.

Model 2

The units of observation for theorists who choose Model 2 are behaviors, events, or situations that are embedded in a context. This may include but is not limited to the person–environment relationship. The theorist is an actively engaged participant, and her theory evolves from theory, practice, and research arenas. The reasoning is connective, the process is collaborative, and the theorist uses dialogues, diaries, experiences, and the self in developing the theory. The goal of the theory is to enhance understanding of and action for changes, and its evaluation is based on the central questions significant to humanity, to the theorist, or to the discipline. The goals for theory development for Model 2 are to increase the visibility of the community reflecting the theory and to provide them with a voice, either their own or that of someone speaking for them.

Some of the same comments made about Model 1 are also appropriate for Model 2. Model 2 does not emanate from one tradition, such as feminist, interpretive, or critical theory. Rather it is informed by these traditions inasmuch as it is informed by nursing history, by nurses' ways of knowing, by the nature of nursing's mission, by the properties of nursing as a human science, and by the practice-orientation of the discipline. Model 2 needs to be created to represent nursing.

CONCLUSION

Nursing's identity as a human science and as a practice-oriented discipline has emerged. We are establishing our unique approaches to knowledge development—approaches that represent our identity as a human science and a practical discipline and approaches that acknowledge the nurses' different propensities for knowing.

It is time for synthesis of the different knowledge identities and the many routes for knowledge development. It is time for further development, utilization, and support of the different models for knowledge development. Models that enhance knowing and understanding, models that evolve from our caring traditions, are mechanisms that support the emerging identity of nursing.

Two models were proposed for the development of knowledge. Some may call these models "paradigms" to guide the formation of communities of scholars and the kind of knowledge developed and structured by them. I prefer to call them models and to offer them as a stimulus for a dialogue about the two major routes in the theoretical journey of theoreticians, researchers, and clinicians. Either could be selected in pursuit of knowledge development in general and theoretical development in particular. They are also offered to consolidate our efforts, to enhance the potential of our speaking with each other in an understandable language, and to focus our knowledge development activities.

As we nurture and support our emerged identity, we need to support more coherent approaches to knowledge development, ones that encompass knowing, understanding, and caring; ones that support the development of models for knowledge development congruent with our mission. Support of such identities includes tangible support from granting agencies as well as publishing support from editors of nursing journals.

By being clear about our mission, our values, and the models we choose to use for knowledge development, we are empowering ourselves to empower our consumers. In order to become clear and to consolidate efforts, we are challenged to further develop and structure knowledge using each model. I believe both models will continue to exist side by side during the decade of the 1990s and perhaps beyond.

REFERENCES

Allen, D. (1985) Nursing research and social control: Alternative models of science that emphasize understanding and emancipation. *Image: The Journal of Nursing Scholarship*, XII(2), 58–64.

Allen, D. (1988) The challenge of gender for the development of nursing science. In V.C. Bridges and N. Wells (Eds.), *Proceedings of the fifth nursing science colloquium: Strategies for theory development in nursing: V.* Boston, MA: Boston University.

Allen, D., Benner, P., and Diekelmann, N. (1986) Three paradigms for methodologies to understand the concept of health. In P. Chinn (Ed.), *Nursing research methodology: Issues and implementation.* Rockville, MD: Aspen Publication.

Belenky, M.F., Clinchy, B.M., Goldberger, N.R., and Tarule, J.M. (1986) *Women's ways of knowing: The development of self, voice, and mind.* New York: Basic Books.

Benner, P. (1984) *From novice to expert: Excellence and power in clinical nursing practice.* Menlo Park, CA: Addison-Wesley.

Benner, P. and Tanner, C. (1987, January) Clinical judgment: How expert nurses use intuition. *American Journal of Nursing*, 87(1) 23–31.

Bernstein, R.J. (1978) *The restructuring of social and political theory.* Philadelphia: University of Pennsylvania Press.

Carper, B. (1978) Fundamental pattern of knowing in nursing. *Advances in Nursing Science/ Practical Oriented Theory, Part 1.* 1(1) 13–23.

Cook, J.A. and Fonow, M.M. (1986) Knowledge and women's interests: Issues of epistemology and methodology in feminist sociological research. *Sociological Inquiry*, 56(1), 2–29.

Dreyfus, H. and Dreyfus, S. (1985) *Mind over machine: The power of human intuition and expertise in the era of the computer.* New York: Free Press.

Duffy, M.E. and Hedin, B.A. (1988) New directions for nursing research. In N.F. Woods and M. Catanzaro (Eds.), *Nursing research: Theory and practice.* St. Louis: C.V. Mosby.

Fry, S.T. (1988) The nature of knowledge. In V.C. Bridges and N. Wells (Eds.), *Proceedings of the fifth nursing science colloquium: Strategies for theory development in nursing: V.* Boston: Boston University.

Gadamer, H. (1979) The problem of historical consciousness. In P. Robinson and J. Sullivan (Eds.), *Interpretive social science—A reader.* Berkeley: University of California.

Habermas, J. (1971) *Knowledge and human interests.* Boston: Beacon Press.

Habermas, J. (1974) *Theory and practice.* Boston: Beacon Press (original work published in 1971).

Habermas, J. (1979) *Communication and the evolution of society.* Boston: Beacon Press.

Hagell, E.I. (1989) Nursing knowledge: A sociological perspective. *Journal of Advanced Nursing*, 14, 226–233.

Harding, S. (1986) *The science question in feminism.* Ithaca, NY: Cornell University Press.

Harding, S. (1987) Introduction: Is there a feminist method? In S. Harding (Ed.) *Feminism and methodology.* Bloomington: Indiana University Press.

Harding, S. (1988) Feminism confronts the sciences: Reform and transformation. In V.C. Bridges and N. Wells (Eds.), *Proceedings of the fifth nursing science colloquium: Strategies for theory development in nursing: V.* Boston: Boston University.

Holter, I.M. (1987) *Critical theory.* Oslo, Norway: Unpublished Master's thesis.

Jacobs-Kramer, M.K. and Chinn, P.L. (1988) Perspectives on knowing: A model of nursing knowledge. *Scholarly Inquiry for Nursing Practice: An International Journal,* 2(2), 129–139.

Jagger, A.M. (1988) *Feminist politics and human nature.* Sussex, UK: Rowman & Littlefield.

Jaspers, K. (1963) *General psychopathology.* Translated by J. Hoenig and M. W. Hamilton. Chicago: University of Chicago Press.

McPherson, K.I. (1983) Feminist methods: A new paradigm for nursing research. *Advances in Nursing Science,* 5(2), 17–25.

McWhinney, I.R. (1989) "An acquaintance with particulars . . ." *Family Medicine,* 21(4), 296–298.

Paterson, J.G. and Zderad, L.T. (1976). *Humanistic nursing.* New York: John Wiley & Sons.

Rose, H. (1983) Hand, brain, and heart: A feminist epistemology for the natural sciences. *Signs: Journal of Women in Culture and Society,* 9(1), 73–89.

Schultz, P.R. and Meleis, A.I. (1988) Nursing epistemology: Traditions, insights, questions. *Image: Journal of Nursing Scholarship,* 20(4), 217–221.

Schutz, A. (1967) The phenomenology of the social world. G. Walsh and F. Lehnert (Trans.). Evanston: Northwestern University Press.

Schwartz, M.A. and Wiggins, O.P. (1988). Scientific and humanistic medicine: A theory of clinical methods. In K.L. White, *The task of medicine: Dialogue at Wickenburg.* Menlo Park, CA: The Henry J. Kaiser Family Foundation.

Sherwin, S. (1987) Concluding remarks: A feminist perspective. *Health Care for Women International,* 8(4), 293–304.

Stacy, J. and Thorne, B. (1985) The feminist revolution in sociology. *Social problems.* 32(4), 301–315.

Travelbee, J. (1963). What do we mean by "rapport"? *American Journal of Nursing,* 63(2), 70–72.

Part 4

Our Epistemology

*P*art Two described and analyzed internal and external factors that have influenced the development and progress of theoretical nursing. Part Three described our discipline as it is known to its members in the late 1980s and early 1990s. Part Four provides a bridge between the past and present in three distinct areas: the sources and resources for theoretical nursing, strategies for development of theories, and criteria by which theories could be described, analyzed, and critiqued. Two themes are apparent in this part: a historical and a more contemporary view in the history of science; and a historical and a more contemporary view in nursing theory. The tension between the opposite poles in these two themes is a healthy and effective tension, so long as work is not stunted while the tension is resolved. Perhaps the tensions, the inconsistencies, and the paradoxes could be considered as integral parts of nursing theoretical progress, and the discipline of nursing and its scientific base could be considered as a process rather than an end result. If this is true, then we can begin to view the effectiveness of an epistemology in its process and in the number of problems in nursing that it has been able to solve.

No attempt is made in this part to discredit one philosophy and promote another; an attempt was made, however, to display our options in the development and progress of theoretical nursing. An attempt was also made to highlight the tensions, to demonstrate what aspects of the two ends of the poles are congruent with nursing and its mission and, finally, to emphasize human aspects of nursing in general and theoretical nursing in particular. These human processes—of the theorist, the nurse, and the client—are an integral part of nursing and its theory. However, certain aspects of empiricism are still significant and useful for nursing.

Chapter 9 addresses conditions essential for theory development, such as nurses as resources of theory and nursing practice as one of the sources for theory, among numerous others. Finally, the chapter focuses on two paradoxes that occupied the field of metatheory for some time: conceptual models versus theories and nursing theory versus borrowed theory.

Chapter 10 describes and analyzes four strategies that have been used in the development of theories in nursing. These are the theory–practice–theory strategy, the practice–theory strategy, the research–theory strategy, and the theory–research–theory strategy. The chapter ends with a proposed strategy offered as another option, a modified practice–theory–research–theory strategy. Exemplars are offered for each strategy to help you to better understand the strategy in actual use.

Chapter 11 reviews previous models used in describing, analyzing, critiquing, and testing theories and proposes a model that is congruent with current trends and philosophies in nursing.

Chapter 9

Sources and Resources: Bedpans and Spinoza

To Spinoza, a 17th-century Dutch philosopher, one of the most significant goals a human being can pursue is knowledge development because knowledge represents power and freedom for humanity. The pursuit of knowledge and the pleasures of understanding were considered by Spinoza to be precursors to permanent happiness, which in turn leads to healthful living. His philosophy integrates mind, body, and nature in articulating the sources and resources of knowledge. He considered some conditions essential for knowledge development, two of which are of concern to us here. He proposed that a high level of understanding of the sources of knowledge and the availability of human beings who are interested and committed to activities related to the processes of development as two essential criteria for knowledge development.

On the sources of knowledge, Spinoza distinguished between four forms of knowledge. The first is "hearsay knowledge," knowing one's birthday because we were told of the day, the time, the circumstances, and who the parents are; the source of that knowledge is not personal experience. The second type of knowledge is perceived through the source of "vague or confused experience." Here, "general impressions" that something has "usually worked" is the source of a great deal of our knowledge, such as knowing that dogs bark, that we will die, and that water extinguishes flame. The third type of knowledge is achieved through "immediate deduction, or by reasoning, one thing is inferred from the essence of another." Specific relationships are absent; therefore, part of the reality is out there to be observed and the other part is logically deduced. Experience may refute this type of knowledge. Hence, the fourth form (which is the highest, incorporates deduction and perception, and combines reality, perception, intuition, and feelings) Spinoza called intuitive knowledge (*scientia intuitiva*). It is not totally unlike the third form of knowledge. It is the kind of knowing that proceeds from "an adequate idea" to the "adequate knowledge of the essence of things" (Copleston, 1963; Durant, 1953).

On human beings in pursuit of knowledge development, Spinoza said

Human being in pursuit of knowledge should be able "1. To speak in a
manner comprehensible to the people and to do for them all things that do
not prevent us from attaining our ends. . . . 2. To enjoy only such pleasures
as are necessary for the preservation of health. 3. Finally, to seek only
enough money . . to comply with such customs as are not opposed to what
we seek." (Spinoza, cited in Durant, 1953, p. 128).

In this chapter the sources and resources of theory as essential components
for theory development are discussed and analyzed. It is assumed that to engage in
some form or another in the theoretical development of the discipline, members of
the discipline should be aware of the sources and resources for theory, utilize them,
and promote them. The conditions related to the sources and resources are necessary but not sufficient for theory development. Other conditions, such as strategies
for the development and evaluation of theories are discussed in Chapters 10 and 11.

SOURCES: FOR THEORY DEVELOPMENT

The Domain Phenomenon

Ideas, questions, and phenomena are the sources of ideas for theory development.
Ideas originate in the mind, and it is through the power of the mind that ideas are
analyzed, separated, and sorted into mere passing thoughts or intellectual ideas
worth pursuing. Early philosophers differed in their discussions of where ideas
come from. John Locke (cited in Nidditch, 1975) used the image of the *tabula rasa*,
the "blank slate," to describe the meaning of ideas. To Locke, experience is the
source of all ideas, reason, and knowledge. Knowledge is founded in experience and
is derived from experience. Locke spoke of observations and reflections as mechanisms for the experiences to be translated into ideas. Experience is not limited to
the external senses, although these sensations are extremely important for knowledge development, but also include internal senses, reflections of the mind. It is the
combination of the discourse between external and internal senses, between observations and reflections, the internal and external dialogue that creates ideas. The
conscious experience, according to Locke, is very significant but inseparable from
the internal experience.

Though the *tabula rasa* idea has long since died, the inseparability of internal
and external sensations is the essence of theory development in nursing. The mind
is ultimately the vehicle through which ideas evolve, yet what external mechanisms
exist for the mind to observe? Nurses have many sources of ideas, sources that have
gone through three distinct stages.

1. The first stage was the total dependence on other disciplines and
   paradigms. A scholarly discipline cannot have its needed
   autonomy and accountability with continuous dependence on
   other disciplines and paradigms as sources of ideas. Such

dependence dictates the significant phenomena or problems instead of allowing the discipline itself to generate its phenomena and problem areas. A focus emanating from educational paradigms promoted the development of theories that explained and predicted phenomena that better answered questions in the educational field, such as theories regarding modularized instruction or teaching and learning strategies. A medical model allowed for observations related to signs, symptoms, illness, and observations.

2. Second, methodology and functions dominated the idea reservoirs of the discipline of nursing. Ideas related to what nurses do and how nurses conduct research led to conceptualizations of nurses' roles and of methods of research (Gortner and Nahm, 1977). The few dissatisfied scholars who continued to consider sources of ideas such as patients and patient care were rejected. They were thought to advocate a single paradigm in nursing—one single explanation of the world, one system of thought and action that would cover everything. That was perceived to be the route to discipline development. The ideas of these scholars were rejected by the majority, and decades went by in which ideas were methodological and functional—research and theory methodologies—rather than substantive. Some perceived the approach of one paradigm for the entire field to be a method of mind control, a stifling approach conducive to insignificant work.

3. Our current stage is the acknowledgment of multiple sources of ideas. This stage allows different philosophical thoughts to live side by side. This is the stage of looking back at all our sources of ideas and using any and all that help to address the problem areas of nursing in order to develop nursing theories.

The phenomena of the discipline are the core source for the needed theoretical development. It is the phenomena that stimulate ideas, questions, and explorations. The phenomena related to understanding, explaining, predicting, and prescribing the caring process that happens between clients and nurses are, and should be, the focus of theoretical work in the discipline of nursing. However, the context and the sources of phenomena that have occupied nurses have been numerous. Each of these sources provide a medium for articulating significant theoretical questions and each lends itself to theoretical analysis and development. Since the context and the source influence the type and the nature of the phenomenon to be considered, it is important for nurses to understand the different sources and to make deliberate choices based on the discipline's mission and priorities.

Extant Nursing Practice

One of the earliest sources of theoretical nursing was the recipient of nursing care and the actual nursing care offered. The writings of Florence Nightingale attest to the significance of the care process for those suffering from disease and from the Crimean war in developing her conceptualization of nursing and its mission. Nightingale's conceptualization of environment as the focus of nursing care, and her admonition to nurses that they need not know all about the disease process, are the earliest attempts at differentiation between the focuses of nursing and medicine. Her concept of nursing, which has been considered more carefully in the 1980s, includes the proper use of fresh air, light, warmth, cleanliness, quiet, and the proper selection and administration of diet, all with the least expense of vital power to the patient. For example, the statement, "Nursing should be to assist the reparative process, and decrease suffering" (Nightingale, 1859), could be subjected to concept development for suffering or the reparative process, or to theory development for the relationship between the reparative process and suffering.

Nightingale's *Notes on Nursing*, in which she articulated phenomena central to the domain of nursing, evolved from extant nursing practice (Nightingale, 1859). The notes were based on her observations and her experience in nursing. They are a living indication of the potential for extant nursing practice to be a source of ideas for theories to describe, predict, and prescribe nursing care. Her focus on environment and health is becoming a more accepted focus of nursing. One cannot help but wonder, if nurses had continued to consider extant nursing practice as the major source of ideas, whether or not the theoretical development of the discipline would have taken a different path. Extant nursing practice as a source of theoretical development was revisited in the late 1980s. The development and analysis of concepts that are related to clinical phenomena are indicators of the acknowledgement of the centrality of nursing practice as a source of theoretical nursing.

Medical Paradigm

Those who followed Florence Nightingale in the development of schools of nursing to educate novices in the art of nursing took her advice regarding the necessity of providing education and apprenticeship to young women who wish to become nurses; however, these followers failed to continue to differentiate the focus and goals of nursing and medicine and failed to further Nightingale's theorization of nursing. Somehow the medical domain of practice, better developed and more powerful, replaced what was starting to become a nursing domain of practice (health: hygiene, environment, and care).

Ideas evolving from the medical domain of practice addressed medical phenomena, signs, symptoms, surgery, medication, illness, and diseases. Early textbooks provide documentation of the context provided to students, which was medicine and surgery. The medical domain with its biomedical theories dictated the questions that may have been asked by nurses. The richness of nursing practice did not provide the impetus for a focus on generalizing, describing, and predicting nursing phenomena or for prescribing nursing care interventions.

The era of total dependence on the medical model neglected the patient as a human being and the environment as significant in the care of ill people. This is well-described by Norris (1982):

> Nursing knowledge, because of nurses' close alliance with medicine, has been traditionally oriented to symptoms. Symptoms represent processes whose end products are failure of bodily systems unless there is medical intervention. It follows that much of the nursing assessment has arisen out of a process of identifying a problem and tracing it back into the medical model where it is considered from the point of view of failure of the human organism. Much of nursing intervention has emerged from attempts to assist in or complement medical intervention and to provide measures that reduce the discomfort caused by the pathology or medical treatment of it. (Norris, 1982, p. 405)

This has resulted in conceptualizing ideas emanating from and impacting on medicine rather than nursing (Allen and Hall, 1988).

Nurses' Experience

Some of nursing care knowledge has been based on personal and group experiences and has been transmitted from generation to generation through apprenticeship, teaching, or textbooks. Ideas generated from experiences of comforting, caring, changing the environment, preparing for hospitalization, preparing for surgery, or preparing for discharge; ideas related to a sense of timing of when to help patients and when not to help patients; and properties and types of interactions are the kinds of ideas that could be developed further into theories. Experience of patients with certain diseases and surgeries were exchanged between the seasoned and the novice, the educator and the student, and the nurse and a colleague. These rich experiences were not articulated into conceptual entities that would have made them more amenable to wider communication, to generalization, to refinement, or to testing. To "know" from individual experiences permits knowledge that is influenced by personal beliefs, personal convictions, and personal experiences to be shared.

It is possible that knowing becomes knowing through a method of "tenacity," in which people hold firmly to their beliefs due to psychological attachment to the thing they presume to know. In the case of nurses, knowing may be repeated experiences, and nurses therefore may refuse to modify their beliefs in the face of new evidence. Fixed beliefs emanating from experiences are then communicated as knowledge through the method of "authority" (Pierce, cited in Kerlinger, 1964, pp. 6–8). To frame ideas and relationships as "authoritative" dictates a decrease in the potential of progress by development or refinement. To develop ideas and relationships as theories allows for further exploration. To speak only from personal experience in patient care is not a scientific sin; but to generalize, to transmit from generation to generation these limited ideas based on personal idiosyncrasies and individual differences, stifles progress in the discipline, limits options for patient care to individuals, and limits experience.

To use experience, however, as a source of ideas to develop concepts and consider relationships prepares those ideas for further exploration, for testing, for generalization, for being challenged and modified. Experiences, when communicated as personal experiences and on an individual basis, do not have the same power of explanation, description, or prediction as experiences that have been raised to a higher level of abstraction and then commitment. Caring for wounds in a certain way, based on one's personal experience, can be an impetus for developing wound-care theory that would describe the wounds, the different modes of caring for them, variables to consider, the proper environment to help the healing process, the materials to use, the outcomes expected, and the relationship between all these.

Experiential accounts of caring have been published over the years in clinical journals. These accounts have been useful for clinicians but ignored by scientists who have claimed a scientific discipline has no place for experiential knowledge. Writings by nurse scholars in the late 1970s and in the 1980s have supported the significance of clinicians' experiences as sources of knowledge. Carper (1978) demonstrated that the nursing literature contains four modes of knowledge, only one of which is empirical; others are aesthetic, personal, and ethical. Benner (1983) acknowledged the clinical know-hows of expert nurses. Nurses' experiences and nursing practice were identified as sources for the discipline's theories and its knowledge (Meleis, 1985). Even when nurses are functioning from a context of a medical model, how that model is modified to become congruent with nursing's mission and goals is a significant question that continues to merit description and investigation.

Extant nursing practice and nursing experience as sources of phenomena for theoretical nursing are different but related. For example, comfort may be described and explained as perceived and experienced by different client populations under different sets of circumstances, resulting in a theory of comfort that addresses the dimensions of comfort, the conditions under which comfort is needed and experienced. The source of this theory is extant nursing practice through nurses promoting comfort to the different populations and nursing experience through nurses observing the different populations' comfort responses to the care delivered. Both sources may increase the scope and the significance of the theory.

Roles

All the sources of ideas that came before the two mentioned previously evolved from practice and pertained to practice. After that, there was a shift of interest to role preparation, which coincided with the 1950s' conceptualization of nursing as a set of functions. Looking for ideas for preparation of nurses for such functional roles as teachers, administrators, consultants, and clinical specialists prompted a shift to disciplines such as education and business administration. Functions within the context of nursing, but derived from other disciplines' theories, became the impetus for investigations and explorations.

Ideas evolving into theoretical propositions were those related to how to prepare for different roles, the effects of different types of unit organizations, or the different types and levels of nursing care delivered. Occasionally patient outcomes were considered, but even then, patient outcomes that were more congruent with other paradigms (*e.g.*, conceptualization of team nursing, nurse satisfaction, and patient satisfaction) were the ideas of the time from which nurses conceptualized nursing. Concepts that emanated from the role preparation paradigm described and predicted effective and efficient functioning as a teacher, administrator, or consultant. Role preparation was not conducive to theoretical development of the discipline; it provided, however, a functional framework for graduate education.

Basic Science

Nurses have relied heavily on paradigms from other fields and disciplines in addition to the medical and role preparation paradigms. The education of nurses at the doctoral level in the fields of sociology, psychology, anthropology, and physiology has prompted a healthy proliferation of ideas. A kind of cross-pollination occurred when systems, adaptation, and stress paradigms, among others, were modified to define and explain nursing phenomena. Peplau (1952), for example, developed an interpersonal theory of nursing using ideas from a psychoanalytical paradigm. Another example is the use of Piaget's theory as a source for developing theories in nursing (Maier, 1969).

Because much of nursing care is predicated on establishing a relationship with patients and on interaction, it becomes important to assess cognitive abilities of patients in order to deliver the appropriate and congruent messages (*e.g.*, patient education). Whereas Piaget's work provided the assumptions and major concepts, propositions specific to nursing care will necessitate concept refinement and derivation. They will also necessitate consideration of variables that may influence cognitive abilities in health care situations. Examples within an area that may be the impetus for theory development based on Piaget are:

- ○ Changes in cognition, before, during, and after nursing or medical interventions;
- ○ Effect of intrusiveness of procedures on altered cognition and on patient responses;
- ○ Clinical therapeutics to deal with the responses in relation to the cognitive level; and
- ○ Clinical therapeutics to change the responses in relation to the cognitive level.

Thus, a theory of cognitive functioning of adults in acute situations may result from a developmental paradigm (Piaget), but it addresses nursing by explaining, describing, predicting, or prescribing nursing phenomena or questions, such as responses to health/illness situations.

Examples of theories deductively evolving from other paradigms but attempting to address nursing phenomena and nursing problems are Johnson's theory (based on a systems paradigm), Roy's theory (based on adaptation, systems, and interaction theory), and Rogers' theory (utilizing systems and developmental paradigms). (See Chapters 13 to 16.)

Ideal Nursing Practice

One other source of ideas for nursing theories has been what Stevens (1984) called the ought-to-be nursing practice, as opposed to the as-is or extant nursing practice.

Some theorists who have developed theories based on the ideal or ought-to-be nursing practice did not use a discovery method; that is, by observing, experiencing, categorizing, and analyzing reality. Instead, they reconstructed reality; they invented what reality should be and how nurses ought to deal with it. When Johnson conceptualized a person as a system of behavior and conceptualized assessment as a process for identifying behaviors, sets, and goals of subsystems, there were no nurses who were assessing reality as such. It was her mental image of what nursing could and should be. A person as an energy field was not a focus of nursing action, nor was a nurse a temporary self-care agent. However, the conceptual images of nursing dealing with a person as an energy field and a nurse as a temporary self-care agent were created by Rogers and Orem, respectively. These nurses combined non-nursing theories, not with actual nursing but with imaginary nursing, or perhaps with nursing as practiced by the few.

Although they were the visionaries in conceptualization, it is this kind of invention that has been problematical for practicing nurses for two decades and may have slowed down the further development and refinement of existing theories and the development of other significant ideas into theories. (Theories developed in the late 1950s and early 1960s were fully acknowledged for discussion and refinement in the 1980s.) Nurses in practice could not reconcile the images of the few with the practice of the many. Theorizing was linked with the ideal (albeit nonexisting) practice, and usefulness of a theory for practice was severely questioned. Both areas, practice and theory, were pushed farther and farther apart.

The Nursing Process

The process of assessment, diagnosis, intervention, and evaluation is another source of ideas for nursing theory. Interest in the nursing process has resulted in numerous conceptualizations of process in nurse–patient relationships and of process in decision making in patient care. Examples are Peplau's, Orlando's, Wiedenbach's, and Travelbee's conceptualizations of components of the nurse–patient interaction process. Other examples are the Harms and McDonald (1966) and Abdellah, Beland, Martin, and Matheney (1961) conceptualization of the decision-making process. Ideas related to problem solving, priority setting, and decision making evolved out of a focus on the nursing process and from questions such as, What are the best approaches to identify needs of patients and to deliver nursing therapeutics?

Nursing Diagnosis

Ideas for theory may emanate from nursing diagnosis. *Nursing diagnoses* are defined as labels given to problems that fall within the domain of nursing. "It is a concise summary, a conceptual statement of the client's health status" (Kim and Moritz, 1982, p. 84). A diagnosis states a conclusion that is based on some order and pattern the diagnostician arrived at through nursing investigation (Durand and Prince, 1966). It incorporates a nurse's judgment. The process of developing theories through the use of nursing diagnosis is in agreement with stages in theory development beginning from concepts.

Jacox identified the first step as a period of specifying, defining, and classifying concepts used in describing the phenomena of the field (Jacox, 1974, p. 5). Therefore, if there is agreement that a first step in theory development is a period of specifying and classifying, and if practice is the arena for theory development, then indeed nursing diagnosis provides a springboard for theory development. Dickoff, James, and Wiedenbach (1968) would classify the result of the process of classifying diagnosis as a step toward a first-level theory. Labeling without description of what is labeled and without propositions for testing is not a theory.

A classification system for nursing diagnosis began with the efforts of the St. Louis University School of Nursing, which sponsored the first conference on diagnosis in 1976 (Gebbie, 1976). The nurses who participated made a decision that theory development in nursing could not begin without the development of and agreement on its terminology. The work of nurses who participated in several of these nursing diagnosis conferences is inspiring and should be the impetus for ideas that could be developed further into theories.

A warning, however, is in order. The taxonomy that evolved out of these two decades of work resulted in a list of diagnoses that are esoteric in language and nonrepresentative of the complexity of human beings. They are nontheoretical or do not emanate from a coherent theoretical perspective, nor is there evidence that they have contributed to clarifying the nursing mission or to improving communication among nurses and with the rest of the health care team (Gordon, Sweeny, and McKeehan, 1980; Shamansky and Yanni, 1983). Nursing diagnoses are only meaningful if we look at diagnosis as a concept denoting a phenomenon (Kritek, 1978). Then questions arise such as:

When does the phenomenon occur?
Why does it occur?
How do we deal with it?
How do we prevent it?
What other conditions occur at the same time?

These are questions that will help in developing theories based on nursing diagnoses. In addition, the extensive reviews of research related to nursing diagnosis (*e.g.*, Gordon, 1985; Kim, 1989) can be the impetus for the development of theoretical synthesis for nursing diagnosis. (see discussion about Theoretical Nursing and Nursing Diagnosis in Chapter 17).

Concepts Clarified and Classified

Delineated and described concepts central to the field of nursing, other than those dealing with diagnosis, constitute another source of ideas for theory development. The sources of knowledge discussed here are the already clarified concepts. Norris (1982) and others delineated and described 15 concepts that are significant in acute care nursing. Norris (1982) reviewed and considered common elements in the concepts and looked for an umbrella concept under which she synthesized all classified concepts. Therefore, the concepts comprised the source for the development of a construct, "basic physiological protection mechanisms." The new synthesis, with relationships between all delineated concepts and with a binding label, underscores a new entity, a nursing perspective. This new synthesis allows for viewing each of the clarified concepts (nausea, vomiting, morning sickness nausea without vomiting, thirst, hunger, insomnia, fatigue, immobility, chilling, itching, disorientation, bed sores, diarrhea, constipation, flatulence, urinary frequency, and perspiration) as a "functional behavioral response that attempts to remove threat" by sounding an alarm or an all-out bulletin announcing some aspect of the law of dynamic homeostasis. Each of the concepts has a protective function. Emotions after responding to protective warnings can be observed and delineated. For example, after vomiting there is a great sense of relief. Some common attributes can bind groups of these responses (*e.g.*, restlessness and insomnia have the common attribute of increased vigilance). With identification of assumptions, linkages, nursing population, types of nursing therapeutics, and nurses' actions, a theory of protection evolved.

Nurses have identified, defined, and clarified many concepts that could be considered sources of ideas for synthesis and further development of theory (Byrne and Thompson, 1978; Carlson and Blackwell, 1978; Kintzel, 1971; Zderad and Belcher, 1968).

Nursing Research and Nursing Theory

A new source of ideas for further development has been available for nurses since the early 1950s. Research already completed and theory already developed are sources of ideas for refinement and further development. Some examples are Barnard's (1980) research on stimulation and development of infants, potentially leading to a set of systematic and coherent propositions, and Lindeman's (1980) work on preoperative teaching, which, together with Johnson's (1972) work, has the potential of becoming a coherent set of propositions about anticipatory guidance. Reviews of research findings related to central nursing concepts or phenomena are significant sources for the development of nursing theory (*e.g.*, those published in *Annual Review of Nursing Research*).

Each of the existing nursing theories is a potential source of ideas for further theorizing. For example, Levine stated that she will develop two theories that she calls "therapeutic intention and redundancy." These theories emanate from her existing nursing theory (Fawcett, 1989, p. 156).

Combined Sources of Ideas

The complexity and contextuality of nursing practice requires a multiplicity of sources for its theories. These sources include clinicians who encounter phenomena that have not been explicated before, researchers who encounter relationships that have not been accounted for in previously developed theories, historians who get a new insight into the development of nursing knowledge, philosophers who question some of the agreed-upon assumptions or who uncover an implicit assumption; all give significant impetus to conceptualization and theorizing. Theory development can proceed from any of those vantage points.

Identifying Domain Paradoxes

Another condition for theoretical development in a discipline is to identify, acknowledge, and accept or transcend the paradoxes that may be related to theory development. Living with paradoxes in a discipline is as effective in the development of its theories as confronting the paradoxes, making a choice, and then moving on with the business of developing the discipline. What is not effective is to pretend there is only one view or to be immobilized with the paradox and to make resolving it the focus rather than the means.

A commitment to theory development was made in nursing by the American Nursing Association in the mid-1960s. However, the debates related to nursing theory may have delayed the process. Much has been written and debated about nursing theory and about the differences for practice between nursing theories and non-nursing theories. Other debates centered around whether nursing needs theory *in* nursing, *of* nursing, or *for* nursing. Others developed a rather strong case for the lack of need of practice theory. Still others showed that nurses borrow all theory. Another group of debaters demonstrated that other practice fields have no theory of their own, and therefore nursing's quest for theories is an unwarranted one.

Theory is not a status symbol or a special honorary card that nursing needs in order to remain in the halls of academia or to achieve professional status. Theory provides the mechanism from which we can organize our observations, focus our inquiry, and communicate our findings. Theory helps to explain, describe, and predict the range of phenomena of interest to nurses that are central in meeting the identified goals and in highlighting gaps in our knowledge. Instead of getting on with the business of developing theories related to our substantive area of practice and advancing nursing knowledge, a good part of two decades (1960–1980) has been spent debating whether nurses are capable of developing theories, whether they should develop theories, or whether theories are even necessary to nursing. On the whole, the theories that were developed in nursing have not been developed further or refined. (There are some exceptions; for example, Roy has been systematic in developing her theory and in proposing refinements and theoretical propositions. See Chapter 13 for analysis of Roy's ideas and for citations.)

In general, theories have become subjects of debate about whether they are philosophies, theories, concepts, metaparadigms, paradigms, grand theories, or, even worse, not theories at all. Out of all these debates more concepts have evolved to describe theoretical thinking in nursing, such as conceptual frameworks, theoretical models, and conceptual models. This evolution only managed to add considerably to the confusion of nurses. The muddle may have delayed the seasoned theoreticians and researchers in their attempts at knowledge development; it has kept the novice from getting involved in the process of theory building, it has confused those outside the discipline who have not understood what nurses are quibbling about, and it has stood in the way of nurses understanding, contributing to, and improving patient care.

In this section, examples of the confusion in the discipline related to its theoretical development are identified and discussed. Only two of the paradoxes that have been the subject of debates in the past are analyzed. These paradoxes were selected for three reasons: they transcend time; their influence on the level of development of theoretical nursing during the 1970s and 1980s is hypothesized to be profound; and understanding these two paradoxes through careful analyses can be useful for analyzing and understanding other contemporary and future paradoxes. These paradoxes symbolize a significant period in the development of the theoretical aspects of the nursing discipline. The full meanings of these debates and their roles in enhancing or constraining the intellectual environment in the discipline have not yet been fully extracted. By reflecting on the meanings of each side of the debates, students of theory and theory development may be able to develop some insights and some visions about forces and constraints in theory development.

Conceptual Models Versus Theory

In one of the first theory classes in the United States, taught at the University of California, Los Angeles in the late 1960s, Dorothy Johnson classified the conceptualizations of nursing that existed at that time as nursing models. It appears that, since then, terms such as *models, frameworks,* or *theories* have been used freely and interchangeably to refer to any conceptualization of nursing reality. An example of a common usage of models is when one is used to denote that the study of a system B is based on the study of a system A, and that all parts of system B correspond to all parts of system A. Then it is said that B is modeled after A, but it does not say there is any causal relationship between A and B. It only means that some of system A's properties are in system B. It also means that the properties of system B that are different from system A's properties need to be identified. Therefore, modeling denotes similarities in most of the pattern and order and in some of the properties. In other words, "when one system is a model of another, they resemble one another in form and not in content" (Kaplan, 1964, p. 263).

Although this is the common use, there are different types of models. The *physical model* duplicates the form and structure but differs in scale; the miniature train and the baby doll who cries, laughs, and sucks are examples of physical models. They are replicas; in other words, laws that govern the original are obeyed by the model. The *semantic model* is built by using similar symbols and could be called a *conceptual analogue.* We use semantic models when we reduce our hypothesis to statistical symbols for the purpose of analysis. A widely used model in nursing is the *formal model.* To develop formal models we resort to deductive logic, deducing from the original theory by using the central components and crucial relationships as a model for data gathering. Formal models exhibit the same properties in components and the same structure, but the context may be different. For example, we may use an epidemiological theory of disease transmission with its components of incubation, contagiousness, and quarantine to describe how nursing theories are transmitted. Whereas correspondence in the formal model is theoretical, there is abstract correspondence between theoretical ideas and empirical observations in the *interpretive model.* Data may be interpreted using an old theory. The model for interpretation combines both data and the old theory.

The notion that nursing conceptualizations are conceptual models evolved out of ideas representing two different assumptions. In the nursing theory course developed by Johnson in the 1960s, the idea that nursing conceptualizations were modeled after guiding paradigms (systems, adaptation, developmental, and symbolic interaction) was introduced. Other writings and analyses were based on the same premise of guiding paradigms. The second idea, that of models, was based on interpretive models and assumed that nursing is the reality and that each of the existing conceptualizations model that reality at different levels of isomorphism. Early designations of nursing thought correspond to the first idea, that conceptualizations are formally modeled after other conceptual schemata (Riehl and Roy, 1974), and later designations correspond to the second idea, that conceptualizations are based on interpretive models (Fawcett, 1989; Fitzpatrick and Whall, 1989).

Use of models also differs in another respect. In some usage, models correspond more to reality: they are less abstract than theories; they contain all variables of the subject matter; and they describe reality more fully. Theories describe fewer variables and are more abstract, but they also correspond more or less to reality (Kaplan 1964). Others considered models as simplified forms of reality. Chin (1961) defined model as "a constructed simplification of some part of reality that retains only those features regarded as essential for relating similar processes whenever and wherever they occur" (p. 201).

Conceptual models and theories have been used synonymously (Dickoff and James, 1968) or definitions for one were used for the other: a set of concepts that are interrelated into a coherent whole and a set of propositions. Johnson (1968a) viewed a model as an "invention of the mind for a purpose" that "is drawn from reality and pertains to reality, but it does not constitute reality" (p. 2). Both sets of definitions could be used to define one or the other, that is, conceptual framework or theory.

Further confusion has arisen because of other interchangeable terms. Conceptual frameworks have been used by some interchangeably with conceptual models and by others interchangeably with theory. Fawcett (1989), among others, dismissed the matter by equating conceptual framework with conceptual model and blamed the difference on semantics. Dickoff and James (1968) defined theory as a mental image being invented for the purpose of describing, relating, and predicting a desired situation. To them, theories are conceptual frameworks; they do not differentiate between the two.

Some attempts have been made to differentiate between theory and conceptual models on such criteria as level of abstraction, degree of explication, level of specificity, types of linkage, and degree to which concepts and assumptions are interdefined (Fawcett, 1989; Fitzpatrick and Whall, 1989; Klein and Hill, 1972, cited in Rodman, 1980). They argued that conceptual frameworks (or models, as they are used interchangeably) are more abstract than theories. They represent a global view of a field—its main concepts and propositions—and therefore provide the blueprint for practice, education, and research (Johnson, 1968a).

Whether or not conceptual frameworks are necessary steps in the process of developing theories has also been debated. Some contend that the conceptual framework is a stepping stone toward theory development (Hill and Hansen, 1960; Nye and Berardo, 1966), a view that has been adapted by some in nursing (Fawcett,

1989). Others question the necessity of conceptual frameworks for development of theory and argue that conceptual frameworks are not necessary steps, nor are they likely to promote or hinder theory development (Rodman, 1980).

The interchangeable use of the different concepts such as conceptual frameworks, models, and theories to describe the same thing has been a problem to the pure semanticists in the field. The attempt to differentiate between them has frequently taken on the dimension of splitting hairs and has only added to the confusion. It is just such confusion that may have contributed to the slow progress and, at times, stilted theory development in nursing and has led to an almost exclusive preoccupation with method and process rather than content and consequences. Instead of addressing the central issues of nursing, we have had to defend its methodology. Theorizing is a painstakingly long process. To minimize the work, to minimize the results by relegating them to the level of "it is only a conceptual framework," decreases the impact of such work and seems to make it not only less threatening but also less significant. The discipline, therefore, tends to be regarded as pretheoretical and, as a result, nursing's contribution is minimized.

There are other disadvantages to the preference of using conceptual frameworks and models when the use of theory would have been much clearer. One such disadvantage could be understood by examining analogous situations—one in which conceptual frameworks and models were used prior to the use of theory and one in which theories were been used from the outset.

Sociology, particularly family sociology, has been unique in believing that conceptual models are distinct from theories. Sociologists have maintained, and nursing scholars have begun to agree, that conceptual models provide a step in the development of theory. However, modern sociologists have since questioned the wisdom of using a conceptual framework to denote the results of theorizing. The skeptics in sociology have pointed out numerous examples in which conceptual frameworks have resulted in theorizing that lacked specification and definition and the slow process of developing propositions for testing (Rodman, 1980).

Physical and natural sciences, on the other hand, do not use conceptual frameworks and models as steps toward development of theory. Instead, they may use the term *developing theory* versus *tested theory*. Notice that many theories (genetic fat theory of obesity, cholesterol theory of cardiovascular diseases, psychoanalytical theory of neurosis) are at different levels of abstraction and different levels of sophistication and have different scopes, different levels of clarity, and varying degrees of understandable definitions; however, they are all called theories.

There are some differences between models, conceptual frameworks, and theory, to be sure. A model has to model another entity, while a theory may or may not model other properties, structures, or functions. Conceptual frameworks may present a set of discrete concepts that are not as interrelated and linked in sets of propositions as we expect from theory. However, this varies, based on the level of development of the theory. Models tend to evoke the idea of empirical positivism mixed with rationalism as a guiding philosophy or a goal, rather than the tool it ought to be. Functions attributed to models as frameworks or directives for the development of research, frameworks for the generation of a hypothesis, guides for data collection, or depositories for research findings or the further development of theory are the same functions attributed to theory.

It is not entirely clear that nursing theorists, in using different labels for their conceptualizations, have done so in any systematic way. For example, in a 1983 text, eight theorists used four different labels when referring to their conceptualizations: theory, model, science, and paradigm (Clements and Roberts, 1983). The similarities and the differences in degree of specificity, level of abstraction, and number of concepts and propositions are not consistent with the labels. One option for utilizing these conceptualizations is to attach the label preferred by the theorist; another option is to use whatever label the user prefers, as long as a definition and rationale are given. Some literature could always be found to document any of the uses.

The perspective of this text is to minimize the differences between conceptual models, frameworks, and theories and to relegate most of these differences to semantics and the confusion created by the many nursing scientists and theoreticians who have been educated in a multitude of fields. The rationale for taking this perspective is not to argue for a new position or to initiate a debate, but rather to cast some doubt on the significance of the differences between theories and conceptual models.

"Theory" is sufficient to describe the conceptualizations that have been proposed by our theorists. The three related aspects claimed to differentiate between theory and conceptual model are definitions, interrelationships, and level of abstraction. The first two, which state that concepts should be defined and interrelated, are considered in the present perspective as a necessity for both theory and conceptual models. The third aspect, level of abstraction, remains an important consideration. Because theories could be classified as grand, middle-range, or single-domain, based on the number of phenomena that the theory addresses, the number of propositions, and the operational level of the definitions, the present perspective proposes this schema to classify nursing theory rather than to relegate the classification system to such different labels as conceptual model, framework, metaparadigm, paradigm, and theory.

Although this perspective is proposed to enhance a common language across disciplines and to divert energy into development and progress in theoretical nursing rather than into circular debates, the final choice of a label is a personal matter and depends on the purpose for which the label is applied. Just as role theory has been proposed and used as a concept, a framework, a model, or a theory in research, practice, and administration in a number of disciplines, and just as the utilizer may consider role theory from a cultural, structural, or intra-actionist perspective, nursing theories could also be utilized in the same way. The manner and the goal of the utilization may help determine the appropriate label.

Based on the perspective proposed here, *nursing theory* is defined as an articulated and communicated conceptualization of invented or discovered reality pertaining to nursing for the purpose of describing, explaining, predicting, or prescribing nursing care. Nursing theory is developed to answer central domain questions.

Nursing Theory Versus Borrowed Theory

For some time now, nurses have been involved in a debate over the types of theory that ought to be developed. They took either practice or basic theory positions. Each side developed a good case as to why one or the other type is possible. The significance of taking one or the other position lies in the idea that the practice theory position encourages forging ahead with theory development and the borrowed theory position discourages nurses from participating in the seemingly futile attempt to develop theories.

The proponents and supporters of the development of practice theory in nursing (Dickoff, James, and Wiedenbach, 1968; Jacox, 1974; Johnson, 1968a; Wald and Leonard, 1964) view nursing theory as a conceptual framework that is invented by the theorist for the ultimate purpose of creating situations to meet desired, preferred end results. Therefore, the ultimate goal for theory development in nursing is to produce a change in a nursing client or a nursing situation that is desired by the nurse or the client. Dickoff and James (1968, p. 200) called this a situation-producing theory.

This is a fourth-level theory; theories at other levels are invented and articulated with the purpose of ultimately leading to this level. The first level is factor-isolating, a level where theories help delineate and describe a phenomenon. The second level is a correlating theory, where factors or concepts are related to depict theories, and the third level is a situation where theories permit prediction and allow promotion or inhibition of nursing care. Each of these levels brings the theorist closer to the goals of nursing that are demonstrated in prescriptive theories, or by the situation-producing level of theory, the fourth level. The development of fourth-level theory is congruent with the purpose of the profession, which ought to be action-oriented as opposed to only academically oriented. Nurses are shapers, not just observers, of reality.

The first-level theory, the factor-isolating theory, is one that helps to articulate and label concepts. The significance of this kind of theory is to enable one to refer back to those concepts that are invented. Without a label we have no concepts; without concepts we have no relationships. Labeling allows for the creation of conceptual entities that become the cornerstones for each subsequent theory level. What Dickoff and James helped nurses to see was the significance of this level of theory, in which they had been engaged long before they began to speak of theory development.

Norris (1975), a "curious nurse clinician," observed numerous incidents of restlessness and noted that, although the term was frequently used in charting, it was not clear how restlessness was identified, when it was identified, why it occurred, and what its consequences were. More important, it was not clear what the nursing intervention should be. Norris' descriptive labeling work is an excellent example of first-level theory according to Dickoff and James (1968). Other examples are Norbeck's (1981) social support study, Norris' (1982) classification of 15 concepts related to basic physiological protection mechanisms, and my own (Meleis, 1975) work on role supplementation and role insufficiency.

Other nurses have proposed organizing nursing around concepts and, in so doing, have provided nursing with numerous identified and labeled concepts (Carlson, 1970; Meltzer, Abdellah, and Kitchell, 1969; Mitchell, 1973). Still others researched labeled concepts in search of validity and reliability (Kim, 1980; Norbeck, 1981; Weiss, 1979). All these are considered first-level theories, an end in their own right, and a beginning of other theory levels when considering Dickoff, James, and Wiedenbach's definitions (1968).

Once concepts are delineated and labeled, a theorist is ready to develop relationships. Correlating theories result from theorists inventing relationships between labeled concepts. These theories are second-level, factor-relating theories. Relating preoperative teaching to postoperative behavior, restless and muscular tension under different conditions, social support and health, or role insufficiency and role supplementation could result in a factor-relating theory.

To predict postoperative behavior by varying preoperative teaching is an instance of third-level, predictive theory. Third-level theory depicts and predicts with a time reference. It is not only relational—as is second-level theory—it is causal, as the theorist discovers that certain conditions lead to others. In fact, all three levels incorporate a discovery of reality but not an invention of reality. None of these three levels purports to change or influence reality. Rather, all lead to the development of the most powerful of theories for a professional practice discipline, the situation-producing theory, which is a fourth-level theory.

One of the significant differences between third- and fourth-level theories is in commitment to a goal. A predictive theory describes what happens, such as postoperative behavior with different strategies of preoperative teaching. In a fourth-level theory, there is a commitment to finding out how it happened. An example could be that certain postoperative behavior is conceived as appropriate behavior to bring about. The theory then proceeds to describe what to do preoperatively to bring about that desired behavior. This level of theory, therefore, has several essential components: (1) an aim or goal specified by the theorist as desirable; (2) a prescription to bring about the desired aim; and (3) a "survey list" to use in future prescriptions.

The survey list is designed to respond to six crucial questions for prescriptive theory:

1. Who or what performs the activity? (Agency)
2. Who or what is the recipient of the activity? (Patiency)
3. In what context is the activity performed? (Framework)
4. What is the end-point of the activity? (Terminus)
5. What is the guiding procedure, technique, or protocol of the activity? (Procedure)
6. What is the energy source for the activity? (Dynamics) (Dickoff, James, and Wiedenbach, 1968, p. 422)

The activities in a prescriptive theory expected to correspond to these questions are agency, patiency, framework, terminus, procedure, and dynamics. Each incorporates internal and external resources as well as the potential for using theories from other disciplines if deemed useful.

All survey questions are asked from the point of view of the goal of the activity and take the prescription into consideration. It is assumed, and practice supports such assumption, that the agent who is expected to perform the prescription does not always hold full jurisdiction over the prescription. A combination of internal resources, such as certain skills, experiences, and techniques, and external resources, such as policies and environment, specifies the agent. In some instances, prescription may be delegated; in others, it may be relegated. A fourth-level theory should include the kinds of agents who are expected to perform the prescription to bring about the desired end result. The authors (Dickoff, James, and Wiedenbach, 1968) proposed a broad concept of *agency* to include all those who have the internal and external resources, and a similar one about patiency. Nurses, physicians, family members, visitors, and so on may be agents performing nursing activities toward nursing goals. Therefore, a theory should specify all possible agents.

Patiency specifies the recipients of the prescriptions with whom agency interfaces for the purpose of bringing about the desired goal. Patiency may designate sick or well people, interacting or noninteracting things or people, animate or inanimate objects, recipients of activities done by registered nurses, and activities done by people other than nurses, but all are bound together by the goal of the activity. Patients are "interactors" with agency and others geared toward the "activity of a desired kind and as possessed of a repertoire of capacities and limitations (much as is the agent) to see a great range of latitude as to ways of producing desired outcomes" (Dickoff, James, and Wiedenbach, 1968).

The agent and the patient in a theory have to be specific in terms of the context within which both occur. The context, called the *framework* by Dickoff and colleagues, requires that the situation-producing theory specify all variables that should be taken into account to bring about the desired goals through an activity produced by an agent and received by a patient. The end product of the activity is the *terminus*, the situation to be produced.

A situation-producing theory also includes the pattern by which the activity is performed. *Procedure* includes the steps to be taken to bring about the desired goal. Procedure, then, includes the arena, the equipment, the type of charting, the type of follow-up, policies to govern it, timing, and the rules-of-thumb governing activity. Although procedures could be detailed, most often they are guidelines and safeguards.

Finally, a nursing theory of the situation-producing type should consider the aesthetic satisfaction of performing the activity and the desire for self-esteem. These are motivating factors in performing and sustaining activities to realize a nursing goal. The more developed the theory, the more likely these two factors are considered. These factors are grouped under what Dickoff and colleagues called the *dynamics* of the theory. When the dynamics are conceptualized adequately, all factors that relate to the agent, such as education, reputation of institution, and rewards, or to patients, such as insurance, will have to be considered in a situation-producing theory.

To understand, explain, predict, and prescribe nursing phenomena and nursing care, nurses should develop practice theories that emanate from the discipline and guide the discipline's actions. There is one significant feature of theory in a practice discipline. Although descriptive, relating, and predictive theories are equally important, nursing practice theory needs to strive for prescriptive theory. Nurses may develop basic theories that describe discovered concepts, relationships related to human beings, nursing situations, nurse–patient interactions, environments, or health; but the ultimate goal is to develop theories to change situations. Therefore, theories that stress change as their goal are practice theories.

Discovery charts a more probable process for the development of basic theories; invention, on the other hand, is a more probable goal of practice theory. Properties or dimensions of transitions, for example, lend themselves to basic theory that describes and explains when transitions are healthy, under what circumstances transitions in health and illness occur, what the consequences of various types and levels of transitions are, and why the variability of consequences exists. What to do to enhance smooth transitions for nursing clients, how to maintain the person–environment harmony in transition, and how to maintain homeostasis and enhance adjustment are questions that lend themselves to practice theories.

Even when theories developed in other disciplines are used to explicate nursing phenomena and nursing problems, the new derivations and new syntheses make them nursing theories. The concept "nursing" does not denote who developed it or where it is used; rather, it reflects the phenomenon that the theory addresses. Nursing theories evolve out of the practice arena or anything that pertains to the practice arena. They are then tested in research. Until the time-consuming job of research is accomplished, face validity of a theory as it pertains to practice should be enough to allow the theory to be one of the blueprints for action.

There are some who challenge the notion that nursing should develop its theoretical base. Their arguments are based on the premise that nursing is a practice discipline and that practice disciplines depend on other disciplines for their theoretical underpinnings. Beckstrand (1978a, 1978b, 1980), for example, takes issue with the contention that nursing is concerned with practice theory. For practice theory to be meaningful, practice knowledge should be different from scientific and ethical knowledge. Beckstrand then examined two aspects of practice knowledge, the knowledge of how to control and how to make changes and the knowledge of what is morally good. She examined these aspects with the question in mind of whether it is possible for practice theory to exist as distinct from science and ethics. The first part of the question needs knowledge of science and the second needs knowledge of what is morally good.

Science, to Beckstrand, seeks to develop the knowledge necessary to change and control. This knowledge, containing law-like relationships, is synonymous with scientific knowledge. Controls are possible in practice situations; however, practice methodology proceeds by valid deductions from scientific laws. Beckstrand then proceeded to show that the field of philosophy known as ethics provides the other body of knowledge that is necessary for practice but that substitutes for practice theory. Both normative ethics and metaethics have relevance to practice, and we can easily borrow and co-opt theories to explain moral obligations and moral values in the discipline. The method of obtaining such knowledge and using it is that of logical reasoning, also a borrowed concept. Nursing utilizes scientific knowledge and logic to meet its ethical goals—all that constitutes the knowledge base of nursing. So, in essence, there is no need for practice theory (Beckstrand, 1978a, 1978b).

Others who agree that nursing does not need its own theory make a case for borrowed theories to describe, explain, and predict phenomena significant to nursing. Family theory, systems theory, and psychological theory are examples of theories that could be borrowed. Johnson, who was the first to use the concept of borrowing (1968a, 1974), defined borrowed theory as "that knowledge which is developed in the main by other disciplines and is drawn upon by nursing" and defined unique theory as "that knowledge derived from the observation of phenomena and the asking of questions unlike those which characterize other disciplines" (Johnson, 1968b, p. 3). However, she warns that any attempts at differentiation are

> hazardous, first of all because the man-made, more or less arbitrary, divisions between the sciences are neither firm nor constant. It appears there is a special unity in knowledge, corresponding to a unity in nature, which defies established boundaries and continuously presses for the larger, more cohesive view. Moreover, knowledge does not innately "belong" to any field of science. It is not exactly happenstance that a given bit of knowledge is discovered by one discipline rather than another, but the fact of discovery does not confer the right of ownership. Viewed in this light, borrowed and unique have no real permanence, or any meaning. (Johnson, 1968b, p. 206)

Johnson, however, differentiated between them in order to make a case for the development of a unique theory of nursing that addresses knowledge of order, disorder, and control and that focuses on phenomena and research questions in a way that is not characteristic of any other discipline (1968a).

Some may agree that applied theory could evolve out of these borrowed theories to describe and explain prediction and prescribe nursing action. These critics make a distinction between basic theory, emanating from other disciplines, and applied theory, based on basic theory, with the exclusive purpose of defining nursing care and patterning interventions with predictable responses. The latter continues to be called borrowed theory by some, which could be considered a fallacy because if we begin with the premise that knowledge is not the exclusive property of any one field and that, eventually, knowledge is for all, "knowledge which we share in common" (Johnson, 1959, p. 199), then knowledge organized into theories in one discipline could freely be used by members of other disciplines. Therefore "borrowing" is really "adapting" or "deriving." Even if we agree that there is such a thing as the borrowing of theories to help in describing, explaining, and predicting phenomena that are significant to nursing, the mere fact that the questions and problems under consideration are nursing questions and problems changes the nature of the so-called borrowed theories. Johnson (1968b) made the point in this way:

> If we continue to observe behavior from the perspective of sociology, anthropology, or psychology; or if we continue to study disease with the aim of elucidating etiologies, properties, or life cycle; or if we continue to inquire into biological functioning or malfunctioning, we will be serving the cause of science but not necessarily the cause of nursing. (p. 209)

Therefore, the nursing perspective guides the reconceptualization of existing theories (Donaldson and Crowley, 1978). Synthesis of so-called borrowed theory with a nursing perspective is essential or the focus of nursing will continue to remain within other disciplines, and, therefore, nursing problems will not be addressed (Phillips, 1977). Barnum (1990) supported this position. She stated that theories from other disciplines must be adapted to the nursing milieu and to the nursing image of a human being to be meaningful for nursing.

The so-called borrowed theories, then, are given new meaning within a perspective appropriate for nursing. Stevens supported Johnson's stand and called knowledge used in different disciplines "shared"; perhaps we should also have shared theories. To say that nursing theories are applied theories based on basic theories borrowed from other disciplines is therefore a myth that only serves to further obfuscate nursing theory. Nursing uses "borrowed theories" originating in other disciplines to describe phenomena belonging to those disciplines, when propositions remain in the context of the borrowed theory. Borrowed theories become "shared theories" when used within a nursing context. Nursing theories describe, explain, and predict domain phenomena.

Nursing needs theories to describe and explain phenomena that are significant in the act and process of nursing, to prescribe effective strategies of care, and to predict outcomes. Theories that were developed in other disciplines are also useful for derivation, integration, and synthesis with the nursing perspective. This process yields nursing theories or theories for nursing practice.

RESOURCES

The sources for theory development are only one essential component in the development of theory. Resources are the second major component. Resources for the theoretical development of the discipline are the nurses themselves and the environment that could nurture and support such development. Each resource will be discussed here.

Being Theoretical

Theoretical thinking, theoretical approaches to viewing situations, and the development of a theoretical identity are essential in engaging in the theoretical development of the discipline. There are myths that surround theory development. Some of these are related to who could and should develop theories. One of these myths is that "idea people" are "ivory-tower types of individuals," that only extremely intelligent people can develop theories. Another myth is that there are theoreticians and there are practitioners; the former cannot practice and the latter cannot theorize.

These myths have greatly influenced the process of conceptualizing in nursing. The intent of this chapter is to demonstrate that, even if the myths had been true at one time, perpetuating them at this time does not promote the discipline of nursing or, more importantly, patient care.

There are no theories without ideas, but there are ideas without theories. Theories evolve from ideas and ideas evolve from hunches, personal experiences, insights, inspirations, intuition, and other's work and experiences. New ideas could be based on the discovery of a new phenomenon, the invention of a new theoretical concept, reintegration of old concepts with new realities, a reformulation of an existing idea, or a new way of organizing old concepts. New ideas also may evolve from asking new questions or even from asking old questions but finding that the old answers no longer answer the questions. The context may have changed and therefore the answers may no longer be adequate.

Ideas are all around us; however, only some ideas develop into theories. Ten conditions may assist in the development of theories, and each of these conditions may be subjected to research investigations.

1. An idea is usually generated by one person, although others may help to nourish it, others may be triggered to follow through, or even two people on opposite sides of the globe may get the same idea simultaneously; however, for each one, the "aha" is a personal matter (Reynolds, 1971). Therefore, a creative person should have the capacity to be alone to develop inner resources (Arietti, 1976).
2. While developers of ideas are intelligent and are found to have high intellectual ability, they are not necessarily brilliant (Reynolds, 1971; Roe, 1951, 1963). They are considered creative and persistent, but not superhuman.
3. These people have an extra sense by which they can differentiate between a good and a bad idea; therefore, they do not spin their wheels on something that will not materialize or on an idea that has no potential for development (Reynolds, 1971).
4. These people have thorough knowledge of the field in which their idea may fit (Meleis and May, 1981). They know the accepted notions surrounding their ideas, and they have a sense of history and context; otherwise, they would not be able to tell whether their discovery, their invention, or their conceptualization is new or whether they have the context within which to place their ideas. "In short, they know when a good idea is a new idea" (Reynolds, 1971, p. 152).
5. They are individuals who are not particularly committed to all the ideas of the field or to those ideas that are held by the scholarly community. Therefore, they are open to new ideas and

are able to stand independent and apart from others (Roe, 1951, 1963). They stand alone to support their own convictions (Armiger, 1974).

6. They are in touch with the phenomenon in some way. They are either deeply engrossed in a clinical area, are committed to researching a particular phenomenon, are trying to synthesize some of the concepts in the field, or are involved in an in-depth study of a particular theory. "No matter what the endeavor, the individuals are deeply engrossed in the subject matter, so deeply that an intuitive or uncommunicable organization of new concepts and their relationships may develop a feeling that later takes form as a theory" (Reynolds, 1971, p. 153).

7. Developers of ideas are willing to take risks.

8. A person whose ideas go beyond the initial idea stage possesses a sense of persistence to work, self-discipline, and an ability for developing a sense of satisfaction that goes with the hard work (Arietti, 1976; Roe, 1951, 1963).

9. Ideas flourish and develop when a person is able to articulate and communicate them to others. Communication of ideas allows for a healthy debate and a healthy critique, both of which are essential for continuous clarification and refinement of ideas. Fear of "idea snatching" may have prevented some good ideas from being communicated and therefore may have kept them from the potential of further development.

10. Whether aware of it or not, a person with an idea that is potentially good has a good sense of intuition and, furthermore, accepts intuition as a significant asset in the development of ideas. To develop that sense a person needs periods of inactivity to daydream, to think freely with no specific structure, and also to be able to suspend judgment until ideas develop (Arietti, 1976). Finally, a person whose ideas go far is usually a person with a good sense of timing.

Nurses with these conditions, wherever they are and in whichever settings, are observing new phenomena, are articulating significant questions and, moreover, have developed their own personal theories about patient care. The difference is that they have not been aware of the significance or the timeliness of these phenomena, relationships, or hunches; or they simply have not discussed or communicated them, which would allow initial hunches to grow, flourish, and attain a systematic theoretical development. For example, the observations (or intuition, or both) of a nurse in a kidney dialysis unit who is consistently able to decide within a few minutes of interaction with patients who come in weekly for dialysis whether or not that patient's dialysis will be completed efficiently and effectively, with or without complication, lend support to the observation that there are indeed some things a nurse considers that help to predict outcomes. This nurse, then, is able to formulate questions about an important phenomenon and may be able to offer a conceptualization of an important aspect of patient care. Other conditions, such as communication or knowledge of the next steps, need to be provided by those in the clinical area who are able to supply these conditions, or provided through collaboration with others who are experienced in development of theories pertaining to practice.

Conditions for theory development, therefore, are: the presence of a cadre of individuals who are firm believers in the significance of theory for nursing practice and who possess the conditions outlined above; and the availability of a theoretically supportive environment.

Theoretically Supportive Environment

Even if a person has the ten characteristics listed previously, she may not be able to engage in the activities and processes inherent in theoretical reflection and development without an intellectually nurturing environment. An intellectually nurturing environment is one that values theoretical nursing, allows time to clarify values, time to articulate and relate ideas, and time to question. It is an environment that permits ambiguity, that does not press for immediate solutions, that allows dissension and does not press for consensus, and that permits philosophical discourse (Meleis and Jennings, 1989; Meleis and Price, 1988; Jennings and Meleis, 1988). What is needed is an environment that acknowledges theoretical abilities and rewards theoretical thinking.

Strategies to develop such environments could evolve from the nature of nursing to complement its natural activities. A team report, for example, could be the medium for questioning and reflecting on clinical phenomena. Members of an administrative team may devote some time for discussing a pressing problem theoretically and from different perspectives. Goals related to theoretical nursing are somewhat different from those related to immediate problem solving. Goals goal related to theoretical nursing are the development of a concept or the analysis of a theoretical perspective. Problem solving, however, focuses on resolving a problem. The point is that creating a supportive environment should not be analogous to creating an environment that is artificial or foreign to an institution; it should fit within an institution's mission and goals and within its daily experiences and functions.

REFERENCES

Abdellah, F.G., Beland, I.L., Martin, A., and Matheney, R.V. (1961) *Patient-centered approaches to nursing.* New York: Macmillan.

Allen, J. and Hall, B. (1988) Challenging the focus on technology: A critique of the medical model in a changing health care system. *Advances in Nursing Science*, 10, 22–34.

Arietti, S. (1976) *Creativity: The magic synthesis.* New York: Basic Books.

Armiger, B. (1974) Scholarship in nursing. *Nursing Outlook*, 22(3), 162–163.

Barnard, K. (1980) Knowledge for practice: Directions for the future. *Nursing Research*, 29(4), 208–212.

Barnum, B.J. (1990) *Nursing theory: Analysis, application, and evaluation* (3rd ed.). Boston: Little, Brown & Co.

Beckstrand, J. (1978a) The notion of a practice theory and the relationship of scientific and ethical knowledge to practice. *Research in Nursing and Health*, 1(3), 131–136.

Beckstrand, J. (1978b) The need for a practice theory as indicated by the knowledge used in conduct of practice. *Research in Nursing and Health*, 1(4), 175–179.

Beckstrand, J. (1980) A critique of several conceptions of practice theory in nursing. *Research in Nursing and Health*, 3(2), 69–80.

Benner, P. (1983) Uncovering the knowledge embedded in clinical practice. *Image*, 15, 36–44.

Byrne, M.L. and Thompson, L.F. (1978) *Key concepts for the study and practice of nursing*. St. Louis: C.V. Mosby.

Carlson, C.E. (Ed.). (1970) *Behavioral concepts and nursing intervention*. Philadelphia: J.B. Lippincott.

Carlson, C.E. and Blackwell, B. (Eds.) (1978) *Behavioral concepts and nursing intervention* (2nd ed.). Philadelphia: J.B. Lippincott.

Carper, B. (1978) Fundamental patterns of knowing in nursing. *Advances in Nursing Science*, 11, 13–23.

Chin, R. (1961) The utility of system models and developmental models for practitioners. In W. Bennis, K. Benne, and R. Chin (Eds.), *The planning of change*. New York: Holt, Rinehart & Winston.

Clements, I.W. and Roberts, F.B. (1983) *Family health: A theoretical approach to nursing care*. New York: John Wiley & Sons.

Copleston, F. (1963) *A history of philosophy* (Vol. 4) *Modern philosophy: Descartes to Leibniz*. Garden City, NY: Image Books.

Dickoff, J. and James, P. (1968) A theory of theories: A position paper. *Nursing Research*, 17(3), 197–203.

Dickoff, J., James, P., and Wiedenbach, E. (1968) Theory in practice discipline: Part 1. Practice oriented theory. *Nursing Research*, 17(5), 415–435.

Donaldson, S.K. and Crowley, D. (1978) The discipline of nursing. *Nursing Outlook*, 26(2), 113–120.

Durand, M. and Prince, R. (1966) Nursing diagnostics: Process and decision. *Nursing Forum*, 5(4), 50–64.

Durant, W. (1953) *The story of philosophy: The lives and opinions of the greater philosophers*. New York: Simon & Schuster.

Fawcett, J. (1989) *Analysis and evaluation of conceptual models of nursing* (2nd ed.). Philadelphia: F.A. Davis.

Fitzpatrick, J. and Whall, A. (1989) *Conceptual models of nursing: Analysis and application* (2nd ed.). Bowie, MD: Robert J. Brady Company.

Gebbie, K. (Ed.) (1976, March 4–7) *Summary of the second national conference: Classification of nursing diagnosis*. St. Louis: C.V. Mosby.

Gordon, M. (1985) Nursing diagnosis. *Annual Review of Nursing Research*, 3, 127–147.

Gordon, M., Sweeny, M.A., and McKeehan, K. (1980) Nursing diagnosis: Looking at its use in the clinical area. *American Journal of Nursing*, 80, 672–674.

Gortner, S.R. and Nahm, H. (1977) An overview of nursing research in the United States. *Nursing Research*, 26(1), 10–33.

Harms, M. and McDonald, F.J. (1966) A new curriculum design: Part III. *Nursing Outlook*, 14(9), 50–53.

Hill, R. and Hansen, D.A. (1960) The identification of conceptual frameworks utilized in family study. *Marriage and Family Living* 22, 299–311.

Jacox, A. (1974) Theory construction in nursing: An overview. *Nursing Research*, 23(1), 4–13.

Jennings, B. and Meleis, A.I. (1988) Nursing theory and administrative practice: Agenda for the 1990s. *Advanced Nursing Science*, 10(3), 56–69.

Johnson, D.E. (1959) A philosophy of nursing. *Nursing Outlook* 7(4), 198–200.

Johnson, D.E. (1968a, April) One conceptual model of nursing. Paper presented at Vanderbilt University, Nashville, TN.

Johnson, D.E. (1968b, May/June) Theory in nursing: Borrowed and unique. *Nursing Research* 17(3), 206–209.

Johnson, D.E. (1974) Development of theory: A requisite for nursing as a primary health profession. *Nursing Research*, 23(5), 372–377.

Johnson, J.E. (1972, November/December) Effects of structuring patients' expectations on their reactions to threatening events. *Nursing Research*, 21(6), 499–504.

Kaplan, A. (1964) *The conduct of inquiry: Methodology of behavioral science.* San Francisco: Chandler.

Kerlinger, F.N. (1964) *Foundations of behavioral research.* New York: Holt, Rinehart & Winston.

Kim, H.S. (1980) Pain theory: Research and nursing practice. *Advances in Nursing Science* 2, 43–59.

Kim, M.J. (1989) Nursing diagnosis. *Annual Review of Nursing Research*, 7, 117–142.

Kim, M.J. and Moritz, D.A. (Eds.) (1982) *Classification of nursing diagnosis: Proceedings of the third and fourth national conferences.* New York: McGraw-Hill.

Kintzel, K.C. (1971) *Advanced concepts in clinical nursing.* Philadelphia, J.B. Lippincott.

Kritek, P. (1978) The generation and classification of nursing diagnosis: Toward a theory of nursing. *Image*, 10(2), 33–40.

Lindeman, C.A. (1980) The challenge of nursing research in the 1980s. In *Communicating nursing research: Directions for the 1980s.* Boulder, CO: Western Interstate Commission for Higher Education.

Maier, H.W. (1969) *Three theories of child development.* New York: Harper & Row.

Meleis, A.I. (1975) Role insufficiency and role supplementation: A conceptual framework. *Nursing Research*, 24(4), 264–271.

Meleis, A.I. (1985) *Theoretical nursing: Development and process.* Philadelphia: Lippincott.

Meleis, A.I. and Jennings, B.M. (1989) Theoretical nursing administration: Today's challenges, tomorrow's bridges. In H.C. Arndt and M. DiVincenti (Eds.), *Dimensions and issues in nursing administration.* Oxford, UK: Blackwell Scientific Publications.

Meleis, A.I. and May, K.M. (1981) Nursing theory and scholarliness in the doctoral program. *Advances in Nursing Science*, 4(1), 31–41.

Meleis, A.I. and Price, M. (1988) Strategies and conditions for teaching theoretical nursing: An international perspective. *Journal of Advanced Nursing*, 13, 592–604.

Meltzer, L.E., Abdellah, F.G., and Kitchell, R. (Eds.) (1969) *Concepts and practice of intensive care for nurse specialists.* Philadelphia: Charles Press Publishers.

Mitchell, P.H. (1973) *Concepts basic to nursing.* New York: McGraw-Hill.

Nidditch, P. (Ed.) (1975) *An essay concerning human understanding.* New York: Oxford University Press.

Nightingale, F. (1859) *Notes on nursing: What it is and what it is not.* London: Harrison.

Norbeck, J. (1981) Social support: A model for clinical research and application. *Advances in Nursing Science*, 3, 43–59.

Norris, C.M. (1975) Restlessness: A nursing phenomenon in search of meaning. *Nursing Outlook*, 23(2), 103–107.

Norris, C.M. (Ed.) (1982) *Concept clarification in nursing.* Germantown, MD: Aspen Systems.

Nye, F. and Berardo, F. (Eds.) (1966) *Emerging conceptual frameworks in family analysis.* New York: Macmillan.

Peplau, H.E. (1952) *Interpersonal relations in nursing.* New York: G.P. Putnam's Sons.

Phillips, J.R. (1977) Nursing systems and nursing models. *Image*, 9(1), 4–7.

Riehl, J.P. and Roy, C. (Eds.) (1974) *Conceptual models for nursing practice.* New York: Appleton-Century-Crofts.

Reynolds, P.D. (1971) *Primer in theory construction.* Indianapolis: Bobbs-Merrill Company.

Rodman, H. (1980) Are conceptual frameworks necessary for theory building: The case of family sociology. *The Sociological Quarterly*, 21, 429–441.

Roe, A. (1951) A psychological study of eminent biologists. *Psychological Monographs*, 65, 1–67.

Roe, A. (1963) *The making of a scientist.* New York: Dodd Mead.

Shamansky, S.L. and Yanni, C.R. (1983) In opposition to nursing diagnosis: A minority opinion. *Image*, 15, 47–50.

Wald, F.S. and Leonard, R.C. (1964, Fall) Towards development of nursing practice theory. *Nursing Research*, 13(4), 309–313.

Weiss, S.J. (1979, March/April) The language of touch. *Nursing Research*, 28(2), 76–80.

Zderad, L.T. and Belcher, H.C. (1968) *Developing behavioral concepts in nursing.* Atlanta, GA: Southern Regional Education Board.

Chapter *10*

Strategies for Theory Development

The aim of nursing science is to develop explanatory and prescriptive theories to understand, anticipate, and control phenomena, events, and situations related directly or indirectly to nursing care. The explanatory and prescriptive theories are based on descriptions of patterns and responses of human beings and environments, or on relationships between human beings and environments within a context of time, environment (societal obligations), and human conditions (including human rights). This aim is congruent with the aims of other sciences that are focused on human beings and their lives (Schensul, 1985).

Thus, the nature of nursing science requires a close relationship between theory, practice, and research. The domain of nursing provides the medium for that connection. Theoreticians, clinicians, and researchers in nursing share the ultimate goal of understanding health care needs of clients and communities who are parts of environments, in enhancing a sense of well-being, in promoting health status, in increasing access and options of health care for clients and communities.

Despite this apparent connection, the recent history of the discipline demonstrates that there has been some tension between theorists, clinicians, and researchers. This tension has been caused by myths and confusion about each others' specialty. Theorists are only "ivory-tower" philosophers who dream up ideas unconnected with practice or research, according to researchers. Researchers, the theorists counter, focus on those small research projects using a more foreign positivist approach to confirm or not confirm disconnected propositions that do not add up to theory. Researchers and theorists are too far removed from clinical practice, say the clinicians. How could they presume that they can describe, explain, or predict outcomes of clinical practice when they have not seen a client for years?

There are some truths in all these positions, but none represents any of the truths in their entirety. The theorists have provided the discipline with a coherent vision of the core of its domain: human beings in constant interaction with their environment. The goals of self-care, adaptation, homeostatis, expanded consciousness, balance, and harmony with environments were articulated by theorists. They proposed concepts that have become the cornerstones of the discipline and about which there has been more agreement than was anticipated in the 1970s. The researchers, on the other hand, have developed instruments for some central concepts, such as wound healing, levels of confusion, social support, and symptom distress. The researchers have tested some theoretical propositions related to clinical practice, such as the determinants of maternal role development, or the determinants of recovery in cardiovascular patients. Clinicians have used theory as the bases for their actions, even when they were not able to articulate what theories they use and under which circumstances.

In the 1980s, there were attempts to complete the practice–theory–research cycle. Mercer, for example, systematically worked on identifying responses to mothering in adult women, in adolescent women, and in women undergoing caesarean and vaginal deliveries (Mercer, 1984; Mercer, Ferketich, May, and de Joseph, 1987; Mercer, Ferketich, May, de Joseph, and Sollid, 1987). Mercer identified clinical issues related to mothering, such as ways in which new mothers establish mothering role cues and timing in the development of these cues. Benoliel's work on psychosocial responses of patients to cancer is another example. Benoliel is a researcher who has engaged in studying clinically relevant questions that are embedded in a theoretical tradition and has developed theoretical propositions from her clinical and investigative work. She also provided guidelines to using her findings and theoretical guidelines in holistic caring for clients who have life-threatening diseases or who are bereaving from losses related to terminal illness (Benoliel and De Valde, 1975; Benoliel, 1977; Benoliel, Tornberg and McGrath, 1984). She bridged the gaps between education, research and practice by providing guidelines for educators for curricular development related to transitions and life-threatening diseases (Benoliel, 1982; Benoliel, 1983). These are only two examples that support the belief that progress in the discipline of nursing is predicated on actualizing the relationship between the scientific, theoretical, clinical, and educational bases.

One assumption that members of the discipline agree on is that disciplines develop through scientific discoveries, and scientific discoveries are useful when they are organized into some coherent wholes. These wholes could be theories or theoretical statements. Theories provide the frameworks that help in describing, explaining, predicting, and prescribing. Therefore, theory construction and development are activities that are essential in all disciplines. In fact, the progress of any discipline is measured by the scope and quality of its theories and the extent to which its community of scholars is engaged in theory development. Completing isolated research projects that are not cumulative or that do not lead to development or corroboration of theories has limited usefulness. Kuhn (1970) contends that disciplines that are in the preparadigmatic stage demonstrate a pattern of research equated with haphazard problem solving; the central questions of the field are not well-identified, and results of the minute research projects do not lead to the theoretical formulation that may explain phenomena, may predict events, situations, or responses, and may help in prescribing interventions.

Activities of theory development are not new to nurses, despite another existing myth that nurses began to learn how to develop theories only in the mid-1970s and early 1980s. Whether they were aware or it or not, clinical nurses have actively participated in conceptualizing aspects of the domain of nursing. These conceptualizations demonstrate attempts at theory development. The earliest such attempts are well-illustrated by Florence Nightingale, who, through the wisdom she gained from her work in the Crimean War, linked health with environmental factors, linked care with systematic data collection, and linked hygiene with well-being. Her efforts resulted in a clear conceptual schema of the client and the goals and the interventions in nursing. Her writings have components of theories that have been tested mainly by epidemiologists. Other aspects of her conceptualization, such as the focus of nursing on environment and health, have been further utilized and developed by other nursing theorists, such as Rogers.

Many more attempts at theory development followed Nightingale's. Some are reported in the literature, and many more may have gone unreported. Any time that concepts are delineated, hunches are developed by linking concepts together to help describe, explain, predict, or prescribe, and those hunches are communicated and used in a number of situations (the genesis of generalization), the beginnings of a theory are formulated. The developer of those hunches has been engaged in a process of theory development. In most instances, the process and product go unreported; therefore, the process is not complete and a theory does not formally develop. A theory is an articulation and communication of a mental image of a certain order that exists in the world, of the important components of that order, and of the way in which those components are connected. The mental image is an abstraction of order in reality as perceived by the theorist. It includes abstract concepts that then provide the potential of being generalized to a number of categorical events or situations. Most probably, then, the many unrecognized efforts in theory development go unrecognized because of a lack of communication and a limited ability to be generalized. But perhaps it was also because of lack of awareness of nurses of their potential to articulate aspects of the discipline theoretically or a reluctance to accept the potential for theorizing in a practice discipline.

The construction of theory in nursing preoccupied the theory literature from the early 1960s to the late 1970s. Metatheoretical writings during that time were focused on suggestions about how to formulate theories, types of theories, and sources for theories. There are several major features that have characterized writing in this area:

1. There was an assumption that processes of theory development were essential for the development of nursing science.
2. There was an assumption that the process of theory development was new to nursing and that nurses had not participated in such activity.
3. Most of the writing about theory development discussed what ought to happen and what strategies should be used. To my knowledge, there has been no analysis of the strategies that actually have been used.
4. There was a tendency to describe processes that were based on other sciences, mainly the physical and social sciences.

5. There was an implicit assumption that there should be one single strategy for theory development; this was particularly evident in the early writings in the field (Hardy, 1978; Jacox, 1974; Johnson, 1974; Newman, 1979). Although I doubt that any of these distinguished authors would have argued against a multiple route to theory development, their written work at that period of time appeared to erroneously give that impression.

6. There was an implicit assumption that theory development was an elitist activity to be engaged in only within the halls of academia. Furthermore, there was an explicit assumption by clinicians that what goes on within the halls of academia had no resemblance to the clinical work that goes on in real life. (Notice the many comments over the years about nursing theory and the lack of clinicians' need for such theory.)

7. There were those who believed that nursing had always borrowed its theory and that nursing was an applied field. To them, there was no need for nursing practice theory because theories from science and ethics were enough to guide nursing (Beckstrand, 1978a, 1978b). Therefore, theory development was a process that was not necessary. These people would have disagreed that the redevelopment, resynthesis, and reintegration of theories were also processes of theory development. Fortunately for nursing, others disagreed with them (Barnum, 1990; Walker and Avant, 1989).

The 1980s were characterized by multiplicity of strategies for theory development. For example, Walker and Avant (1989) proposed different beginning points for theorizing concepts, statements or theories, different approaches for derivation, synthesis, or development. The 1980s also were characterized by multiplicity of research approaches that would inevitably lead to different types of theories (Allen, Benner, and Diekelman, 1986). The development of concepts important to nursing and central to its domain was another significant feature of the decade. Examples these concepts are self-neglect (Reed and Leonard, 1989), environment (Stevens, 1989), dyspnea (Carrieri, 1984) cachexia (Lindsey, Piper and Stotts, 1982) and comfort (Arruda-Neve, Meleis, and Larson, in review).

There is agreement among those who have discussed theory development that the proper domain for theory development in nursing is nursing practice and situations or events related to responses or anticipated responses to health and illness. Current and future theoretical work will focus on further development of concepts emanating from the domain of nursing and its mission. Central domain concepts are environment, sense of well-being, interaction, coping with transitions, and nursing therapeutics, among others. Theory development may also occur in the functional areas of administration and teaching and learning.

A review and analysis of the literature of theory in nursing, including concept development, yields four major strategies of theory development. These are:

theory–practice–theory; practice–theory; research–theory; and theory–research–theory. A fifth strategy, practice–theory–research–theory, is recommended as an ought-to-be strategy, to be utilized by itself or in combination with any of the others. Each of the strategies is presented and discussed in this chapter.

THEORY–PRACTICE–THEORY STRATEGY

The theorist who utilizes this strategy begins the process of theorizing by selecting a theory to use in practice. This strategy is based on several premises:

○ There is an existing theory that can help in describing and explaining nursing phenomenon; however, the theory assumptions are not completely congruent with the assumptions that guide nursing.
○ The theory is not entirely useful in helping nurses meet their goals in nursing practice. The theory does not define phenomena in ways that are useful for the integrity of the nurse–practice–act definitions.
○ The theory does not directly help in defining actions for nurses. The focus of the theory is different from the focus needed for nursing practice.
○ The theory does not provide adequate definitions of the central concepts of nursing.
○ Concepts are essential in giving some order to situations and events.

One other important premise is that theories and concepts guide what we see. These concepts are results of early experiences, educational background, or theoretical bent. The interactionist theorists look at a nurse–patient situation and choose to focus on interaction, role-taking, symbols, and roles where the psychoanalytic theorist may see denial, repression, latent hostility, maternal or paternal conflict. Before we had a concept called "burnout," we did not see burnout, even though the syndrome undoubtedly existed. We did not have a label to give that constellation of behaviors; we did not have a reservoir in which we could connect and deposit those seemingly discrete feelings of apathy, demonstrations of irritability and impatience. Therefore, we did not articulate it as burnout. For example, there is no burnout described by people living in the Middle East; that is, there is no such concept even though the behaviors may exist and may have always existed. Undoubtedly, new circumstances develop for which observers then may articulate and label new concepts or redefine existing concepts.

This strategy for theory development speaks only to those circumstances in which we see the world through a well-established theory with delineated concepts. It is that theory then that guides actions and dictates how we see nursing and how we act in the world.

There are many examples in the nursing literature that demonstrate the use of this strategy in theory development. (See Table 10-1 for a summary of examples of theory–practice–theory.) Peplau's (1952) theory of interpersonal relations in nursing was based on psychoanalytical theory that she used as a framework to describe psychiatric nursing practice. Her theory of nursing reflects psychoanalytical concepts and her psychiatric nursing clinical expertise. Johnson's (1980) view of the client as consisting of subsystems of behavior and her theory about assessments and diagnoses of nursing problems as occurring due to imbalance, overload, or deprivation are based on biomedical and systems paradigms. Her background in pediatric care, her continuous interest in clinical nursing, and the paradigms guiding her nursing world resulted in her theory of nursing. Johnson's view of a client with subsystems of behavior is analogous to, but not equal to, the biomedical system. Her notion of homeostasis as a goal of nursing is parallel to Parsons' (1951) idea of homeostasis of social systems. The structure and function of Johnson's subsystems are modeled after the structure and function of Parson's social systems. The result is a theory of nursing that describes a nursing client, explains some of the actions of the client and the nurse and, perhaps, could in the future predict further action.

Some may say these are borrowed theories. Barnum (1990) disagreed. She stated that "borrowed theories remain borrowed as long as they are not adapted to the nursing milieu and the nursing image of man. Once such theories have been adapted to the nursing milieu, it is logical to refer to these boundary overlaps as shared knowledge rather than as borrowed theories" (p. 95). The strategy discussed here is based on the assumption that theory development in nursing is based on derivation of theories developed in other disciplines as well as on unique nursing knowledge. Dickoff and James (1968) contended that theories from biology, psychology, and sociology are "building blocks . . . in the mansion of nursing theory" (p. 202). A new meaning is given to the guiding theory or paradigm, a new meaning that is pertinent to nursing. Norbeck (1981), Mercer (1981), Millor (1981), and Meleis (1975) are all examples of authors who used a theory or viewed nursing through

Table 10–1
Examples of Theory–Practice–Theory: Clinical and Paradigmatic Origins of Selected Nursing Theories

Theory	Practice	Theory
Psychoanalytic theory	Psychiatry	Peplau
Systems theory	Pediatrics	Johnson
Adaptation theory	Pediatrics	Roy
Existentialist	Psychiatry Adult/Med Surg	Travelbee Paterson and Zderad
Biomedical systems	Med Surg	Orem Henderson Abdellah Maslow

another paradigm and developed a conceptualization of social support, maternal role attainment, child battering, and role supplementation, respectively, describing and explaining behaviors related to nursing care.

There are other modifications of this strategy, of which Roy and Roberts (1981) and Paterson and Zderad (1988) are examples. Roy viewed nursing from systems, adaptation, and interactionist paradigms. Her theory combines those paradigms with nursing practice and the result is the person as an adaptive system or with two internal control systems, the regulator and the cognator subsystems. The activities of these subsystems are demonstrated through four adaptive modes (effectors): the physiological mode, the self-concept mode, the role-function mode, and the interdependence mode. The development of the modes, particularly the self-concept, the role-function, and the interdependence modes, are derived from an interactionist sociological paradigm as exemplified by self-concept, role, and symbolic interactionist theories. Paterson and Zderad's (1988) uniqueness evolved out of using existentialist philosophy as the paradigm for the development of their nursing theory. There are several common processes in the development of theories through this strategy:

- ○ Knowledge of non-nursing theories and of a practice field;
- ○ Analysis of theory and practice area (analysis is a process by which the object of analysis is reduced into components and each component is defined and evaluated, theories are reduced to assumptions, concepts, and propositions, and practice is described through exemplars and case models);
- ○ Use of assumptions, concepts, and propositions of theory to describe the clinical area;
- ○ Redefinition of assumptions, concepts, and propositions to reflect the domain of nursing (redefining may also include modifications of some aspects of theory); and
- ○ Construction of theories involving development of explanation of exemplars representing the redefined assumptions, concepts, and propositions (assumptions, concepts, and propositions reflect a centrality in original theory).

An example of these processes is provided by considering Johnson's theory of behavioral subsystem. Johnson used Parson's concept of behavioral system, redefined it from a nursing perspective as "all patterned, repetitive and purposeful ways of behaving that characterize each man's life, are considered to comprise his behavioral system" (Johnson, 1980, p. 209). She then identified seven subsystems, labeled each, and discussed the relationship between each subsystem and the whole system. There are several characteristics of a theory that evolve from this strategy. The parent theory is well described and parallels the new practice-based theory. Concepts, attributes, properties, and descriptions are similar in both theories. The context for the evolving theory is differentiated from the context of the parent theory.

Table 10–2
The Clinical Theorist (Theory–Practice–Theory) and the Clinician
Who Uses Theory (Theory–Practice)

Theory–Practice–Theory	Theory–Practice
Goal	
Development; strategies for development	Application; strategies for application
Strategies	
Analyses; synthesis; comparison; refinement; extension; mental processes; reflection; creation	Analyses; description; interpretation; application
Uses	
Understand; know; develop	Understand; know
Evaluation	
Authenticity; congruency; context for discovery; context for justification; other criteria for evaluation of theory	Authenticity; congruency; context for justification
Person	
Clinical theorist	Clinician

Finally, it might be helpful to differentiate between the *clinical theorist* and the *clinician who uses theory*. The clinical theorist is the person whose goals include the refinement and development of theory. The clinician who uses theory has a goal of application of theory. The clinical theorist is engaged in practice and in the development or refinement of theory. She uses such processes as analyses, syntheses, comparisons, refinements, extensions, and reflections as well as other mental processes. She uses the process of theory development to understand, to know, or to further develop some coherent generalizations that go beyond the present situation. The clinician who uses theory uses mainly clinical strategies to apply theories for the purpose of understanding and knowing. The differences and similarities are presented in Table 10-2.

PRACTICE–THEORY STRATEGY

Conceptualizations that evolve from practice and that are based on experiences in the clinical field are developed using practice–theory strategy. There are several premises upon which this strategy is built:

1. Whatever theories that exist are not useful in describing the phenomenon of interest to the person. We may not know, for example, what is providing comfort to nursing clients, how comfort is defined, how it is achieved, who is expected to participate in providing it, what are the different ways in which it is manifested, and what is feasible and what is not feasible in comforting patients in various stages of health-illness. Answers to these questions could be articulated conceptually by clinical experts through descriptions of models of comforting acts derived from their practice.
2. The person is able to develop theories; there are resources to support the process of developing theories.
3. The phenomenon is significant enough to pursue, as developing knowledge about a phenomenon is a long process.
4. There may be clinical understanding and wisdom about the phenomenon, but that understanding has not been articulated into a meaningful whole.

The clinician begins the process of theory development with a nagging question that evolves from a practice situation. The insight is grounded in the practice situation, and the result has the potential for understanding other similar situations through the development of a set of propositions. The strategy depends on observations of new phenomena in a practice situation, development of sensitizing concepts, and labeling, describing, and articulating properties of these concepts. The properties are the subconcepts included in them, the boundaries, the definitions, the examples, the meaning, and so forth. Walker and Avant (1989) called this strategy *concept synthesis* and defined it as "a strategy for developing concepts based on observation or other forms of empirical evidence. . . . A concept synthesis is data based" (p. 51). This strategy involves labeling and linking concepts to form propositions.

The development of theory using this strategy is heavily based on the work of Glaser and Strauss (1967). While collecting data, the theorist keeps diaries, observes, analyzes similarities and differences, and develops concepts and then linkages. The grounded theory approach is credited to sociologists Schatzman and Strauss (1973) and Glaser and Strauss (1968), who have done a great deal to articulate the process and share its nuances, providing us with a multitude of examples to demonstrate its utility. It is a strategy not entirely foreign to nursing; the Yale School of Nursing developed a school of thought in theory development that is parallel to the work done by Glaser and Strauss.

Theories evolving from the Yale approach are those related to interpersonal relations and interactions in nursing, as viewed by Orlando, Travelbee, and Wiedenbach (see Chapter 14). These theorists developed their ideas by being totally immersed in clinical work, either giving care themselves or observing care being given. They used a variety of methods to collect their clinical data, such as case studies, interviews, and observations. It appears that they then isolated the central phenomenon of nursing related to the client's interaction with the nurse and those phenomena related to the development of nurse–patient relationships. Categories emerged, concepts were labeled, and beginning propositions were developed.

These were theories based upon and evolving from clinical practice, with the intention of describing and explaining extant nursing practice. One may presume that the theorists did not use any existing paradigm or theories. This may or may not be true. An equal presumption may be that these theorists had an interactionist background, prompting them to see nursing practice in one particular way. This strategy is most useful for clinicians, particularly when they deliberately begin to use the process to develop theories and articulate and communicate them. (Backscheider (1971) offers a useful example of this process.)

One of the most significant processes used by the pre-1980s theorists who demonstrated this strategy is their knowledge of their clinical areas. They had the resources to identify exemplars and to compare and contrast different exemplars. They may have used the same components defined and discussed in this chapter under the heading "practice–theory–research–theory strategy." However, without more information published about their strategies, it is not possible to use their work as an example of the modified practice–theory method.·

Theorists using this strategy in the late 1980s tended to describe the processes involved in theorizing. An example of this strategy is that provided by theorists who were interested in describing noncompliant behaviors. Clients who do not follow and "comply" with prescribed regimens have been labeled noncompliant or difficult. Neither concept adequately describes the roles of intention and environment in not adhering to a regimen. Reed and Leonard (1989) proposed the concept of *self-neglect*, which is defined as intentional neglect in spite of available resources. The authors described a clinical situation that prompted their conceptualization, reviewed existing theories, compared and contrasted self-neglect with other like concepts, such as suicide and noncompliance, and provided more clinical exemplars to refine the properties and attributes of the concept.

RESEARCH–THEORY STRATEGY

Theory development is considered exclusively as a product of research by empiricists, postempiricists, and postpositivists. Therefore, according to this perspective, the strategy *par excellence* is research–theory. Theorists who adhere to this strategy believe that theories evolve from confirmed or refuted research findings. Reynolds (1971) refers to this strategy in the construction of theories as the "Baconian approach." It is also most commonly known as the inductive method. Reynolds proposed four steps to this strategy.

1. Select a phenomenon that occurs frequently and list all the characteristics of the phenomenon.
2. Measure all the characteristics of the phenomenon in a variety of situations (as many as possible).
3. Analyze the resulting data carefully to determine if there are any systematic patterns among the data worthy of further attention.

4. Once significant patterns have been found in the data, formalization of these patterns as theoretical statements constitutes the laws of nature (axioms, in Bacon's terminology). (p. 140)

This method was, in the past, suggested as a favored approach to theory development in nursing by some. Theories here are referred to as scientific theories and are developed.

> Because isolated facts are of little interest to scientists, they try to put the knowledge of their respective fields together in such a way that the various events or phenomena with which they are concerned are systematically related to one another. A biologist, for example, wants to know not only about cells, species, and adaptation, but also how all of these are related to each other and to other biological phenomena. Scientific knowledge is systematically organized into "theories." The purpose of a scientific theory is to describe, explain, and predict a part of the empirical world. (Jacox, 1974, p. 4)

The strategy presupposes two significant conditions: that there is agreement in the field on the major concepts that should concern its community of researchers, and that each research concerns itself with a manageable number of variables with patterns that are easily detectable. Social science research could not guarantee these conditions (Reynolds, 1971); nursing is similar in some ways. Until the 1980s, there was very little agreement on the central questions in the field. Therefore, isolated research projects were launched to explore questions that were either tangentially related to the mission of nursing or the answers to which were central to other disciplines.

As nurses begin to agree that nursing deals with human beings who are in constant interaction with their environment, they also begin to appreciate all the complexities inherent in these phenomena. The boundaries of even the most operationalized variables in nursing are not as totally distinct as is usually expected from those who elect to use this strategy. In addition, although patterns could be and are being detected from findings, the feat is not an easy one. We are left with many completed, distinct research projects answering minute questions that are either not central to nursing or are not translatable to patterns that could eventually be connected to theory. Therefore, the steps and conditions of this strategy are not entirely congruent with the state of the art in nursing or with its focus on human responses.

The proponents of this strategy believe there is truth out there in real life that can be captured through the senses and can be verified or falsified. Repeated verification is an indication of truth and should prompt the development of scientific theories. Nurse researchers who have used this strategy in developing theories are Johnson (1972), Barnard (1973), Lindeman and Van Aernam (1973), and Johnson and Rice (1974).

Not all proponents of this method advocate sensory data as the basis of truth, and not all of them speak of validation and falsification. The grounded theorists have proposed another approach within this strategy that is based on discovery of concepts and identification of patterns, processes, and explanations. The design proposed by Glaser and Strauss (1968) is that of field study, in which not only theories evolve from research but the research question also evolves from the data gathered. The sole purpose of research, as proposed by this group of field researchers, is the development of theory. Numerous theories have been developed using the second approach, the grounded theorists' approach (Fagerhaugh, 1974; Stern, 1981). A similar approach was used by Smith (1981) in conceptualizing health as described through family modalities, including clinical, role-performance, adaptation, and eudaemonistic modes.

This research–theory method is best exemplified by Lindeman, who advocated the development of theory from research in her keynote address to the Western Society for Research in 1980. Lindeman used her own research to illustrate the research–theory process; it is used here as an exemplar of research–theory strategy for theory development.

The Research–Theory Method: Exemplar by a Researcher: Carole A. Lindeman (1980)*

The first study, designed to determine the value of preoperative teaching, led to the conclusion that structured preoperative teaching significantly improved the adult surgical patient's ability to cough and deep breathe postoperatively and also significantly reduced the mean length of hospital stay.

A second study was conducted to determine the most efficient way to implement a structured preoperative teaching program. That study, "The Effects of Group and Individual Preoperative Teaching," led me to conclude that group teaching was as effective and more efficient than individual teaching. These findings and those from the first study were consistent with educational research and theory. However, other results from that second study could not be explained by existing theory and continued to trouble me. Those results were:

1. Site of incision does interact in a significant way with teaching method. Subjects receiving group instruction and having "other" incisions had a shorter length of hospital stay than the same group receiving individual instruction. Ventilatory function scores were not different for the two groups. Interpretation required consideration of psychosocial factors in contrast to the physiological factors associated with the stir-up regime.
2. Age, per se, does not alter postoperative ventilatory function when preoperative teaching and practice are provided. Mean postoperative values on ventilatory function tests were not significantly different for subjects in the various age ranges. In fact, older subjects having major procedures did significantly better than their younger counterparts.

---

* Quoted by permission from the author and publisher. Lindeman, C.A. (1980) The challenge of nursing research in the 1980s. In *Communicating nursing research: Direction for the 1980s*. Boulder, CO: Western Interstate Commission for Higher Education.

3. Smoking history, per se, does not affect postoperative ventilatory function, length of hospital stay, or number of analgesics administered when preoperative teaching and practice are provided. There were no significant differences between smokers and nonsmokers.

According to the medical literature, these were factors associated with high risk groups. However, when these so-called "high risk" patients received structured preoperative teaching, their postoperative ventilatory function measures were comparable to other patients. The conceptual/theoretical framework for the research did not explain these results. I was left with a big unanswered "Why?"

Before pursuing those unanswered questions, I conducted a third study dealing with the effects of preoperative visits by operating room nurses. Although a large array of dependent variables were included, the data led to the conclusions that the preoperative visit was useful to the operating room nursing personnel for creating a safe, effective, and efficient intraoperative experience, but it did not produce measurable health status benefits for the patient. Coming from an educational psychology framework, I focused on the content of the teaching encounter as a way to explain why the one intervention, structured preoperative teaching, produced measurable benefits and the second intervention, preoperative interview, did not. I concluded that patients could learn and recall psychomotor behaviors taught in the preoperative period, but material that only served a cognitive structuring process, if learned, would not be retained.

However, I was then involved in a fourth study that refuted my interpretation and led me to propose a different set of theoretical statements. The fourth study was a descriptive study of significant nursing interventions in the preoperative and intraoperative periods and postoperative welfare. The study used Donabedian's structure, process, and outcome framework; however, due to observations made in our pilot study, we added patient baseline data to the overall framework. Much to my surprise, the data showed that patient baseline and organizational data were more strongly correlated with patient welfare than were specific nursing interventions.

I continued to mull over the conclusions from these various studies in an attempt to bring order to the data. Although each study by itself had been useful in making decisions about nursing practice, it seemed that they would be more useful if the results—the expected and the unexpected—could be tied together in some meaningful way in the form of nursing practice theory.

It is difficult, if not impossible, to describe one's thought processes as data and concepts are analyzed. Let it suffice to say that I continued to focus on three concerns:

1. A nursing intervention relating to skill development had a significant impact; a nursing intervention involving cognitive structuring did not.
2. Interactions between the patient and the intervention were not totally predictable and, in fact, were quite surprising.
3. Interactions between the institution and the intervention were not totally predictable.

Emerging from these data, from observations made during the research, and from my further analysis was the conclusion that patient welfare is [affected] by three major sets of variables: organizational, content of care, and patient characteristics. It also seemed clear to me that the critical variable is the patient, with nursing care only effective to the extent that it facilitates the patients' management of their own care.

Having identified the major concepts, the next step in this inductive process involves formulation and validation of relational statements.

The following statements have validity in terms of the research cited earlier:

1. The recipient of health care is the single most important variable in determining actual health status.
2. Those organizations having a potential for enhancing self-health-care management are most likely to have a positive influence on actual health status.
3. Those interventions having a potential for enhancing self-health-care management are most likely to have a positive influence on actual health status.
4. Characteristics of the care-giver as a person are not significant in determining actual health status.
5. The presurgical nursing interventions designed to enhance the self-health-care management abilities of the patient will influence postoperative health status.

Within this inductive process, I am now at the point of theory construction. To complete this step of the process I have had to reconsider the nature or definition of nursing. Without this broader perspective, any theory would exist in limbo. Its ability to predict and its test in reality would remain unknown. Again, for my own efforts, I have conceptualized nursing as a profession that exists because society has needs for health care. These needs generate from three factors: environmental and social factors, disease factors, and health factors. Those health issues or needs that arise because of the interaction of these three factors are the primary focus of nursing. Included are such issues as child abuse, maternal attachment, teenage suicide, the chronically ill, and so forth. Nursing may also assist other professionals by coordinating or implementing components of their plan of care. The social workers, nutritionists, physicians, psychologists, and others all have a role in dealing with issues generating from one or more of these three factors. I personally believe that nursing does have a unique and independent practice role, and it is defined in terms of the point of interplay of these factors.

Now, back to theory development. My next step is to analyze already completed research in terms of the five relational statements presented earlier. I need to consider patients other than presurgical. I need to explore settings other than acute care. I need to explore further interventions—those that relate to health maintenance more than disease prevention. I need to re-examine my major construct, "self-health-care management," in terms of the label—does it truly and clearly communicate the nature of the variable? Is it really the variable producing the observable effects? Only when a review of this nature is completed will I be ready to construct a formal theory that can then be tested, modified, and expanded by other researchers and scholars.

THEORY–RESEARCH–THEORY STRATEGY

The difference between this strategy and research–theory strategy lies in the use or nonuse of theory as a guiding framework for the research questions. Theorists who begin the research by defining a theory and determining propositions for testing and then go steps further to modify and develop the original theories are considered utilizers of this strategy. Although many researchers use processes that are similar to the ones that theorists may use, there are some significant differences between researchers and theorists utilizing this strategy. The researcher using theories aims at testing, confirming, refuting, or replicating theories. She uses theory as a framework for operational definitions for variables and statements, and she uses mental processes, problem solving, and interpretive processes to describe findings. The theorist who uses research as a means for the development of theory ends investigation with a refined, modified, or further developed coherent theoretical explanation of theory. The impact on the discipline is different and is needed for different purposes. The theorist researcher's findings are specific to selected phenomena and selected findings while the theorist's impact may be through integrated theoretical statements that explain and predict a wider range of phenomena (Table 10-3).

The processes used for theory–research–theory are:

1. A theory is selected that is compatible with the domain of nursing to explain the phenomenon of interest.
2. Concepts of the theory are redefined and operationalized for the research.
3. Findings are synthesized and used to modify, refine, or develop the original theory.
4. In some instances, the result may be a new theory.

PRACTICE–THEORY–RESEARCH– THEORY STRATEGY

Nursing practice is one of the most significant and neglected sources for theory development. Theorists who use this strategy assume the significance of the relationship between practice, theory, and research, and assume that there is a role that each plays in the development of nursing theory. The theorist also assumes, implicitly or explicitly, that viewing clinical situations is done with the cumulative wisdom of previous clinical situations as well as with whatever theories or frameworks the individuals may have in their repertoires. The person, theorist, clinician, or researcher in a human science is also an integral part of these experiences. Even when an attempt at distancing between the nursing theorist and client is premeditated and carefully implemented and guarded, the infiltration of previous experiences or theories in shaping the clinical situation is inevitable. These previous experiences are part of a nursing perspective. All these factors are the context that shapes what we see, how we see it, and how we analyze it.

Table 10–3
Differences between Theory–Research–Theory Strategy and
Theory–Research Strategy

Theory–Research–Theory	Theory–Research
Goal	
Test, refine, develop theory; openness to options for further developments	Test, accept, refute, replicate; aim to conclude
Uses	
A framework for research and for modification of theory; define concepts for future use; generate new propositions; explain, define questions	A framework for research; define variables and questions; prove/disprove
Strategies	
Mental processes; creative, abstract, reflective thoughts; interpretation; synthesis; intuitive leaps	Mental processes; problem solving; interpretation
Evaluation	
Theoretical thinking; conceptual definitions; other theory analyses criteria	Variable definitions; validity; reliability; other research criteria
Impact on Discipline	
Through integrated theoretical statements that explain and predict with a wider scope	Through selected scientific findings that explain and predict specifics
Future	
Generates more propositions; inspires	Provides support for existing propositions and for clinical actions

Phenomena seen from a nursing perspective are not seen in exactly the same way as phenomena seen from a sociological perspective. A nursing perspective is focused on health, comfort, care, the nursing process, and other domain concepts. Nurses are concerned with phenomena that will eventually make a difference in some aspect of health care. Therefore, in nursing, one describes or explains a phenomenon through a health/illness and person–environment response perspective. Different perspectives offer "unique ways of viewing the world or phenomenon" (Donaldson and Crowley, 1978). A perspective "defines the nature and limits of inquiry into phenomena" (Donaldson and Crowley, 1978). Another assumption for this strategy is that there is some kind of reality that exists out there, and there is a pattern and order in the universe around us, as well as paradoxically, for a certain degree of uniqueness. Because we live in an orderly, nonrandom world, this order is comprehensible to a certain extent and within a context. That concept of uniqueness deserves a pause.

If each event or process of a phenomenon were absolutely unique or occurred randomly, without order or pattern, there could be no generalization, albeit a contextual one. Without some degree of generalization there is no science, because all sciences attempt to generalize about recurrent phenomena. Scientists, unlike philosophers, must also assume some logical connection between perceivable events as well as a certain degree of predictability. Nurses have been focusing on uniqueness in practice to individualize care. However, we must consider seriously Ellis' (1982) admonition against using the uniqueness of man as a crutch to avoid patterning and order, the essential components of theory and science. Uniqueness reminds us to consider patterns of diversity and individuality, which, when considered, could add to the complexity and richness of theory. Therefore, uniqueness and patterning are also significant premises upon which this strategy is based.

With this caveat and with the necessity of considering the rich contextual background in mind, it may seem difficult to isolate a beginning point for this strategy. However, like the previous strategies, there are some essential, but not sufficient, stages and processes that may facilitate theorizing attempts. These stages and processes are delineated in the following sections.

Stages and Processes in Theorizing

There are no recipes for the development of theory; there is no one way of doing it, nor is there a way by which the richness and the haphazardness of the process can be fully captured. Theorizing is not reducible to a linear set of components or to neat and tidy sets of processes. A conceptualization could happen all at once, or it could take years and never quite evolve into a useful integrated view of reality. There are, however, six stages and several processes that are useful in engaging in the whole activity of theorization, whether theorization is used as a framework for research, for data interpretation, for concept development, for statistical model building, or for the development of a theory. The stages are: (1) taking in, (2) description of phenomenon, (3) labeling, (4) concept development, (5) statement development, (6) explicating assumptions, and (7) sharing and communicating. Although these stages and processes are presented here linearly and consequentially, they could occur simultaneously, out of sequence, or in conjunction with other yet undelineated stages. It is useful for students of theory to deliberately and consciously experience each of these stages, even when such experiences are based on just rehearsals.

Taking In
Taking in is a process of sizing up a situation that has attracted our attention for whatever reason, whether that reason is cognitive, affective, objective, or sub-

jective, whether it is a hunch or just an uneasy feeling. Taking in has several characteristics. A phenomenon may attract and hold the attention of the observer, making her pause to think about it and reflect on its nature. This **attention-grabbing** may happen when the phenomenon is occurring, or it may evolve retrospectively. A clinician may air the room whenever she changes a dressing without pausing to think about the relationship of increased fresh air in the room and healing. That action or its consequences may have been occurring regularly but, because it has not grabbed her attention, she has not been able to develop it further. Attention-grabbing includes observations, mental labor, and personal involvement, all so closely intertwined that it is hard to reduce them to linearity as to what happens first and what happens second.

Observation is a very complex process, more of a sensory experience than merely seeing. Accurate observation is difficult because of the tendency for selective observations and selective inattention. To know when one is observing with the eyes and when one is observing through mental activity helps to clarify and distinguish dimensions of observation (Zderad and Belcher, 1968). Both activities are part of attention-grabbing and are essential in developing theories, but they need to be distinguished. We cannot totally separate what we observe from what we want to see or what we observe from our experiences; nor do we want to. However, we can allow ourselves to observe what we do not know, what we, at this time, do not understand, and what is out of the realm of our experience. Observation occurs both with the "naked eye" and within a "matrix of theory." Beveridge (1957) reminds us that:

> Accurate observation of complex situations is extremely difficult, and
> observers usually make many errors of which they are not conscious.
> Effective observation involves noticing something and giving it significance
> by relating it to something else noticed or already known; thus it contains
> both an element of sense-perception and a mental element. It is impossible to
> observe everything, and so the observer has to give most of his attention to a
> selected field, but he should at the same time try to watch out for other
> things, especially for anything odd. . . . Powers of observation can be
> developed by cultivating the habit of watching things with an active, inquiring
> mind. (pp. 104–105)

A deliberate attempt needs to be made to experience and practice naked-eye observations as well as observations within the matrix of theory or those guided by a paradigm. Observation is not a new skill to nurses; it has been the cornerstone of practice. As King (1975) put it:

> Direct observation has been a primary function of nurses for centuries.
> Nurses collect voluminous data in their daily activities to gain immediate
> factual information to plan and give nursing care. They have been trained to
> make observations and to measure selected physiological and behavioral
> parameters of human beings to answer immediate questions. (p. 26)

After the initial serendipitous identification of a phenomenon from a clinical setting, or from careful review of research studies, the attention grabbing is followed by **attention-giving**. Attention giving is a more deliberate process. It is a process that includes careful delineation of situations or events that have the potential of demonstrating the phenomenon under consideration. Situations or incidents selected for observation should vary in order to consider different aspects of phenomena. An example may illustrate this process. A primary health care worker in Cali, Colombia, noticed over the years that *per diem* maids tend to ignore all attempts to bring them to the clinic early in their pregnancy for prenatal care. She also noticed that they tended to bring their sick children to the emergency room with the very first sign of any mild illness. The discrepancy between getting prenatal care and getting pediatric care grabbed her attention. The health care worker may then choose to give this matter her attention and deliberately look into the differences between the two clinics, the meanings attached to pregnancies and offsprings and to preventive and curative care, or she may choose to consider the environment of both clinics, or a number of alternatives depending on the interest, the goals, and the previous experiences of the theorist.

> Sometimes a question—a patient's, a colleague's, one's own—may call attention to some phenomenon and provoke thinking. The beginning may be the absence of an expected response experienced by the nurse with surprise, anger, disappointment, or relief. These subjective responses may be used as clues to the nature of the phenomenon itself. (Zderad, 1978, p. 40)
>   It is looking at the experience with wide-open eyes, with knowledge, facts, theories held at bay; looking at the experience with astonishment. Concentrating on the experience is absolutely necessary. Becoming absorbed in the phenomenon without being possessed by it is equally important (Oiler, 1982, p. 180).

During the taking-in stage, a dialogue with oneself, with one's theoretical journal, with others, or with all these may be helpful in delineating the phenomenon to further pursuit. The dialogue may include the following questions:

> What is it that is attracting the attention of the observer?
> Where does it happen?
> Is it similar to or different from happenings under different sets of
>   circumstances?
> Under what conditions does the observer sense it, see it, hear it,
>   observe it, read it, or touch it?
> Can the observer describe it? What is the description?
> Can the observer document it with model cases and prototype
>   situations?

The objective of completing the taking-in stage with the two processes of attention grabbing and attention giving is to delineate a phenomenon for further theoretical development.

Description of Phenomenon

The interest in some problem, question, situation, or event—theoretical or clinical—gnaws at the observer for some time. Our early theorists began their theoretical formulations with a nagging problem based on experience, observation, and thinking that was related to organization of nursing curricula and the nature of the substantive knowledge that should be included in nursing courses. Some specific questions that baffled them were, What is nursing? and What is nursing's mission? The combination of their questions and their clinical backgrounds resulted in several theories that have helped us distinguish the boundaries of our discipline. These theories have attempted, and succeeded in some ways, to provide some abstract concepts and propositions that can be generalized to different areas of specialization in nursing.

Nursing has gone beyond the beginnings of being concerned only with the global questions that preoccupied our colleagues in theory. The discipline of nursing is capable of focusing its inquiry and the goals for developing theories to phenomena surrounding health, transitions, interactions, nursing clients, and nursing therapeutics.

The observer should attempt to respond to the following questions in defining the phenomenon:

> What is the phenomenon?
> When does it occur?
> What are the boundaries of the phenomenon?
> What does it share with a larger class of phenomena?
> Does the phenomenon vary? Under what circumstances?
> Is the phenomenon isolated in reality?
> Does it have a function? Are there multiple factors associated with it?
>   Does it serve an explanatory purpose?
> Does it refer to a long-term behavior, to characteristic or habitual
>   modes of behaving, or to patterns of behavior detectable in
>   repeated or similar acts?
> Is the phenomenon related to time and place?
> Is the phenomenon related to some theoretical framework, to one's
>   basic philosophy of nursing or manner of being? In what way?

This sums up what the phenomenon is and where and when it occurs. All this will help in describing a phenomenon.

A description of a phenomenon may be first articulated in question form. An interest in sleeplessness in intensive care units may prompt one of the following questions (Landis, 1983):

> Why do patients experience periods of lack of sleep in intensive care
>   units?
> What are the properties of sleeplessness or wakefulness in intensive
>   care units?
> Is sleeplessness an adaptive coping style or a maladaptive one?

Others' interests or clinical focuses may prompt other types of questions, such as:

What processes do nurses go through to decide whether or not to
  provide pain medication for patients experiencing pain?
What are the properties of effective transition into the sick or well
  role?
What are effective and ineffective transitions?
What are the predictors of occurrence of premenstrual stress?
What is a stressful menopausal experience?
Why do certain immigrant groups seem to be more consistently
  "satisfied" with health care than others?
What types of social support do different subcultural groups need
  during illness?

Once the general problem area is identified, a set of questions are then asked
to determine whether the problem of interest falls within the domain of nursing.
They include:

In what way is the phenomenon related to nursing's substantive
  knowledge process?
In what way would understanding the phenomenon help in explaining
  some aspect of nursing care?
Can you think of some questions around that phenomenon, the
  answer to which would be significant to nursing?
How is the phenomenon related to the social policy statement of
  what nursing is?
Are there some biases that you could identify: background of the
  researcher, presence of the researcher?
Did the investigator provide contrasting observations, thereby
  demonstrating contexts in which phenomena are observed or not
  observed?
Are there repetitive patterns?

A phenomenon is not a thing in itself; it is not what exists, but rather it is
organized around perceptions. When experience and sensory and intuitive data
become coherent as a whole, and prior to attachment of any meaning, we have a
phenomenon. A phenomenon, then, is an aspect of reality colored by the perception
of the viewer of that reality. A phenomenon remains merely a phenomenon as long
as we attach no cognitive, intuitive, or inferential interpretation. For example,
separate and repetitive observations of the appearance of newly immigrated groups
occurring more often in emergency rooms than in the regularly scheduled outpa-
tient clinics is a beginning observation that may evolve into a phenomenon. When
one observes that individuals belonging to the immigrant group tend to miss scheduled appointments and appear at unscheduled times, a vague pattern begins to
emerge. When the observer further hears an individual from the same or another
immigrant group rejecting the pace of life in the United States and complaining
about having to plan activities and events so far in advance, then the vague pattern

begins to form into a shape. The form could be concerns about planning, disenchantment with structured existence, or various abilities to deal with emergencies in preference to maintenance. The observer can then ask questions, can observe, can read, can structure situations in which planning is considered a norm (*e.g.*, birthing preparation, rehabilitation, and discharge), and can therefore ascertain whether indeed a pattern is still apparent.

Delineation of phenomena is achieved through the analysis of models or exemplars. Model situations are vivid examples of the phenomenon and help to describe it. A model situation depicts reality in its prototype, its ideal form, and it allows demonstration of what the phenomenon is and where it exists (Chinn and Jacobs, 1987).

Labeling

Labeling is a stage that comes somewhere in the process of theorizing, and the label may change several times in the process. The function of labeling is to communicate succinctly, to relate to the written literature, to help to delineate what further observations to obtain, and to reduce a phenomenon that is usually described in a paragraph to a concept or statement. Labeling is more than selecting a Label X to describe Phenomenon Y. Labeling allows for semantic analysis (Scheffler, 1958). Semantic analysis permits the theorist to consider the normative use of the term as well as other more esoteric uses of it. Labeling is associated with a kind of defining that ranges from a dictionary definition to a more complex definition that takes the perspective of the theorist into consideration. The label, "preference for spontaneity," emerged from further consideration of Middle Eastern immigrants' health and illness behaviors to denote their lack of enthusiasm about planning, preference for dropping-in over making appointments, preference for missing appointments, and preference for showing up in the delivery room with no prenatal care (Olesen and Meleis, manuscript in progress). A label and semantic analysis bring the theorist closer to concept development.

There are some criteria to be considered in labeling concepts. Lundberg (1942) suggests Eubank's (1932) criteria:

> (1) They are always used in the same sense whenever employed, (2) they are reasonably precise, (3) each "contains only one cardinal idea," and (4) they are fundamental or essential to the complete interpretation of their particular field.

Labeling a concept is a highly individualized experience, and it involves interpretations of the phenomenon. It includes hunches, opinions, and speculations. A labeled phenomenon is a concept or a statement, but it is predefined theoretically and operationally.

Concept Development

Somewhere in this process of theorizing, and not in linear progression, a concept begins to emerge. Concepts evolve out of a complex constellation of impressions, perceptions, and experiences. Conception in Kantian terms is an organized perception. Phenomena are perceived, and only when they are organized and labeled do they become concepts. Concepts are a mental image of reality tinted with the theorist's perception, experience, and philosophical bent. They function as a reservoir and an organizational entity and bring order to observation and perceptions. They help to flag related ideas and perceptions without going into detailed descriptions.

Several processes are useful in concept development. These are defining, differentiating, delineating antecedents and consequences, modeling, analogizing, and synthesizing. **Defining** depends on the label that was given to the phenomenon. Therefore, the labeling stage should be carefully considered; premature labeling may prompt the theorist to review unrelated literature. Defining a concept helps to delineate subconcepts and dimensions of the concept. During the process of defining concepts theoretically and operationally, the theorist is smoothing rough edges, clarifying ambiguities, enhancing precision, and relating concepts to some empirical referents.

Lundberg (1942) also suggests that:

> Operational definitions, then, are merely definitions which consist as far as possible of words clearly designating observations of events and performable and observable operations subject to corroboration. Thus, they may consist of (1) "physical manipulations," such as reading the weight on a weight scale, (2) "objective verbal designations of these manipulations," or (3) "verbal designations of symbolical or mental operations," such as the definition of "preference for spontaneity."

Operational definitions of concepts in nursing have to be referenced in practice and put into context in reality. Otherwise, they would not be useful for nurses (Jacobs and Huether, 1978). Human responses, one of the units of analysis for nursing theorists, may not always lend themselves to the same corroboration expected in the physical sciences and strived for by social scientists, nor should they.

Differentiating is a process of sorting in and sorting out similarities in and differences between the concept being developed and other like concepts. In developing the concept of transition as a central concept in nursing, Chick and Meleis (1986) discussed the similarities and the differences between the priorities of the concepts of transition and change. Similarly, Reed and Leonard (1989) described how they saw the differences between self-neglect, the concept under development, and suicide and noncompliance. The importance in utilizing the process of differentiation is in accessing related bodies of literature and in further refining the attributes of the concept under development.

In **delineating antecedents**, the theorist is attempting to define the contextual conditions under which the concept is perceived and is expected to occur. Antecedents to transitions that are of interest to the domain of nursing have been defined as events such as recovery, death, immigration, amputation, diagnoses of chronic illnesses, pregnancy, and admission to hospital (Chick and Meleis, 1986). The theorist may ask, So what?, in attempting to identify the consequences of the concept. Consequences are those events, situations, or conditions that are related to and preceded by the concept under development.

To **delineate consequences**, a theorist can practice listing every concept or statement that, in her opinion, or as manifested in research findings, may result from the concept. It is important to deliberately attempt to delineate positive as well as negative consequences. Consequences of transition may be disorientation, confusion, growth, changes in body image, changes in self-concept, and role sufficiency (Meleis, 1975).

Modeling is the process of defining and identifying exemplars to illustrate some aspect of the concept. Exemplars could be clinical referents or research referents. Several types of models are used, each to illustrate different aspects of a concept. A same model is one that illustrates the concept in its entirety. A contrary model is a situation, a group, or an incident in which a contrasting aspect of the concept is absent or is present under a different set of contextual conditions. A population that is not in some major transition may be compared with one that is undergoing a significant transition, which may provide the contrary model. A like model and a contrary model help the theorist in articulating, demonstrating, and highlighting the differences between situations, events, and clients in which the phenomena related to the concept are demonstrated and not demonstrated, thus increasing the potential for clarifying it further. Paterson and Zderad (1988) described a technique of explanation through negation to help in describing the phenomena. Presenting another related phenomenon that does not describe the phenomenon under development helps in sharpening the clarity of that phenomenon.

> A phenomenon cannot be described completely by negation but it may be
> clarified to some extent by saying what it is not. For instance, empathy is not
> sympathy; it is not projection; it is not identification. (p. 90)

Analogizing is a process by which a deliberate choice is made to describe the concept under development through another concept or phenomenon that is sufficiently like the one under study but that has been studied more extensively, explored more systematically, and therefore is better understood than the concept under study. If the phenomenon or the concept are alike but represent different domains, and we understand one more than the other, then perhaps the better understood phenomenon will help shed some light, raise better questions, and offer greater insight into the lesser understood phenomenon. An example of analogizing is the use of fables or fictional stories to illustrate the concept. One example of analogizing that I used is of aliens from other times and planets to illustrate the need for international collaboration in knowledge development (Meleis, 1987).

Synthesizing is a process of bringing together findings, meanings, and properties that have been amplified by each of the processes described previously. Synthesizing includes, but is not limited to, describing future steps in theorizing.

Statement Development

The development of a concept may be an end result for some theorists and an interim stage for others that leads to further development through statement development, or research implementation. However, concept development may not be possible because the situation calls for statement development. The questions that we may be facing in nursing as a human science are: Is concept development the only avenue to development of theory? Is it possible that the building block for nursing theories are statement development?

Statement development is a stage during which explanations related to the phenomenon are provided. The explanations link the concepts, antecedents, consequences, and assumptions. Statements are developed to describe, to explain, to prescribe, or to predict. They are developed as an end result or to synthesize other statements for research purposes.

To develop statements, several questions may be helpful. Examples of these questions are:

> In what ways can we further explicate the concept being considered?
> In what ways are nursing clients' health and environment affected by the concept?
> What are some potential consequences of the concept?
> What are some corollaries of the concept?

Propositions are tentative statements about reality and its nature. They describe relationships between events, situations, or actions. Propositions could be developed to describe the properties of the concepts; these descriptive propositions are called *existence propositions* (Zetterberg, 1963). They are factor-isolating propositions (Dickoff, James, and Wiedenbach, 1968), and the end result is therefore descriptive theory, as essential to science as any other theory. Consider, for example, descriptive theory of the atom and its significance to our knowledge of the atom.

Propositions may also be relational, describing the association between concepts or causal relationships between concepts (Reynolds, 1971). The process of developing propositions is also a process of identifying the central questions related to the concept. Propositions provide the central answers that help to explain, describe, or predict nursing reality. The more refined, developed, and advanced the relationship statements are, the more they are able to describe and predict the nature of the relationship, the direction of the relationship, and the strength of the relationship (Chinn and Jacobs, 1987).

Organizing propositions is one of the processes in the propositional stages. Organization of propositions could be accomplished through different channels. Propositions may be arranged to represent process of concept discovery and process of formation of a proposition. In this case, a chronological organization is achieved. A second way is to organize propositions around the central concepts in the theory. A third method is to organize propositions in terms of significance for testing, beginning with those whose test represents the central questions of the theory. Other ways are to organize around independent variables or around dependent variables. Ordering propositions enhances their usefulness and their aestheticism (Zetterberg, 1963).

Explicating Assumptions

During every stage of the process the observer pauses, reflects, and questions both implicit and explicit assumptions. To regard periods of wakefulness as sleeplessness, the observer has made an assumption that certain periods of wakefulness are disruptive and that disturbed behavior may result in sleeplessness. Imagine that the observer is beginning from an opposite point of view (*i.e.*, that wakefulness promotes healing); observation will be more open to positive consequences, to what promotes wakefulness, and so on. Therefore, reflection on and analysis of one's views, beliefs, and theoretical underpinnings will help delineate assumptions of the developing theory.

Sharing and Communicating

None of these stages and processes are entirely new to nurses, whether they are clinicians, theorists, or researchers. What may have made it appear new in the 1980s was the growing acceptance of conceptualization as a significant aspect of knowledge development in nursing. This acceptance is demonstrated in the journals that are devoted to conceptual development of the discipline and in the increasing productivity in metatheory and theory writing. No theorization process is complete without opportunities to share and communicate it with colleagues. Theorizing may happen in isolation, but it does not grow in isolation. Sharing and communicating goes beyond writing and publication. It should be defined as a daily happening in the lives of clinicians, theorists, and researchers.

Instead of staging opportunities for sharing and communicating conceptualizations, redefining existing opportunities and resources may enhance this process of sharing and communicating. Clinical conferences may be redefined to include a theoretical journal sharing hour. Faculty meeting time may be reorganized to permit discussion for evolving concepts or statements; students may use part of their class time for a juice or sherry hour to freely discuss phenomena of interest.

Tools for Theory Development

Theory development includes a mental process that incorporates analysis, discovery, formulation, and validation of uniformities. These may come as a result of sensory observation or as a consequence of logical or rational analysis of the problem or the phenomenon. They may also result from intuitive reasoning, from an insight that occurs over an extended period of time, or from a "click" that comes as quick as lightning. The thought processes can be spontaneous or premeditated—the timing is never predictable (Sorokin, 1974)—but a conscious effort to look at the phenomenon or the questions is infinitely more helpful in bringing the process to closure. It does not guarantee the "click," but it increases the chances.

Just as the process of researching is enhanced by knowledge of substantive content, knowledge of research methodology, experience, and ability to critique research, all processes of theory development are supported and enhanced by knowledge of what constitutes theory, knowledge of what major issues are confronting theorizing, the ability to critique theory, knowledge of existing theories, and knowledge of major pitfalls in the development of theory. Knowledge of the context for theory such as the clinical area is essential. Theorizing is a process that is refined through a deliberate experience. The processes of reflecting, analyzing, questioning, relating, thinking, writing, changing, and communicating are integral parts of philosophical analysis, essential to theory development, and a prelude to and a consequence of research. Keeping a theory diary or journal, in which observations, reflections, and relationships are systematically logged, helps the theorist to sort out thoughts, develop documentation, and synthesize empirical reasoning with intuitive reasoning.

Norms utilized to enhance science are useful in enhancing theory development. Merton (1979) identified a number of these norms, two of which are pertinent here: the norms of communality and organized skepticism. Communality encourages nurses to share developing ideas and expose beginning theories for review by peers to help sharpen the theory and to allow the norm of organized skepticism to prevail. This latter norm "requires detached scrutiny of work according to empirical and logical criteria" (Meleis and May, 1981). Dialogues with colleagues in practice, in theory, and in research promote other ways of looking at concepts—other angles and other perspectives.

Another essential tool that has been discussed in the nursing literature is that of intuition. *Intuition* is defined as reaching some decision or conclusion without the conscious or apparent availability of information (Rew, 1986; Westcott, 1968). Rew (1986) defines the attributes of intuition as follows: "Knowledge of a fact or truth, as a whole; immediate possession of knowledge; and knowledge independent of the linear reasoning process" (p. 23). Whether this tool is intuition or the expert speaking (Benner, 1984), recent writings encourage allowing that inner voice to surface, to believe in it, and to trust it (Rew, 1986; Agan, 1987; Rew and Barrow, 1987).

Closely related to intuition are introspection and reflection. Silva (1977) reminded us "to value truths arrived at by intuition and introspection as much as those arrived at by scientific experimentation" (p. 62). Reflection is a process of thinking that may or may not be bound by the need for problem solving.

CONCLUSION

Knowing and experimenting with strategies for theory development increases theorizing abilities but does not guarantee the development of theory, nor should it. A probable result of such knowledge is the integration of philosophical processes with empirical processes, resulting in a more integrated knowledge. The rift between scientists and philosophers that marked the era of empirical positivism is decreasing. Our early philosophers believed that science is based totally on philo-sophical processes, our scientists believed that it is based on the intellectual labor inherent in the philosophical processes. This chapter demonstrated this later process as an essential one for embarking on research, for interpreting research. Both processes are processes of theorizing. The end result may or may not be a theory; the end result may be clarification of a concept or the articulation of a number of propositions that may be an extension of another theory. Systematic research is an essential step in the process to complete the practice–theory–research loop. Eventually, a theory will have to respond to the analytical and critical criteria presented in the next chapter.

REFERENCES

Agan, R.D. (1987) Intuitive knowing as a dimension of nursing. *Advances in Nursing Science,* 10(1), 63–70.

Allen, D, Benner, P., and Diekelman, N.L. (1986) Three paradigms for nursing research: Methodological implications. In P.L. Chinn (Ed.), *Nursing research methodology: Issues and implications.* Rockville, MD: Aspen Systems.

Arruda-Neve, E.N., Meleis, A.I., and Larson, P. (In review) Comfort of Hispanic patients: A concept analysis.

Backscheider, J. (1971) The use of self as the essence of clinical supervision in ambulatory patient care. *Nursing Clinics of North America,* 6(4), 785–794.

Barnard, K. (1973) The effect of stimulation on the sleep behavior of the premature infant. In M.V. Batey (Ed.), *Communicating nursing research, collaboration and competition.* Boulder, CO: Western Interstate Commission of Higher Education.

Barnum, B.J. (1990) *Nursing theory: Analysis, application, and evaluation* (2nd ed.). Boston: Little, Brown & Co.

Beckstrand, J. (1978a) The notion of a practice theory and the relationship of scientific and ethical knowledge to practice. *Research in Nursing and Health,* 1(3), 131–136.

Beckstrand, J. (1978b) The need for a practice theory as indicated by the knowledge used in conduct of practice. *Research in Nursing and Health,* 1(4), 175–179.

Benner, P. (1984) *From novice to expert: Excellence and power in clinical nursing practice.* Menlo Park, CA: Addison-Wesley.

Benoliel, J.Q. (1977) Social characteristics of death as a recorded hospital event. *Communicating Nursing Research,* 8, 245–265.

Benoliel, J.Q. (1982) Educating nurses for community-based care of advanced cancer patients. AACE Abstracts. *Medical and Pediatric Oncology,* 10(1982), 30A–31A.

Benoliel, J.Q. (1983) The historical development of cancer nursing research in the United States. *Cancer Nursing,* 6(4), 261–268.

Benoliel, J.Q. and De Valde, S. (1975) As the patient views the intensive care unit and the coronary care unit. *Heart and Lung,* 4(2), 260–264.

Benoliel, J.Q., Tornberg, M.J., and McGrath, B.B. (1984) Oncology transition services: Partnerships of nurses and families. *Cancer Nursing,* 7(2), 131–137.

Beveridge, W.I.B. (1957) *The art of scientific investigation.* New York: W.W. Norton.

Carrieri, V.K., Janson-Bjerklie, S., and Jacobs, S. (1984) The sensation of dyspnea: A review. *Heart and Lung,* 13(4), 436–447.

Chick, N. and Meleis, A.I. (1986) Transitions: A nursing concern. In P.L. Chinn (Ed.), *Nursing research methodology*. Boulder, CO: Aspen.

Chinn, P.L. and Jacobs, M.K. (1987) *Theory and nursing: A systematic approach*. St. Louis: C.V. Mosby.

Dickoff, J. and James, P. (1968) A theory of theories: A position paper. *Nursing Research*, 17(3), 197–203.

Dickoff, J., James, P., and Wiedenbach, E. (1968) Theory in practice discipline: Part 1. Practice oriented theory. *Nursing Research*, 17(5), 415–435.

Donaldson, S.K. and Crowley, D. (1978) The discipline of nursing. *Nursing Outlook*, 26(2), 113–120.

Ellis, R. (1982, July/August) Conceptual issues in nursing. *Nursing Outlook*, 30(7), 406–410.

Eubank, E.E. (1932) *The concepts of sociology*. Lexington, MA: D.C. Heath.

Fagerhaugh, S.Y. (1974, October) Pain expression and control on a burn care unit. *Nursing Outlook*, 22, 645–650.

Glaser, B.G. and Strauss, A.L. (1967) *The discovery of grounded theory: Strategies for qualitative research*. Chicago: Aldine.

Glaser, B.G. and Strauss, A.L. (1968) *Time for dying*. Chicago: Aldine.

Hardy, M.E. (1978) Practice oriented theory: Part 1. Perspectives on nursing theory. *Advances in Nursing Science*, 1(1), 37–48.

Jacobs, M.K. and Huether, S.E. (1978) Nursing science: The theory-practice linkage. *Advances in Nursing Science*, 1(1), 63–74.

Jacox, A. (1974) Theory construction in nursing: An overview. *Nursing Research*, 23(1), 4–13.

Johnson, D.E. (1974) Development of theory: A requisite for nursing as a primary health profession. *Nursing Research*, 23(5), 372–377.

Johnson, D.E. (1980) The behavioral system model for nursing. In J.P. Riehl and C. Roy (Eds.), *Conceptual models for nursing practice* (2nd ed.). New York: Appleton-Century-Crofts.

Johnson, J.E. (1972, November/December) Effects of structuring patients expectations on their reactions to threatening events. *Nursing Research*, 21(6), 499–504.

Johnson, J.E. and Rice, V.H. (1974, May/June) Sensory and distress components of pain. *Nursing Research*, 23(3), 203–209.

King, I.M. (1975) A process for developing concepts for nursing through research. In P.J. Verhonick (Ed.), *Nursing Research* (Vol. 1) Boston: Little, Brown & Co.

Kuhn, T.S. (1970) The structure of scientific revolutions. In Neurath, O. (Ed.), *International encyclopedia of unified science* (2nd ed.). (Vol. 2) Chicago: University of Chicago Press.

Landis, C. (1983) Sleeplessness in intensive care unit: A developing concept. Paper presented in N202A at the University of California, San Francisco.

Lindeman, C.A. (1980) The challenge of nursing research in the 1980s. In *Communicating nursing research: Direction for the 1980s*. Boulder, CO: Western Interstate Commission for Higher Education.

Lindeman, C.A. and Van Aernam, B. (1973) Nursing intervention with the presurgical patient: The effects of structured and unstructured preoperative teaching. In F. Downs and M. Newman (Eds.), *A source book in nursing research*. Philadelphia: F.A. Davis.

Lindsey, A., Piper, B., and Stotts, N. (1982) The phenomenon of cancer cachexia, review. *Oncology Nursing Forum*, 9(2), 38–42.

Lundberg, G.A. (1942) *Social research*. New York: Longman's Green.

Meleis, A.I. (1975) Role insufficiency and role supplementation: A conceptual framework. *Nursing Research*, 24(4), 264–271.

Meleis, A.I. (1987) Pandemic images: Knowledge development for empowerment. Keynote address given at Sigma Theta Tau, San Francisco.

Meleis, A.I. and May, K.M. (1981) Nursing theory and scholarliness in the doctoral program. *Advances in Nursing Science*, 4(1), 31–41.

Mercer, R. (1981, March/April) A theoretical framework for studying factors that impact on the maternal role. *Nursing Research*, 30(2), 73–77.

Mercer, R. (1984) Predictors of maternal role attainment at one year post birth. *Western Journal of Nursing Research*, 6(3), 62.

Mercer, R., Ferketich, S., May, K., and de Joseph, J. (1987) A comparison of maternal and paternal responses during pregnancy. *Proceedings Council of Nurse Researchers Conference*, Arlington, VA, October 13–16, American Nurses' Association.

Mercer, R., Ferketich, S., May, K., de Joseph, J., and Sollid, D. (1987) Maternal and paternal responses in high- and low-risk pregnancies. Symposium. *Proceedings Sigma Theta Tau International Biennial Conference*, San Francisco, November 10, Sigma Theta Tau International.

Merton, R.K. (1979) *The sociology of science: An episodic memoir.* Carbondale and Edwardsville: Southern Illinois University Press.

Millor, G.K. (1981) A theoretical framework for nursing research in child abuse and neglect. *Nursing Research*, 30(2), 78–83.

Newman, M.A. (1979) *Theory development in nursing.* Philadelphia: F.A. Davis.

Norbeck, J. (1981) Social support: A model for clinical research and application. *Advances in Nursing Science*, 3, 43–59.

Oiler, C. (1982) The phenomenological approach in nursing research. *Nursing Research*, 31(3), 178–181.

Olesen, V. and Meleis, A. (Manuscript in progress) Spontaneity: A social phenomenon observed in Middle-Eastern immigrants.

Parsons, T. (1951) *The social system.* New York: Free Press.

Paterson, J.G. and Zderad, L.T. (1988) *Humanistic nursing* (2nd ed.). New York: National League of Nursing.

Peplau, H.E. (1952) *Interpersonal relations in nursing.* New York: G.P. Putnam's Sons.

Reed, P.G. and Leonard, V.E. (1989) An analysis of the concept of self-neglect. *Advanced Nursing Science*, 12(1), 39–53.

Rew, L. (1986) Intuition: Concept analysis of a group phenomenon. *Advances in Nursing Science*, 8(2), 21–28.

Rew, L. and Barrow, E.M. (1987) Intuition: A neglected hallmark of nursing knowledge. *Advances in Nursing Science*, 10(1), 49–62.

Reynolds, P.D. (1971) *Primer in theory construction.* Indianapolis: Bobbs-Merrill Company.

Roy, C. and Roberts, S. (1981) *Theory construction in nursing: An adaptation model.* Englewood Cliffs, NJ: Prentice-Hall.

Schatzman, L. and Strauss, A.L. (1973) *Field research: Strategies for a natural sociology.* Englewood Cliffs, NJ: Prentice-Hall.

Scheffler, I. (1958) *Philosophy and education.* Boston: Allyn and Bacon.

Schensul, S.L. (1985) Science theory and application in Anthropology. *American Behavioral Scientist*, 29(2), 164–185.

Silva, M.C. (1977) Philosophy, science, theory: Interrelationships and implications for nursing research. *Image*, 9(3), 59–63.

Smith, J. (1981) The idea of health: A philosophical inquiry. *Advances in Nursing Science,* 3(3), 43–50.

Sorokin, P. (1974) How are sociological theories conceived, developed and validated. In R.S. Denisoff, O. Callahan, and M.H. Levine (Eds.), *Theories and paradigms in contemporary sociology.* Itasca, IL: F.E. Peacock.

Stern, P.N. (1981) Solving problems of cross-cultural health teaching: The Filipino childbearing family. *Image,* 13, 47–50.

Stevens, P. (1989) A critical social reconceptualization of environment in nursing: Implications for methodology. *Advanced Nursing Science,* 11(4), 56–68.

Walker, L.O. and Avant, K.C. (1989) *Strategies for theory construction in nursing* (2nd ed.). New York: Appleton-Century-Crofts.

Westcott, M.R. (1968) *Antecedents and consequences of intuitive thinking.* Final report to U.S. Department of Health, Education, and Welfare. Poughkeepsie, NY: Vassar College.

Zderad, L.T. (1978) From here-and-now to theory: Reflections on how. In J.G. Patterson, *Theory development: What, why, how?* New York: National League for Nursing.

Zderad, L.T. and Belcher, H.C. (1968) *Developing behavioral concepts in nursing.* Atlanta, GA: Southern Regional Education Board.

Zetterberg, H.L. (1963) *On theory and verification in sociology,* rev'd ed. Totowa, NJ: Bedminster Press.

A Model for Evaluation of Theories: Description, Analysis, Critique, and Testing*

Nurses have always evaluated theories. They evaluated theories to apply to practice, to develop curricula, to use in teaching, to operationalize for research, or to utilize in daily decision making. These evaluations may be deliberate, systematic, criteria-based, objective, conscious, and elaborate, or they may be subjective, experiential, quick, and based on a limited set of criteria. Both types of evaluations are essential; neither type is sufficient by itself.

Evaluation of theory is an essential component of nursing practice and of knowledge development, for the following reasons:

1. To decide which theory is more appropriate to use as a framework for research, teaching, administration, or consultation;
2. To identify effective theories in exploring some aspect of practice or in guiding a research project;
3. To compare and contrast different explanations of the same phenomenon;
4. To enhance the potential of constructive changes and further theory development;
5. To identify epistemological approaches of a discipline through attention to the sociocultural context of the theorist and the theory;
6. To assess the ontological beliefs in a discipline;
7. To identify schools of thought in a discipline;

---

*This chapter is adapted, with considerable changes, from an earlier manuscript written by A.I. Meleis and published in Chaska, N. (1982) *The nursing profession: Time to speak.* New York: McGraw-Hill, 1982.

8. To affect changes in clinical practice, to define research priorities, and to identify content for teaching and guidelines for nursing administration;
9. To have nursing frameworks to justify nursing to the public;
10. To identify strategies for theory development;
11. To define a discipline's domain; and
12. To be a critical consumer of theories.

Before going any further in reading this chapter, I suggest you take a few minutes to identify one or two theories (nursing or non-nursing) that you have used in your work or personal life. For example, you may identify role theory as a framework for your research on women's daily activities in a nursing home and their health; endorphin theory linking stress with exercise; or Maslow's theory in understanding patient's needs. The next set of questions to ask and reflect on are: Why did you select to use these theories in your work? Why not other theories that may provide a different set of equally plausible explanations? To complete this exercise, you should be able by now to identify the criteria you used in making a decision about what theory to use.

Over a 25-year span, I have asked students, faculty, clinicians, and administrators in the United States as well as in several other countries these questions. In reviewing the answers and analyzing their content, a number of criteria emerged. Now, compare your criteria with those identified next.

Personal: Individuals who use this criterion discuss their personal comfort in using the theory, their intuitive choices, and the theory's congruency with their philosophical view of life.

Mentor: There are those who use a theory because they were mentored by a theorist. They spoke of personal influence, respect, personal contact, and educational experience.

Theorist: Who the theorists are, their standing in the field, their status, and how well they are recognized were among the reasons that a theory was selected.

Literature support: Others identified the availability of extensive writings about the theory that gave them assurance of the level of significance of the theory and the status it holds.

Sociopolitical congruency: The congruency between the theory implementation process and the sociopolitical as well as the economic climate was another criterion often identified by audiences. These people spoke of a climate that supports one theory over another because, for example, it did not necessitate structural changes, it required minimal preparation, or it was imposed by administration.

Utility: The ease by which theory was understood and applied prompted a group of users to select a certain theory over another.

Although these criteria are neither all inclusive nor representative of all nurses, definite themes evolved and are experientially supported. The decision to use one theory and not another involves both subjective and objective processes. The decision process could be considered as falling on two continua, each ranging from low to high. Thus, a decision could be both highly objective and highly subjective, low on subjectivity and on objectivity, or could be one of numerous other options in between.

The subjectivity in theory selection is as important as the objectivity. We can select a theory based on well-defined criteria; therefore, the decision becomes highly objective. However, if the theory's assumptions are not congruent with ours, or if we are not convinced by the theorist's experiential background, or if we are not comfortable with other work done by the theorist, the decision process becomes subjective. On the other hand, a selection may be based on one's having worked with the theorist and, without making a decision per se, on one's continuing to utilize the theory. A highly objective decision with low subjectivity could result in theory use that is not as true to the theory premises and propositions; and perhaps vice versa.

The objective evaluation and critique of theories is as complex as the subjective evaluation. To simplify any evaluation, we must break it down into components. For example, when a research project is critiqued, the analysis is done along structural criteria, such as the introduction, conceptual framework, research questions and hypotheses, methodology, results, discussion, conclusions, and limitations. The critique is then completed by looking for clarity, significance, timeliness, and documentation, among other criteria. To analyze and critique theories objectively, numerous criteria have been recommended by a number of authors. In fact, analysis and critique of theories have preoccupied many nurse meta-theorists over a period of time that even preceded the diligent theory development efforts.

Two disciplines have profoundly influenced evaluation of nursing theory: sociology and psychology. The result has been a synthesis of criteria from these disciplines, at times too empirically based and at other times too critical of our theories. When we adhered to some of these criteria, we tended to discount nursing theories, relegating them to the category of individual subjective philosophical expositions. Although some of these criteria are appropriate for the discipline of nursing, others emerge that directly relate to and represent nursing. The rationale for the requirement for a different set of criteria is that nursing, a scientific and a humanistic field, has a domain that encompasses human beings and deals with complex sets of variables; therefore, the criteria for theory evaluation should take into consideration its theory complexity and context.

Each one of the evaluation models offered in nursing literature addressed one aspect of a theory to the exclusion of others. For example, Johnson (1974) focused on a congruence of theory mission with goals relegated by society to nurses (social congruence, utility, and significance). Earlier, in an unpublished manuscript on requirements of an effective model, Johnson (1970) offered a set of requirements that focused on the mission of nursing practice: goals of action, patience, the actor's place and role, source of difficulty, intervention focus, and mode and consequences of care. Although Johnson also addressed the necessity of explicit and consistent structure (assumption and values) and content (nursing's unique goal, ability to be generalized, restrictiveness, continuity, and specificity), other utility criteria were not included, such as research utility and potential for theoretical propositions. Johnson pioneered the development of a set of objective requirements for effective models in nursing and the use of internal and external requirements. Her evaluation model was not published, however, and was therefore limited in exposure and refinement.

Barnum (1990) proposed evaluative criteria that are appropriate for internal criticism (internal construction of theory) and external criticism (which considers theory in its relationships to human beings, nursing, and health). The criteria for internal criticism are clarity, consistency, adequacy, logical development, and level of theory development. The criteria for external criticism are reality conversion, utility, significance, discrimination, scope of theory, and complexity (Barnum, 1990, pp. 85–99). These are useful judgment criteria, particularly when used with descriptive and analytical criteria offered in the model proposed in this chapter.

Similar criteria are offered by Ellis (1968), who delineated seven criteria for what she considered significant theories: a broad scope, complexity, testability, usefulness, identification of implicit values, generation of information, and use of meaningful terminology. Hardy (1974) organized her criteria around the concept of "adequacy": meaning, logical, operational, empirical, and pragmatic. She also believed that adequate theories should have the ability to be generalized, should contribute to understanding, and should be able to predict. It is indeed a challenge to find theories in any discipline to meet all these criteria simultaneously. At worst, the criteria provide serious theory developers with milestones toward which they should strive.

Lest theory developers get discouraged by the rigorous criteria, Duffey and Muhlenkamp (1974, p. 571) offered the following modest set of questions by which theories can be evaluated:

> Does the theory generate testable hypotheses?
> Does the theory guide practice?
> How complete is its subject matter?
> Did the theorist make her biases explicit?
> Does the theory have propositions, and are relationships explicit?
> Is it parsimonious?

Chinn and Jacobs (1987) offered a refreshingly different approach to evaluating theories that was based more on criteria for evaluation of psychological theory. They recommended evaluating theories by considering five criteria: clarity (semantic clarity, semantic consistency, structural clarity, and structural consistency), simplicity, generality, empirical applicability, and consequences. A list of questions was offered to help the evaluator make an objective decision about the level of the criteria (pp. 137–147).

Fawcett (1988), dissatisfied with previously developed evaluation criteria because of the seeming overlap between criteria for evaluating theories and those more appropriate for evaluating conceptual frameworks, offered an analytical and evaluative framework. The framework separates questions for analysis from those intended for evaluation. For analysis, Fawcett proposed a consideration of the historical evolution of the model, approach to model development, content, and source of concern. For the evaluation, she proposed evaluation (judgment based on criteria) of explicitness of assumptions, degree of comprehensiveness of content, logical congruence, ability of the model to generate and test theories, how much the model contributes to knowledge development in nursing, and social considerations (pp. 41–52). Although these were proposed as criteria for evaluating conceptual models, the same criteria could be used in analyzing and evaluating theories.

I encourage you to review as many of these proposals for evaluation as is possible. The criteria reflect the level and sophistication of our knowledge at different stages of development of nursing as a scientific discipline. In reviewing the different criteria, several trends emerge:

- ○ Theories are described, analyzed, and tested.
- ○ There are internal and external criteria for evaluating theories.
- ○ The internal descriptive criteria include assumptions, concepts, relationships, and definitions.
- ○ The internal critical criteria include some areas of agreement, such as consistency, clarity, and logical development.
- ○ Evaluation criteria take into consideration the fit between the theory and external criteria (human beings, society, prevailing paradigms), not only the intrinsic criteria.
- ○ There has evolved a more accepting attitude toward a shift from the rigor of empiricism to the more realistic rigor of potential for testability.
- ○ There is wider acknowledgment of the complexity of evaluation criteria (the two sides of simplicity, the many meanings of complexity, etc.) and, therefore, wider acceptance of multiple criteria.
- ○ There is less prejudice toward descriptive theories.

The model proposed here takes these trends into consideration, draws on many of the previously delineated criteria, and further acknowledges that even when systematic criteria are advanced to ensure objective analysis and critique, objectivity is not guaranteed, nor should it be. Individuals may differ on how they use criteria, and perceptions of meaning of criteria may be influenced by individual variations and by context variations. It is also acknowledged here that some criteria may be conflicting; that to enhance simplicity, complexity may suffer; and that to advocate a wider scope, accuracy for deviant cases or opposing situations may be jeopardized.

The proposed model defines *evaluation* as encompassing description, analyses, critique, and testing. By using this model, a reviewer acknowledges extant evaluations that have been completed by nurse theorists, researchers, and clinicians, among others. The model is also based philosophically more on a historical view of science than on an empirical view. Therefore, it proposes to analyze the central questions that are solved by the theory, the role of the background of the theorist in the development of the theory, and the sociocultural context of the theory, the theorist, and the discipline. In other words, human processes are considered an integral part of theory description, analysis, critique, and testing (Laudan, 1977).

DESCRIPTION

Before embarking on theory evaluation, the reviewer should recognize and identify the boundaries of the review. Boundaries include degree of exposure to theory, length of time devoted to understanding theory, and type of work done with theory (*e.g.*, having taught theory, used it in practice, used it in research, worked with the theoretician, or any number of other alternatives). In doing so, the reviewer attempts to separate objective and subjective rationales.

An initial thorough reading and scanning of the central work of a theorist helps to identify the central questions the theorist is attempting to answer. For example, a central question for developmental theorists is how human beings mature. More often than not, it is not entirely clear in nursing theory what questions the theorists are attempting to answer. The central questions of the theory are answered in the form of the theory propositions. Propositions are the crux of a theory. From propositions, questions emerge that guide exploration and research. Identification of propositions at the outset helps make the job of delineating assumptions and concepts an easier one. It is not a linear process, but a cyclical one in which concepts may be identified, followed by pertinent propositions, followed by more concepts and pertinent assumptions, and so on. This entire process of identifying assumptions, concepts, and propositions addresses the structural components of the theory. (See Table 11-1 for a summary of theory description.)

Structural Components

A theory begins with a set of "givens" that either have been empirically tested or accepted by a number of other theories or previous research. These "givens" are the *theory assumptions*. They could evolve from a philosophical standpoint, from ideological positions, from ethical considerations, from cultural heritage, from social structure, or from previously tested and supported hypotheses. Assumptions also represent one's values. Assumptions of a theory are not subject to testing by the same theory; rather, they lead to a set of propositions that are to be tested. They are the basis from which we can determine the point of view of the theorist. In nursing

Table 11–1
Theory Description

Criteria	Unit of Analysis
Structural components	Assumptions
	Concepts
	Propositions
Functional components	Focus
	Client
	Nursing
	Health
	Nurse–patient interactions
	Environment
	Nursing problem
	Nursing therapeutics

theories, there are assumptions about nursing, human behavior, life, death, health, and illness.

Early writing in theory provides *implicit assumptions*; these are statements that are not identified as *explicit assumptions* by the theorist. Explicit assumptions are identified by authors as their assumptions. Implicit assumptions are imbedded in the writings; they are statements not identified as assumptions, yet they are central for the development of theory propositions or answers to questions. They are statements that are considered by the reviewer to be significant in the development of the theory. The idea that a patient has the right to learn about the gravity of his illness is an implicit assumption in our Western society, whereas the reverse is an implicit assumption in Middle-Eastern cultures. A proposition built on this assumption responds to the question of what is the most effective way to impart the information about the grave diagnosis to the patient. Another proposition would question whether a relationship exists, for example, between certain strategies for giving information about diagnosis and rate of recovery. The rationale for the proposition is only understood when assumptions underlying it are delineated.

As theorists in nursing become more systematic in their theory development efforts, more explicit assumptions are stated, and fewer assumptions are left implicit. The plethora of literature that has discussed theory critique and theory development should be credited with the constructive changes demonstrated in the updated, further developed, or new theories evolving in nursing. Roy, for example, in further developing her theory, followed a more systematic approach in which she identified assumptions and carefully related many of the concepts to the assumptions, thereby providing theoretical propositions with better potential for testability (Roy and Roberts, 1981).

When identifying the internal structure of a theory, one should use a description that involves a careful search of the inherent assumptions; at the same time, one should not overlook the implicit ones. The more effective theories are those in which authors explicitly state the assumptions guiding their thinking. The more explicit the premises of the theory are, the less ambiguity there is when interpreting its conditions and goals.

The internal structure of a theory could be further described by delineating the concepts upon which the theory is built. Descriptive properties used in relation to concepts are clarity, conceptual definitions, observable properties, and boundaries; concepts are also described as being primitive (*i.e.*, concepts that originated in this particular theory) or derived (*i.e.*, concepts that were derived from other theories). Hage (1972) provided criteria to help determine whether concepts in a theory are primitive or derived. The introduction of a concept in theory with no definition—because the concept has an agreed-upon meaning, has simple definitions, has an intuitively obvious definition, or has been defined elsewhere—designates a primitive concept. The definition of the derived concept is within the theory and is based on the primitive terms. The definitions of the primitive terms are outside the theory (Hage, 1972, pp. 111–115).

The usage of primitive and derived concepts in this book differs from Hage's usage. *Primitive concepts* are those concepts introduced in the theory as new and therefore defined within the theory. *Derived concepts*, on the other hand, are concepts from outside the theory that have taken on a different meaning within the theory. For example, in Meleis (1975), role is a derived concept, and role supplementation is a primitive concept, that is, a new concept with a new definition.

Concepts are also evaluated along the abstract/concrete dimension. The degree of generality determines the abstract/concrete level. The more general a concept is, the more it transcends time and geography, the higher the level of abstraction. Concepts have also been classified along the general variable/nonvariable dimension (Hage, 1972). Nonvariable concepts in nursing are sex, ethnic background, religion, and marital status. Examples of variable concepts (general variables) are sex-role orientation, level of well-being, degree of cultural identity, and level of sick role. It becomes apparent that each nonvariable could be converted into a general variable.

There are several advantages to having general variables (Hage, 1972). General variables allow more precise classification and allow for variations that are more congruent with variations in reality. Classification of a patient as male or female yields some significant data and a certain degree of predictability of structure and function of a few of the biological systems. However, sex-role orientation, a general variable, may help us to more precisely describe clients and predict their patterns of rehabilitation.

Just as assumptions and concepts are delineated, sometimes simultaneously and at other times cyclically, theory propositions also should be delineated and described. A *proposition* is a descriptive statement of the properties and dimensions of a concept or a statement that links two or more concepts together. Propositions provide the theory with the powers of description, explanation, or prediction. A theory that has more assumptions than propositions is a theory with limited power. It indicates that we have to agree to too many conditions for a few descriptions or predictions. If we consider the relationship of assumptions and propositions in a ratio form, an inverse relationship (with the number of propositions being higher than the number of assumptions) allows for more explanatory power.

There are different types of propositions, each type having a different purpose. *Existence propositions* are constructed around one phenomenon and therefore only describe and assert the existence of this one phenomenon. Propositions with the power of explanation, on the other hand, link concepts; therefore, they are expected to have two or more concepts. They are formulated to explain and assert something pertaining to the reality embodied in the theory. These are *relational propositions*, which encompass many types of propositions, such as those that just describe the existence of a relationship, those that describe the direction of such a relationship, and those that can predict the relationship, the direction of the relationship, and the conditions under which that relationship may or may not occur.

Further description of a proposition could be done along dimensions specified by Zetterberg (1963, pp. 69–71). This is best illustrated by using an example of a two-concept proposition derived from Johnson's subsystem theory:

> The higher the level of met functional requirements of the affiliated
> subsystem of the Middle Eastern immigrant, the greater the recovery rate.

A *reversible proposition* would have "and vice versa" at the end of the statement, therefore requiring two testings, one with the condition of "met functional requirements" and prospectively considering recovery rate, and the other beginning with different levels of recovery rate and then retrospectively considering levels of "met functional requirements."

A second dimension is whether the proposition is *deterministic* or *stochastic*. Nursing has a predisposition toward more stochastic propositions that incorporate a probability condition, rather than "if X then always Y," which is deterministic and improbable in a humanistic science. A stochastic proposition, albeit a probabilistic one, would be:

> The higher the level of met functional requirements of the affiliated
> subsystem, the more probable is a greater recovery rate.

A third dimension is whether the proposition is *sequential* or *coexisting*. A sequential proposition assumes that one variable occurred before the other variable. Propositions in nursing lend themselves more to coexisting propositions when describing existing relationships and to sequential propositions when engaged in theorizing about interventions and consequences of intervention. This dimension characterizes theorizing that is central and essential to nursing.

A fourth dimension is demonstrated in the relationships between concepts. This relationship may be sufficient (if X, then Y, regardless of anything else) or contingent (if X, then Y, but only if Z) (Zetterberg, 1963, p. 71). Humanistic sciences cannot strive to produce sufficient propositions. Propositions in nursing theory include numerous variables and probabilistic relationships.

A last dimension identifies whether the relationship is necessary or can be substituted. A necessary relationship is "if X, and only if X, then Y." A substitutable relationship is "if X, then Y; but if Z, then also Y." Like other concepts in nursing, greater recovery rate is contingent on a number of variables and not only on "met functional requirements of one subsystem"; therefore, a substitutable proposition is more appropriate. To increase the explanatory power of such a proposition and then the predictive power, all other concepts related to recovery rate could be identified. For example:

> The higher the level of met functional requirements of the affiliated
> subsystem of the Middle Eastern immigrant, the greater the recovery rate.
> The higher the level of met functional requirements of the aggressive
> subsystem, the greater the recovery rate.

Thus, propositions in nursing may be reversible, stochastic, coexisting, contingent, and substitutable. Attention to each dimension provides for a way to describe the propositions and for deliberately developing propositions along these dimensions; this may help in enhancing the power of contextual explanations, if that is what the theorist wishes to do. This labeling also allows appropriate assessment of the propositions and their power of explanation and predictability. The clarity and systematization of propositions are also considered when we analyze the selected ordering and sequencing of propositions.

This first level of description is structural. The next level involves description of theory in terms of the function of the theory. This level considers the concepts of the nursing domain.

Functional Components

Unlike a structural analysis of a theory, a functional assessment of a theory carefully considers the anticipated consequences of the theory and its purpose. A functional analysis is focused on the relationship between the theory's assumptions, concepts, and propositions and those of the domain. (Again, refer to Table 11-1 for a summary of theory description.)

Concepts of the Domain

Theory is described around questions central to the discipline of nursing, including the following:

○ Who is acted upon? This is the major question that begins to address the function of theory. Does the theory identify the focus of the theory as the client, family, community, or society, or does the theory consider the target as one to the exclusion of others? The target of action here denotes both the target of assessment and the target intervention; the target in nursing should be the client (in the broadest sense) in health or illness.

- ○ What definitions does the theory offer for nursing, client, health, nursing problems, environment, and nurse–patient interactions? Are definitions explicit and clear?
- ○ Does the theory offer a clear idea of what the sources of the nursing problem are, whether the sources lie within or outside of the individual?
- ○ Does the theory provide any insights in the form of intervention for nursing? Are the variables to be manipulated well-delineated? Is it clear what the points of entry are for a nursing intervention? Is the focus of intervention justifiable within the theory? Points of entry could vary from manipulating outside stimuli (Johnson, 1968) to interactions and transactions between client and nurse (King, 1971) to behaviors within systems (Auger, 1976).
- ○ Are there guidelines for intervention modalities? Are they specified? Is there potential for the evolution of such intervention modalities?
- ○ As a nursing theory, does it provide guidelines for the role of the nurse?
- ○ Are the consequences of nurses' actions articulated in the theory? Are they intended or unintended, positive or negative, anticipated and delineated? Is there a plan for dealing with such consequences?

These criteria are generally consistent with those offered by others, including Dickoff, James, and Wiedenbach (1968) and Barnum (1990).

ANALYSIS

Analysis is defined as a process of identifying parts and components and examining them against a number of identified criteria. Analysis includes concept and theory analysis.

Concept Analysis

Concept analysis is a useful process in the cycle of theory development as well as in theory evaluation. Concept analysis may occur at many different points in the process of evaluation and development. Wilson (1969) proposed several steps and techniques in analyzing concepts. These steps do not necessarily have to be completed in this order.

1. Definition, identification, and description of the different dimensions and components of the concept. For example, we proposed "transitions" as a central concept in nursing; we have defined the concept as "those periods in between fairly stable

states, a passage from one life phase, condition, or status to another" (Chick and Meleis, 1986). We have identified some of its components and dimensions as process, disconnectedness, perception of transition, and patterns of response.

2. Comparison of the concept to others with similar properties and dimensions in order to establish its boundaries (Walker and Avant, 1988; Norris, 1982). Transition, for example, can be differentiated from the general concept of change sufficiently to make it useful in alerting nurses to relevant aspects of the life contexts of clients. In this case, transition is seen as a special case of the general phenomenon of change (Chick and Meleis, 1986).

3. Description of some of the antecedents to the concept and of some of the consequences (Lindsey, Piper, and Stotts, 1982), and matching some of these descriptions with what occurs in nursing practice. Examples of antecedents of transition are illness, recovery, loss, birthing; examples of consequences are distress, role performance changes, and disorientation.

4. Development, description, and analysis of exemplars or model cases. This step may include empirical results that are related to the concept.

5. Development, description, and analysis of contrary cases to normative cases. Situations in which the concept appears only occasionally or appears under a new set of conditions are called borderline cases and are also useful in analyzing concepts.

The process of concept analysis may include *semantic analysis*, which is analysis of linguistic meanings of the label given the concept; analysis of *logical derivation*, which is the logical progression of identifying, supporting, and labeling a concept; and *context analysis* of the concept, which includes the conditions under which the concept is manifested. Any inferences about concept should be analyzed for their sources, whether they are logically or empirically derived.

Each one of these steps is a test of the occurrence of the concept. These tests are both conceptual and clinical, but they are not tests as defined by empiricists. They are, however, equally necessary tests and equally important steps in the process of testing concepts that involve the development of empirically valid and reliable research instruments.

Theory Analysis

While concept analysis is a process that could occur early in the process and cycle of theory development and theory testing, theory analysis is a later process. (See Table 11-2 for a comparison of theory analysis and concept analysis.) Theory analysis involves taking into consideration important variables that may have influenced the development of the theory and its current structure. In analyzing theories, consider several criteria: the theorist, paradigmatic origins, and internal

Table 11–2
Analysis

Analysis	Criteria	Units of Analysis
Concepts	Differentiation from others	Definitions
	Semantic	Antecedents
	Logic	Consequences
	Context	Exemplars
Theories	The theorist	Educational background
		Experimental background
		Professional network
		Sociocultural context
	Paradigmatic origins	References, citations
		Assumptions
		Concepts
		Propositions
		Hypotheses
		Laws
	Internal Dimensions	Rationale
		System of relations
		Content
		Beginnings
		Scope
		Goal
		Context
		Abstractness
		Method

dimensions. These criteria provide for a better understanding of choices of central theory questions, goals of theory, the theory phenomena, and strategy of theory development; these criteria also set the stage for the critique.

The Theorist

A comprehensive analysis of theories includes a careful consideration of the author of the theory. Areas for exploration include experiential background, educational background, employment, and reconstruction of the professional and academic networks that surrounded the theorist while the theory was evolving. Such an analysis may include mentors, students, and sponsors when appropriate. This analysis helps in identifying influencing factors on the theory's inception and on its further development. Very often, clarifications in a theory, redefinitions, or extensions are directly or indirectly related to a new mentor relationship, a new degree, an employment move, or other variables that contribute to shifts in orientation.

Analysis helps to uncover external and internal factors influencing a theorist, such as the beliefs held by the theorist, the patterns of reasoning, and their origins. This may lead to a better understanding of the human parameters involved in theory development, an essential component of a historicist's conception of science (Silva and Rothbart, 1984).

This segment of analysis could be done in a number of different ways, including through a review of all that has been written by the theorist and all that has been written by others about the theorist, through direct communication with the theorist, and through communication with mentors and students. A review may also focus on only one aspect or more of the theorist (Fulton, 1987). Analyzing the theorist's background will help to clarify internal dimensions, which follows as the next order of business in analyzing theories.

Consideration of who the theorists are as people, as nurses, as educators, as clinicians, and as theorists was the subject of analyses during the 1980s. These analyses took the form of short reviews (for example, Marriner-Tomey, 1989) or elaborate videotapes (see Chapter 19). These analyses are indications of the value the discipline places on the contributions of these theorists, the significance of knowing the theorist behind the theory for further understanding of the theory and for enhancing the potential for others to model their theoretical work and actions.

Paradigmatic Origins of Theory

Theoretical thinking in nursing evolves from a prototype theory or can be traced to theories utilized in other fields. Examples of such theories are those of Johnson, who derived her theory from the premises of the systems paradigm (Parsons, 1949; Riehl and Roy, 1980, pp. 207–216) and Paterson and Zderad (1988), who based their work on the existentialist philosophy. Therefore, for a careful consideration of this component, the theory analyst should become conversant with paradigmatic origins of the theory under consideration and address those origins in the analysis.

To identify the paradigm from which the theory may have evolved or other theories that may have influenced the development of the current theory, the review considers the following:

References, bibliography provided;
Background of theorist, educationally and experientially; and
Sociocultural context that may have influenced the development of
the theory.

Analysis of the theory in relationship to these components provides answers to three major questions:

1. Is the theory derived from and built upon a specific paradigm?
2. What are the origins of the paradigm?
3. Why was this particular paradigm used?

More specifically, on what prototype theory or paradigm did the theorist build the conceptual structures? How extensively is the original paradigm or theory used?

Is the use of paradigm obvious to the reviewer, made explicit or implicit by the writer? Does the theorist present the rationale for selection of the theory or parts of the theory used? From where do theory inadequacies originate, prototype theory or nursing theory? Are the problems detected those of borrowed theory or are they the result of translation? Does nursing theory improve on prototype theory? How congruent or incongruent is the use of components of prototype theory with nursing theory? How different or similar are the definitions to prototype theory definitions? Are goals the same? Is justification for variance included? Are there other nursing theories derived from the prototype theory? What are they?

Internal Dimensions

The components of the internal structure act as guidelines to describe a theory, as discussed under Theory Description. Dimensions described in this section help in analyzing theories to enhance understanding of the approaches used to develop the theory, in delineating gaps in the theory, and in giving perspective to why some omissions are not necessarily gaps in the theory but in some instances are merely what the theory intended to be. This will soon become clear. The dimensions described next provide the necessary lexicon to describe a theory.

The first dimension to consider is the *rationale upon which the theory is built*. Questions to consider in describing the theory along this dimension include: Are components of the theory united in a chain-link fashion? Is it a theory of the factor type? Is the theory developed around concepts and thus a concatenated theory? Or is it based on certain sets of relationships that are deduced from a small set of basic principles and therefore hierarchical in nature? The concatenated theory has fewer explanations that converge on a central point and therefore embodies existence propositions, whereas the set of relationships theory embodies an interpretive model (Kaplan, 1964).

The second dimension to consider is that of *system of relations*. Questions to be asked are: Do relations explain elements or do elements explain relations? A monadic approach in theory construction considers single irreducible units, as opposed to a field approach, which considers its unit of analysis in terms of a number of other mini-units. An example of the monadic approach is cell theory, and an example of the field approach is a theory of personality in terms of roles. A monadic approach is one in which the attributes and properties of the phenomenon are the focus of the theory. A field approach focuses on the relationships between the phenomena and thus explains the phenomena by the relationships. Therefore, a theory of a human being as a subsystem of behavior would be monadic and a theory of human environmental interaction would be a field theory.

Content of the theory is a third descriptive dimension (Kaplan, 1964). Content is distinguished by the range of laws and group of individuals to which the theory refers. A theory could be classified as molar or macrotheory, or as molecular or microtheory. Organizational theories in sociology are macro in content, whereas role theory is micro. This dimension considers the range of relationships in the theory and the set of individuals to which the relationships refer. When a theory considers the human being in totality, it is a macrotheory. When the theory addresses needs during illness, it is a microtheory. Therefore, Rogers' work (1970) is an example of macrotheory whereas Orem's (1985) is an example of microtheory.

At what point a theorist begins articulating ideas and whether a theorist addresses a theory of extant nursing practice or one of ideal nursing practice specifies another dimension, namely that of *theory beginnings* (Kaplan, 1964). A constructive beginning is hypothetical and is intended to build up a picture of more complex phenomena, whereas a principle theory beginning is more empirically grounded (discovered). A theory with a constructive beginning tends to be more complete, clear, and adaptable and tends to consider relationships hypothetically; the latter is more analytical and addresses the "is" rather than the "ought to be." It is more perfect and better substantiated.

A theory with a constructive beginning is also called a deductive theory because it emphasizes a conceptual structure deduced from another conceptual structure (Duffey and Muhlenkamp, 1974). Its laws are logically interrelated. It is through such deductive logic that some theories are derived. The major criticism of deductive theories is the lack of empirical support until they are tested in research. The principle theory beginning is also called the inductive beginning. It, on the other hand, consists essentially of summary statements or empirical relations. An example of the former (deductive theory) in nursing is Rogers' (1970) theoretical conceptualization of man in his symphonic harmony with the environment. Her theory evolved from principles of physics, thermodynamics, and evolution, among others. An example of the latter (inductive theory) is a conceptualization of issues surrounding dying, evolving from Glaser and Strauss's (1965) and Benoliel's (1967) work, even though these have not been formally labeled as nursing theory.

Many theorists have addressed the *scope of theory* and its significance in describing the capability of the theory. The basic question that considers a theory's scope is: How many of the basic problems in nursing or any of its specialities could be addressed by the same theory? The significance of scope stems from the notion that theories having wider scope tend to be more general and last longer (Kuhn, 1970). In addition, the significance of a theory increases as its scope broadens (Ellis, 1968). Therefore, to answer questions related to scope, we also address generality. Theories with a very wide scope are also called "grand theories," as opposed to "single-domain theories," which could be placed at the other end of a scope continuum.

The major criticism associated with both ends of the scope continuum (*i.e.*, grand theories and single-domain theories) involves the attempts of grand theories to explain everything surrounding a set of phenomena, which is also why they may be limited in their power to explain (a major criticism of Parsons' (1949) attempts at a theory of sociology). *Single-domain theories* address only simple, abstract, isolated facts and principles. The empiricist and methodologist, Robert Merton (1964), is credited with advocating middle-range theories, thus avoiding those criticisms. *Middle-range theories* consider a limited number of variables, have a particular substantive focus, focus on a limited aspect of relationship, are more susceptible to empirical testing, and could be consolidated into more wide-ranging theories.

In nursing, Jacox (1974), following Merton's ideas, urged the development of middle-range theories for limited aspects within the discipline of nursing, such as pain alleviation or promotion of sleep. A major criticism of middle-range theories is that they lead to fragmentation of a discipline when the discipline has no agreed-upon phenomenon. Middle-range theories are more appropriate now in nursing, particularly after we have identified and broadly agreed upon the boundaries of nursing knowledge and nursing domain concepts.

Questions to ask when considering the *goal of a theory* are: Why was the theory developed? What is its aim and intent? Theories are constructed to describe, to explain, to predict, or to prescribe. A descriptive theory gives information related to phenomena under consideration but does not make a claim beyond that, nor does it tell us what to expect in the future. When a beginning linkage and description of relationships between derived concepts are provided, the theory becomes an explanatory theory. Correlative studies to test explanatory theories provide empirical evidence in support of these theories. Another goal explicated in some theories is that of prediction. A predictive theory encompasses propositions of an "if . . . then" nature in a consequential manner. The ultimate goal in nursing is to prescribe; therefore, prescription is another theory goal. Theories might have all of these goals, or they may explicate only one goal or another. At this time in the developmental history of nursing theory, it is essential that a theory represent each of the goals.

The *context of a theory*, in which the central phenomenon is addressed, is yet another dimension for theory evaluation. Johnson (1959) called attention to the need in nursing for theories addressing knowledge of order, knowledge of disorder, and knowledge of control. The knowledge of order addresses phenomena that are central to objects, events, and interactions in a healthy context. They describe regularities in such phenomena. They describe the normal state and natural scheme of things. They provide baseline data. An example of such knowledge is provided by Auger (1976) in her explication of Johnson's (1968) normal patterns of a person's behavior within systems of behavior. Knowledge of disorder, on the other hand, recognizes a context of disorder within which nurses deal. An attempt to develop such knowledge, not yet bound together in a theoretical schema, was manifested in the first conference on classification of nursing diagnosis (Gebbie, 1976) and in subsequent conferences. To prescribe a course of action that, when implemented, could change the sequence of events in a desired way is to have knowledge of control. Examples of theories addressing such knowledge are Orem's self-care theory (1979) and Meleis (1975) and Meleis, Swendsen, and Jones' role supplementation (1980) theories, among others. Theories could also address knowledge of process, which includes the nursing process and nurse–patient interactions (Paterson and Zderad, 1988).

Abstractness, another theory dimension, is evaluated by length of reduction and deduction between its propositions. A highly abstract theory requires more steps to reduce the chain "connecting the theoretical terms with the observable ones" (Kaplan, 1964, p. 301). It is a theory with wide spaces between its propositions and a conceptual schema that is highly removed from reality but still pertains to it. If abstractness is put on a continuum from high abstractness to low abstractness, Rogers and Johnson would be at the high end and Orem at the low end.

Finally, the *method of theory development* should be carefully assessed. Barnum (1990) proposed that there are four methods utilized in developing theories. One can assess these methods by considering the reasoning upon which the theory is built, the system of action, and the plan for progression. A dialectical method is exemplified by Rogers' work (Barnum, 1990) and is based on Hegel's dialectical process. It speaks to the fusion of opposites (Newman, 1979). It emphasizes relationship with a whole and, in fact, each whole explains parts and each part is a whole explaining other parts. A dialectical method encompasses contradictions, apposition, and dilemmas, but order evolves out of the interaction among all of them. Erickson's developmental theory (1963) is an example of resolution of conflict and crisis in the process of moving into the next level of development. A dialectical method defies Aristotelian logic, which is another method of theory development—the logical method. This is a method in which the parts are organized to describe the whole systematically and categorically. A theory of this nature offers a description of each part, and the whole is more and different than the sum total of all parts. Barnum (1990) considers the theories of Johnson and Roy in this category.

The other two methods of theory development, according to Barnum (1990), are problem theories and operational theories. Both appeal more to common sense, use persuasion in supporting ideas, and utilize their experiences in theory development. Problem theories (Henderson, 1966; Nursing Theories Conference Group, 1980) are organized around nursing problems, while operational theories (Orem, 1985) are organized around methods of intervention.

CRITIQUE OF THEORY

Critique is defined by *Webster's Third New International Dictionary* as "critical examination or estimate of a thing or situation with the view to determining its nature and limitations or its conformity to standards."* Several criteria are essential in critiquing theory. These are relationships between structure and function, diagram of theory, circle of contagiousness, usefulness, and external components. Each is defined and presented below.

Relationship Between Structure and Function

In critiquing a theory according to criteria listed next, the critic considers the relationship between the structure and the function (Table 11-3). This is accomplished by making a critical assessment and judgment of the relationship between the different components of the theory, such as assumptions, concepts, propositions, and domain concepts. In doing so, the critic cannot judge the logic inherent in the development of a dialectic theory by the same criteria used when judging a

---

* By permission. From *Webster's Third New International Dictionary* ©1986 by Merriam-Webster Inc., publisher of the Merriam-Webster® dictionaries.

Table 11–3
Theory Critique—Relationship between Structure and Function;
Diagram of Theory; and Circle of Contagiousness

Criteria	Units of Analysis
Relationship between structure and function	Clarity
	Consistency
	Simplicity/complexity
	Tautology
	Teleology
Diagram of theory	Visual and graphic presentation
	Logical representation
	Clarity
Circle of contagiousness	Geographical origin of theory and geographical spread
	Influence of theorist versus theory

logical theory; rather, the method used dictates the critique. Several criteria could be taken into consideration, such as clarity, consistency, simplicity/complexity, and tautology/teleology.

Clarity
Clarity is defined on a continuum ranging from high to low. It denotes precision of boundaries, a communication of a sense of orderliness, vividness of meaning, and consistency throughout the theory. Clarity is also defined by Chinn and Jacobs (1987) as "lucidness and consistency" (p. 137). Clarity is demonstrated in assumptions, concepts, and propositions as well as in domain concepts. To have clarity in concepts is to have theoretical and operational definitions that are consistent throughout the theory, are presented in a parsimonious way, and are consistent with theory assumptions and propositions. Questions such as, Are concepts operationally defined? and Do they seem to have content and construct validity?, help to determine concept clarity. Propositional clarity is manifested in a coherent and logical presentation of propositions and systematic linkages between the theory concepts. The criterion of clarity varies within a range from high clarity to low clarity.

Consistency
The boundaries between clarity and consistency are not easily determined. The degree to which a congruency exists between the different components of a theory describes its consistency. The fit between assumptions and concept definitions, between concepts as defined and their use in propositions, and between concepts and clinical exemplars can all be considered determinants of consistency.

Simplicity/Complexity

Another criterion with which to critique a theory is its level of simplicity/complexity. The more phenomena the theory considers, the more potential relationships it could generate, and the more complex the theory is (Ellis, 1968). Simplicity of a theory is more desirable if it focuses on fewer concepts and few relationships that may enhance its utility. Complexity of a theory may be a desirable criterion if the complexity enhances the number of explanations and predictions the theory offers. Therefore, simplicity in the face of very complex contextual reality is as unadvisable as complexity in theory would be when the theory explains a limited number of relationships. Chinn and Jacobs (1987) advocate simplicity in theory that has been tested and as a means for generating ideas and hypotheses, but question the value of simplicity in untested theory.

Tautology/Teleology

Clarity, consistency, and simplicity/complexity of a theory could also be described through tautology and teleology. A general assessment of *tautology*—the needless repetition of an idea in different parts of the theory—is considered. Tautology decreases the clarity of the theory. A careful consideration of causes and consequences, which are kept separate, avoids teleology. *Teleology* occurs when the definition of concepts, conditions, and events uses consequences rather than properties and dimensions. When defining concepts by consequences only, the theorist introduces new concepts to define existing ones. This practice leaves the original concept undefined. Teleology is another dimension in the relationship between structure and function. The critic, therefore, should consider questions such as: Does the theory have logical coherence? Are definitions of nursing phenomena concise? Is it a teleological theory?

Diagram of Theory

Clarity of theories and models are further enhanced by visual representation of the theory. Major questions to be addressed in relation to this component are: Was the theory visually and graphically presented? Did graphic presentation enhance understanding of different components of the theory? More specifically: How clear is the visual representation? Is it an accurate representation of the text? Does it include major concepts? Are linkages clear? Are linkage directions indicated? Is representation logical? Are there overlaps? Are there gaps? Is representation a substitute for words and explanation or is it a supplementation? Is the diagram clear and well-defined? Is there a correspondence between diagram and concepts and propositions in the text? Do the diagrams enhance understanding of the text?

Circle of Contagiousness

The final test of any theory is whether or not it is adopted by others (Table 11-3). The units of analysis here are geographical location and type of institution. Theories in nursing have been utilized within the geographical areas from which they emanated. Rogers' theory is used at New York University and tested by Rogers' students;

Johnson's is used in Los Angeles and tested by her students. Therefore, when the theory begins to cross several concentric circles from its origin, its circle of contagiousness increases, and we can infer that the theory is receiving more acceptability, uninfluenced by the theorist.

The critic should review the literature, indexes, and citations for answers to questions such as: Where has the theory been used or where is it being used both geographically and institutionally? What is it used for (research, education, administration, clinical practice, etc.)? How influential was the theorist in prompting the implementation of the theory? Where was it first introduced? What happened in the interim? Has the theory been considered and utilized crossculturally and transculturally? A critique of the circle of contagiousness of a theory is made in conjunction with the usefulness of theory.

Usefulness

A critique of the usefulness of a theory encompasses four areas: its potential for usefulness in practice, research, education, and administration. (Table 11-4):

Usefulness in Practice

A thorough review and assessment of theory has to consider its potential for operationalization and utilization in nursing practice. A practitioner who is considering utilizing a theory in some practice area should assess the theory in terms of its function: its goals, consequences, and potential for practice. Therefore, the theory should be able to respond to these questions or have a framework to help the clinician respond to them: Does the theory provide enough direction to affect

Table 11–4
Theory Critique—Usefulness

Criteria	Units of Analysis
Practice	Direction
	Applicability
	Generalizability
	Cost-effectiveness
	Relevance
Research	Consistency
	Testability
	Predictability
Education	Philosophical statement
	Objectives
	Concepts
Administration	Structure of care
	Organization of care
	Guidelines for patient care
	Patient classification system

practice? Does it have a framework for prescription? Does the theory include abstract notions that are not applicable to practice? Does the level of abstraction or understandability render it applicable or inapplicable? Does the theory cover all areas of nursing? Should it? Does the theory currently apply to practice? Who pays for utilization of the theory in practice? Is it cost-effective? Is it a timely nursing practice theory? In other words, does it have relevance for the way nursing is practiced today? Where does the theory fit in terms of nursing process? Is the theory understandable to the practitioner? What is the assessment of practitioners of the theory as to its uniqueness and its esoteric language? To what extent can we manipulate its phenomena? How does it relate to diagnosis-related groups (DRGs)?

Usefulness in Research

The *raison d'etre* of theories is to guide and be guided by research; therefore, a critique of a theory should include questions related to assessment of a theory's potential for testability. The concepts and propositions should eventually be related in a consistent manner to a systematic set of observable or testable data. Otherwise, if a theory remains untested, its usefulness is in question. Schrag (1967) emphasizes the significance of a theory's potential for research, which he calls "the empirical adequacy" of a theory, and this potential is realized through congruence between "theoretical claims and empirical evidence." He asserts that credibility refers to the "goodness of fit between claims and existing evidence, while predictability estimates how well the claims will hold true in the future" (Schrag, 1967, p. 250).

Theories are established on current information; it usually is up to the future to provide evidence that corroborates them or demands their information. Although the aim of research is not to establish the absolute truth of the theoretical propositions, it is essential that it begins to indicate a degree of confidence based on empirical evidence. It is noteworthy that, to any unsophisticated reviewer, any supportive corroboration between theory and data uncovered through research is bound to give support to the entire theory structure, however premature that might be. The reverse could also be true. Therefore, the type and extent of empirical corroboration should be skeptically considered by answering several questions, including: What specific theory propositions did the research consider? Were these central or peripheral propositions? Was the research undertaken to provide empirical validity to concepts or relationships? Was theory used to generate testable propositions or to interpret findings? Were explicit theory assumptions considered in designing methodology?

While it is significant to the theory critique to note that theories are tested on a piecemeal basis, the critic should still consider finding responses to the following questions: Does the theory build on previous research? Was research done using the theory? What propositions were being tested? How reproducible is the research? Can the findings be generalized? What research designs have been used? Why? How appropriate are they? Can prescriptive and predictive (experimental and quasi-experimental) studies be designed? Are the research results relevant to other fields? Is the research used appropriately? Do the theories state what research is to be completed to support central theory propositions?

The research potential or testability of a theory should not be critiqued lightly. As Berthold (1968) and Ellis (1968) stressed, the ultimate criteria for evaluating a theory's usefulness are whether it generates predictions or propositions concerning relevant events and whether it stimulates new observations and insights that could subsequently be corroborated. Units of analysis for testability are theoretical and operational definitions, theoretical propositions, availability of references in nursing reality, ongoing research, and completed research.

Has there been empirical verification of its properties? How consistent are its propositions with other theories and laws? Is there evidence for corroboration (Schrag, 1967)? Finally, one can detect any spuriousness in the theory's components as manifested in logical or research determination of whether or not dependent variables are potentially related to other independent variables.

Usefulness for Education

The beginning evaluation of nursing theories for their potential to offer guidelines for nursing curricula and programs coincided almost completely with the development of most of the theories that we now consider to be nursing theories. In fact, as we analyze the rationales and the goals of a good number of the nursing theorists, nursing education invariably prompted the search for a coherent presentation of what nursing is about. Nursing theories grew out of dissatisfaction with what Barnum (1990) called the disease/body systems curriculum model. Invariably, a growing uneasiness prompted a shift to a needs-orientation, such as that offered by Henderson (1966) and Abdellah (1969), and with it a rejection of biological systems of the diseases as a framework. Unfortunately, the shift to a nursing conceptualization was a premature one because it occurred simultaneously with the theory being developed, and therefore many faculty members suffered from the pitfalls of the developing theory.

The National League for Nursing criteria for a conceptual framework to guide curricula was both a blessing and a menace to our curricula. The blessing was the reorientation of faculty to nursing theory, while the menace emanated from the prematurity of the use of nursing theories. Nursing theories could provide the major premises upon which a curriculum is built, yet I believe that it is not feasible to develop an entire program on just one conceptualization of nursing. For example, theories about teaching and learning, about the learner, and about the environment are complementary to nursing conceptualizations.

Usefulness in Administration

Use of nursing theory in administration is considered in terms of the structure and organization of care. Theories ought to provide the potential for guiding and describing nursing care. Nursing theories are expected to guide care of clients and are not expected to provide the administrator with guidelines for administration or for leadership style. Analysis shows how useful theory can be for provision of guidelines in patient care on a large scale. Does it help the patient classification system? How congruent is the mission of nursing as articulated by theory with the mission as articulated by different nursing organizations? Does the theory provide any specific guidelines for theory implementation on an organizational scale? Does it provide assistance in determining criteria for quality control?

Other criteria for evaluation of theories for nursing administration were identified by Buchanan (1987). These include the congruency of theory with professional standards such as licensing requirements, as well as standards stipulated by such accrediting bodies as the American Nurses Association and the American Hospital Association. Theories selected by administrators should also be congruent with the legal structure governing nursing functions in the different countries.

External Components

Finally, the theory should be assessed against several external criteria. These are: personal values, other professional values, social values, and social significance (Table 11-5).

Personal Values
Ellis (1968) and Johnson (1987) emphasized the importance of recognizing values inherent in theories and in making them explicit. A critical consideration of values should account for those values of the theorist and the critic. In the latter, the fit between the theorist's and critic's personal and professional values should be considered. It is through such careful assessment that biases can be delineated.

Congruence With Other Professional Values
A similar assessment of the values espoused in the theory should be made of the values of other professions. Health care professionals will be able to enhance patient care through collaboration and complementarity of value systems. Awareness of such complementarity or competition in professional values enhances the potential of the development of a collaborative working schema to close the professional value gaps (Johnson, 1974).

Table 11–5
Theory Critique—External Components of Theory

Criteria	Units of Analysis
Personal values	Theorist implicit/explicit values
	Critic implicit/explicit values
Congruence with other professional values	Complementarity
	Esotericism
	Competition
Congruence with social values	Beliefs
	Values
	Customs
Social significance	Value to humanity

Congruence With Social Values
Beliefs, values, and expectations of different societies and cultures within societies shape and direct the type of theory that is most useful. Although self-help, self-care (at its different levels), and individuality are goals congruent with some cultures' value systems, they are the antithesis of those espoused in others. Therefore, theories with such goals and consequences would be incongruent and inappropriate to some societies and should be avoided. Careful critical assessment of societal values and theory values is an integral part of a thorough theory critique. Questions should be addressed such as: Is the role of the nurse within the model congruent with the role of the nurse as perceived by society? Are actions and outcomes congruent with societal expectations of nursing? (Johnson, 1974; 1987)

Social Significance
In our attempt to enhance nursing science and articulate the discipline of nursing, we must not neglect the significance of its practice to humanity and society. The philanthropic Bacon's profound words of the 18th century still hold true today:

> Lastly, I would address one general admonition to all; that they consider what are the true ends of knowledge, and that they seek it not either for pleasure of mind, or for contention, or for superiority to others, or for profit, or fame, or power, or any of these inferior things, but for the benefit and use of life; and that they perfect and govern it in charity. For it was from lust of power that the angels fell, from lust of knowledge that man fell; but of charity there can be no excess, neither did angel or man ever come in danger by it. (Bacon, in Ravetz, 1971, p. 436)

A critic philosophically should ask whether the goals and consequences of theory make a substantial and valued difference in lives of people. (Consider questions from the perspective of clients and from the perspective of other health professionals.) The critic should also ask whether intended and unintended consequences are carefully considered (Johnson, 1974; 1987).

THEORY TESTING

The definition of theory testing has been the subject of questioning in nursing (Chinn, 1984; Chinn, 1986; Silva, 1990). It has also been equated with evaluation of theories and considered the most significant goal in developing, accepting, and utilizing theories. It is considered here as one component of theoretical evaluation of the discipline. To equate testing with evaluation and to consider it the only significant goal for theory development is to ignore all the descriptive, analytical, and critical commentaries on theories that have been published and that have added to our understanding of theories and are significant for knowledge development. (Refer to writings in *Advances in Nursing Science, Nursing Outlook, American Journal of Nursing,* and *Journal of Advanced Nursing* during 1970–1980 for extensive examples of writings describing, analyzing, and critiquing theories and theoretical thoughts.) To equate testing with evaluation is also to reduce theoretical knowledge to the context of justification and to exclude the context of discovery with its process orientation.

Theory testing is a systematic process of subjecting theoretical propositions to the rigor of research in all its forms and approaches, and consequently the use of the results to modify or refine the research propositions. Theory testing presumes the complete cyclical relationship between theory, research, and theory. Theory testing is neither a static process nor an end result. The dynamic testing process begins with theory development and continues with testing and more development of theory, pausing long enough to reflect and go through the cycle again.

Theory testing is not a single entity. It has many dimensions needing many different approaches. Silva (1990) reviewed tests of nursing theories and identified four perspectives: tests to verify theories through empirical methods; tests to verify theories through personal experiences; tests to verify theories through analysis; and tests to verify theories through practical application. Earlier, in a review of 62 studies in which the use of theories of Johnson, Roy, Orem, and Rogers guided the studies, Silva (1986) found three ways in which theory testing was used. In 24 studies, there was a *minimal* use of the theory other than in identifying it as a framework for the study. She labeled 29 of the studies, which used the theories as a way to organize their review of literature or to select their instruments, as *insufficient*. Only 9 of the 62 studies qualified in the third category of *adequate* use of theories. These were studies in which the hypothesis testing and findings were integral to the theory and actually provided evidence to modify, accept, or reject theory propositions.

Silva proposed the third category as the type of test that should be the goal for nurses in the development of the discipline. She further attributed this lack of empirical testing to the pressure on nurse investigators to use a conceptual framework for their studies without clear guidelines on what is involved in testing, to the highly abstract theories and lack of precise measures and the subsequent "lack of tolerance to methodological imperfections," and finally to an inability to systematically retrieve theory-based research.

Testing of theory should include proposition testing as defined by Silva (1986). However, considering the type of theories that nurses are continuously developing, that is, theories that illuminate the discipline, it would be inadvisable at any point in the developmental process of a discipline that is based on human science, to limit its investigative powers to a narrow view of theory testing. Currently, there are at least six approaches to theory testing in nursing. These are:

1. Testing the utility of nursing theory: Research developed to evaluate the use of theory in practice, teaching, or administration falls under this category. Units of analysis for this category are the individual nurse, teacher, student, or administrator. The intent of this type of research is to determine the feasibility of the use of theory by the group of individuals using the theory. This research

tests the learner's ability to recall, comprehend, evaluate, and use the theory. Results of such tests relate to and enhance adult learning theories or cognitive theories rather than nursing practice theories (*e.g.*, Jacobson, 1984).

A variation of this category is testing the difference between the use of the different existing theories. Jacobson (1984), for example, used a semantic differential scale to define some of the differences among King, Orem, Rogers, Roy, and Wiedenbach theories as perceived by users. Eight factors emerged to account for 49% to 56% of the variation between the theories as perceived by users. The factors are sophistication, dynamism, clarity, usefulness, focus, utility, scope, and scientific rigor. This approach to testing a model was critiqued conceptually and methodologically by Nicoll, Meyer, and Abraham (1985). Pertinent to the current discussion, suffice it to say that, in their view, nursing models are to be evaluated individually in terms of their content. An external evaluation, from their perspective, is incongruent with the nature of models as specific to a certain context and thus ineffectual in advancing nursing knowledge.

Tests designed to compare the feasibility of implementing different theories are useful if they are problem- and context-specific. For example, using Johnson's theory and King's theory to assess and diagnose the nursing care needs of an immigrant patient undergoing a kidney transplant, then comparing the processes and contents of assessment, could help in understanding learners' abilities to use the theories and to compare the efficiency and effectiveness of the theories in defining the priority needs of the patient.

2. Testing propositions from other disciplines: Research in this category is designed to test propositions from theories that were developed in other disciplines. Nursing literature has numerous examples of this type of research. Tests related to theory utilization also fall under this category because they are designed to address proposition related to educational theory. Other examples are research to test propositions evolving from systems theory, adaptation theory, role theory, and stress theory. An example of a test of theories from other disciplines is that of Maslow's theory (Davis-Sharts, 1986).

3. Testing propositions from other disciplines as they relate to nursing: Research in this category involves, more specifically, testing propositions as they relate to a nursing phenomenon or testing propositions that are of interest to nursing. Examples of this research include studies designed to test role strain in nursing faculty (Meter and Agronow, 1982; O'Shea, 1982) and in women

(Woods, 1985a, 1985b), based on role theory, and studies to test concepts from other disciplines (Wewers and Lenz, 1987).

4. Testing nursing concepts: Research in this category is designed to develop a measurable concept by identifying corresponding variables. The objective of testing in this category is to develop a valid and reliable means by which the concept is tested. Validity means that the instrument, the tool, or the means by which the concept is measured indeed measures that concept, and the extent to which it is used provides data compatible with other relevant evidence (Diers, 1979). Reliability means that these instruments consistently measure the same concept. The development of valid and reliable instruments, tools, or means by which concepts could be measured is one of the priorities in the development and testing of nursing theories. Examples include Lush, Janson-Bjerklie, Carrieri, and Lovejoy (1988); Nield, Kim, and Patel (1989); Carrieri, Janson-Bjerklie, and Jacobs (1984), and Derdiarian and Forsythe (1983).

5. Testing nursing propositions: Research in this category is designed to test theoretical propositions that are derived from nursing theories. There are three major types of propositions tested in nursing:

   ○ Existence propositions: These relate two or more concepts to demonstrate their existence. Research designed to test existence of propositions merely demonstrates that the two concepts exist concurrently. Descriptive studies of levels of self-care of oncology patients are one example, others may relate levels of self-care to degree of anxiety. Correlational tests are most suitable analytical models for this type of research.
   ○ Predictive propositions: Tests designed to explore predictive propositions demonstrate the effect of one concept on another. Such propositions are modeled after the question: What will happen if . . . ? For example, studies designed to test interactional theories propositions asked: What will happen if patients are given an opportunity to express their feelings of anxiety before surgery? (Dumas and Leonard, 1963)
   ○ Prescriptive propositions: Research designed to test nursing interventions use principles from evaluation research. The objective is to find out how effective is the intervention in bringing about the desired goals. Examples are Smith (1986) who tested Rogers' principle of integrality and Mentzer and Schorr (1986) who tested Newman's proposition linking situational control and perception of duration of time.

6. Testing through interpretation: Theory may also be tested by using it as a framework for interpretation. This may support, refine, or extend a theory.

CONCLUSION

Theory development and evaluation are cyclical, continuous, and dynamic processes. One cannot exist without the other. Theory evaluation includes description, concept analysis, theory critique, and theory testing. These processes are based on the view that science is a human process that includes not only valid findings but also observations, agreements, useful solutions to problems, and the theorists, their experiences and credibility.

Theory evaluation is central to the development of theory; it is the responsibility of every clinician, academician, and administrator. If each does her share, we are then assured of the continuous growth of a body of knowledge to guide research and practice.

The theory evaluation model provided here could be used as a whole or in parts to evaluate theories. One evaluator could not complete a full theory evaluation by using all components of the model. An evaluator may choose to focus on any one of description, analysis, critique, or testing or on one part of any of these components. A careful analysis of the theorist and her contributions is as valuable in advancing knowledge as testing one proposition of a theory. Each offers members of the discipline different findings. Analyses focused on the theorist provide strategies for the development of theories and theorists, as well as forces and constraints that promote scholarship. Tests focused on accepting or rejecting propositions or generating propositions help in explaining, describing, and predicting substantive content of the field.

Despite the many critics who have been skeptical of Kuhn's attempts to delineate criteria that govern choices of good theory and have labeled them as futile, and because "the decision of a scientific group to adopt a new paradigm cannot be based on good reasons of any kind, factual or otherwise," (Shapere, 1966) Kuhn continued to assert that, indeed, we can delineate such criteria and that accuracy, consistency, broad scope, simplicity, and fruitfulness in research are essential as objective criteria for judging competing theories (Kuhn, 1977, p. 321). However, Kuhn also maintained that "every individual's choice between competing theories depends on a mixture of objective and subjective factors, or of shared and individual criteria." (p. 325) The subjective factors are based on idiosyncratic factors and are therefore dependent on individuals' preferences and personalities. Both subjective and objective factors have a place in our understanding of the philosophy of science.

The discussion provided here emphasized the objective criteria. It provided criteria for theory description, analysis, critique, and testing in an attempt to decrease the margin of subjectivity and to enhance that of objectivity. The goal is not to avoid subjectivity altogether, but to give objective criteria a fair chance. The model of theory critique (Fig. 11-1) is designed not only to provide the basis for understanding the internal structure of theory but also the social, intellectual, and structural context that surrounds its development. It delineates a comprehensive framework for all the norms and parameters against which theories ought to be analyzed and critiqued.

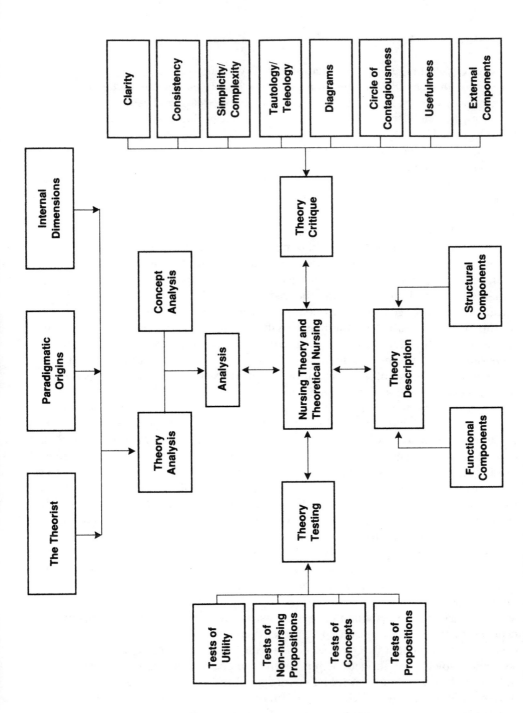

Figure 11-1. A model for theory evaluation.

When using the delineated criteria for evaluating theories, it is important to note that theories may be superior in some points and evolving in other aspects. No one theory will satisfy or be able to address all criteria. Styles of inquiry and personal preferences for theory design affect the configuration and function of theory. Throughout the analysis, one should not lose track of the ultimate purpose of theory, which is to systematize data and provide its users with a unique insight into the matter at hand. Nor should we underestimate the test of time. It is finally the temporal dimension that will determine which theory is adequate and useful and therefore survives and dominates.

REFERENCES

Abdellah, F.G. (1969, September-October) The nature of nursing science. *Nursing Research*, 18, 390–393.

Auger, J.R. (1976) *Behavioral systems and nursing*. Englewood Cliffs, NJ: Prentice-Hall.

Benoliel, J.Q. (1967) *The nurse and the dying patient*. New York: Macmillan.

Berthold, F.S. (1968) Symposium on theory development in nursing. *Nursing Research*, 17(3), 196–197.

Buchanan, B.F. (1987) Conceptual models: An assessment framework. *Journal of Nursing Administration*, 17(10), 22–26.

Carrieri, V.K., Janson-Bjerklie, S.J., and Jacobs, S. (1984) The sensation of dyspnea: A review. *Heart and Lung: The Journal of Critical Care*, 13(4), 436–447.

Chick, N. and Meleis, A.I. (1986) Transitions: A nursing concern. In P.L. Chinn (Ed.), *Nursing research methodology*. Boulder, CO: Aspen.

Chinn, P.L. (1984) From the editor. *Advances in Nursing Science*, 6(2), ix.

Chinn, P.L. (1986) From the editor. *Advances in Nursing Science*, 6(2), viii.

Chinn, P.L. and Jacobs, M.K. (1987) *Theory and nursing: A systematic approach*. St. Louis: C.V. Mosby.

Davis-Sharts, J. (1986) An empirical test of Maslow's theory of need hierarchy using hologeistic comparison by statistical sampling. *Advances in Nursing Science*, 9(1), 58–72.

Derdiarian, A.K. and Forsythe, A.B. (1983) An instrument for theory and research development using the behavioral systems model for nursing: The cancer patient. Part 2. *Nursing Research*, 32(5), 260–266.

Dickoff, J., James, P., and Wiedenbach, E. (1968) Theory in practice discipline: Part 1. Practice oriented theory. *Nursing Research*, 17(5), 415–435.

Diers, D. (1979) *Research in nursing practice*. Philadelphia: J.B. Lippincott.

Duffey, M. and Muhlenkamp, A.F. (1974) A framework for theory analysis. *Nursing Outlook*, 22(9), 570–574.

Dumas, R.G. and Leonard, R.C. (1963) The effect of nursing on the incidence of postoperative vomiting. *Nursing Research*, 12(1), 12–15.

Ellis, R. (1968) Characteristics of significant theories. *Nursing Research*, 17(3), 217–222.

Erikson, E. (1963) *Childhood and society* (2nd ed.). New York: W.W. Norton.

Fawcett, J. (1988) *Analysis and evaluation of conceptual models of nursing*. Philadelphia: F.A. Davis.

Fulton, J.S. (1987) Virginia Henderson: Theorist, prophet, poet. *Advances in Nursing Science*, 10(1), 1–17.

Gebbie, K. (Ed.) (1976, March 4–7) *Summary of the second national conference: Classification of nursing diagnosis.* 1310 South Boulevard, St. Louis, MO 63104.

Glaser, B.G. and Strauss, A.L. (1965) *Awareness of dying.* Chicago: Aldine.

Hage, J. (1972) *Techniques of problems of theory construction in sociology.* New York: John Wiley & Sons.

Hardy, M.E. (1974) Theories: Components, development, evaluation. *Nursing Research,* 23(2), 100–107.

Henderson, V. (1966) *The nature of nursing.* New York: Macmillan.

Jacobson, S.F. (1984) A semantic differential for external comparison of conceptual nursing models. *Advances in Nursing Science,* 6(2), 58–70.

Jacox, A. (1974) Theory construction in nursing: An overview. *Nursing Research,* 23(1), 4–13.

Johnson, D.E. (1959) The nature of a science of nursing. *Nursing Outlook,* 7(5), 291–294.

Johnson, D.E. (1968, April) One conceptual model of nursing. Paper presented at Vanderbilt University, Nashville, TN.

Johnson, D.E. (1970, Winter) Requirements of an effective model. For N203, Class in Theory, University of California, Los Angeles.

Johnson, D.E. (1974) Development of theory: A requisite for nursing as a primary health profession. *Nursing Research,* 23(5), 372–377.

Johnson, D.E. (1987) Evaluating conceptual models for use in critical care nursing practice. *Dimensions of Critical Nursing Care,* 6(4), 195–197.

Kaplan, A. (1964) *The conduct of inquiry: Methodology of behavioral science.* San Francisco: Chandler.

King, I. (1971) *Toward a theory for nursing.* New York: John Wiley & Sons.

Kuhn, T.S. (1970) The structure of scientific revolutions. In Neurath, O. (Ed.), *International encyclopedia of unified science* (2nd ed.) (Vol. 2). Chicago: University of Chicago Press.

Kuhn, T.S. (1977) *The essential tension.* Chicago: University of Chicago Press.

Laudan, L. (1977) *Progress and its problems: Toward a theory of scientific growth.* Berkeley: University of California Press.

Lindsey, A.M., Piper, B.F., and Stotts, N.A. (1982) The phenomenon of cancer cachexia: A review. *Oncology Nursing Forum,* 9(2), 38–42.

Lush, M.T., Janson-Bjerklie, S., Carrieri, V.K., and Lovejoy, N. (1988) Dyspnea in the ventilator-assisted patient. *Heart and Lung,* 17(5), 528–535.

Marriner-Tomey, A. (1989) *Nursing theorists and their work* (2nd ed.). St. Louis: C.V. Mosby.

Meleis, A.I. (1975) Role insufficiency and role supplementation: A conceptual framework. *Nursing Research,* 24(4), 264–271.

Meleis, A.I., Swendsen, L., and Jones, D. (1980) Preventive role supplementation: A grounded conceptual framework. In M.H. Miller and B. Flynn (Eds.), *Current perspectives in nursing: Social issues and trends.* St. Louis: C.V. Mosby.

Mentzer, C.A. and Schorr, J.A. (1986) Perceived situational control and perceived duration of time: Expressions of life patterns. *Advances in Nursing Science,* 9(1), 12–20.

Merton, R. (1964) *Social theory and social structure,* rev'd ed. London: Free Press of Glencoe.

Meter, M.J. and Agronow, S.J. (1982) The stress of multiple roles: The case for role strain among married college women. *Family Relations,* 31(1), 131–138.

Newman, M.A. (1979) *Theory development in nursing.* Philadelphia: F.A. Davis.

Nicoll, L.H., Meyer, P.A., and Abraham, I.L. (1985) Critique: External comparison of conceptual nursing models. *Advances in Nursing Science,* 7(4), 1–9.

Nield, M., Kim, M.J., and Patel, M. (1989) Use of magnitude estimation for estimating the parameters of dyspnea. *Nursing Research*, 38(2), 77–80.

Norris, C.M. (1982) *Concept clarification in nursing*. Rockville, MD: Aspen Systems.

The Nursing Theories Conference Group. (1980) *Nursing theories: The base for professional nursing practice*. Englewood Cliffs, NJ: Prentice-Hall.

Orem, D.E. (1985) *Nursing: Concepts of practice* (3rd ed.). New York: McGraw-Hill.

O'Shea, H.S. (1982) Role orientation and role strain of clinical nurse faculty in baccalaureate programs. *Nursing Research*, 31(5), 306–310.

Parsons, T. (1949) *The structure of social action*. New York: Free Press.

Paterson, J.G. and Zderad, L.T. (1988) *Humanistic nursing*. New York: National League for Nursing, Pub. No. 41-2218.

Ravetz, J. (1971) *Scientific knowledge and its social problems*. New York: Oxford University Press.

Riehl, J.P. and Roy, C. (Eds.) (1980) *Conceptual models for nursing practice* (2nd ed.). New York: Appleton-Century-Crofts.

Rogers, M. (1970) *An introduction to the theoretical basis of nursing*. Philadelphia: F.A. Davis.

Roy, C. and Roberts, S.L. (1981) *Theory construction in nursing*. Englewood Cliffs, NJ: Prentice-Hall.

Schrag, C. (1967) Elements of theoretical analysis in sociology. In L. Gross (Ed.), *Sociological theory: Inquiries and paradigms*. New York: Harper & Row.

Shapere, D. (1966) Meaning and scientific change. In R.G. Colodny (Ed.), *Mind and cosmos: Essays in contemporary science and philosophy*. University of Pittsburg Series in the Philosophy of Science (Vol. 3) Pittsburg: University of Pittsburg Press.

Silva, M.C. (1990) Testing of nursing theory: Four perspectives on meaning. *Proceedings of NLN's first national conference on measurement and evaluation*. New York: National League for Nursing.

Silva, M.C. and Rothbart, D. (1984) An analysis of changing trends in philosophies of science on nursing theory development and testing. *Advances in Nursing Science*, 6(2), 1–13.

Silva, M.C. (1986) Research testing nursing theory: State of the art. *Advances in Nursing Science*, 9(1), 1–11.

Smith, M.J. (1986) Human-environment process: A test of Rogers' principle of integrality. *Advances in Nursing Science*, 9(1), 21–28.

Stevens, B.J. (1984) *Nursing theory: Analysis, application, and evaluation* (2nd ed.). Boston: Little, Brown & Co.

Walker, L.O. and Avant, K.C. (1988) *Strategies for theory construction in nursing* (2nd ed.). Norwalk, CT: Appleton & Lange.

Wewers, M.E. and Lenz, E.R. (1987) Relapse among ex-smokers: An example of theory derivation. *Advances in Nursing Science*, 9(2), 44–53.

Wilson, J. (1969) *Thinking with concepts*. London: Cambridge University Press.

Woods, N.F. (1985a) Employment, family roles, and mental ill health in young married women. *Nursing Research*, 34(1), 4–10.

Woods, N.F. (1985b) Relationship of socialization and stress to perimenstrual symptoms, disability, and menstrual attitudes. *Nursing Research*, 34(3), 145–149.

Zetterberg, H.L. (1963) *On theory and verification in sociology*, rev'd ed. Totowa, NJ: Bedminster Press.

Part 5

Our Pioneers

*P*art Five is devoted to a discussion of nursing theories in relation to present-day nursing theory and practice. The intent of this part is to emphasize several themes introduced in other parts and to develop them further by providing interpretive examples. The first theme is that nursing theories have evolved out of a sociocultural context, were influenced by the educational and experiential background of the theorists, and cannot be understood or adequately analyzed without a consideration of these influences. The second theme is that existing theories are not competitive but are complementary and may be used by the same person for different purposes or by different people for different purposes. The third theme is that theories can be viewed, interpreted, and used in many different ways and are not restricted to the purposes for which they were developed.

Theory users and their interpretations of theories are significant to the progress of a discipline. A final theme, not directly or explicitly presented in this part, but one that could be indirectly derived, is that progress in the discipline of nursing is measured by the development of theories, research, the theorists, the researchers, and the number of central problems that can be answered by existing theories.

Chapter 12 includes two methods by which nursing theories can be viewed. The first is to analyze theories in terms of their paradigmatic origins, time and period of development, central questions, and central concepts. The second method considers the theories in terms of current agreed-upon concepts.

Chapters 14 through 16 describe, analyze, critique, and provide examples of tests of nursing theories that were selected to represent some of the domain concepts. The model proposed in Chapter 11 is used to guide the presentation of each of the theories. The description, analysis, critique, and examples of tests presented here are preliminary and condensed. They are offered to assist you in embarking on your own critical analysis. The extensive bibliography offered in Chapter 19 is intended to support readers who may choose a more thorough analysis and critique of theories. I also encourage you to consider other domain concepts and other nursing theories. Although the theories are organized around domain concepts, the description is general and encompasses as much of the theorists' conceptualizations as possible.

Chapter *12*

Nursing Theory: An Elusive Mirage or a Mirror of Reality

Nursing theories mirror different realities. Throughout their development, they reflected the nursing interests of the time, the sociocultural context, and the theorists' educational and experiential backgrounds. When we consider all the theories together and hold them up to the realities of nursing practice, a number of other images are then formulated. The images are not always distinct images, well-formulated images, or true mirror images; however, they are not mirages or figments of the imagination of the theorist either. They reflect some realities of nursing at the time of development, and they are helping to shape the realities of our time.

This chapter provides several ways in which theories can be viewed. These ways are neither mutually exclusive nor inclusive. They are presented to stimulate other innovative ways in which to view and classify nursing theories. The purpose of these different views and classifications is twofold. First, the more ways in which we can analyze any phenomenon, the more potential there is for seeing different images and details that are not readily apparent when only viewed from one perspective. The second purpose is related to the first: utilizing theories for different uses is enhanced by the many different perspectives from which we view the theories. It is like seeing the image of a garden in a mirror with many flowers, many colors, and many beds, then moving the mirror closer to a bed of California poppies and seeing the rich orange-yellow cups swaying in the fine breeze, then keeping the mirror in position and stepping back a few feet to get another look, to discover the different shades of color blending with the green of the stems. Each of the images depends on where the mirror is in relation to the garden and where the viewer is situated in relation to the mirror and the garden.

The first section of this chapter provides an analysis of nursing theories that were developed between 1950 and 1970 according to the images of nursing of that time (Fig. 12-1). In the second section, theories are classified according to the roles that nurses may play. Roles played by nurses are to a large extent determined by the theoretical perspective guiding their practice. In the third section, theories are

Figure 12–1. Chronology of nursing theorists.

classified according to how they will be evaluated in this book. In the fourth section, areas of agreement are presented. Whether these are the same images or the same classifications that the theorists saw when they developed their theories is neither discussed nor debated here. What is becoming apparent is that the theories together offer a number of images—translated into concepts—that both are reflected in the theories and reflect nursing practice. How they are classified is also reflected in other's hindsight.

Nursing theories have been classified by their paradigmatic origins into

the developmental models, models based on the developmental theories of Erikson (1963), Freud (1949), Maslow (1954), Peplau (1952), C. Rogers (1959), and Sullivan (1953) and based on the behaviorist school (Bijou and Baer, 1961). Among the systems models are found the adaptation system model of Roy (1970), the triad system of Howland and McDowell (1964), the life process system of M. Rogers (1970), and Johnson's behavioral system model (1968). . . . Then, in addition, there is another type of model for nursing-

Table 12–1
Schools of Thought in Nursing Theories—1950–1970

Needs Theorists	Interaction Theorists	Outcome Theorists
Abdellah	King	Johnson
Henderson	Orlando	Levine
Orem	Paterson and Zderad	Rogers
	Peplau	Roy
	Travelbee	
	Wiedenbach	

practice, called an interaction model, since its conceptual system is dependent on symbolic interaction theory. The most well-known models in this group are those of Orlando (1961) and Wiedenbach (1964). (Johnson, 1974, p. 376)

In the first section of this chapter, twenty years of theorizing are analyzed using Johnson's pioneering insights (that is, the paradigmatic origins of theories as one dimension) as well as a number of other dimensions. These include the time period of theory development, temporal dimensions focusing on different sociocultural contexts, central theory questions, and central concepts. This analysis resulted in three distinct patterns or schools of thought (Table 12-1). Each school of thought will be presented in the following discussion. Members of each school of thought will be compared in terms of their views of nursing, focus of nursing, goals of nursing, nursing problems, and nursing therapeutics. The central roles that nurses are expected to play when adopting a particular school of thought to practice are then compared.

IMAGES OF NURSING, 1950–1970

The First School of Thought: Needs

This school of thought includes theories that were developed in response to the question, What do nurses do? Answers to this question focused on a number of theorists describing functions and roles of nurses. Conceptualizing functions led the theorists to consider a nursing client in terms of a hierarchy of needs. When any of these needs are unmet and when a person is not able to fulfill his own needs, then nursing care is needed. Nurses then function by providing necessary action to help patients meet their needs.

Peplau preceded Henderson by providing a theoretical construct of what nursing is. Hers was a theory designed to give focus to psychiatric nursing. Therefore, although intrapsychic needs dominated her theory, her interest and experience in psychiatric nursing led to her introduction of nurse–patient interpersonal relationships as another focus in nursing. Henderson's theory, in keeping with the intraperson focus of the time and not deviating completely from medical science, was conceived to describe all nursing care in terms of the needs of patients.

This school of thought, of need deficits or nurse functions, also included Abdellah and Orem. One may refer to this group as the *need* or *deficit school of thought*, not medical in orientation but based on Maslow's hierarchy of needs and influenced by Erickson's stages of development (neo-Freudian and still not too far removed from medicine). This school of thought has also been referred to as the Columbia school of thought; all or most of the theorists who focused on needs either graduated from or worked at Columbia University. Although the theorists may not attribute the development of their theories to their work or association with Columbia, it is worth noting that they have a common educational background. Perhaps others may wish to explore the influence of Columbia Teachers College on nursing theory development. Judging from the number and caliber of international students who graduated from there, Columbia Teachers College may have had a significant influence on the development of theoretical nursing in other countries as well.

As Tables 12-2 through 12-6 indicate, the needs theorists provided us with a view of a human being that was slightly different but very close to the view provided by the biomedical model. The hierarchy of needs begins with physiological needs and safety needs and progresses to include other higher-level needs, such as belonging, love, and esteem needs. Neither Henderson nor Abdellah considered self-actualization needs as within the province of the nurse (as manifested in the omission rather than the commission); Orem added development of self-care requisites in her updated writing.

The focus of this school of thought, then, is on problems and needs of patients as seen by health care providers and on the role of nurses to assess these needs, to fulfill the need requisites. When lower needs are met, more mature needs may

Table 12–2
Needs Theorists—A View of Nursing

Theorists	Definition of Nursing
Abdellah	Use of problem solving approach to deal with 21 problems related to needs of patients
Henderson	Helping with 14 activities contributing to health or recovery, help the individual become independent of assistance
Orem	Self-care agency to meet individual's need for self-care action in order to sustain life and health, recover from disease or injury, and cope with the effect

Table 12–3
Needs Theorists—Focus of Nursing

Theorists	Focus of Nursing
Abdellah	Problem solving approach to 21 nursing activities, sustenal, remedial, restorative, preventive, self-help, need deficit or excess
Henderson	Assistance with 14 daily activities or needs
Orem	Deficit between self-care capabilities and self-care demands of patients

Table 12–4
Needs Theorists—Goals of Nursing

Theorists	Goals of Nursing
Abdellah	Help individual meet health needs and adjust to health problems
Henderson	Completeness or wholeness and independence of patient to perform daily activities
Orem	Eliminate deficit between self-care capabilities and demand

Table 12–5
Needs Theorists—Nursing Problems

Theorists	Nursing Problems
Abdellah	Condition faced by patient for which a nurse can assist, overtly and covertly (21 problems)
Henderson	Patient's lack of knowledge, strength, or will to carry out 14 activities
Orem	Deficiency in 8 universal, 2 developmental, and 6 health deviation requisites/needs.

emerge (Peplau, 1952). Perceptions of clients, a focus on environment, and the role of nurse–patient interactions in dialogues and intervention are not fully developed (see Table 12-7).

Table 12–6
Need Theorists–Nursing Therapeutics

Theorists	Nursing Therapeutics
Abdellah	Preventive care (hygiene, safety, exercise, rest, sleep, body mechanics)
	Sustenal care (psychosocial care)
	Remedial care (provision of oxygen, fluid, nutrition, elimination)
	Restorative care (coping with illness and life adjustment)
Henderson	Complementing and supplementing knowledge, will, and strength of patient to perform 14 daily activities and to carry out his medical prescriptions
Orem	Wholly compensatory system (nurse performs all self-care for patient)
	Partly compensatory system (nurse and patient perform patient self-care)
	Supportive-educative system (nurse helps in overcoming any self-care limitations)

Table 12–7
Needs Theorists—A Summary

Focus	Problems
	Nurses' function
Human being	A set of needs or problems
	A developmental being
Patient	Need deficit
Orientation	Illness, disease
Role of nurse	Dependent on medical practice
	Beginnings of independent functions
	Fulfill needs requisites
Decision making	Primarily health care professional

A Second School of Thought: Interaction

A second question was then beginning to be formulated, not totally ignoring the first question but complementary to it. Whereas the first question that guided earlier theorists was, What do nurses do?, the second question evolving from the Yale University School of Nursing was, How do nurses do whatever it is they do? Answers to the "how" question focused on the interaction process. Peplau was the pioneer in that group (1952), yet her answer was more congruent with the prevailing interest at the time in psychoanalytic theory and closer to the biomedical model of man. It is significant when studying the history of ideas to note the connection between the first school of thought at Teacher's College and the second one at Yale. The Yale, or *interactionist school of thought*, school grew out of the needs approach, with some of the concepts still prevailing in both; this will be demonstrated in the following discussion. The conceptualization of Imogene King, also a graduate of Teacher's College, evolved out of interest in the "how" of nursing care.

Interaction theories were conceived in the late 1950s and early 1960s and viewed nursing as an interaction process with a focus on the development of a relationship between patient and nurse. These theories grew out of the social milieu in the country and sociocultural forces in nursing that existed at that time, including the following:

- ○ This was the post-Sputnik era.
- ○ There was a focus on such values as human integrity, as promoted by President Kennedy.
- ○ The Cuban crisis may have promoted return to focus on humanity and relationships in fear of outside invasion.
- ○ The beginning formation of hippie groups, communal living, and the flower children indicated a definite need for intimacy and human relations.
- ○ Technological advances continued, but with a growing distaste for mechanization and dehumanization.

What was happening in nursing at that time? Nursing was undergoing some significant changes:

- ○ Federal monies to improve curricula and education of nurse researchers was available.
- ○ A need for integrated curricula arose, freeing psychiatric nurses to identify core concepts to integrate throughout nursing curricula and allowing them to observe and reflect on the process of nursing care in all nursing subspecialties.

Tables 12-8 through 12-13 present theories of the interactionists. Although some continued to address the needs of the patient, all interactionists focused their attention on the process of care and on the ongoing interaction between nurses and clients. Their theories were based on interactionism, phenomenology, and existentialist philosophy.

What did we learn from the interactionists? (This is also described in Table 12-13.)

- ○ Nursing is a deliberate process that can be elucidated.
- ○ Nursing encompasses help and assistance.
- ○ Nursing is an interpersonal process occurring between a person in need of help and a person capable of giving help.

Table 12–8
Interaction Theorists—A View of Nursing

Theorists	Definitions
King	A process of action, reaction, and interaction whereby nurse and client share information about their perceptions of the nursing situation and agree on goals
Orlando	Interaction with patients who have a need or response to suffering individuals or those anticipating helplessness
	Assistance to individual to avoid, relieve, diminish, or cure sense of helplessness
Paterson and Zderad	A human dialogue, intersubjective transaction, a shared situation, a transactional process, a presence of both patient and nurse
Peplau	Therapeutic interpersonal, serial, goal-oriented process
	A health-focused human relationship
Travelbee	An interpersonal process, an assistance to prevent, cope with experiences of illness and suffering, and to find meaning in these experiences
Wiedenbach	Sensing, perceiving, validating patients need for help, ministering help needed in a deliberate, goal-oriented way

Table 12–9
Interaction Theorists—Focus of Nursing

Theorists	Focus of Nursing
King	Nurse–patient interactions that lead to goal attainment in a natural environment
Orlando	Care for the needs of the patients who are distressed, with consideration for perception, thought, and feeling through deliberate action
Paterson and Zderad	Patient is a unique being
	Patient's perception of events
	Both patient and nurse are the focus
Peplau	Nurse–patient relationship and its phases
	Orientation, identification, exploitation, and resolution
	Harnessing energy from anxiety and tension to positively defining, understanding, and meeting productively the problem at hand
Travelbee	Interpersonal relations, finding meaning in suffering, pain, and illness
	Self-actualization
Wiedenbach	Patient's perception of condition, care, action

Table 12–10
Interaction Theorists—Goals of Nursing

Theorists	Goals of Nursing
King	Help individuals maintain their health so they can function in their role
Orlando	Relieve distress, physical and mental discomfort Improve sense of well-being
Paterson and Zderad	Develop human potential, more well-being for both patient and nurse
Peplau	Develop personality, making illness an eventful experience Forward movement of personality and other ongoing human processes in the direction of creative, constructive, productive personal and community living
Travelbee	Cope with an illness situation and find meaning in the experience Assist patient to accept humanness
Wiedenbach	Meet the needs of an individual experiencing need for help

Table 12–11
Interaction Theorists—Nursing Problems

Theorists	Nursing Problems
King	When nurse and patient do not perceive each other, the situation, or communicate information, transactions are not made, goals are not attained
Orlando	Distress due to unmet needs
Paterson and Zderad	Persons with perceived needs related to the health/illness quality of living
Peplau	Unsuccessful or incomplete learning of life tasks Energy used in tensions and frustrations due to unmet needs, opposing goals—giving rise to conflict, aggression, anxiety Discomfort, anxiety, doubt, guilt, obsession, compulsion
Travelbee	Lack of support in nurse–patient relationship Not finding meaning in illness, transitory discomfort, anguish, malignant despair, apathetic indifference
Wiedenbach	Person with need for help (unmet needs due to physical or inadequate environment)

Table 12–12
Interaction Theorists—Nursing Therapeutics

Theorists	Nursing Therapeutics
King	Goal attainment, transaction, perceptual validation
Orlando	Deliberate nursing process not automatic
Paterson and Zderad	Humanness—use of nurse's self, existentially nurturing, being, relating, meeting, maximum participation
Peplau	Development of problem-solving skills through the interpersonal process (educational, therapeutic, and collaborative)
Travelbee	Use of nurse's self, original encounter, emerging identities, empathy, sympathy, rapport
Wiedenbach	Ministration of help, validation, rational, reactional, and deliberate

- The nurse, to be able to give help, should clarify her own values, use the self in a therapeutic way, and be involved in the care.
- Care is not a mechanistic act but a humanistic act.
- The humanistic interactionist nurses used existential philosophy, symbolic interaction, and developmental theories to develop their conceptions of nursing.
- They defined illness as an inevitable human experience; if one learns to find meaning in it, it will become a growing experience.

Table 12–13
Interaction Theorists—A Summary

Focus	Nurse–patient interactions
	Illness as an experience
Human being	Interacting being
	A set of needs
	Can validate needs
	Human experience with meanings
Patient	Helpless being
	A human experience with meaning
Orientation	Illness/disease
Role of nurse	Deliberate helping process
	Self as a therapeutic agent
	Use of the nursing process
Decision making	Primarily health care professional
	Validated by clients

They differ from the previous group who defined illness as a deviation to be corrected.

○ They defined nursing as caring, assisting (all others), and helping to find meaning—actions that increase human potential and better well-being.

○ They all indicated that the nurse needs systematic knowledge to help her in assessing, diagnosing, and intervening.

○ The nursing process is well-developed by these theorists.

○ Properties, antecedents, and consequences of interactions are well-developed, and all are centered around forming relationships and relieving distress.

○ Beginning movement leads toward the patient becoming an equal partner in the nursing process.

○ The interactionist nurse considers uniqueness, dignity, and worth values of patients as important in the development of wellness. A view of an autonomous individual with individual established norms was beginning to emerge. Help, it was emphasized, was to be tailored to individual needs.

○ Properties of interaction as validation (Wiedenbach), meeting (Orlando), being totally present, and relating (Paterson and Zderad) are delineated and defined by this group of theorists.

○ The theories concede that perception of the patient is important in assessing illness and its meaning.

○ The major nurse–patient interaction relationship goal is derived from their observation that the person in need of help becomes distressed; the purpose is to prevent or deal with this distress.

○ The interactionist theorist reminds us that the nurse is a human being who needs to self-reflect in order to understand her own values. Without such understanding, the nurse will not be able to be a human being who cares, gives care, establishes connections, and helps patients relieve their distress.

○ The theorists tentatively introduced the notion of effect of environment on patients. To them, unmet needs of the patient develop because of:

   ○ Physical limitations (from incomplete development, temporary or permanent disability, or restrictions in environment); and
   ○ Adverse reactions to inadequate environment (Orlando).

○ This group of theorists reintroduced the significance of nurses' intuition and subjectivity in the nursing act.

○ Some common assumptions guided the development of the interactionist theories. These are:

   ○ The integrity of an individual has to be maintained;
   ○ Individuals have self-awareness and are therefore able to identify their needs;

- ○ Individuals strive toward actualization;
- ○ Events in life are human experiences inevitable and essential in helping to move to the next stage in development; and
- ○ The nurse cannot separate herself as an individual from the act of care—the nurse is an integral part of care.

- ○ Interaction theorists provided nursing with a new perspective:

  - ○ There is a reciprocal assessment process;
  - ○ Patient perspective is significant in health care;
  - ○ Situation determines needs and care; and
  - ○ Patients are helpless and suffer due to illness.

A number of concepts were identified by the interaction theorists as central to nursing. These concepts remain to be significant components of interaction in nursing:

Sensing;
Perceiving;
Validating;
Existential transactions;
Goal orientation of interaction; and
Nurses' self-development.

Interaction theories neither addressed nor focused on:

A more complete view of a human being (human beings are interacting beings with a minimal focus on biopsychocultural focus); and
A view of the environment, except tangentially in some instances.

A Third School of Thought: Outcome of Nursing

The third question that the nurse theorist asked is the "why" of nursing care. While not ignoring the "what" and the "how," this group of theorists attempted to conceptualize the outcome of nursing care and then proceeded to describe the recipient of care. Two of the most influential theorists in this group are Dorothy Johnson and Martha Rogers. They graduated from Harvard and Johns Hopkins, respectively, but did most of their work at opposite ends of the North American continent—New York and Los Angeles. This East/West school of thought is referred to in this book as the *outcome school of thought.*

Johnson influenced theoretical thinking in nursing, and her theory will influence nursing more in the future than it did in the past as the goals of nursing become more congruent with stability than change (Hall, 1983). Rogers, on the other hand, has helped to shape nursing research that is based on theoretical thinking. Neither theory is as developed as that of Sister Callista Roy who, as nursing director of Mount St. Mary's, had the faculty resources to implement her theory into courses and content, thereby helping in turn to operationalize the theory further. Both

Table 12–14
Outcome Theorists—A View of Nursing

Theorists	Definitions of Nursing
Johnson	External regulatory force acting to preserve the organization and integration of patient's behavior at an optimal level when behavior is a threat to social, physical health or illness
Levine	Patient advocacy, devotion to humanity and self-respect of patient, perception and support for personal and individualized needs, compassion, commitment, and protection
Rogers	Humanistic science for maintaining and promoting health, preventing illness, caring for and rehabilitating the sick and disabled
Roy	Theoretical system of knowledge viewing client as biopsychosocial being (ill or potentially so) who adapts to changing environment
	Nurse acts through nursing process to promote adaptation

Johnson and Rogers, with faculty members of the University of California, Los Angeles, and New York University, respectively, have also partially operationalized their theories, but not to the same extent. The publications of Roy on uses of theory in practice have enhanced the use of her theory in several schools of nursing. Myra Levine, who views the goal of nursing as conservation of energy, also belongs in this group.

This group of theorists (Tables 12-14 through 12-18) conceptualized the goal of nursing care as bringing back some balance, stability, and preservation of energy or enhancing harmony between the individual and the environment. They based their

Table 12–15
Outcome Theorists—Focus on Nursing

Theorists	Focus of Nursing
Johnson	Man as a behavioral system with subsystems, each having a structure, a function, and functional imperatives (drive, set, behavior) and each requiring protection, stimulation, and nurturance
Levine	Four principles guide conception of human being (energy, personal, structural, and social integrities) and their organismic responses (fear, inflammation, stress, sensory)
	Nursing is conservation of energy and integrities
Rogers	Life processes of human beings, unitary person–environment energy fields, complementarity, resonance, and helicy
Roy	Focal, contextual, and residual stimuli and their effect on the cognator and regulator mechanisms, in turn effecting four adaptive modes: physiological, self-concept, role function, and interdependence

Table 12–16
Outcome Theorists—Goals of Nursing

Theorists	Goals of Nursing
Johnson	Behavioral system balance, subsystems that function efficiently and effectively
Levine	Conservation of energy and integrities (personal, structural, social), restoration of well-being and independent activity
Rogers	Promote symphonic interaction and harmony between man and environment Strengthen coherence and integrity of human field
Roy	Promote person's adaptation in physiological needs, self-concept, role function, and interdependence

Table 12–17
Outcome Theorists—Nursing Problems

Theorists	Nursing Problems
Johnson	Structural functional stress in one subsystem (insufficiency, discrepancy) and between subsystems (incompatibility, dominance)
Levine	Response to fear, response to stress, inflammatory response, sensory response
Rogers	Disruptions in organization and structure of interacting human environment fields
Roy	Ineffective coping mechanisms causing ineffective responses that disrupt the integrity of the person

Table 12–18
Outcome Theorists—Nursing Therapeutics

Theorists	Nursing Therapeutics
Johnson	Inhibition, constriction, supplementation, protection, nurturing (supportive/maintenance, teaching, counseling, and behavior modification)
Levine	Therapeutic—alter course of adaptation Supportive—maintain course of adaptation
Rogers	Repatterning of human environment fields or assistance in mobilizing inner resources
Roy	Manipulation of focal, residual, and contextual stimuli with patient's zone of positive coping

Table 12–19
Outcome Theorists—A Summary

Focus	Energy
	Balance, stability, homeostasis presentation
	Outcome of care
Human being	Adaptive and developmental being
Patient	Lack of adaptation
	Systems deficiency
Orientation	Illness, disease
Role of nurse	External regulatory mechanism
Decision making	Primarily health care provider

conceptualizations on system, adaptation, and developmental theories. They directed their focus on the outcome of care. Their view of a human being and the nursing client incorporated the need theorists' conceptualization of the human being. (The goals of subsystems of behavior of Johnson's theory and adaptive modes by Roy have parallels in the hierarchy of needs by Henderson, nursing functions by Abdellah, and universal needs by Orem.) Although they spoke of harmony with the environment, stability, conservation of energy, and homeostasis as potential outcomes, the consequences are at a high level of abstraction, limiting utility of theories in outcome measures. The outcome theories provide nursing with a well-articulated conception of a human being as a nursing client and of nursing as an external regulatory mechanism (Table 12-19).

NURSING THEORIES CLASSIFIED

Nursing theories are further classified in this text in terms of the primary focus in the theory. In classifying theories for analysis, it is assumed that each classification system adds more understanding to each theory. Correspondence between each of the classification systems is neither presented nor discussed in this text. You may wish to consider the relationship between the different classification systems.

In reviewing the theories for classification, central domain concepts, central questions the theory addresses, and the areas that seem to be most developed were some of the conditions used as a guideline for theory classification. Four central focuses emerged from this review: clients, person–environment interactions, interactions, and nursing therapeutics. Although theories may appear to fit in more than one of these areas, my decision to place a theory in a particular area in this text was based on the *primary* focus in the theory.

Johnson, Roy, and Neuman focused their theoretical development on the *client* or the client system. These theories provide a comprehensive analysis of the client as seen from a nursing perspective. Although health and environment may have been discussed in various degrees, these concepts do not appear to be as well developed or as central to these theories. Hence, Johnson, Roy, and Neuman were classified as client-focused theories, and they appear in Chapter 13, "On Nursing Clients."

Rogers' central focus in her theory is on the relationship between clients and their environment. Clients in Rogers' theory are the environment-client, and one cannot be assessed in isolation from the other. Hence, Rogers theory was classified under person–environment interactions and is analyzed in Chapter 14, "On Environment."

The properties, the components, and the nature of the interactions between clients and nurses were the focus of several theoretical formulations. King, Orlando, Paterson and Zderad, Travelbee, and Wiedenbach concentrated on nurse–patient interactions and considered them the focus of nursing. These theories are evaluated in Chapter 15, "On Interactions."

What nurses should do and under what circumstances these actions should be delivered were the focus of theoretical formulations in Levine and Orem's theories. These theories are therefore evaluated as theories that could provide nurses with frameworks for *intervention*. Unlike client-oriented theories that are more effective in providing nurses with a framework for assessment, intervention theories provide nurses with guidelines for intervention. These theories are evaluated in Chapter 16, "On Nursing Therapeutics."

ROLES NURSES PLAY

The preceding analyses suggest that nurses focus on different aspects of care at different times or for different purposes. Nursing is not exemplified by one group of theories more than another at all times. Rather, the situation may dictate when nursing should focus on needs, interaction, or outcomes. Newman (1983) makes the following point:

> One of the factors determining the applicability of a theory is the temporal
> frame of reference. For example, if one is viewing a relatively short time
> frame, the adaptation model might apply, whereas in a longer time frame,
> phenomena would be apparent that could not be explained by adaptation
> alone. (p. 391)

Nurses play different roles at different times, and the nursing theories have helped to suggest the different roles that nurses play. Need-oriented nurses are actively doing and functioning; they rely on problem solving, they carefully plan their interventions, and they evaluate their work mainly (but not only) by the activities performed.

Interaction-oriented nurses rely on the process of interaction and include themselves in the sphere of other actions; they use themselves therapeutically and evaluate their actions primarily in terms of interactions. Interaction-oriented nurses rely more on counseling, guiding, and teaching—helping clients find meanings in their situations—and less on doing and functioning. Among the interactionists are the existentialists who focus on the human potential. That potential includes for both the nurse and the client the goal of authentic being and the process of creating options and openness to present and future experiences.

Outcome-oriented nurses focus on the goals of maintaining and promoting energy and harmony with the environment and enhancing the development of healthy environments. Outcome nurses do not include themselves as therapeutic agents; they enact the healing roles but do not necessarily consider authentic being as essential in healing. (See Table 12-20).

AREAS OF AGREEMENT AMONG AND BETWEEN THEORISTS AND SCHOOLS OF THOUGHT

Nursing theories have been considered in terms of their contrasting and competitive views. In the first section of this chapter, an attempt was made to address how they may complement each other as theories and as different schools of thought. In this section, areas of agreement among the various schools of thought are identified.

- ○ Nursing theories offer a beginning articulation of what nursing is and what roles nurses play.
- ○ Nursing theories offer a view of the philosophical underpinnings in nursing (*e.g.*, interaction, phenomenology, and existentialism).
- ○ Nursing theories provide descriptions of how to help patients become comfortable, how to deliver treatment with the least damage, and how to enhance high-level wellness.
- ○ Nursing theories offer a beginning common language and a beginning agreement about who the nursing care recipients are.
- ○ It is obvious that we should not view the recipients only through biological glasses (as biological systems) or psychological glasses (as id, ego, and superego), but rather through holistic glasses. Nursing clients are more than the sum total of their psychological, sociological, cultural, or biological parts.
- ○ Recipients of care respond to events in a holistic way.
- ○ The recipient is a member of a reference group set, and interventions are only meaningful if the whole unit is considered.
- ○ Recipients have needs, and nursing assists them in meeting those needs.

The theories have other themes in common. These emerge when one considers images evolving from the theories when compared with nursing realities. In this process, several concepts emerge as central to nursing. These are addressed in the following conclusion.

Table 12–20
Roles Nurses Play According to Different Theories

Theorists	Roles Nurses Play	Image
Needs Theorists		
Abdellah	Problem solver and performer of 21 physiological and psychosocial activities for the patient	They provide an image of a nurse who is active and busy working and a patient who is striving for independence. The nurse's work is focused on doing a deliberate and well-planned activity.
Henderson	Complementing, supplementing knowledge	
	The will to perform daily activities	
Orem	Temporary self-care agent for universal health deviation and development of self-care needs	
Interaction Theorists		
King	Goal attainer or else!	They provide an image of a nurse as present-oriented, situational, a humanist, a process-oriented professional whose interest is the interaction and, for some, also the person. The nurse, to some, is also important in the interaction.
	Teach, counsel, guide, give care, gather information, set mutual goals	
Orlando	Deliberate, repetitive, and situational interactions	
Paterson and Zderad	Existentialist and phenomenological nurturer of the human potential (self and patient)	
Peplau	Freudian helper	
	Stranger who works hard to become a surrogate	
Travelbee	Meaning finder (more than a dictionary meaning) and existentialist	
Wiedenbach	Deliberate helper who focuses on extrasensory perception and does not forget to validate the process	
Outcome Theorists		
Johnson	The external manipulator: external regulatory force to preserve organization and integration of patient's behavior	They provide an image of the nurse as goal setter, a futurist, environmentalist, who has extrasensory and energy preservation powers.
	Controller	
Levine	Conservator of all	
Rogers	The environmental nurse, the symphony player: promotion of person–environment interaction	
	The healer without touch	
Roy	The pace setter: external regulatory force to modify stimuli affecting adaptation to create four modes of adaptation	

CONCLUSION

The domain of nursing deals with people who are assumed to be in constant interaction with their environment and yet have unmet needs, are not able to care for themselves, or are not adapting to the environment due to interruptions or potential interruptions in health. The domain of nursing focuses on therapeutics to help in meeting the needs of the person and to enhance adaptation capability, self-care ability, health, and well-being. Theory and research are the processes by which the domain concepts and problems are developed, validated, and communicated. Practice, education, and administration are the means by which the domain goals are implemented.

REFERENCES

Bijou, J.W. and Baer, D.M. (1961) *Child development: A systematic and empirical theory.* New York: Appleton-Century-Crofts.

Erikson, E.H. (1963) *Childhood and society* (2nd ed.). New York: W.W. Norton.

Freud, S. (1949) *An outline of psychoanalysis.* New York: W.W. Norton.

Hall, B. (1983) Toward an understanding of stability in nursing phenomena. *Advances in Nursing Science*, 5(3), 15–20.

Howland, D. and McDowell, W.E. (1964, Winter) Measurement of patient care: A conceptual framework. *Nursing Research*, 13(1), 4–7.

Johnson, D.E. (1968) One conceptual model of nursing. Paper presented at Vanderbilt University, Nashville, TN.

Johnson, D.E. (1974) Development of theory: A requisite for nursing as a primary health profession. *Nursing Research*, 23(5), 372–377.

Maslow, A.H. (1954) *Motivation and personality.* New York: Harper & Row.

Newman, M. (1983) The continuing revolution: A history of nursing science. In N. Chaska (Ed.), *The nursing profession: A time to speak.* New York: McGraw-Hill.

Orlando, I.J. (1961) *The dynamic nurse–patient relationship.* New York: G.P. Putnam's Sons.

Peplau, H. (1952) *Interpersonal relations in nursing.* New York: G.P. Putnam's Sons.

Rogers, C. (1959) A theory of therapy, personality, interpersonal relations as developed in a client-centered framework. In J. Koch (Ed.), *Psychology: A study of a science* (Vol. 3) New York: McGraw-Hill.

Rogers, M.E. (1970) *An introduction to the theoretical basis of nursing.* Philadelphia: F.A. Davis.

Roy, C. (1970, March) Adaptation: A conceptual framework for nursing. *Nursing Outlook*, 18, 42–48.

Sullivan, H. (1953) *The interpersonal theory of psychiatry.* New York: W.W. Norton.

Wiedenbach, E. (1964) *Clinical nursing: A helping art.* New York: Springer-Verlag.

Chapter 13

On Nursing Clients

The work of three theorists emerges as significant developments in the conceptualization of the nursing client. Central questions for these theorists are: Who is the nursing client? In what ways does a nursing client benefit from nursing care? What is the outcome of care? The three theorists are Dorothy Johnson, Sister Callista Roy (a mentor and her student), and Betty Neuman. Johnson asserted in all her metatheory as well as theory publications that what differentiates nursing from medicine and other health sciences is its perspective of a nursing client as a behavioral system. To Roy, a client is an adaptive being with two subsystems for adapting—the regulator and cognator mechanisms—and four adaptive modes. The human being as represented by central structure, lines of defense and resistance, becomes a client according to Neuman when threatened or attached by environmental stressors. This chapter offers a description, an analysis, and a beginning critique of the three theorists' conceptualizations.

Dorothy Johnson

THEORY DESCRIPTION

The early questions with which Dorothy Johnson concerned herself pertained to what knowledge base nurses needed for nursing care (1959a). Nursing care to her did not depend on medical care, nor was its goal recovery from illness or more desirable health practices. She labeled nursing's responsibilities that are related to medical care and better health "delegated medical care" and "health care," respectively (1961). Although nurses also performed functions related to "delegated medical care" and "health care," the essence of nursing, its central mission, should lie in "nursing care," which Johnson considered ill-defined with no well-delineated theoretical framework. When the latter is defined, when the specific goals are articulated, then we will be able to speak of a science of nursing (1959b).

Johnson's conceptualization of nursing, then, is based on the premise that nursing has a unique, independent contribution to health care that is distinct from its delegated dependent contributions (1964). All contributions delegated to and unique to patient care and cure are significant but, as professionals, nurses are obligated to articulate and communicate to the public their primary mission and their nursing goals, as well as their secondary mission that is delegated from medicine. The public is aware of the latter but less aware of the former. A client, to Johnson, behaves in an integrated, systematic, patterned, ordered, and predictable way. Behavior is goal-oriented, and goals are an organizing framework for all behavior. Behavior is the sum total of biological, social, cultural, and psychological behaviors.

Johnson (1980) conceptualized a nursing client as a behavioral system, with behaviors of interest to nursing organized into seven subsystems of behavior (Table 13-1). Each one of the subsystems has a structure, function, goal, and set. The structure of a behavioral subsystem is analogous to the anatomy of a biological subsystem. It identifies the components and the subcomponents by which we can identify the subsystem of behavior.

First is the *drive* or the *goal* of the subsystem. Goals or drives are universal; however, the strength of the goal may differ and, in fact, may fluctuate in the same person from strong to weak. Goals have different meanings in different people or at different times in the same person. Another parameter on which goals may differ is the object of the goal. For example, when observing the eating behavior of a Middle Eastern immigrant, an inference may be made that the goal of eating is to achieve appetite pleasure or to internalize an external environment (universal drive). The variety of the food and the total absorption into the act of eating (to the exclusion of external environment) may demonstrate the strength and the meaning of the eating behavior. The object is the type of food preferred by Middle Eastern immigrants— usually highly salty, high in protein, and free of pork and alcohol.

A second structural component is the *set*, which is the ordinary, regular, normal behavior a client resorts to in order to meet the goal of the subsystem. For example, pureed vegetable soup is a type of food normally eaten by Middle Eastern immigrants in an illness situation. Another example of set is a Middle Eastern immigrant's preference to have a room full of visitors at all times to meet his affiliative needs, which happens to be the usual way this particular person has of handling the stress of hospitalization. Therefore, expecting and maintaining a large group of family members at the bedside is a normal pattern of behavior for this particular person.

Choices represent to Johnson another component in the structure of a subsystem. Choices represent the available repertoire of options that a person has to meet particular goals. Choices are regulated by sex, age, cultural background, and socioeconomic status, among other variables. To meet the needs of procreation without a commitment to a partner—for example, through artificial insemination—is an option within the repertoire of some women and not of others, based on their perception of their own choices.

Finally, the goal, set, and choice are complemented by directly observing the *behavior* of the client. The behaviors that bring about desired goals and whether or not the normal patterns of behavior are appropriate under the circumstances of the

Table 13–1
The Subsystems of Behavior—Johnson*

Achievement Subsystem

The function is mastery or control of either some parts of environment or of self in such areas as physical, creative, mechanical, social, and intellectual skills. These are measured against some acceptable yardstick.

Affiliative Subsystem

Inclusion into relations, intimacy, relating, bonding with the ultimate function of survivial.

Aggressive Subsystem

Modes used to protect and preserve oneself from dangers, whether real or imaginary.

Dependence Subsystem

Used interchangeably with attachment; the ultimate function being approval, attention, or recognition and physical assistance through assistance from a repertoire of others.

Eliminative Subsystem

Difficult to differentiate from the biological elimination system. It incorporates modes of behavior in the excretion of wastes, addresses when, how, why, and under what conditions a person externalizes what is internal and what needs to be expelled.

Ingestive Subsystem

Similar to digestive biological system but incorporates when, why, how, and under what normative conditions the internalizing of external environment takes place. Its function is "appetitive satisfaction."

Sexual Subsystem

Recognizes strong similarity to biological system but considers all other behaviors that are related to subsystem (*e.g.*, gender–role identity, courting, mating). The function is procreation and gratification.

* *Based on Grubbs, J. (1980) An interpretation of the Johnson behavioral system model. In J. P. Riehl and C. Roy (Eds.),* Conceptual models for nursing practice, *2nd ed., pp. 217–254. New York: Appleton-Century-Crofts; and based on Johnson, D. E. (1980) The behavioral system model for nursing. In J. P. Riehl and C. Roy (Eds.).* Conceptual models for nursing practice, *2nd ed. New York: Appleton-Century-Crofts.*

health/illness situation are examples of observations and analyses that may be useful. Behaviors are also compared and contrasted with available options for the individual.

Each of the subsystems also has a *function* that is analogous to the physiology of biological systems. The goal of the subsystem that is part of the structure is not entirely distinct from its function.

Subsystems, and indeed the client system, continue to grow, develop, and remain viable. Therefore, Johnson questioned what assistance subsystems may need to be able to do so, and her answer was "certain functional requirements" (1980, p. 212) that can be met by the individual or by others when the individual cannot meet such requirements. These functional requirements are:

1. Protection from unwanted, disturbing stimuli;
2. Nurturance through giving input from environment (food, friendship, caring); and
3. Stimulation by experiences, events, behavior that would "enhance growth and prevent stagnation" (Johnson, 1980, p. 212).

Subsystems continue to maintain themselves as long as both the internal and external environments are orderly, organized, and predictable, and as long as each of the goals is met. When there is a disturbance in structure, in function, or even in the functional regimen (even though the structure and function may not have been affected), nursing care is indicated. Nursing has the goal of maintaining, restoring, or attaining a balance or stability in the behavioral subsystem or the system as a whole. Nursing acts as an "external regulatory force" to modify or change the structure or to provide ways in which subsystems fulfill the structure's functional requirement (Johnson, 1980, p. 214).

Johnson based her theory on a number of explicit and implicit assumptions (Table 13-2). The theory specifies that the behavior of the person who is ill is the object of nursing care. Therefore, nursing's specific contribution to patient welfare is fostering efficient and effective behavioral functioning in the patient during and following illness (Johnson, 1980, p. 207).

Nursing makes its contribution through identification of a behavioral subsystem or subsystems that are threatened or could potentially be threatened by illness or hospitalization. In Johnson's theory, the source of difficulty is clearly within the subsystem or within the functional requirements, whether or not manifested in structure, in function, or in the functional requirements. Johnson's assumptions are explicit and clear. The theory provides useful definitions of person, health, nursing problem, and nursing therapeutics, and no definitions for nursing process, interactions, or environment. Definitions are highly abstract; however, extensions offered by Auger (1976) and Holaday (1980) provide clear operationalization of definitions of person and of nursing therapeutics. One of the potential problem areas in clarity is the use of some concepts with different meanings, one more acceptable and less esoteric than another (such as ingestion and elimination) that, when considered from a biological standpoint, denote a different meaning (Tables 13-3 and 13-4).

Table 13–2
Assumptions—Johnson

Explicit Assumptions*

○ Behavior is the sum total of physical, biological, and social factors/behaviors.
○ "The behavior of an individual evident at any given point in time is the product of the net aggregate of consequences of these factors over time and at that point in time."
○ "When these regularities and constancies are disturbed, the integrity of the person is threatened and the functions served by such order are less than adequately fulfilled."
○ A person is a system of behavior characterized by repetitive, regular, predictable, and goal-directed behaviors that always strive toward balance.
○ There are different levels of balance and stabilization. Levels are different at different time periods.
○ Balance is essential for effective and efficient functions of the individual (a minimum of energy expenditure, maximum satisfaction, and survival).
○ Balance is developed and maintained within the subsystem or the system as a whole in order to maintain adaptation and environment.
○ Changes in structure or function of a behavioral subsystem is related to dissatisfied drive, lack of functional requirements, or changes in environmental conditions.

Implicit Assumptions

○ A person could be reduced to small components to be studied.
○ A person as a system is the sum total of its parts (*i.e.,* subsystems).
○ All behaviors can be observed through sensory data.

* *This section is based on D. Johnson's class notes from the University of California, Los Angeles, 1970 and Johnson, 1968a.*

The consequences that Johnson alluded to are adjustment and adaptation. An unintended consequence that was not discussed by Johnson is unwarranted dependence on others for meeting the needs of the subsystem. The theory does not address the potential of such dependence.

Johnson did not clearly identify theoretical propositions in her published work, but she has discussed the implications of her theory for nursing research in a number of theory and research conferences. Her position has been that appropriate, cumulative research in nursing is only possible when we agree on the mission and goals of nursing (1974). Propositions in Johnson's theory are existence propositions. Existence propositions (Zetterberg, 1963) in this case lead to factor-isolating theories (Dickoff, James, and Wiedenbach, 1968) (Table 13-5).

Table 13–3
Concepts—Johnson

Behavior	Structural	Internal Regulation
Subsytems of	Components	External Regulation
Behavior	Goal	Restore
Affilliative	Set	Maintain
Ingestive	Choice	Attain
Eliminative	Action	Stability
Aggressive	Function	Instability
Sexual	Functional Requirements	
Dependence	Protection	
Achievement	Stimulation	
	Nurturance	

Table 13–4
Definition of Domain Concepts—Johnson

Nursing	An external regulatory force that acts to preserve the organization and integration of the patient's behavior at an optimal level under those conditions in which the behavior constitutes a threat to physical or social health or in which illness is found (Johnson, 1980, p. 214).
Goal of nursing	Restore, maintain or attain behavioral integrity, system stability, adjustment and adaptation, efficient and effective functioning of system (1980, p. 214).
Health	Efficient and effective functioning of system; behavioral system balance and stability.
Environment	Identified internal and external environments, but provided no specific definition.
Human being	A bio-psycho-social being who is a behavioral system with seven subsystems of behavior.
Nursing client	A bio-psycho-social being as a behavioral system threatened by loss of order, predictability, or stability due to illness or potential illness. "All patterned, repetitive, purposeful ways of behaving that characterize each man's life are considered to comprise his behavioral system." (Johnson, 1980, p. 209).
Nursing problem	Instability in the system or one of the subsystems due to functional or structural stress: a) inadequate drive satisfaction; b) inadequate fulfillment of the fucntional requirements; c) changes in environmental conditions (Grubbs, 1980, p. 224).
Nursing process	Not addressed.
Nurse–patient relations	Not addressed.
Nursing therapeutics	Regulate and control: a) providing protection, nurturance, or stimulation to subsystems; b) by external mechanisms restricting, defending, inhibiting, or facilitating (Johnson, 1961; 1980).
Focus	Responses of person to stress, the reduction of stress, and the support of natural defenses and adaptive processes (1961, p. 66).

Table 13-5
Potential Propositions—Johnson

Person

1. Behavior is orderly, systematic, and organized around seven subsystems of behavior. Each subsystem of behavior is identifiable by structure, goal, set, choice, behavior by function, and by a number of functional requirements.
2. Internal regulatory mechanisms affect the structure, function, and functional requirements in the subsystem of behavior of the entire system.
3. Behavioral subsystem disorders are manifested in disturbances in structure, function, or functional requirements in each subsystem. Behavioral subsystem disorders are differentiated into insufficiency in one of the subsystems, dominance in one or more of the subsystems, or incompatibility between two or more of the subsystems.

Environment

1. External regulatory mechanisms affect each subsystem of behavior, and the entire system is demonstrated by structure function and the subsystem functional requirements.

Health

1. Health, a behavioral system balance or stability, is manifested in the effective and efficient attainment of the goals and functions of each subsystem of behavior as judged by the nurse and mediated by the right of the patient.
2. Balance could be determined through manifestations of general harmony with and between the behavioral systems.

Nursing Process

1. Johnson's theory does not yield any theoretical propositions related to the nursing process. Assessing and diagnosing, using Johnson's theory, brings about efficient and effective nursing care.

Interactions

1. Johnson's theory does not yield any theoretical propositions related to the nursing process except when we consider subsystem interactions.

Nursing Therapeutics

1. Nursing is an external force that functions through control or modification of external regulatory mechanisms for the purpose of achieving balance and stability as demonstrated by efficient and effective functioning.
2. Nursing therapeutics are differentiated into nurturance, stimulation, and maintenance.
3. Nursing therapeutics deal with insufficiency, dominance, and incompatibility.

THEORY ANALYSIS

The Theorist

Dorothy Johnson, a pediatric nurse by training, received her bachelor of science degree from Vanderbilt University School of Nursing in Nashville, Tennessee and a master of public health degree from Harvard University. She spent the balance of her nursing career as a professor of pediatrics at the University of California, Los Angeles, where she influenced the lives and theoretical identities of many faculty members, administrators, and students alike. Her interest in sociology and psychology influenced the development of her theory.

Johnson worked with students in the master's program. Although some wrote master's theses and many went on to further education, the focus of the program for which she held a primary responsibility in pediatrics was on preparing clinical specialists in the program. Perhaps that may explain the paucity of research related to her theory.

Paradigmatic Origins

Johnson stated that her theory is a product of philosophical ideas, sound theory and research, her clinical experiences, and many years of thinking, discussing, and writing (Johnson, 1978). There were several sources for her theory. First and foremost, her conception of a person as a system of behavior is analogous to the concept of a person as a biological system differentiated into a set of biological systems, such as cardiovascular, skeletal, endocrine, digestive, and so on. Just as each biological subsystem is differentiated by a structure demonstrated in anatomical dissection, a behavioral system has a structure when abstractly dissected. A structure has several components: a goal, a set, a choice, and behavior. Biological subsystems have functions and so do behavioral subsystems. Physiology speaks to biological subsystem functions. Both sets of subsystems have functional requirements.

Johnson's assumptions are congruent with general systems theory assumptions, and concepts consistently evolve from Johnson's systems assumptions. For example, functioning of systems, interdependency of subsystems, balance in subsystems, regularity and constancy of behaviors, energy, boundaries, and disequilibrium are concepts defined by Bertalanffy (1968). Some concepts were used by Johnson with consistent meaning. Johnson considered integration, wholeness, organization, interaction, and integration of a human being as subsystems, all of which are derived from systems theory. The impact of her writings on nursing science in general and on theory in particular underwent a revival in the 1980s. More writing in theory in the 1980s demonstrated the profound impact of her 1950s renaissance theory ideas.

Johnson's theory is also based on a systems paradigm, as perceived from a sociological background. One sees the influence of Talcott Parsons (1951) on her writing in more than one way, but especially in her attempt to conceptualize all nursing as dealing with a person as a system of behavior. Parsons attempted to conceptualize one theory to encompass all sociology. He perceived the science for the Social System Analysis, the social system representing society as the focus of sociological explorations. Components of the structure of a social system—goal, set, choice, and behavior—are the same in Johnson's theory as in Parsons' theory.

Johnson relied on practice to provide the impetus for her theory, on sociology to provide the paradigm, and on psychology to support the validity of the derived concepts, such as Ainsworth's (1972) on affiliation and Feshback's (1970) on aggression.

Internal Dimensions

Johnson's theory embodies an analytical model of what a nursing client is and what the problems that result from this conceptualization are. It is a theory that is developed to answer the questions: What is nursing? and When does a person become a nursing client? Therefore, the answers focus on concepts, and it is a concatenated theory. It is based on a field system of relations focusing on the ill or potentially ill person. It revolves around a concept.

Johnson's theory has a constructive beginning that is a hypothetical conceptualization of a human being from a nursing perspective. It is based on a parallel conceptualization of a human being as a set of biological subsystems. It is also analogous to the conceptualization of Parson's (1951) social system in terms of a structure, function, goals, set, choices, action, functional imperatives, and the goal of stability for the subsystems. Therefore, Johnson's is a deductive, hypothetical theory.

Although Johnson's goal was that her ideas would describe and explain all behaviors that are within the domain of nursing and of all action (therefore to be a macrotheory of nursing), it is a useful microtheory of the client in nursing as a behavioral system. It is a middle-range theory addressing normal and abnormal patterns of behavior in the nursing client. It has a broad scope as it describes and explains a wide range of problems related to assessment of clients (all drives, needs, regulators affecting behavior).

It is interesting to note that, while Johnson advocates that nursing should develop knowledge of control (1968a), the phenomena that she addresses and develops are related to knowledge of order and somewhat to the beginnings of knowledge of disorder.

THEORY CRITIQUE

Johnson's theory provides nursing with a sufficiently broad scope to include a number of diverse areas of nursing. However, the theory is limited to nursing's concern for the ill, hospitalized person and less congruent with nursing's orientation toward health (*e.g.*, Johnson, 1987).

Johnson offers the nursing practice a concept, broad in scope, of a person as a system of behavior; this concept helps in organizing assessment of normal patterns of behavior and deviations from normalcy of internal and external mechanisms that may influence subsystems. Although the theory includes concepts of nursing problems and nursing therapeutics, these concepts are highly abstract in Johnson's work. The extensions offered by Auger (1976), and somewhat by Grubbs (1980), provide an operationalization of definitions of a person and nursing therapeutics. Johnson's theory helps explain the component of a person's behavior that is of interest to nursing. Knowledge of order (normal patterns of behavior) and knowledge of disorder (abnormal patterns of behavior) is synthesized from social, behavioral, and natural sciences. The theory provides, in abstraction, broad guidelines to knowledge of control; the theory's complexity, however, stems from its high abstraction.

The nursing process used by many educational and nursing service institutions was not addressed in Johnson's theory because Johnson focused on a theory of human behavior responses to the stress of illness. Grubbs (1980) demonstrated how Johnson's client assessment theory could be used in conjunction with the nursing process.

The major utility of this theory lies in its framework for the assessment component of the nursing process. Auger and Dee (1983) used it as a guideline to develop a patient classification system. The system provided nursing and hospital administration with the capability to establish levels of staffing based on patients' needs. Clinicians used Johnson's theory as a basis for the development of a classification system that was helpful in providing patients in psychiatric units with purposeful care (Dee and Auger, 1983). The classification system could be used in other settings (Dee, 1986).

Several other analyses were reported in the literature documenting the utility of the theory in practice. Holaday (1980) discussed how the theory was used in pediatrics for assessment and in conjunction with other theories for intervention. Small (1980) used the theory to interpret her research and as a framework for caring for visually impaired children. As a consequence of the theory, the authors found it helpful in providing a framework for diagnosis, in selecting interventions, and in evaluating outcomes. Rawls (1980) described and evaluated the utility of the theory in caring for patients with amputations.

Johnson's theory is focused on individual care, it is better suited for long-term care, and the complexity of the model requires a professional nurse with sound grounding in a number of sciences. It provides an effective guide for assessment and a frame for diagnosis and intervention. However, patterns of behavior that require the care of the nurse are yet to be identified, defined, and developed.

Johnson has profoundly influenced theoretical thinking since 1959, but sparse publication of her theory has limited the radius of contagiousness of her ideas. Johnson always maintained that curricula of nursing should be guided with a well-evaluated conceptualization of nursing (Johnson, 1989). Within that belief system, several curricula emanated from her theory. Most of the application work was done at the institution where Johnson taught—the University of California, Los Angeles (implementation began about 1964). However, the mobility of her colleagues and students has helped in implementing her theory in educational programs at the University of Colorado, Denver (Hadley, 1970), the University of Hawaii, Honolulu, and the Vanderbilt University, Nashville.

The utilization of Johnson's theory in the United States was based on an operationalization of the theory into the University of California, Los Angeles curriculum and on the fact that Wu (1973) and Auger (1976) developed and published their books, extending Johnson's ideas. The combination of these two books provided the beginning student with knowledge of order that replaced the old fundamentals of nursing. Those fundamentals were based on the medical model and were taught to beginning students. No published material is available to describe the painstaking efforts of the University of California School of Nursing faculty in translating Johnson's ideas into a curriculum—a curriculum that was later emulated with refinements in Hawaii and Colorado. Later, in the 1980s, Harris (1986) chronicled the utilization of Johnson's theory as a framework for the curriculum at the University of California, Los Angeles.

External Components

In her theory, Johnson diligently identified the assumptions, defined most of the nursing domain concepts, and provided guidelines for utilization in conjunction with the nursing process. The assumptions and conceptualizations are congruent with current professional values regarding the uniqueness of nursing, its separateness and interdependence. Also, the view of stability is becoming accepted as a world view for nursing. However, the theory's focus on the individual and disorder is incongruent with nursing's claim to health maintenance and promotion and to nursing's interest in aggregates as seen in the concept of community health.

Johnson was one of the first nursing scholars to identify the significance of congruence between nursing goals and societal expectations (1974, p. 376). She continued over the years to emphasize that the client and the public are the ultimate judges of the nursing mission. The theory grew out of her conviction that improvement in care is the ultimate goal. The studies done by Grubbs (1980), Holaday (1981), and Small (1980) assume such congruence and speak to patients' satisfaction of care. However, as with all other theories, such congruence between public expectations and nurses' stated goals needs to be explored. Perhaps the public's interest in health and in health care commensurate to its cost is in the best interest of nurses and will augment nurses' views of their mission with the public's view of nursing's goals. Until then, it is safe to assume that a theorist who spoke vehemently for improved patient care and for the significance of the public view in shaping the nursing mission has translated those views into her theory.

THEORY TESTING

Johnson, in presenting her theory, invariably spoke of the significance of theory in guiding research (1968b). She admonished that research using her theory should focus on identifying and explaining "the behavioral system disorders which arise in connection with illness, and . . . develop the rationale for and means of management" (1968b, p. 6).

Damus (1980) explored the validity of theory in practice and collected observations related to behavioral system disorder in posttransfusion hepatitis patients. Her study demonstrated a positive relationship between behavioral and physiological disequilibrium and a relationship between nursing diagnosis and nursing intervention. More important, this study lent support to the idea that, indeed, the "source of subsystem disorders can be identified and predicted" and also lent unequivocal support to the usefulness of the theory in nursing practice (1980, p. 287).

Holaday's study of achievement in well and chronically ill children (1974, 1981) and Porter's (1972) on stimulation of premature infants lend validity to notions of the subsystem, its utility, and isolation in patient care. Holaday completed two research studies related to the affiliative subsystem of behavior (1981, 1982) and the achievement subsystem (1974). In the first, the cry of the chronically ill infant received a different pattern of maternal response than the cry of the well infant. The set goal components of the subsystems provided the interpretation for the mother's responses to the cry.

Five research tools were developed to measure perceived quality of nursing care and perceived behavioral changes of cancer patients, based on Johnson's theory. The first patient indicators of nursing care were developed to record "incidences of readily observable physiological complications acquired by institutionalized patients" and to measure quality of care (Majesky, Brester, and Nishio, 1978, p. 365). They were based on Johnson's assumption that the occurrence of a complication is a manifestation of a person's "ability to cope with stresses on the behavioral systems" (p. 365). Therefore, to monitor behavioral changes, a nurse can derive the status of a person on a health/illness continuum. The 105 items of potential complications representing infection, immobility, and fluid imbalance were subjected to validity screening and reliability testing.

The second research tool, the Derdiarian behavioral system model, resulted in 193 items categorized to represent each subsystem of the behavior, which are useful for identifying perceived changes due to cancer (Derdiarian, 1983; Derdiarian and Forsythe, 1983; Derdiarian, 1984). These attempts are useful beginnings of factor-isolating, categorizing, and providing empirical descriptions of some central concepts in the theory.

The third research tool was a projective test developed by Lovejoy (1983; 1985) to assess family functioning as perceived by leukemic children. The fourth instrument was developed and validated by Dee (1986) as a classification instrument for psychiatric patients. The fifth was developed by Bruce, Hinds, Hudak, Mucha, Taylor and Thompson (1980) to measure the quality of outcomes for renal disease patients. Each of these tools has the potential for further support of theory and its utility.

These tools demonstrate the usefulness of the theory in the assessment of nursing problems. One of the requirements for subsystem survival is the provision of stimulation. In an attempt to identify the needs of premature infants, Porter (1972) explored the relationship of sensory stimulation and growth and development of premature infants. Subsequent to this study, others have provided evidence that indeed infants demonstrated marked growth and development when premature infants are stroked frequently and when infants are handled frequently.

Attributions of success to internal and external variables differentiated between chronically ill and normal children. The chronically ill children tended to attribute success and failure to outside variables and normal children tended to attribute the same to internal variables. Holaday (1974) interpreted the results to indicate disequilibrium in the achievement subsystem. Both studies lend more empirical clarity to two of Johnson's subsystems. The dependency subsystem also received some investigative attention (Stamler and Palmer, 1971). These studies support the presence of subsystem conceptual boundaries.

Other studies are based on psychiatric patients (Dee, 1986) or have developed and published a description of indicators in patient care that are central to nursing (Majesky, Brester and Nishio, 1978). The potential in these studies is tremendous because the researchers are attempting to delineate patient care outcomes based on nursing interventions.

Outcomes of behavioral system stability are still complex and highly abstract. Factor-isolating studies and exemplars are needed to delineate different states of stability. The theory's clarity is demonstrated in its view of the person and its lack of clarity is viewed in outcomes. Nursing service administrations have used the theory to develop nursing assessment forms for history, nursing admission, and discharge. The questions in the forms evolve from a behavior system framework that characterizes this theory (Dee, 1986; Dee and Auger, 1983).

Theories can be used as a framework for interpretation. A good example of this use is provided in the research of Holaday (1981, 1982, 1987) that was described previously. Holaday found that maternal responses to ill infants were characterized by quick response time and immediacy; mothers were in close vicinity of infants at all times; and the mothers' interventions were multiple rather than singular. In other words, mothers tended to pick up the ill infant, rock, pat, and give a pacifier, as compared with just picking up the well infant. Mothers of the ill infants did not discriminate between different types of cries as well as did mothers of the well infants (*e.g.*, cries due to pain or restlessness). Holaday interpreted her results using Johnson's components of the behavioral subsystems theory that is set-goal, which was narrow in the case of the ill children. In other words, mothers of chronically ill children responded to every cry with no discrimination. With this theory-based interpretation, nursing implications according to Holaday (1981; 1987) were for helping mothers with their set-goal of the affiliative subsystem, that is, the subsystem that focuses on relations.

Johnson's theory was used internationally as a framework to describe perceived rights for disclosure of information related to each subsystem of behavior. Two factors emerged to be significantly related to perceptions of rights for disclosure. These factors correspond to the achievement, ingestion, and elimination subsystems. The findings support these subsystems' functions of the need for mastering the environment through information and the need for incorporating information regarding patients' concerns (Naguib, 1988).

Sister Callista Roy

THEORY DESCRIPTION

The central questions of Sister Callista Roy's theory are: Who is the focus of nursing care? and What is the target of nursing care?; and to a lesser extent, When is nursing care indicated? As with other current theories in nursing, the outcome of nursing care received limited consideration in Roy's descriptive theory.

Roy's first ideas appeared in 1964 in a graduate course paper written at the University of California, Los Angeles. Roy published these ideas in 1970, and subsequently, different components of her framework crystalized during the decades of the 1970s and 1980s. Over the years, Roy identified the assumptions upon which her theory is based (Table 13-6). More recently, the theory incorporated humanistic assumptions regarding the dignity of human beings and the role of nurses in promoting integrity in life and death. Roy also made the client appear more visible in

Table 13-6
Assumptions—Roy

Explicit Assumptions (Roy, 1980)
- The person is a bio-psycho-social being.
- The person is in constant interaction with a changing environment.
- To cope with a changing world, the person uses both innate and acquired mechanisms, which are biological, psychological, and social in origin.
- Health and illness are one inevitable dimension of the person's life.
- To respond positively to environmental changes, the person must adapt.
- The person's adaptation is a fucntion of the stimulus he is exposed to and his adaptation level.
- The person's adaptation level is such that it comprises a zone indicating the range of stimulation that will lead to a positive response.
- The person has four modes of adaptation: physiological needs, self-concept, role function, and interdependence. (Roy, 1980, pp. 180–182).
- "Nursing accepts the humanistic approach of valuing other persons' opinions and viewpoints" (Roy, 1984, p. 36). Interpersonal relations are an integral part of nursing (Roy, 1984, p. 36).
- There is a dynamic objective for human existence with the ultimate goal of achieving dignity and integrity (Roy, 1984, p. 38).

Implicit Assumptions
- A person can be reduced to parts for study and care.
- Nursing is based on causality.
- Patients' values and opinions are to be considered and respected.
- A state of adaptation frees an individual's energy to respond to other stimuli (Roy, 1984, p. 38).

---

the care process, although this visibility is more philosophical in nature and less operationalized in practice.

Roy's assumptions in general are in agreement with current views in nursing regarding adaptations, human beings, and nursing. Her implicit assumptions attest to the totality of the individual as manifested in behavior, active participation of individuals in life, and an individual's potential for self-actualization. New humanistic values have been identified in Roy's theory (1984; 1987; 1988). The principles of humanism are creative power, holism, subjectivity, purposefulness in life, interpersonal relations, and activity. Although others have tended to view the holistic nature of the theory (Mastal and Hammond, 1980), it was not until 1984 that Roy emphasized the holistic nature of a person and the humanistic care of nurses. In 1987 and 1988, these humanistic values were described.

According to Roy's theory, a person—a bio-psycho-social being, an adaptive system, a human being—is in constant interaction with a changing environment; therefore, a person is continually changing and attempting to adapt. When he is not adapting positively and is therefore manifesting ineffective responses, he is of concern to nursing; however, once a person manifests effective behavior, he no longer needs nursing attention. A person uses both innate and acquired mechanisms to ready himself to adapt to his environment (Andrews and Roy, 1986).

A person is conceptualized as having two subsystems for adapting. These are the regulator and cognator mechanisms. The regulator mechanism works primarily through the autonomic nervous system to organize a reflex action that prepares the individual to respond and adapt to the environment. The major parts of the regulator subsystem are the neural, endocrine, and perception-psychomotor parts (Roy and McLeod, 1981). The regulator mechanism receives stimuli from the internal and external environments, both of which are basically chemical or neural, and receives all input into the central nervous system. Body responses observed by the nurse are effects of autonomic responses, responsiveness of endocrine glands, and the perception process. The latter is altered by cultural and social factors (external stimuli) and "must remain in short-term memory long enough for a psychomotor choice or response to be made" (Roy and McLeod, 1981). The bodily responses, brought about through the chemical–neural–endocrine channels, are fed back as additional stimuli to the regulator system (Roy, 1984, pp. 28–36).

The second mechanism is the cognator subsystem, which identifies, stores, and relates stimuli so that a symbolic meaning can be attached to the behavior. The cognator mechanism is composed of several parts and corresponding processes: (1) perceptual/information processing manifested in the processes of selective attention, coding, and memory; (2) learning, manifested in imitation, reinforcement, and insight; (3) judgment, which involves the process of problem solving and decision making; and (4) emotion, which is manifested in defenses to seek relief and affective appraisal and attachment. These processes are influenced by internal and external stimuli and affect the psychomotor choice of response of orientation, approach, avoidance, flight, or hiding as demonstrated in the form of spoken or unspoken words. Failure in either the regulator or the cognator mechanisms result in maladaptation (Roy, 1984).

All input is channeled through the processes of the regulator and the cognator and produce responses through four effector modes: physiological needs, self-concept, role function, and interdependence. The two subsystems are related to each other through perception and are related to each effector mode differently. Whereas the regulator is related predominantly to the physiological mode,

> . . . since very little is known physiologically about the process of perception
> formation, memory, and choice of psychomotor responses, the other modes
> of self-concept, role function, and interdependence must relate to the
> meaning of a given perception for the individual human system. The meaning
> of the perception will, therefore, influence the body response. (Roy and
> McLeod, 1981, p. 67)

On the other hand, the cognator subsystem is related to all adaptive modes. Processes such as selective attention, imitation, problem solving, and appraisal influence nutritional intake in the physiological mode, role function, self-concept, and interdependence. Likewise, within each mode, all cognator processes could be manifested; for example, attachment, reinforcement, and memory are integral parts of role cues selected by a person. The physiological mode is a result of the needs of individuals for physiological integrity. This mode allows individuals to respond physically to their environment. There are five basic needs and fair regulator processes in this mode. The physiological needs are activity and rest, nutrition, elimination, oxygenation, and protection. The regulator processes are described as the senses, fluids, and electrolytes, neurological functions, and endocrine functions.

The self-concept mode is related to the need for psychic integrity. Self-concept is defined by a person through significant others, and it includes perceptions of the physical and personal selves. The physical self is manifested in body sensations (feelings and experience) and image (view of self). The components of the personal self are self-consistency (continuity of self), self-ideal (expectations), and the moral–ethical–spiritual self (values) (Andrews and Roy, 1986; Roy, 1987).

The role function and interdependence of the modes are focused on the need for social integrity. Role is viewed in Roy's theory as a set of expectations of individuals toward each other. She classified roles as primary (based on age, sex, and development), secondary (acquired through relations with others and made permanent), and tertiary (activities that are more temporary) (Andrews and Roy, 1986). The interdependence between individuals is expressed in ability to love, to respect, to value, and to receive love, respect, and value.

Stimuli affecting modes and mechanisms are identifiable as focal stimuli (those that are immediate in an individual's life), residual stimuli (attitudes and previous experiences), and contextual stimuli (all other stimuli, *e.g.*, heat, aggravating a rash, or noise that is irritating to a person in pain).

In early writings, Roy and McLeod (1981) proposed that a theory of the person as an adaptive system (*i.e.*, regulator and cognator mechanisms) should be used in conjunction with the Roy adaptation model. This was later modified and synthesized so there was no differentiation between the model and the theory (Roy, 1984). A person is conceptualized as an adaptive system that includes input (stimuli adaptation level), control processes (the regulator and the cognator as coping mechanisms), effectors (four modes), and output (adaptive and ineffective responses) (Roy, 1984, p. 30). See Table 13-7.

Later developments in Roy's theory have helped to clarify her view of a person. However, some concepts remain ambiguous and overlapping. Although concepts are mainly derived from other paradigms, the primitive ones (regulator and cognator) are not as precisely identified and defined. Concept boundaries are not clear. For example, effector modes and focal stimuli overlap (there is overlap in some effector modes, such as in interdependence role, self-concept, and role function). There is also overlap between adaptive modes and mechanisms, and there is lack of clarity in the definitions, as others have discussed (Mastal and Hammond,

Table 13-7
Concepts—Roy

Adaptation	Physical, personal, moral–
Adaptation level	ethical–spiritual self
Adaptation zone	Self-consistency
Adaptive response	Self-ideal/self-expectancy
Client: An Adaptive System	Learning
Biological	Inner cell of self-concept
Anatomy	Self-esteem
Physiology	Adaptive Modes
Psychological	Regulator process
Perceiving	The senses
Learning	Neurological function
Acting	Endocrine function
Social	Fluid and electrolyte
Family	Role Function
Community	Expressive
Work Group	Instrumental
Society	Primary role
Adaptive System	Secondary role
Cognator	Tertiary role
Regulator	Role function
Adaptive Stimuli	Position
Focal	Role performance
Contextual	Role mastery
Residual	Social integrity
Physiological Modes	Interdependence
Activity and rest	Nurturing
Nutrition	Affectional adequacy
Elimination	Significant other
Oxygenation	Support systems
Psychological Modes	Receptive behaviors (love, respect, value)
Self-concept	Contributive behaviors (love, respect,
Psychic integrity	value)

1980). Environment and internal stimuli remain operationally undifferentiated (Tiedeman, 1983).

Roy and McLeod (1981) and Roy and Roberts (1981) have provided a useful systematic presentation of all possible links between variables resulting in a multitude of theoretical propositions. This is clearly a theory that lends itself to the development of more propositions. The propositions provided by the theorist are theoretically sound, structurally adequate, systematic, and relational. The researcher's task is in operationalizing propositions for research projects. The propositions tend to focus on biological events (physiological response, intact neural pathways) rather than nursing phenomena. The propositions are linear and bivariate, but Roy is striving for nonlinear and multivariate relationships (Roy and Roberts, 1981, p. xiv).

Roy's theory has a high descriptive and explanatory power of the individual as an adaptive system, but the theory has limited predictive and prescriptive power. The descriptive and explanatory potential could be further enhanced with existence propositions. This is the task most needed for the further development and refinement of this theory. While Roy has attempted to establish the theoretical validity of each coping system and effector mode, work now should proceed to establish their empirical validity.

THEORY ANALYSIS

The Theorist

After receiving a master of science degree in pediatric nursing, Sister Callista Roy, who was a pediatric nurse by training, proceeded to study sociology at the University of California, Los Angeles, where she received her doctorate in 1976. The impetus of her theory was inspired by her having been the advisee and student of Dorothy Johnson. Her first manuscript, conceptualizing man as an adaptive system, was based on Helson's (1964) theory of adaptation level and was written for Johnson's graduate class on conceptual models in nursing. Later influenced by Ralph Turner, the sociologist, Roy derived her explication of self-concept and role function.

Forces in the development of her model have been her administrative position at Mount St. Mary's College, which allowed her the further development of theory in curricula and allowed her utilization of the expertise and the support of faculty members who taught at that institution. Sister Callista Roy is an eloquent speaker and a prolific writer, with a great deal of energy that has helped spread her ideas nationally and internationally. After completing a postdoctoral fellowship at the University of California, San Francisco School of Nursing (where she was trained as a clinical scholar on a Robert Wood Johnson fellowship in 1985), she embarked on a new phase in her research/practice theory career. As a clinical scholar and while in the program, she has utilized her theory in a clinical neurology setting.

Paradigmatic Origins

Roy's theory is a synthesis of concepts developed outside the domain of nursing and redefined within the context of nursing. Although Helson's adaptation level theory appears to be the impetus for the central concept in this theory—adaptation as a process—Roy clearly and admittedly was also influenced by her mentor and teacher, Dorothy Johnson. Johnson conceptualized a person as a behavioral system with seven subsystems, and Roy conceptualized a person as a system with two subsystems as coping mechanisms and four modes of coping. The similarities continue to encompass goals of nursing (homeostasis), focus (external regulatory mechanisms), the patients (maladaptive or potentially maladaptive people), and later, a person with ineffective behavior.

Roy's doctoral education in sociology and her work with Ralph Turner influenced her development of the role, interdependence, and self-concept (an interactionist approach) as effector modes.

> One's self-concept is defined by interaction with others. One-to-one
> interactions between individuals are characterized by the use of verbal and
> nonverbal symbolic communication. (Roy and Roberts, 1981, p. 205)

To be specific, Roy's theory evolved from a synthesis of concepts from the adaptation, systems, and interactional paradigms. There are parallels between the list of concepts with the physiological modes, Johnson's subsystems of behaviors, Henderson's activities of daily living, and unmet needs (*e.g.*, rest, elimination, circulation).

The development of Roy's theory progressed rather rapidly to meet curricular needs of Mount St. Mary's College in Los Angeles. Therefore, some sense of urgency, and the backgrounds of existing faculty, may have contributed to some of the seemingly fragmented and overlapping concepts. The expediency may have created content to be used in a curriculum rather than content that would enhance the development of nursing knowledge through questioning and refinement. All these influences and forces have been acknowledged in later writings (Andrews and Roy, 1986).

Internal Dimensions

Roy's theory is a moderately abstract, logically deductive microtheory of the nursing client developed around descriptions of concepts; thus, it is a concatenated theory developed around adaptation and its modes. Roy uses a field approach with units of analysis in terms of other mini-units. The theory has a broad scope. It attempts to address a broad range of problem areas related to the client who has demonstrated ineffective responses to internal and external stimuli. The goal of the theory is to conceptualize the nursing client, in Roy's early writings, as four coping modes, and in later writing, as a system with two subsystems—the regulator and the cognator—and even later as input, two subsystems, four effector modes, and output

(Roy, 1984). Roy and Roberts (1981) proposed the Roy theory as "a nursing practice theory . . . which is the knowledge of disorder" (p. 24), but in fact it provides a framework to organize knowledge that addresses modes and mechanisms of adaptation as well as ineffective behavior.

THEORY CRITIQUE

Roy's theory evolved out of mental imagery of what nursing is, who the nursing client is, and what the goal of nursing care is. It was deductively derived from other theoretical formulations but was not based on previous research findings, nor did it generate many published research findings (Roy, 1976, p. 691; Roy and McLeod, 1981). During twenty years of development of theory, Roy has clarified her own philosophic assumptions and discussed them (Roy, 1988). Some of her assumptions could be propositions and therefore could be tested. One example is the conceptualization of human beings with four coping modes. Furthermore, which behaviors are components of what mode of coping need also be subjected to evaluation. Roy acknowledges such directions in formulating propositions (Roy, 1980).

Roy is given a great deal of credit as a theorist who has systematically attempted to develop theoretical propositions to enhance the potential of research. Nevertheless, the propositions are based more on neurological and biological sciences. Some of these propositions tend to reduce the person to responding to chemical or neural stimuli through neural inputs (Roy and Roberts, 1981, pp. 62–66). The perspective is demonstrated in attention to central concepts and attention to careful articulation of assumptions congruent with the nature of nursing. Clarity of the concepts could be enhanced by theoretical distinctiveness, operational definitions, valid empirical referents, and reliable data. Clarity of a theory in nursing could be enhanced by explicit relatedness between central concepts of the theory.

The few studies conducted utilizing Roy's theory were directed to exploring and further developing concepts that are not as central to the theory, such as perceptions of the nursing clients. However, perception of the patient was not a central concept of the early conceptualization of man. Therefore, the earliest research projects focused on perceived adaptation levels of the elderly client (Idle, 1978) and perceptions of decision making (Roy, 1977) rather than on empirically describing systems, effectors, or ineffective responses. When developing her theory later, perception emerged as a concept that links the regulator and cognator mechanisms (Bunting, 1988). Others, such as Randall, Poush-Tedrow, and Van Landingham (1982) provided support for the centrality of perceptions. Roy acknowledged and supported the notion of client involvement in their care:

> According to this nursing model, the person is to be respected as an active participant in his care. . . . The goal arrived at is one of mutual agreement between the nurse and patient. Intervention[s] are the options that the nurse provides for the patient. (Roy and Roberts, 1981, p. 47.)

Roy's theory was used to develop research instruments, to describe responses to different health/illness concepts, and to evaluate interventions. Tools were developed to measure perceptions of adaptation levels (Idle, 1978); perceptions of powerlessness in decision making (Roy, 1979); health care outcomes for cancer patients (Lewis, Firsich, and Parsell, 1978, 1979); and regaining functional abilities after delivery (Tulman and Fawcett, 1988).

What the theory lacks in research utilization, it more than compensates for in practice, education, and administrative utility. The theory has synthesized theory with process of clinical judgment adequately and has offered an excellent check list for assessment of variables responsible for the problematic behavior (*i.e.*, focal, contextual, and residual stimuli) and the setting of priorities for action. Although there is no systematic evidence of effect of use of the theory on staff or educators, many personal testimonies across the country attest to a sense of direction and organization when the theory has been used. The theory offers less direction in prescribing.

In developing and testing an assessment tool based on Roy's theory, Wagner (1976) indicated, in her findings, the lack of boundaries between role function, interdependence, and self-concept modes, but demonstrated the theory's utility in a variety of diverse practice settings. The theory was used in assessing and planning care for patients in surgical settings (Roy, 1971), in community settings (Schmitz, 1980), in obstetric and pediatric settings; in short, in distributive and episodic settings (Wagner, 1976). The setting that created the most difficulty was the intensive care setting (Wagner, 1976). The theory has demonstrated its usefulness in assessing gerontology patients (Janelli, 1980; Farkas, 1981), young children (Galligan, 1979), cardiac patients (Gordon, 1974), postpartum patients (Kehoe, 1981), and cesarean fathers (Fawcett, 1981a). It has been useful in neonatal care (Downey, 1974) and in demonstrating depression and life satisfaction among a group of retired people (Hoch, 1987).

In all these studies, the utility of a check list to identify normal behavior and deviations from normal behavior was demonstrated, and the potential of the theory in identifying outcome criteria to be used for quality assurance was also been demonstrated (Laros, 1977). At the same time, however, they demonstrated a lack of concept boundaries, a severe limitation of the theory's framework for understanding person–environment interactions, and a lack of direction for clinical therapeutics.

The circle of contagiousness of the theory in education is wide and extensive compared with other theories. For educational settings faced with the need for the development of a conceptual framework for curricula, the availability of a theory that has been operationalized at Mount St. Mary's College School of Nursing, including the textbooks and literature to use, made for enthusiastic adoption of the theory. Roy's theory has been used in eleven of the United States (27 schools) and also in Canada and Switzerland (Fawcett, 1984). The theory has also been used in specialty curricula (Brower and Baker, 1976).

Clinical setting administrators have also attempted a further operationalization of the theory in several settings. In each instance, it provided a framework for assessment of patient needs in each of the modes and a ready-made, usable classification system for the stimuli. Recording patient care needs was rendered more organized and simple, and there were indications of increased patient satisfaction and expanded professional practice (Mastal, Hammond, and Roberts, 1982; Laros, 1977).

All concepts related to the physiological mode, or effectors, are concrete and are most directly related to observable data; data related to this mode tend to predominate the findings. Perhaps this is partially because concepts from the other three modes are generally abstract, less operationalized, and beset with unclear boundaries. The concepts are theoretically defined but lack both boundary validity and operational definition. Adaptation, the consequence of nursing care—a process and an end result—lacks both theoretical and operational definition and validity. Exemplars of adapted patients and patients with ineffective behavior (process and product) could help in beginning to develop theoretical definition.

Concepts are tautological, such as focal stimuli, which are also identified behaviors in each of the modes. The view of a person as an open interacting system and the view of input and output appear to be inconsistent, even though Roy, in her later writing, incorporated both input and output within her conceptualization of a person. On the whole, Roy used a field approach and logical method in the development of her theory, and she defined units in terms of other mini-units.

External Components of Theory

Society and other health care professionals would agree that nursing deals with the physiological needs of the patient and the goal of adaptation in that mode, but there may be less agreement on the role of nursing in relation to other modes. Perhaps this is due to decreased clarity of those modes or the focus of the health care system on biological and physiological aspects of care. The systematic assessment potential that Roy's theory offers is congruent with the prevailing view of the need for an organized system in assessment and intervention and utility of the nursing process in patient care.

The simplicity of the theory and the available operationalized teaching-oriented literature enhanced its wide geographic spread but limited its more thoughtful and inquisitive utilization; coping mechanisms of cognator and regulator are limited in utility due to lack of clarity. The complexity of the propositions has hampered its operationalization for research. Educators and clinicians in search of a coherent way to present and discuss their care or teaching found the theory useful and provided more face validity to the concepts of the theory. Researchers, on the other hand, either ignored the theory or found the complexity of the propositions and their physiological perspective cumbersome or unrepresentative of the nursing perspective, so they turned to other perspectives. For whatever reasons, creative energies centered around face validity studies rather than on construct, criterion validity, or relational research.

The strength of Roy's theory lies in its exemplary nature of theory development. The theory evolved out of a belief that nursing has a unique contribution to patient care and that the recipient of care is an open adaptive system. After structurally identifying major components of theory, assumptions, and concepts, Roy proceeded to develop the functional components (*i.e.*, utility in education, practice, and research). Then she backtracked and systematically identified theory propositions. The theory is ready for some systematic research.

THEORY TESTING

Studies were conducted by Roy during her postdoctoral Robert Wood Johnson fellowship at the University of California, San Francisco, to determine head injury patients' cognitive processes and to test different propositions of the theory. This research is not yet documented in the literature. Others have used the theory to describe responses to chronic illness (Pollock, 1986); perceptions of stressors of children in an intensive care unit (Munn and Tichy, 1987); the needs of spouses of surgical patients (Silva, 1987); and the differences between recovery rates in the functional abilities of postpartum vaginal and cesarean delivery patients (Tulman and Fawcett, 1988).

The effects of interventions that were designed within an adaptation framework were evaluated in several studies. Examples are evaluation of effects of using a birth chair on mothers and infants (Cottrell and Shannahan, 1986; 1987) and of prenatal education on unplanned cesarean birthing (Fawcett and Henklein, 1987). Fawcett's (1981b) research in identifying the needs of cesarean parents is an example of significant research offering support to Roy's modes of adaptation as a primary assessment framework. Levels of adaptation have been an elusive consequence but a most significant aid in understanding the nursing care process and its intended goals. The study of Lewis, Firsich, and Parsell (1979), geared toward developing an instrument to measure the adaptation level of chemotherapy patients, is a step in the right direction in the empirical definition of adaptation. Relationships between study variables and theory concepts need further analysis (Tables 13-8 and 13-9).

Table 13–8
Definition of Domain Concepts—Roy

When nursing is needed	The adaptive system of a person who is ill or has the potential of illness "when unusual stresses or weakened coping mechanisms make the person's usual attempts to cope ineffective."
Goal of nursing	To enhance the adaptation of the patient in the four modes to free energy to respond to other stimuli. Freed energy promotes healing abilities and wellness (Roy & Roberts, 1981). "To promote adaptation" (Roy, 1984, p. 36) and "to decrease ineffective responses" (Roy, 1984, pp. 37–38).
Health	A state of adaptation that is manifested in free energy to deal with other stimuli. A process of promoting integrity (Roy, 1984, p. 39).

(continued)

Table 13–8 (*Continued*)

Environment	Internal and external stimuli. There are three classes of stimuli: the focal stimuli immediately confronting a patient; contextual, all stimuli; residual pertinent stimuli, but cannot validate effect on current situation. In other words, it is "all conditions, circumstances, and influences surrounding and affecting the development and behavior of persons and groups" (Roy, 1984, p. 39).
Human being	Functions holistically (Roy, 1984, p. 36), highest possible fulfillment of human potential (Andrews and Roy, 1986).
Nursing client	A person, family, group, or community. Bio-psycho-social adaptive systems with two processor subsystems that are mechanisms for adapting or coping—the regulator and the cognator. The system has four affectors of adaptation, or the adaptive modes: physiological needs, self-concept, role function, and interdependence (Roy & Roberts, 1981, p. 43). A holistic, adaptive system (Roy, 1984, p. 36).
Nursing problem	The source of difficulty is coping activity that is inadequate to maintain integrity in the face of a need deficit or excess (Roy, 1980, p. 184).
Nursing process	A "particular format" used in nursing that utilizes the problem-solving approach. It comprises the six steps of assessment of behaviors, assessment of influencing factors, nursing diagnosis, goal-setting, intervention, and evaluation (Roy, 1984, pp. 42–62).
Nurse–patient relations	Acknowledged in 1984 as important, but not defined. Defined in 1987 through nursing process.
Nursing diagnosis	"Changes in internal or external environment can trigger need deficits or excesses. Within the appropriate adaptive mode, coping activation is stimulated. When the coping mechanism is ineffective in meeting the demand, ineffective behavior results" (Roy & Roberts, 1981, p. 47). "The behavior with its predominant stimulus" (Roy & Roberts, 1981, p. 47).
Nursing therapeutics	Traditional techniques such as comfort measures or health teaching, or entirely new activities that have not been discovered, all with the goal of promoting adaptation (Roy & Roberts, 1981, pp. 47–48).
Focus	On persons, groups, families, communities, or societies with ineffective behavior, and on manipulation of stimuli so that they would fall within the patient's zone of positive coping. Increase, modify, decrease internal or external stimuli. Traditional interventions such as providing comfort or health teaching, or new undiscovered interventions (Roy, 1984, p. 28).

Table 13-9
Propositions—Roy

○ Nursing actions can increase a person's adaptive responses.
○ Nursing actions can decrease a person's ineffective adaptive responses.
○ People interact with changing environment in an attempt to achieve adaptation and health.

Betty Neuman

THEORY DESCRIPTION

The central questions for Betty Neuman are: How can nurses organize the vast knowledge needed to deal with complex human situations that require nursing care? and How do nursing clients interact, adjust to, and react to stress? Neuman considers her theory as wellness-oriented and as a holistically focused conceptualization of client and nurse responses and actions (Neuman, 1989a). Neuman articulated a number of basic assumptions about client systems, environmental stressors, responses to stress, lines of resistance and defense health, energy, and wellness (Neuman, 1989a, p. 17-22). These explicit assumptions are described in Table 13-10. Central concepts of her theory are included in Table 13-11.

Table 13-10
Assumptions—Neuman*

---

1. Nursing clients are dynamic; they have both unique and universal characteristics and are in constant energy exchange with environments.
2. The relationship between client variables—physiological, psychological, sociocultural, developmental, and spiritual—influence a client's protective mechanisms and determine a client's response.
3. Clients present normal range of responses to the environment that represent wellness and stability.
4. Stressors attack flexible lines of defense, then normal lines of defense.
5. Nurses' actions are focused on primary, secondary, and tertiary prevention.

* These assumptions are based on Neuman (1979a).

Table 13–11
Concepts—Neuman

Variables
    Physiological
    Psychological
    Sociocultural
    Developmental
    Spiritual
Flexible line of defense
Normal line of defense
Lines of resistance
Basic structure/energy resources
Stressors
    Intrapersonal
    Interpersonal
    Extrapersonal
Environment
    Internal
    External
    Created
Health
    Wellness
    Stability
Prevention
    Primary
    Secondary
    Tertiary
Reconstitution
Theory of Optimum Client System Stability

To Neuman, nurses deal with clients as a whole. Nursing clients are people who are anticipating stress or who are dealing with stress (Neuman and Young, 1972). Nurses focus their attention on those responses that could be labeled stressful responses. These responses are then within the domain of nursing. In nursing whole human beings, the nurse diagnoses the level of stability, internal and external environmental stressors, and the effect of stressors on a client's system stability. Levels of stability can be determined through analysis of lines of defense, lines of resistance, basic structure energy resources or survival factors, and the five interacting, dynamic variables: physiological, psychological, sociocultural, developmental, and spiritual (Neuman, 1989a). The spiritual aspects of Neuman's theory were absent in her earlier work (Neuman, 1982); they were added to other variables and developed in her 1989 conceptualization of the composite client system. To Neuman, a client system is a whole system. A client is a physiological, psychological, sociocultural, developmental, and spiritual being.

The *client system*, also referred to as the client, is defined in terms of a core structure and a series of concentric circles in addition to the five previously mentioned variables. The core structure includes basic survival factors that are universal and that characterize all species as well as all unique features of a particular client system. The basic universal survival factors are the innate and genetic factors and natural strengths and weaknesses of the system. Therefore, according to Neuman, this component of the universal core structure is where the innate factors that regulate temperatures, the genetic response patterns, and any innate strengths or weaknesses in all body organs are found. However, this core structure also contains unique aspects of a client system that characterize a person, such as cognitive abilities. A client's response patterns are determined and regulated by this core structure. Both universal and unique features of a client system are described by Neuman as normal temperature range, genetic structure, response pattern, organ strength and weakness, ego structure, and "knowns" or commonalities (1989a, pp. 27–29).

A client system is also described through two lines of defenses, a flexible one and a normal one (Neuman, 1982). All environmental stressors first attempt to attack the flexible line of defense. It is visually represented in Neuman's diagrams as the outermost circle surrounding the basic core structure of energy sources; the line is depicted as broken to signify its flexible nature. It is a buffer to a client's normal line of defense, also known as the "client's normal or stable state." The function of this line of defense is to fight the invasions of stressors or to fight the reactions to stressors. Neuman (1989a) describes this line of defense as

> . . . accordionlike [sic] in function. As it expands away from the normal
> defense line, greater protection is provided; as it draws closer, less protection
> is available. It is dynamic rather than stable and can be rapidly altered over a
> relatively short time period or in a situation like a state of emergency or a
> condition like undernutrition, sleepless, or dehydration. (pp. 28 and 29)

The function of the flexible line of defense as a buffer to the normal line of defense is rendered ineffective by some stressors, singularly or in groups. The stressors will then attack the normal line of defense, and when that in turn becomes ineffective in warding off the effect of the stressor to penetrate the core structure or allowing reactions to stress to occur, then a response to stress will be manifested. Responses are described as instability or illness.

The normal line of defense is another component of the client system. It is vital in protecting the basic core structure and the integrity of the system. "This line represents what the client has become, the state to which the client has evolved over time or the usual wellness level" (Neuman, 1989a, p. 30). Although not quite as flexible as the flexible line of defense, the normal line of defense still has the capability of expanding or contracting over time. It is depicted with a solid circle surrounding the next layer of the client system, which is the lines of resistance. This is where the system stability and integrity are manifested, and this is where the normal patterns of wellness levels for the client system are found. Its dynamic nature is apparent in its ability to remain stabilized in dealing with stressors.

Stressors singularly or in groups could continue to penetrate the client system, heading for its basic structure and energy resources. Before the stressor is allowed to influence the basic core of a client system, however, it has to penetrate what Neuman calls lines of resistance. These lines involuntarily activated are three broken concentric circles surrounding the core of a client system. As a stressor succeeds in penetrating the normal line of defense, the lines of resistance are activated. "These resistance lines contain certain known and unknown internal factors that support the clients' basic structure and normal defense line, thus protecting system integrity" (Neuman, 1989a, p. 30).

Neuman provides the "mobilization of white blood cells" as an example of activation of a line of resistance. If lines of resistance succeed in warding off stressors, that is "reversing the reaction to stressors," then the client system reconstitutes its energy resources and basic structure (Neuman, 1989a, p. 31). If lines of resistance fail, then energy will be depleted. The degree of energy depletion goes from minimal to death.

Each one of these concentric circles has a major function. The flexible line of defense shields the normal line of defense; the normal line of defense is a buffer to each of the lines of resistance; and all these lines combine function to prohibit the stressor from invading the core structure of a human being. All the lines combined also protect the core structure from reacting to stress. Each defense and resistance line varies according to such variables as age and development.

To Neuman, stressors are all environmental, and they have the potential for disrupting the stability of the client system (1989a, p. 50). Stressors attempt to penetrate the flexible and normal lines of defense, and the results are positive or negative responses. How a client system responds to stress is determined by the resistance demonstrated through lines of defense and resistance and by the dynamic relationship of five variable areas. The five variable areas are: physiological, which describe bodily structure and function; psychological, which are related to mental processes and relationships; sociocultural, which relate to social and cultural functions; developmental, referring to life development processes; and spiritual, referring to the spiritual belief system. Neuman (1989a) maintained that the spiritual component has not been well-developed in nursing.

To answer her central questions about nursing, Neuman (1974, 1989a) demonstrated that a systems/stress theory of human beings would help nurses organize the vast knowledge amassed about human beings and their environments. An elaborate depiction of stressors and their penetrating abilities and of human beings and their natural and acquired resistance abilities emerged as the framework that nurses could use in describing their clients' problems and the territory for nursing intervention.

As outlined in Table 13-12, nurses also assess stressors in the environment. Environments are internal, external and created, and all may influence a client system in a circular fashion. Client system and environment relate reciprocally, and the outcome of this relationship is corrective or regulative for the client system. The internal environment is intrapersonal, the external environment includes the interpersonal and extrapersonal components, and the created environment is a compos-

Table 13–12
Definition of Domain Concepts—Neuman

Nursing	Is concerned with all and potential stressors. Deals with assessment of effect and potential effects of environmental stressors (Neuman, 1989a, p. 34).
Goal of nursing	To keep client's system stable. To assist clients to adjust, which is a requirement for optimum wellness level (1989a, p. 34).
Health	"Facilitate optimum wellness for the client through retention, attainment or maintenance of client system's stability" (1989a, p. 25). Health is wellness. It is a point on a continuum running from greatest negentropy to maximum entropy (1989a, p. 25).
Human being	A physiological, psychological, sociocultural, developmental, and spiritual being. Represented by central structure, lines of defense, and lines of resistance.
Nursing client	A human being who is threatened with, or who is attacked by, environmental stressors.
Environment	"All internal and external factors or influences surrounding the identified client or client system." Three types of environments were identified: internal, external, and created. The stressors are part of the environment. The internal environment is contained within the boundaries of the client system. The external environment contains forces outside a client system. The created environment denotes a client's unconscious mobilization of such structural components as energy factors, stability, and integrity. (1989a, pp. 31–33)
Nursing problem	A whole client system threatened with or actually manifesting responses to stressors.
Nursing process	Neuman describes three central steps: nursing diagnoses, nursing goals, and outcomes (1989a, pp. 39–41).
Nurse–patient relations	Not discussed.
Nursing intervention	Prevention is the intervention identified by Neuman. There are three components in her intervention typology: primary, secondary, and tertiary. Reconstitution is part of tertiary prevention.

ite of the intrapersonal, interpersonal, and extrapersonal components. Neuman described the internal and external environments in the following way:

> The internal environment consists of all forces or interactive influences internal to or contained solely within the boundaries of the defined client/client system. It correlates with the model intrapersonal factors or stressors. The external environment consists of all forces or interactive influences external to or existing outside the defined client/client system. It correlates with both the model's inter and extrapersonal factors or stressors. (Neuman, 1989a, p. 31)

The created environment is dynamic and is an interface that exists and connects the internal and external environments. Although the created environment may be created unconsciously by a client, it acts as a reservoir for the existence or for the maintenance of the integrity of the client system. The expressions related to this environment are conscious or unconscious or both. The environment infiltrates all systems and all structures, it is purposeful, and it protects the functions of client/client systems.

> The insulating effect of the created-environment changes the response or possible response of the client to environmental stressors, for example, the use of denial or envy (psychological), physical rigidity or muscular constraint (physiological), life cycle continuation of survival patterns (developmental), required social space range (sociocultural), and sustaining hope (spiritual). (Neuman, 1989a, p. 32)

The created environment's goal is the unconscious stimulation of the client's health. It includes self-esteem, values, beliefs, and energy exchanges. Therefore, care-givers should explore ideas, beliefs, and fears as much as they explore symptoms and other causal factors. Finally, we should remember that energy is continuously flowing between client and environment. The care-giver's assessment and intervention is for the purpose of bringing optimal stability, which is the best possible state of wellness. Determining levels of wellness is accomplished through a consideration of client energy levels (Neuman, 1989a, p. 33). When more energy is expended than generated, the client system moves to entropy or illness. As more and more energy is needed to expend and less and less energy is being generated, death may result. Neuman defined entropy as "a process of energy depletion and disorganization, moving the system toward illness or possible death." (Neuman, 1989a, p. 48)

The goal of the care-giver is to maintain or to bring about the system's stability. This process is called by Neuman a process of *reconstitution*. Reconstitution brings the system a state of stability or wellness that is higher or lower than the previous state. Nursing actions are described in terms of prevention. Prevention is primary, secondary, and tertiary. Preventive aspects of care that occur before the stressors invade the client system are primary. Primary prevention identifies potential stressors and augments positive coping and function. When stressors attack the client system, nurses then mobilize and support internal and external responses, protect the core structure, facilitate treatment, and continue with any needed primary prevention. These actions are described by Neuman as secondary prevention (Neuman, 1989a, p. 21; Neuman, 1989b, p. 56).

Neuman describes the development of a theory that evolved from her theory of nursing; the theory is called the theory of optimal client system (Neuman and Koertvelyessy, 1986, cited in Neuman, 1989a, p. 46). Other theories could be developed as well. Neuman's theory has the potential for many theoretical propositions. A number of propositions are described in Table 13-13.

Table 13–13
Propositions—Neuman

- ○ Primary prevention prevents stressors from penetration of flexible line of defense.
- ○ Primary prevention prevents stress responses.
- ○ Secondary prevention enhances wellness and decreases stress.
- ○ By supporting strengths of clients's systems and conserving their energy, nurses can increase level of wellness.

THEORY ANALYSIS

The Theorist

Betty Neuman is a community mental health nurse who received her bachelor's degree in nursing in 1957 and master's degree in nursing in 1966 from the University of California, Los Angeles. She started her teaching job in 1966 (when we became office mates at UCLA) and was charged with coordinating the community mental health consultation clinical specialist program.

Although the UCLA faculty were busily operationalizing and implementing Johnson's theory at that time, Neuman was uninvolved in this process. She was concerned about the development of a framework to describe the consultation role of nurses, one that could help students describe and explain their actions and the rationale for their actions. The result of that concern was the development of her theory of a client who is in need of health care. Since the role of community mental health consultant is not necessarily exclusively a nursing role, this may explain why Neuman maintains in her writings that her theory is designed for use by any health professional.

Neuman has worked as a teacher, a consultant, and a writer, and has maintained a small private practice as a licensed marriage and family counselor. She taught programs in stress reduction and in self-help for retarded children. Neuman received a doctorate degree from Ohio University in 1985. Currently, she continues to lecture, write, and consult, and she is a consultant for the Neuman Systems Model implementation trustee group (Neuman, 1989c, p. 453).

Paradigmatic Origins

There are several paradigmatic origins for Neuman's theory. The origin is explicitly identified by Neuman as systems theory as conceptualized by Bertalanffy (1968). Neuman utilized Caplan's (1964) preventive functions, which she used in teaching the master's program in community mental health to define the levels of actions of nurses (Neuman, 1989c). Other origins identified by Neuman are Chardin's (1955) conceptualization of wholeness; Putts' (1972) application of systems theory in nursing; ideas about adaptation and environment (Neuman, 1989a, p. 12); Marxist ideas of synthesis of man and environment (Cornu, 1957); Gestalt psychology (Edelson, 1970), in which the interaction of people and their environments are described, and Selye's (1950) ideas about stress and bodily responses. Neuman relied heavily on these sources, which are all equally appropriate for utilization by mental health workers. It is the multiplicity of Neuman's sources that provides the breadth in her theory.

Internal Dimensions

This is a highly abstract and a deductive theory constructed from hypothetical beginnings, and it was derived from a number of paradigms. The theory is hierarchical, evolving from a set of principles describing relationships between lines of defense, lines of resistance, basic structure, and energy resources. Neuman's is a field theory that explains the relationship of a client system to the environment, and it is a macrotheory that attempts to describe client system relationships with environment and nurse actions in all client situations. The theory has a broad scope in which Neuman attempted to describe the domain of nursing (and health care in general). It could be classified as a macrotheory that describes the domain of nursing and explains what nurses ought to do in providing primary, secondary, and tertiary prevention.

Neuman's theory was constructed to provide her with a framework for teaching community mental health consultation in a graduate program. It was constructed as a framework in order to synthesize the different theories that she believed are essential for use by a community mental health consultant. Examples of such theories are crisis theory, Gestalt theory, and stress and adaptation theory. Neuman's theory was also developed to identify nurse's actions and the focus of such actions. It provides a comprehensive description of nursing clients and a framework to describe nursing interventions. It describes knowledge of order; that is, it provides a descriptive account of the normal structure of client's systems and of patterns of attack of stressors. It does not provide the user with the necessary descriptive scheme for patterns of responses to stress.

Neuman's theory is logically developed, as demonstrated in her conceptualization of a client system as having several parts, with these parts interacting and relating to form a larger whole (Stevens, 1984). Interventions also have parts and levels. Primary, secondary, and tertiary prevention are identified, but it is not clear why other intervention actions are excluded, or, if included, where they should be within the conceptual scheme of interventions. Many nurses would question the rationale for including all nursing interventions within a prevention framework. There are other critical questions of the theory. Neuman addresses antithetical and mutually exclusive concepts without addressing their complementarity and supplementarity. Examples are stability and dynamism, the conscious and unconscious environments, and holism and isolated responses (*e.g.*, psychological responses of denial). The relationship between these opposites and ways by which they are synthesized have not been addressed.

One of the strengths of this theory is Neuman's use of clear diagrams. These diagrams are printed in practically all of her publications. They make the theory visually appealing and enhance its clarity.

THEORY CRITIQUE

Neuman clearly identified some assumptions on which her theory is built (Fawcett, 1989). There are some implicit assumptions not well defined, such as valuing individuality of clients (Lancaster and Whall, 1989, p. 262). Although this is a theory with a potential to use families and communities as clients, Neuman does not identify assumptions related to such potential. Values inherent in nursing in relationship to the role of patients in maintaining and promoting health are not addressed.

The central concepts of theory lack clarity. For example, the relationship between health and wellness and between health and the World Health Organization's mandate for health for all by the year 2000 are used interchangeably, without careful attention to the different meanings inherent in each.

Neuman (1989c) describes a wide circle of contagiousness for her theory that spans the United States and international countries. Use of her theory encompasses all program levels and a variety of nursing sources. Neuman details an impressive list of utilizers of her theory during the decades of the 1970s and 1980s (Neuman, 1989c, pp. 460–466). This extensive utilization prompted the development of slide shows, videotapes, and the Neuman Systems Model Trustee Group, Inc., which is charged with the task of seeing that her theory flourishes and continues to be used accurately.

The utility of Neuman's theory has been demonstrated in many ways (Campbell and Keller, 1989). Neuman (1989b) describes patient situations in which her theory could be used in suicide counseling, and Lillis and Cora (1989) provide an analysis of the use of Neuman's theory in a case study. Neuman's theory has been used in community health nursing settings (Beddome, 1989; Benedict and Sproles, 1982), as a framework for family assessment (Reed, 1989), as a guide for assessing and intervening in dysfunctional families (Herrick and Goodykoontz, 1989), in caring for patients in hospital settings (Burke, Capers, O'Connell, Quinn, and Sinnott, 1989), as a framework for perinatal nursing (Dunn and Trepanier, 1989), for assessment of renal patients (Breckenridge, 1989), as a framework for patients recovering at home from myocardial infarction (Ross and Bourbonnais, 1985; Smith, 1989), and for nursing during the acute stage of spinal cord injury (Sullivan, 1986).

Buchanan (1987) offers a modification of the theory for use with aggregates, families, and communities. She clarified and added an extension to each of the central theory concepts; however, the major additional contribution appears to be the collaborative decision-making process. These additions are congruent with Neuman's rationale for the development of her ideas, which is the development of a framework to be used by different members of the health care team. The extensions are also congruent with the theory assumptions. The theory's potential application to caring of people with different cultural heritages was discussed by Sohier (1989).

Neuman's theory is reported to have guided the development of curricula in Neuman's college (Mirenda, 1986), as well as being utilized as a framework for programs in transition from associate to baccalaureate programs (Lowry and Jopp, 1989; Sipple and Freese, 1989), and as a framework for cooperative (two-school) baccalaureate programs (Nelson, Hansen, and McCullagh, 1989). The faculty and administrators in most of these programs found Neuman's theory clear; it provided a holistic vision of nursing—a clear nursing perspective, and it provided an emphasis on client's perceptions—a useful framework for analysis of clients.

One example of this evaluation is in Nelson, Hansen and McCullagh (1989). Mrkonich, Hessian, and Miller (1989) describe using Neuman's theory as a framework for three accredited baccalaureate nursing programs that are situated in private, religious, and liberal arts colleges. The authors report that the theory's use was enhanced by its common language, which facilitated communication between health care professionals (p. 93). They also credit the theory for its potential to stimulate research and further development of theory (Mrkonich, Miller and Hessian, 1989). Mirenda (1986) described the Neuman college nursing process tool that was developed to be used by students in assessing nursing clients. The tool is reported to help students use Neuman's theory clinically.

Neuman's theory is used as a framework for demonstration of the process of concept development. The richness of the diagrammatic representation of the theory concepts and relationships has helped faculty members in one college devise visual representation to assist students to learn about conceptual models (Johnson, 1989).

There are many indications of the theory's international use. Examples of are provided by Ross, Bourbonnais, and Carroll (1987) and Bourbonnais and Ross's (1985) descriptive accounts of the theory's utility for the fourth and final year of a baccalaureate program in Canada. Story and Ross (1986) demonstrated the theory's effective utility in the development and implementation of a framework for clinical learning experiences for nursing with families of the elderly at home. These authors also discussed the feasibility of using multiple nursing theories within the same curriculum to guide different learning experiences.

Similar examples of utility in curricula were provided by many others. These examples were collected by Neuman in a book of readings (Neuman, 1989a). This collection demonstrates the extensive utility of her theory for baccalaureate programs and associate degree programs as well as for a framework for multi-level planning.

The theory's utility in administrative practice has also been demonstrated. It was used as a framework for community health administration (Drew, Craig, and Beynon, 1989), and it was used as a framework for the reorganization of structure and function of the nursing department at Jefferson Davis Memorial Hospital

(Hinton-Walker and Raborn, 1989). Kelley, Sanders, and Pierce (1989) describe the utility of the theory in guiding nurse administrators in their management and leadership roles in educational and practice settings. They also report the development of a tool for assessing and evaluating "conditions upon which the nurse administrators' goals are established and modified" (p. 129).

The Neuman Systems Management Tool, well described and illustrated, is tailored to provide administrators with a guide for actions and decisions within three minutes of use. No reports of validity or reliability of the tool were provided. Others report its use in the development of nursing care plans (Capers and Kelly, 1987) as well as in planning and implementation of the theory in nursing practice (Capers, O'Brien, Quinn, Kelly and Fenerty, 1985).

External Components of Theory

Neuman's theory is congruent with values about holism in nursing and the reciprocal relationship between environments and client systems. The theory is also highly useful for nurses who tend to speak in terms of prevention rather than treatment or intervention. The focus of the theory on involvement of clients and on assessment that includes defense and resistance is an acceptable nursing focus. The theory is particularly useful for nurses who believe that all health care professionals share the same goals and actions. In proposing the universality of assessment and intervention among the different health professionals, Neuman failed to identify the unique contributions of nurses to the health care team.

THEORY TESTING

Neuman's theory has generated limited research. One of the theory's propositions—that primary prevention inhibits the impact of the stress of surgery—was tested by Ziemer (1983). The study results failed to support the theoretical proposition. Although there is a potential for utilizing the theory as a framework for research, the limited use of Neuman's theory in research raises many questions about its descriptive and explanatory powers. However, Harris, Hermiz, Meininger and Steinkeler (1989) report increasing empirical utilization of Neuman's theory.

Louis and Koertvelyessy (1989) surveyed schools of nursing to determine the use of nursing models in curricula and research. The questionnaires contained specific information related to the use of Neuman's theory. The response rate of 38% was analyzed, and the results indicated that 92% of the responding schools used one of 26 nursing models in their graduate programs as a framework. The respondents identified 41 different models studied by graduate students. Neuman's was one of the most cited models. The authors of the survey report were able to identify 38 research studies that used Neuman's theory. They concluded that the studies were descriptive and that most of the concepts of Neuman's theory were studied, with the exception being the spiritual variable. The researchers used the theory as an outline of the phenomenon, as a framework for the methodology, and as a framework for interpretation and for implications. The report did not include information on the nature of the studies, the findings, or the implications of the findings on Neuman's theory or nursing practice. No citations were provided.

Despite the limitations of Neuman's theory in stimulating research, the utility of the theory in the clinical and educational spheres has been amply documented.

REFERENCES

Johnson

Ainsworth, M. (1972) Attachment and dependency: A comparison. In J. Gewirtz (Ed.), *Attachment and dependency*. Englewood Cliffs, NJ: Prentice-Hall.

Auger, J.A. (1976) *Behavioral systems and nursing*. Englewood Cliffs, NJ: Prentice-Hall.

Auger, J.A. and Dee, U. (April, 1983) A patient classification system based on the Behavioral System Model of Nursing: Part 1. *The Journal of Nursing Administration*, 13, 38–43.

Bertalanffy, L. von (1968) *General systems theory: Foundations, development, application*. New York: George Braziller.

Bruce, G.L., Hinds, P., Hudak, J., Mucha, A., Taylor, M.C., and Thompson, C.R. (1980). Implementation of ANA's quality assurance program for clients with end-stage renal disease. *Advances in Nursing Science*, 2(2), 79–95.

Damus, K. (1980) An application of the Johnson behavioral system model for nursing practice. In J.P. Riehl and C. Roy (Eds.), *Conceptual models for nursing practice* (2nd ed.). New York: Appleton-Century-Crofts.

Dee, U. and Auger, J.A. (1983, May) A patient classification system based on the Behavioral System Model of Nursing: Part 2. *The Journal of Nursing Administration*, 13, 18–23.

Dee, U. (1986) Validation of a patient classification instrument for psychiatric patients based on the Johnson model for nursing. Unpublished doctoral dissertation. San Francisco: University of California.

Derdiarian, A. (1983) An instrument for theory and research development using the behavioral systems model for nursing: The cancer patient, Part I. *Nursing Research*, 32(4), 196–201.

Derdiarian, A. (1984) An investigation of the variables and boundaries of cancer nursing: A pioneering approach using Johnson's behavioral systems model for nursing. In *Proceedings of the 3rd International Conference on Cancer Nursing*. Melbourne, Australia: The Cancer Institute/Peter MacCallum Hospital and the Royal Melbourne Hospital.

Derdiarian, A. and Forsythe, A.B. (1983) An instrument for theory and research development using the behavioral systems model for nursing: The cancer patient, Part II. *Nursing Research*, 32(4), 260–267.

Dickoff, J., James, P., and Wiedenbach, E. (1968) Theory in a practice discipline, Part 1. Practice oriented theory. *Nursing Research*, 17(5), 415–435.

Feshback, S. (1970) Aggression. In P. Mussen (Ed.), *Carmichael's manual of child psychology* (3rd ed.). New York: John Wiley & Sons.

Grubbs, J. (1980) An interpretation of the Johnson behavioral system model. In J.P. Riehl and C. Roy (Eds.), *Conceptual models for nursing practice* (2nd ed.). New York: Appleton-Century-Crofts.

Hadley, B.J. (March, 1970) The utility of theoretical frameworks for curriculum development in nursing: The happening at Colorado. Paper presented at WICHEN General Session, Honolulu, Hawaii.

Harris, R.B. (1986) Introduction of a conceptual model into a fundamental baccalaureate course. *Journal of Nursing Education*, 25, 66–69.

Holaday, B. (1974) Achievement behavior in chronically ill children. *Nursing Research*, 23(1), 25–30.

Holaday, B. (1980) Implementing the Johnson model for nursing practice. In J.P. Riehl and C. Roy (Eds.), *Conceptual models for nursing practice* (2nd ed.). New York: Appleton-Century-Crofts.

Holaday, B. (1981) Maternal response to their chronically ill infants' attachment behavior of crying. *Nursing Research*, 30(6), 343–347.

Holaday, B. (1982) Maternal conceptual set development: Identifying patterns of maternal response to chronically ill infant crying. *Maternal Child Nursing Journal*, 11(1), 47–58.

Holaday, B. (1987) Patterns of interaction between mothers and their chronically ill infants. *Maternal Child Nursing Journal*, 16(1), 29–45.

Johnson, D.E. (1959a) A philosophy of nursing. *Nursing Outlook*, 7(4), 198–200.

Johnson, D.E. (1959b) The nature of a science of nursing. *Nursing Outlook*, 7(5), 291–294.

Johnson, D.E. (1961) The significance of nursing care. *American Journal of Nursing*, 61(11), 63–66.

Johnson, D.E. (1964, June) Is there an identifiable body of knowledge essential to the development of a generic professional nursing program? Paper presented at First Interuniversity Faculty Work Conference Nursing Council, NEBHE, Stowe, VT.

Johnson, D.E. (1968a) Theory in nursing: Borrowed or unique. *Nursing Research*, 17(3), 206–209.

Johnson, D.E. (1968b, April) One conceptual model of nursing. Paper presented at Vanderbilt University, Nashville, TN.

Johnson, D.E. (1974) Development of theory: A requisite for nursing as a primary health profession. *Nursing Research*, 23(5), 372–377.

Johnson, D.E. (1978) State of the art of theory development in nursing. In *Theory development: What, why, how?* New York: National League for Nursing.

Johnson, D.E. (1980) The behavioral system model for nursing. In J.P. Riehl and C. Roy (Eds.), *Conceptual models for nursing practice* (2nd ed.). New York: Appleton-Century-Crofts.

Johnson, D.E. (1987) Evaluating conceptual models for use in critical care nursing practice. *Dimensions of Critical Care Nursing*, 6(4), 195–197.

Johnson, D.E. (1989) Some thoughts on nursing. *Clinical Nurse Specialist*, 3(1), 1–4.

Lovejoy, N. (1983) The leukemic child's perceptions of family behaviors. *Oncology Nursing Forum* 10(4): 20–25.

Lovejoy, N. (1985) Needs of vigil and nonvigil visitors in cancer research units. In *Fourth Cancer Nursing Research Conference Proceedings*. Honolulu: American Cancer Society.

Majesky, S.J., Brester, M.H., and Nishio, K.T. (1978) Development of a research tool: Patient indicators of nursing care. *Nursing Research*, 27(6), 365–371.

Naguib, H.H. (1988) *Physicians', nurses', and patients' perceptions of the surgical patients' educational rights*. Unpublished doctoral dissertation: University of Alexandria, United Republic of Egypt.

Parsons, T. (1951) *The social system*. New York: Free Press.

Porter, L. (1972) The impact of physical-physiological activity on infants' growth and development. *Nursing Research*, 21(3), 210–219.

Rawls, A.G. (1980) Evaluation of the Johnson behavioral model in clinical practice. *Image*, 12, 13–16.

Small, B. (1980) Nursing visually impaired children with Johnson's model as a conceptual framework. In J.P. Riehl and C. Roy (Eds.), *Conceptual models for nursing practice* (2nd ed.). New York: Appleton-Century-Crofts.

Stamler, C. and Palmer, J.O. (1971) Dependency and repetitive visits to the nurse's office in elementary school children. *Nursing Research,* 20(3), 254–255.

Wu, R. (1973) *Behavior and illness.* Englewood Cliffs, NJ: Prentice-Hall.

Zetterberg, H.L. (1963) *On theory verification in sociology* (rev ed.). Totowa, NJ: Bedminster Press.

Roy

Andrews, H.A. and Roy, C. (1986) *Essentials of the Roy adaptation model.* Norwalk, CT: Appleton-Century-Crofts.

Brower, H.T. and Baker, D.J. (1976) Using the adaptation model in a practitioner curriculum. *Nursing Outlook,* 24(11), 686–689.

Bunting, S.M. (1988) The concept of perception in selected nursing theories. *Nursing Science Quarterly,* 1(4), 168–174.

Cottrell, B. and Shannahan, M. (1987). A comparison of fetal outcome in birth chair and delivery table births. *Research in Nursing and Health,* 10, 239–243.

Cottrell, B. and Shannahan, M. (1986) Effect of the birth chair on duration of second stage labor and maternal outcome. *Nursing Research,* 35(6), 364–367.

Downey, C. (1974) Adaptation nursing applied to an obstetric patient. In J.P. Riehl and C. Roy (Eds.), *Conceptual models for nursing practice.* New York: Appleton-Century-Crofts.

Farkas, L. (1981, March) Adaptation problems with nursing home application for elderly persons: An application of the Roy adaptation nursing model. *Journal of Advanced Nursing,* 6, 363–368.

Fawcett, J. (1981a) Assessing and understanding the cesarean father. In C.F. Kehoe (Ed.), *The cesarean experience: Theoretical and clinical perspectives for nurses.* New York: Appleton-Century-Crofts.

Fawcett, J. (1981b) Needs of cesarean birth parents. *Journal of Obstetric, Gynecologic, and Neonatal Nursing,* 10, 371–376.

Fawcett, J. (1984) *Analysis and evaluation of conceptual models of nursing.* Philadelphia: F.A. Davis.

Fawcett, J. and Henklein, J. (1987) Antenatal education for cesarean birth: Extension of a field test. *Journal of Obstetric, Gynecologic, and Neonatal Nursing,* 16, 61–65.

Galligan, A.C. (1979) Using Roy's concept of adaptation to care for young children. *American Journal of Maternal Child Nursing,* 4(1), 24–28.

Gordon, J. (1974) Nursing assessment and care plan for a cardiac patient. In J.P. Riehl and C. Roy (Eds.), *Conceptual models for nursing practice.* New York: Appleton-Century-Crofts.

Helson, H. (1964) *Adaptation-level theory: An experimental and systematic approach to behavior.* New York: Harper & Row.

Hoch, C. (1987). Assessing delivery of nursing care. *Journal of Gerontological Nursing,* 13(1), 10–17.

Idle, B.A. (1978) SPAL: A tool for measuring self-perceived adaptation level appropriate for an elderly population. In E.E. Bauwens (Ed.), *Clinical nursing research: Its strategies and findings* (Monograph series No. 2) Indianapolis: Sigma Theta Tau.

Janelli, L.M. (1980) Utilizing Roy's adaptation model from a gerontological perspective. *Journal of Gerontological Nursing,* 6(3), 140–150.

Kehoe, C.F. (1981) Identifying the nursing needs of the postpartum cesarean mother. In C.F. Kehoe (Ed.), *The cesarean experience: Theoretical and clinical perspectives for nurses.* New York: Appleton-Century-Crofts.

Laros, J. (1977) Deriving outcome criteria from a conceptual model. *Nursing Outlook*, 25, 333–336.

Lewis, F., Firsich, S.C., and Parsell, S. (1978) Development of reliable measures of patient health outcomes related to quality nursing care for chemotherapy patients. In J.C. Krueger, A.H. Nelson, and M.O. Wolanin, *Nursing research. Development, collaboration, utilization.* Germantown, MD: Aspen.

Lewis, F.M., Firsich, S.C., and Parsell, S. (1979) Clinical tool development for adult chemotherapy patients: Process and content. *Cancer Nursing*, 2(2), 99–108.

Mastal, M.F. and Hammond, H. (1980) Analysis and expansion of the Roy adaptation model: A contribution to holistic nursing. *Advances in Nursing Science*, 2(4), 71–81.

Mastal, M.F., Hammond, H., and Roberts, M.P. (1982) Theory into hospital practice: A pilot implementation. *Journal of Nursing Administration*, 12(6), 9–15.

Munn, V.A. and Tichy, A.M. (1987) Nurses' perceptions of stressors in pediatric intensive care. *Journal of Pediatric Nursing*, 2, 405–411.

Pollock, S. (1986). Human responses to chronic illness: Physiologic and psychological adaptation. *Nursing Research*, 35(2), 90–95.

Randall, B., Poush-Tedrow, M., and Van Landingham, U.J. (1982) *Adaptation nursing: The Roy conceptual model applied.* St. Louis: C.V. Mosby.

Roy, C. (1971) Adaptation: A basis for nursing practice. *Nursing Outlook*, 19(4), 254–257.

Roy, C. (1976) *Introduction to nursing: An adaptation model.* Englewood Cliffs, NJ: Prentice-Hall.

Roy, C. (1977) *Decision-making by the physically ill and adaptation during illness.* Unpublished doctoral dissertation, University of California, Los Angeles.

Roy, C. (1979) Relating nursing theory to education: A new era. *Nurse Educator*, 4(2), 16–21.

Roy, C. (1980) The Roy adaptation model. In J.P. Riehl and C. Roy (Eds.), *Conceptual models for nursing practice* (2nd ed.). New York: Appleton-Century-Crofts.

Roy, C. (1984) *Introduction to nursing: An adaptation model* (2nd ed.). Englewood Cliffs, NJ: Prentice-Hall.

Roy, C. (1987) Roy's adaptation model. In R.R. Parse, *Nursing science: Major paradigms, theories, and critiques.* Philadelphia: W.B. Saunders.

Roy, C. (1988) An explication of the philosophical assumptions of the Roy adaptation model. *Nursing Science Quarterly*, 1(1), 26–34.

Roy, C. and McLeod, D. (1981) Theory of the person as an adaptive system. In C. Roy and S.L. Roberts, *Theory construction in nursing: An adaptation model.* Englewood Cliffs, NJ: Prentice-Hall.

Roy, C. and Roberts, S.L. (1981) *Theory construction in nursing: An adaptation model.* Englewood Cliffs, NJ: Prentice-Hall.

Schmitz, M. (1980) The Roy adaptation model: Application in a community setting. In J.P. Riehl and C. Roy (Eds.), *Conceptual models for nursing practice* (2nd ed.). New York: Appleton-Century-Crofts.

Silva, M.C. (1987) Needs of spouses of surgical patients: A conceptualization within the Roy adaptation model. *Scholarly Inquiry for Nursing Practice: An International Journal*, 1, 29–44.

Tiedeman, M.E. (1983) The Roy adaptation model. In J.J. Fitzpatrick and A.L. Whall (Eds.), *Conceptual models of nursing: Analysis and application.* Bowie, MD: Robert J. Brady Company.

Tulman, L. and Fawcett, J. (1988) Return of functional ability after childbirth. *Nursing Research*, 37(2), 77–81.

Wagner, P. (1976) Testing the adaptation model in practice. *Nursing Outlook*, 24(11), 682–685.

Neuman

Beddome, G. (1989) Application of the Neuman systems model to the assessment of community-as-client. In B. Neuman, *The Neuman systems model* (2nd ed.). Norwalk, CT: Appleton & Lange.

Benedict, M.B. and Sproles, J.B. (1982) Application of the Neuman model to public health nursing practice. In B. Neuman, *The Neuman systems model: Application to nursing education and practice*. Norwalk, CT: Appleton-Century-Crofts.

Bertalanffy, L. (1968) *General system theory*. New York: George Braziller.

Bourbonnais, F.F. and Ross, M.M. (1985) The Neuman systems model in nursing education: Course development and implementation. *Journal of Advanced Nursing*, 10(2), 117–123.

Breckenridge, D.M. (1989) Primary prevention as an intervention modality for the renal client. In B. Neuman, *The Neuman systems model* (2nd ed.). Norwalk, CT: Appleton & Lange.

Buchanan, B.F. (1987) Human environment interaction: A modification of the Neuman systems model for aggregates, families, and the community. *Public Health Nursing*, 4(1), 52–64.

Burke, Sr., M.E., Capers, C.F., O'Connell, R.K., Quinn, R.M., and Sinnott, M. (1989) Neuman-based nursing practice in a hospital setting. In B. Neuman, *The Neuman systems model* (2nd ed.). Norwalk, CT: Appleton & Lange.

Campbell, V. and Keller, K.B. (1989) The Betty Neuman health care systems model: An analysis. In J.P. Riehl-Sisca, *Conceptual models for nursing practice* (2nd ed.). Norwalk, CT: Appleton & Lange.

Capers, C.F. and Kelly, R. (1987) Neuman nursing process: A model of holistic care. *Holistic Nursing Practice*, 1(3), 19–26.

Capers, C.F., O'Brien, C., Quinn, R., Kelly, R., and Fenerty, A. (1985) The Neuman systems model in practice: Planning phase. *Journal of Nursing Administration*, 15(5), 29–39.

Caplan, G. (1964) *Principles of preventive psychiatry*. New York: Basic Books.

Chardin, P.T. (1955) *The phenomenon of man*. London: Collins.

Cornu, A. (1957) *The origins of Marxian thought*. Springfield, IL: Charles C. Thomas.

Drew, L.L., Craig, D.M., and Benyon, C.E. (1989) The Neuman systems model for community health administration and practice: Provinces of Manitoba and Ontario, Canada. In B. Neuman, *The Neuman systems model* (2nd ed.). Norwalk, CT: Appleton & Lange.

Dunn, S.I. and Trepanier, M. (1989) Applications of the Neuman systems model to perinatal nursing. In B. Neuman, *The Neuman systems model* (2nd ed.). Norwalk, CT: Appleton & Lange.

Edelson, M. (1970) *Sociotherapy and psychotherapy*. Chicago: University of Chicago Press.

Fawcett, J. (1989) *Analysis and evaluation of conceptual models of nursing* (2nd ed.). Philadelphia: F.A. Davis.

Harris, S.M., Hermiz, M.E., Meininger, M., and Steinkeler, S.E. (1989) Betty Neuman: Systems model. In A. Marriner-Tomey, *Nursing theorists and their work*. St Louis: C.V. Mosby.

Herrick, C.A. and Goodykoontz, L. (1989) Neuman's systems model for nursing practice as a conceptual framework for a family assessment. *Journal of Child and Adolescent Psychiatric and Mental Health Nursing*, 2(2), 61–67.

Hinton-Walker, P. and Raborn, M. (1989) Application of the Neuman model in nursing administration and practice. In B. Henry, C. Arndt, M. Di Vicenti, and A. Marriner-Tomey, *Dimensions of nursing administration: Theory, research, education, practice*. Boston: Blackwell Scientific Publications.

Johnson, S.E. (1989) A picture is worth a thousand words: Helping students visualize a conceptual model. *Nurse Educator*, 14(3), 21–24.

Kelley, J.A., Sanders, N.F., and Pierce, J.D. (1989) A systems approach to the role of the nurse administrator in education and practice. In B. Neuman, *The Neuman systems model* (2nd ed.). Norwalk, CT: Appleton & Lange.

Lancaster, D.R. and Whall, A.L. (1989) The Neuman systems model. In J.J. Fitzpatrick and A.L. Whall, *Conceptual models of nursing: Analysis and application* (2nd ed.). Norwalk, CT: Appleton & Lange.

Lillis, P.P. and Cora, V.L. (1989) A case study analysis using the Neuman nursing process format: An abstract. In B. Neuman, *The Neuman systems model* (2nd ed.). Norwalk, CT: Appleton & Lange.

Louis, M. and Koertvelyessy, A. (1989) The Neuman model in nursing research. In B. Neuman, *The Neuman systems model* (2nd ed.). Norwalk, CT: Appleton & Lange.

Lowry, L.W. and Jopp, M.C. (1989) An evaluation instrument for assessing an associate degree nursing curriculum based on the Neuman systems model. In J.P. Riehl-Sisca, *Conceptual models for nursing practice* (3rd ed.). Norwalk, CT: Appleton & Lange.

Mirenda, R.M. (1986) The Neuman systems model: Description and application. In P. Winstead-Fry (Ed.), *Case studies in nursing theory*. New York: National League for Nursing.

Mrkonich, D.E., Hessian, M., and Miller M.W. (1989) A cooperative process in curriculum development using the Neuman health care systems model. In J.P. Riehl-Sisca, *Conceptual models for nursing practice* (3rd ed.). Norwalk, CT: Appleton & Lange.

Mrkonich, D.E., Miller, M., and Hessian, M. (1989) Cooperative baccalaureate education: The Minnesota intercollegiate nursing consortium. In B. Neuman, *The Neuman systems model* (2nd ed.). Norwalk, CT: Appleton & Lange.

Nelson, L.F., Hansen, M., and McCullagh, M. (1989) A new baccalaureate North Dakota-Minnesota nursing education consortium. In B. Neuman, *The Neuman systems model* (2nd ed.). Norwalk, CT: Appleton & Lange.

Neuman, B. (1974) The Betty Neuman health-care systems model: A total person approach to patient problems. In J.P. Riehl and C. Roy, *Conceptual models for nursing practice*. New York: Appleton-Century-Crofts.

Neuman, B. (1982) *The Neuman systems model: Application to nursing education and practice*. Norwalk, CT: Appleton-Century-Crofts.

Neuman, B. (1989a) The Neuman systems model. In B. Neuman, *The Neuman systems model* (2nd ed.). Norwalk, CT: Appleton & Lange.

Neuman, B. (1989b) The Neuman nursing process format: Family case study. In J.P. Riehl-Sisca, *Conceptual models for nursing practice* (3rd ed.). Norwalk, CT: Appleton & Lange.

Neuman, B. (1989c) In conclusion—In transition. In B. Neuman, *The Neuman systems model* (2nd ed.). Norwalk, CT: Appleton & Lange.

Neuman, B. and Young, R.J. (1972) A model for teaching total person approach to patient problems. *Nursing Research*, 21(3), 264–269.

Putt, A. (1972) Entropy, evolution and equifinality in nursing. In J. Smith (Ed.), *Five years of cooperation to improve curricula in western schools of nursing*. Boulder, CO: Western Interstate Commission for Higher Education.

Reed, K.S. (1989) Family theory related to the Neuman systems model. In B. Neuman, *The Neuman systems model* (2nd ed.). Norwalk, CT: Appleton & Lange.

Ross, M.M. and Bourbonnais, F.F. (1985) The Betty Neuman system model in nursing practice: A case study approach. *Journal of Advanced Nursing*, 10(3), 199–207.

Ross, M.M., Bourbonnais, F.F., and Carroll, G. (1987) Curricular design and the Betty Neuman systems model: A new approach to learning. *International Nursing Review*, 34(3), 75–79.

Selye, H. (1950) *The physiology and pathology of exposure to stress*. Montreal: ACTA.

Sipple, J.A. and Freese, B.T. (1989) Transition from technical to professional-level nursing education. In B. Neuman, *The Neuman systems model* (2nd ed.). Norwalk, CT: Appleton & Lange.

Smith, M.C. (1989) Neuman's model in practice. *Nursing Science Quarterly*, 2(3), 116–117.

Sohier, R. (1989) Nursing care for the people of a small planet: Culture and the Neuman systems model. In B. Neuman, *The Neuman systems model* (2nd ed.). Norwalk, CT: Appleton & Lange.

Stevens, B.J. (1984) *Nursing theory: Analysis, application, evaluation* (2nd ed.). Boston: Little, Brown & Co.

Story, E.L. and Ross, M.M. (1986) Family centered community health nursing and the Betty Neuman systems model. *Nursing Paper*, 18(2), 77–88.

Sullivan, J. (1986) Using Newman's model in the acute phase of spinal cord injury. *Focus Critical Care*, 13(5), 34–41.

Ziemer, M.M. (1983) Effects of information on postsurgical coping. *Nursing Research*, 32(5), 282–287.

Chapter 14

On Human Being– Environment Interactions

When Martha Rogers asked the central question of her theory, What is the focus of nursing?, the answer was readily human being–environment interchange. Human beings and the environment are both unitary, irreducible, four-dimensional, negentropic energy fields that are identifiable by pattern and organization. Neither unitary human being nor unitary environment can be discussed, considered, or understood in isolation from the other. They are interrelated in an irreducible way. This fresh look at environment, unique in nursing and quite different from other theorists' views of environment, made it easy to consider Rogers as a significant force in our conceptual understanding not only of environment but of human being– environment interactions. Rogers' theory is described, analyzed, and critiqued in this chapter under the domain concept of environment. Some tests of the theory proposition are also included. I also encourage you to look at Florence Nightingale's work for a conceptualization of environment as well as other theorists' conceptualizations of environment.

Martha Rogers

THEORY DESCRIPTION

Rogers, a nurse leader and significant nursing theorist, specifically identified her theory as a conceptual system of nursing intended to stimulate the development of nursing theories. Nursing theories, Rogers maintains, could only be developed as a result of nursing research that is completed within the conceptual system she conceived. In later work, Rogers relabeled her conceptualization as the science of unitary man (1980a), and then, even later, as a paradigm for nursing (Rogers, 1983a). She also changed the word "man" to "human being."

Examples of theories that may evolve from Rogers' paradigm are a "theory of accelerating evolution," a "theory for paranormal phenomenon," and "rhythmical correlates of change" (1980a; 1987). Consistent with the premises of this book and based on the arguments developed in Chapter 9 on conceptual frameworks and theory, Rogers' conceptualization will be treated here as a theory. As has been done with each theory, the analysis and critique are provided to enhance understanding of the theory, to explain its role in the development of nursing's domain, and to encourage the further utilization, refinement, and development of the theory.

The central questions that Rogers attempted to answer are: What is the focus of nursing? Who is the nursing client? What knowledge is needed to develop the science of nursing? Rogers' conceptualization of nursing as a unique science is based on several explicit assumptions, presented in Table 14-1, and it encompasses several major concepts, presented in Table 14-2.

Most of Rogers' concepts are unique to her conceptualization. The concept of a unitary human being, with which Rogers' name is becoming known, is a primitive concept. All other concepts are derived from a general systems theory (pattern,

Table 14–1
Assumptions—Rogers

Explicit Assumptions

- Nursing is concerned with the life process of a human being, which is irreversible, along a space–time continuum (Rogers, 1970, p. 59).
- The focus of the science of nursing is the unitary human being, his innovative wholeness, and his integral and continuous relationship with the environment. That relationship involves energy and matter exchange. Matter is energy (1970, pp. 47, 54).
- There is pattern and organization in the wholeness of the unitary human being, but causality cannot explain it (1970, pp. 53, 65).
- Conceptual systems are preludes to theories, and theories are tested in real life with a feedback to theories. The cycle is continuous, open, and changeable based on changes in knowledge (1970, pp. 83–88).
- Unitary human beings are characterized by the ability to use abstraction, imagery, language, thought, sensation, and emotion (1970, p. 73).
- Reality does not exist but appears to exist as expressed by human beings (1980, p. 333).
- Nursing is based on a humanistic and not a mechanistic model (1970, pp. 87, 138).
- Generalization can only occur from a study of the whole but not any of the parts in isolation.
- Human behavior demonstrates reason and feelings (1970).
- Unitary man possesses the ability to join in the process of change deliberately and with probability (1983b, p. 222, 1986).
- The human field and its environmental field are postulated to be coextensive with the universe (1983b, p. 222).

Table 14–2
Concepts—Rogers

Unitary human being Energy field	Life process Rhythmicity
Unitary environment Energy field	Self-regulation Negentropy

Energy field
    Open
    Pattern and organization
    Four dimensionality
	Evolutionary emergence
	Unitary human development
	    Helicy
	    Resonancy

Unidirectionality	Integrality
Sentience	
Thought	

organization, negentropy), physics (electrodynamic), an evolutionary theory (life process, helicy), and adaptation theories (homeostasis, adaptation). Her concepts are abstract, general, conceptually defined, and documented, but they lack operational referents, which may explain the slow utilization of the theory by nurse practitioners. See Table 14-3.

Table 14–3
Definition of Domain Concepts—Rogers

Nursing	A learned profession, a science of unitary human beings, and the art of "imaginative and creative use of this knowledge in human service" (Rogers, 1980b, p. 122). It is concerned with living and dying. Fields of practice span the gamut of in and out of hospital, community, and the moon.
Goal of nursing	To bring and promote symphonic interaction between a human being and his environment through participation in a process of change. This is done to "strengthen the coherence and integrity of the human field and to direct and redirect patterning of the human and environmental fields" (1970, p. 122). Maximum health potential (p. 86). "Meaningful life and meaningful transition from life to death" (1970, p. 125).
Health	Health and illness are not dichotomous but continuous, are part of the same continuum, and are an expression of the life process; they are socially defined. Health is "characteristics and behaviors emerging out of the mutual, simultaneous interaction of the human and environment fields" (1980b). One can extrapolate that Rogers' view of health could be the greater developmental coherence that evolves from human being–environment energy fields that are novel, emerging, and more diverse in pattern and organization. Health and illness are not differentiated, nor are there any norms of health (Madrid and Winstead-Fry, 1986).

(continued)

Table 14–3 (Continued)

Environment	"An irreducible, four-dimensional, negentropic energy field, identified by pattern and manifesting characteristics different from those of the parts and encompassing all that is other than any given human field" (1983b, p. 222).
Human being	"An irreducible, four-dimensional, negentropic energy field identified by pattern and manifesting characteristics that are different from those of the parts and which cannot be predicted from knowledge of the parts" (1983a, glossary). Unitary human being develops through three principles: helicy, resonancy, and complementarity.
Nursing client	Human being–environment relationship (1970, p. 127).
Nursing problem	Not specifically addressed because Rogers believes labels of problems and illness are tentative and based on societal definition. Problems may denote changes in wave patterns and organization and in rhythmical correlates of change (1980a, pp. 334–335). Disharmony or lack of integrity in human being–environment energy fields.
Nursing process	Not specifically addressed. However, what Rogers says about scientific process applies here: "The subjective world of human feelings must be incorporated into so-called 'objective science'" (1970, p. 87).
Nurse–patient relations	Not addressed.
Nursing therapeutics	"Repatterning of man and environment for more effective fulfillment of life's capabilities" (1970, p. 127). Beliefs in innovative therapeutic modalities such as therapeutic touch (1985).
Focus	"Activities of daily living" must be considered within the context of the opportunities for human being–environment interchange that would stimulate the "flow of repatterning commensurate with the openness of nature" (1970, p. 123). Unitary human being in interaction with unitary environment.

To Rogers, a unitary human being is an energy field in constant interaction with the environment, which is also an energy field and a unitary one. Energy fields are more than the sum total of their parts, which may be physical, social, psychological, or biological in nature; they are open for exchange and extend to infinity. Energy fields are identifiable through dynamic-nonstatic wave patterns and organization that changes from "lower frequency, longer wave pattern to high frequency, shorter wave pattern" based on the principle of resonancy. Energy fields are four-dimensional, transcend time and space, and therefore have imaginary boundaries that are unique and changeable (Rogers, 1980a; 1983b; 1986).

Change is innovative and probabilistic. The goal of change is the further differentiation of human and environmental fields from lower to higher diversity. Change is based on continuous interaction between a unitary human being's energy field and the environmental energy field. Human development was cited as a goal

(1970) and rejected later (Malinski, 1986). The end point is not balance or equilibrium; rather, while there is no end point, there is a harmony that evolves and manifests in mutuality or integrality of person–environment–energy fields. These states of integrality, if we can call them states, are identified through patterns. Pattern to Rogers is:

> . . . an abstraction. It gives identity to the field. The nature of the pattern changes continuously. Each human field pattern is unique and is integral with its own unique environmental field pattern. (Rogers, 1986, p. 5)

Rogers postulated three principles to describe the patterns of human being and environment interactions and change (Rogers, 1986). To understand the nature, direction, and power of change, one has to consider motion and changes in energy fields through these principles: resonancy, helicy, and integrality. *Resonancy* describes the direction of change from lower to higher wave patterns. The principle of *helicy* postulates that change manifested in increasing diversity and nonrepeating rhythmicity is continuous. *Integrality* describes the nature and the process of the relationship between the human and energy fields, which is a continuous and a mutual process. Rogers also postulated that human beings are thinking beings who are capable of intimate involvement within a continuously changing environment.

THEORY ANALYSIS

The Theorist

It is difficult to think of the New York University nursing program without thinking of Martha Rogers. It is equally impossible to consider environment as a central concept in nursing without immediately thinking of Florence Nightingale and Martha Rogers. Both have left their imprints on nursing in more ways than one, but certainly on theoretical nursing and, more particularly, on the meaning of environment and its centrality to nursing.

Martha Rogers is one of the pioneers who envisioned a science of nursing in the late 1950s and early 1960s and advocated nursing having its own body of knowledge. She maintained that the science of nursing is unique and is not a synthesis of all sciences—it is more than that. Although synthesis may occur, the result is an integrated whole, as different from the parts as a unitary human being is different from the sum total of its parts. Martha Rogers began advocating that view in 1952.

Rogers received a diploma in nursing from Knoxville General Hospital School of Nursing, Knoxville, Tennessee, in 1936. She went on to earn a bachelor of science degree from George Peabody College, Nashville, in 1937. From Teachers' College she received a master's degree in nursing in 1945, and she also received a master's degree in public health from Johns Hopkins University in 1952 (Rogers, 1983b).

Rogers completed the requirements for her doctorate degree in science at Johns Hopkins one day in 1954, got on a train and, one day later, was head of the nursing program at New York University. One of her first acts was to teach doctoral student seminars. She noted that the dissertation students in nursing were part and parcel of dissertation seminars in the education department. Rogers' belief in the uniqueness of nursing and its science prompted her to design a separate seminar for the nursing students. She quickly realized that the parameters of that unique knowledge had not been identified as yet. That became Rogers' mission in nursing (Winstead-Fry, 1984).

As an advocate of diversity, Rogers demonstrates it in her personal life through her love of music and science fiction; in her writing, which incorporates philosophy, music, futurology, and physics; and the special talent with which she combines wit, humor, science, and art in speaking about nursing. Martha Rogers is one of the few scholars in nursing who will transcend her time and the profession.

Paradigmatic Origins

Rogers developed her theory from a number of paradigms; concepts were synthesized into what is now a whole around unitary human being, unitary environment, energy fields, and continuous interaction with the environment as an energy field. Understanding of Rogers' theory is enhanced by the study of general systems theory (Rogers, 1985). The constant interaction between human beings and environment, the interrelationships of the energy field, and the openness of both to continuous exchange of matter and energy are based on Bertalanffy's (1968) definition of an open system. Although Rogers uses some of the terminology of systems theory, she denies the study of subsystems and isolated behavior as representing the whole of the unitary human being. Rogers also draws on the assumptions and concepts of the general systems theory in two other ways: the unitary human being as an organization of the whole, which is more than the sum of the parts; and the individuality and uniqueness of human beings as reflected in this pattern and organization and in their wholeness. Furthermore, Rogers uses the concept of negentropy—a general systems theory concept—to develop helicy, which is the "continuous innovative, probabilistic, increasing diversity of human and environmental field patterns characterized by nonrepeating rhythmicities" (Rogers, 1980a). Negentropy is a property of both the human being and his environment.

Physics and electromagnetic theory provide some of the basic premises and concepts of Rogers' theory. The energy field of unitary human being and the environment are dynamic, are irreducible, are unbound, extend to infinity, and are identifiable by waves and patterns. Physicists provide the rationale for the existence of such energy fields and for understanding of resonancy as the "continuous change from lower frequency to higher frequency wave patterns" in human and environmental fields (Rogers, 1980b, p. 2).

The electrodynamic theory of life (Burr and Northrop, 1935) was used by Rogers as the link between physics and life processes in nursing. Rogers used the tenets of evolution theory to explain the increase in diversity, differentiation, complexity, and patterning in developing human and environmental behaviors. A unitary human being is always in the process of "becoming" rather than "being"; at any point, he is more than he has been because all his previous actions, experiences, interactions, and being are incorporated into his present being. A unitary human being is a homeodynamic being and is not homeostatic (Rogers, 1980c). The process is therefore evolutionary toward more complexity; and dynamic equilibrium, which characterizes adaptation theory, is not possible as a goal in life.

Rogers has been influenced by the early Greek philosophers and modern theory and philosophy. Her writings draw on Burr and Northrop (1935), Chardin (1961), Polanyi (1958), and Lewin (1964), among others. In addition, she drew on her vast fiction reading, interest in classical music, and modern physics to describe her concept of nursing science.

Internal Dimensions

Rogers used the dialectic method of reasoning in developing her theory, due to the fact that higher level principles are subsumed under lower level concepts (Barnum, 1988). The theory is basically concatenated and has a hypothetical constructive beginning, evolving from synthesis of concepts from a number of fields, the core of which are a number of concepts that are central to nursing. These are unitary human being, unitary environment, energy field, open system, patterns, four-dimensionality, and unitary human development. The relationships between concepts are still at a very tentative stage.

Rogers' theory is a deductive theory that is monadic with several irreducible units, but it is macro in content and wide in scope as it purports to describe life processes that result from person–environment–energy field interaction. The intent of the theory is to explain and predict, but currently it is descriptive of the life process of the unitary human being and deals with knowledge of order. The theory does not offer conceptual guidelines for knowledge of disorder or control. The concepts lead to description of patterns, rhythmicities, and symphonic harmony.

THEORY CRITIQUE

Nursing is expected to describe the life process of unitary human beings and their environments, which are expressed in health and illness, and to attempt to explain and predict the nature and direction of the development of both. "The aim of nursing is to assist people in achieving their maximum health potential . . . their maximum well-being within the capability of each person" (Rogers, 1970, pp. 86, 135). Rogers defined the goal of professional nursing as follows:

> Professional practice in nursing seeks to promote symphonic interaction
> between man and environment, to strengthen the conference and integrity of
> the human field, and to direct and redirect patterning of the human and
> environment fields for realization of maximum health potentials. (Rogers,
> 1970, p. 122)

A nurse utilizing Rogers' theory works on mobilizing individual or family resources, heightening her integrity, and strengthening the human being–environment or family–environment relationships (Rogers, 1988).

The scope of Rogers' theory is broad and has the potential to encompass the phenomena of the domain of nursing. However, while it articulates the central phenomena, it does not define practice, nor does it attempt to do so. The theory appears too abstract; concepts—while defined theoretically—do not lend themselves readily to the practice arena or to measurable variables for research. Rogers never claimed her conceptualization to be a theory, and her thinking and ideas preceded all current attempts at theory building. This may be why she has not offered a systematic operationalization of her concepts for utilization in practice and research. Nevertheless, the notion of considering the individual as a whole and the focus of nursing on the human being–environment relationship is quite appealing to nursing and lends itself to a theory of human being–environment interaction.

Others have extended Rogers' theory and have postulated that the characteristics of a unitary human being could be related to needs and activities of daily living. Since unitary human beings can feel, exchange, be awake, move, choose, value, and relate, a group of nurses (theoreticians, clinicians, and researchers) have developed such a conception and delineated a number of nursing diagnoses according to these characteristics (Kim and Moritz, 1982). See Table 14-4.

Table 14–4
Characteristics of Unitary Human Being–Rogers

Factor I. Interaction	Factor II. Action
A. Exchanging	A. Valuing
1. Eating and drinking	1. Philosophical beliefs about health,
2. Eliminating	human interactions, and spirituality
3. Breathing	B. Choosing (human beings knowingly
4. Giving and receiving	makes choices—wise, unwise, or
B. Communicating	detrimental)
1. Verbal	1. Judgement and decision-making
2. Nonverbal	capacity regarding alternatives,
C. Relating	consequences, commitments
1. Spacing	C. Moving
2. Touching	1. Mobility (rhythm and patterns)
3. Eye contact	Factor III. Awareness
4. Belonging	A. Waking (sleep behavior, patterns, and
5. Referencing	quality)
6. Family response to patient illness	B. Feeling (as perceived and as manifested)
	C. Knowing (health knowledge,
	abstractions, motor skills)

(Adapted from Lucy Field and Margaret Newman, Clinical application of the unitary man: Case study analysis. In Kim, M.J. and Moritz, D.A. (Eds.) (1982) Classification of nursing diagnosis: Proceedings of the third and fourth national conferences. New York: McGraw-Hill Book Co.; copyrighted by the C.V. Mosby Co., St. Louis.

Diagnoses such as noncompliance (choosing), anxiety (feeling), respiratory dysfunction (exchanging), impairment of mobility (moving), spiritual concern (valuing), alternations in sleep/rest activity (waking), and alterations in patterns of sexuality (relating) have been defined in relation to a unitary human being (Kim and Moritz, 1982; Rossi and Krekeler, 1982, pp. 276–277).

Several writers have demonstrated some of the theory's utility in practice. Madrid and Winstead-Fry (1986) proposed a useful assessment framework derived from Rogers' focus on patterns. One component of this framework is living in the relative present, experiencing comfort with the past and present of the individual. Shared communication, a sense of rhythm (a flow in daily life), a connection to environment (a sense of place in a community), personal myth (a sense of self identity), and system integrity (survival) are other components of the assessment framework. For each of the components, the authors offer a range of intervention options.

Whelton (1979) synthesized Rogers' theory with nursing process theory in delivering care to patients with decreased cardiac input and impaired neurologic function. Others have demonstrated the theory's principles in therapeutic touch (Krieger, 1976) and in conceptualizing hyperactivity in children within the framework of synergism as being merely changes in a person's pattern of interaction with the environment (Blair, 1979). Rogers herself provided the potential for understanding aging and hyperactivity (1980a) by her theory. Minimal sleep needs of the hyperactive child are seen by Rogers as a response to increasing complexity and diversity of wave patterns and frequency of environmental fields; therefore, hyperactivity, if not viewed from unitary human being–environment interactions, tends to be labeled as a disease.

Despite all these attempts at clinical operationalization and utilization, the general sentiment in practice, education, and administration remains the same. The potential is there in the theory, but the incomplete nature of it, the esoteric concepts and the level of abstractness, and the overlap between concepts due to lack of definition all render Rogers' theory's use limited in practice. Not only is it difficult to operationalize and measure characteristics and actions of unitary human beings and energy fields, but one is also faced with the limitations of the existing English language in describing the four-dimensionality of a human being and the influence of the tremendous acceleration of change on humanity (Rogers, 1980a). Rogers' approach, however, is more meaningful in the 1990s than it was in the 1960s, 1970s, or 1980s.

External Components of Theory

A decade ago, Rogers' theory was an unknown; it was esoteric and not reflective of nursing. The changes in prevailing views of health, developments in physics, and the movement toward holism have facilitated nurses' acceptance to further explore her theory. The focus of nursing is now on the unitary human being who is in constant interaction with the environment. There is indication that nursing practice is more positive about the potential of Rogers' theory (Rossi and Krekeler, 1982).

Each nurse–patient interaction is an interaction of energy fields that evolves into repatterning and reorganizing waves in the direction of increasing differentiation and diversity. Each encounter is unique; it moves forward and becomes more complex. Feelings, thoughts, experiences, and awareness of the nurse and patient and their environments blend together, each one emerging not totally the same as before. Repatterning is a new pattern evolving from a previous pattern that requires investigation into the "nature of field patterns and organization." These views are valued by nurses, consumers, and, indeed, more and more by other health professionals.

THEORY TESTING

Gill and Atwood (1981) attempted to use Rogers' theory as the basis for a study of wound healing in animals, but were legitimately criticized by Kim (1983) for reductionism, causality, and inappropriate use of the animal model. Others have succeeded in explaining some of Rogers' propositions without resorting to reductionism or mechanistic approaches. For example, Rogers' proposition that unitary human beings/environments are dynamic fields of energy, always sending and receiving messages that change both the human and environment fields in complexity and diversity, has been tested and has received some support (Katz, 1971). Although Katz, a graduate of New York University, did not link her findings to Rogers' theory per se, her findings lend support to this proposition. Katz's experimental subjects, premature infants who were subjected to a patterned regimen of auditory stimulation from tape recordings of the maternal voice, achieved greater motor and tactile adaptive maturation.

Porter's (1972) findings support Katz's (1971) and Rogers' proposition that environmentally imposed motions speed up infant growth and development. Goldberg and Fitzpatrick (1980) hypothesized that movement therapy for institutionalized individuals, as a holistic nursing intervention derived from Rogerian theory, would improve psychological well-being as demonstrated in morale and in attitudes toward aging. The hypothesis was supported, lending further support to Rogers' theoretical propositions. Heidt (1981), testing another intervention based on Rogerian premises, found that subjects who received nursing intervention through therapeutic touch had greater reduction in posttest anxiety scores than those who received it through casual or no touch.

Other studies reformulated and deduced a theorem regarding environmental disruption and sleep/wakefulness rhythms and tested it on a general population and a clinic population. More specifically, the theorem stated:

> Persons experiencing a deviation in the rhythmic relationship with their environment will manifest greater complexity and diversity in their sleep/ wakefulness patterns than persons who are not experiencing a deviation in the rhythmic relationship with their environment. (Floyd, 1983, p. 43)

Although the findings demonstrated a significant difference in "increasing diversity" (total wakefulness time was greater for rotating shift workers than for nonrotating shift workers), there was minimal support for "increasing complexity" (rotating shift workers slept less than nonrotating shift workers). The study lends support to the theorem but raises some questions when the study used a clinical sample. Floyd's (1983) study represents an example of the potential innovation in testing Rogers' propositions and the significance of systematic study of propositions emanating from nursing theory.

Developmental stages and time orientation were the focuses of another study based on Rogerian theory that concluded that there is "support for the developmentally-based nature of specific dimensions of temporality" (Johnston, Fitzpatrick, and Donovan, 1982, p. 120). These studies, together with Newman's (1979; 1986) theory of health, are based on the interrelationships between time, space, consciousness, and movement, and are fine extensions of Rogers' ideas.

Despite such progress, there are still major gaps in our methodology for unitary human beings/unitary environments and their energy fields. Should such gaps in our present knowledge halt all research investigations utilizing Rogers' theory? Is it possible to develop investigations accounting for all Rogers' premises and concepts with our present limited knowledge? The answer is "no" to both questions. As demonstrated previously, researchers who have been inspired by Rogers' theory and theoretical propositions have found innovative ways to test and support some theory propositions without adhering to or accounting for all assumptions and principles of the theory. For example, well-being in Goldberg and Fitzpatrick's (1980) study was measured in terms of psychological well-being rather than in terms of the greater developmental coherence that involves human being–environment energy fields, as Rogers would emphasize.

A valuable resource that contains a comprehensive analysis of tests completed on Rogers' theory is edited by Malinski (1986). This compilation, in addition to a review of literature based on Rogers' theory, may indicate several conclusions about the theory, including the following:

- ○ A world view is emerging in nursing that is congruent with Rogers' principles (Malinski, 1986).
- ○ There are some universal questions about Rogers' world view (Meleis, 1988).
- ○ Research work that utilizes Rogers' principles is increasing (Benonis, 1989; Quinn, 1989; Schodt, 1989).
- ○ Existing methodological approaches are not entirely useful in investigating principles postulated in her theory (Smith, 1986, 1988; Phillips, 1989; Moccia, 1985), and therefore, "there is an essential need for methodological studies aimed at development, validation, and evaluation research tools and strategies for the unitary science framework" (Cowling, 1986, p. 74).
- ○ There is a definite evaluation in the types of studies completed to test or further develop Rogers' principles (Ference, 1986; Fitzpatrick, 1988; Clarke, 1986).

Ference (1986) describes the mid-1960s studies, which are mainly doctoral dissertations, as studies of human development; in the 1970s the studies revolved around the principle of complementarity that was later relabeled integrality. Concurrently, several of Rogers' students studied body image in an attempt to explain human and environment fields. The variable of time dominated investigations in the mid-1970s, for example, Newman (1989) researched perception of time in relationship to gait tempo. According to Ference (1986, p. 38), "these studies helped future researchers to define the meaning of time in a space-time context."

Other studies during that period, according to Ference (1986), focused on locus of control, field independence, and differentiation. Several instruments unique to Rogers' theory have been developed. Two have been reported. These are the Human Field Motion Test (Ference, 1986) and the Human Field Power Test (Barrett, 1986).

Work is continuing to develop more instruments and test theories, for example:

> Several students have developed measures to explore aspects of Rogers'
> model or to measure theories that they have derived from the model. Helen
> Ference developed the Human Field Motion Scale and Elizabeth Barrett
> developed a measure and theory of power that is nonsexist, both based on
> Rogers. Additional work has been done on meditation, a scale to measure
> development as defined by Rogers, and several studies of creativity,
> differentiation, and parent/child interaction are underway. (Winstead-Fry,
> 1984)

Another significant test of any theory is the extent to which it has stimulated theoretical published discourse. Rogers' theory inspired the development of other theories, such as Newman's theory of health (Newman, 1986). Others, particularly graduate students from Wayne State University, Case Western Reserve University, Rochester University, Boston University, and New York University are engaged in researching propositions derived from Rogers' theory. Rogers' theory has been operationalized for educational settings. The curriculum of nursing at New York University is not the only one based on Rogers' theory. It has been used to develop curricula at Duquesne, College of Mount St. Vincent, and Fairleigh Dickinson University (Winstead-Fry, 1984).

Rogers' theory is complex, is somewhat tautological (she acknowledges an overlap between concepts), and has an aura of coherent truth but the reality of a challenge in operationalization. Although difficult for the American practitioner, it is understandable in the international arena. Its view of humanity and environment and the lack of separation between mind and body is congruent with the Eastern view, and it is expected that its circle of contagiousness will increase more rapidly than ever anticipated in the decade ahead. It is congruent with professional values in nursing and with the emerging perceptions of humanity.

REFERENCES

Barnum, B.J.S. (1988) *Nursing theory: Analysis, application, and evaluation* (3rd ed.). Boston: Little, Brown & Co.

Barrett, E.A.M. (1986) Investigation of the principle of helicy: The relationship of human field motion and power. In V.M. Malinski (Ed.), *Explorations on Martha Rogers' science of unitary human beings*. Norwalk, CT: Appleton-Century-Crofts.

Benonis, B.C. (1989) The lived experience of recovering from addiction: A phenomenological study. *Nursing Science Quarterly*, 2(1), 37–43.

Bertalanffy, L. von (1968) *General systems theory: Foundations, development, application*. New York: George Braziller.

Blair, C. (1979) Hyperactivity in children: Viewed within the framework of synergistic man. *Nursing Forum*, 18, 293–303.

Burr, H.S. and Northrop, F.S.C. (1935) The electro-dynamic theory of life. *The Quarterly Review of Biology*, 10, 322–333.

Chardin, T. (1961) *The phenomenon of man*. New York: Harper Torchbooks.

Clarke, P.N. (1986) Theoretical and measurement issues in the study of field phenomena. *Advances in Nursing Science*, 9(1), 29–39.

Cowling, W.R. (1986) The science of unitary human beings: Theoretical issues, methodological challenges, and research realities. In V. Malinski (Ed.), *Explorations on Martha Rogers' science of unitary human beings*. Norwalk, CT: Appleton-Century-Crofts.

Ference, H. (1986) The relationship of time experience, creativity traits, differentiation, and human field motion. In V. Malinski (Ed.), *Explorations on Martha Rogers' science of unitary human beings*. Norwalk, CT: Appleton-Century-Crofts.

Fitzpatrick, J. (1988) Theory based on Rogers' conceptual model. *Journal of Gerontological Nursing*, 14(9), 14–16.

Floyd, J.A. (1983) Research using Rogers' conceptual system: Development of a testable theorem. *Advances in Nursing Science*, 5(2), 37–48.

Gill, B.P. and Atwood, J.R. (1981) Reciprocity and helicy use related to EFT and wound healing. *Nursing Research*, 30(2), 68–72.

Goldberg, W.G. and Fitzpatrick, J.J. (1980) Movement therapy with the aged. *Nursing Research*, 29(6), 339–346.

Heidt, P. (1981) Effect of therapeutic touch on anxiety level of hospitalized patients. *Nursing Research*, 30(1), 32–37.

Johnston, R.L., Fitzpatrick, J.J., and Donovan, M.J. (1982) Developmental stage: Relationship to temporal dimensions (Abstract). *Nursing Research*, 31(2), 120.

Katz, V. (1971) Auditory stimulation and developmental behavior of the premature infant. *Nursing Research*, 20(3), 196–201.

Kim, H.S. (1983) Use of Rogers' conceptual system in research: Comments. *Nursing Research*, 32(2), 89–91.

Kim, M.J. and Moritz, D.A. (Eds.) (1982) *Classification of nursing diagnosis: Proceedings of the third and fourth national conference*. New York: McGraw-Hill.

Krieger, D. (1976) Healing by the laying on of hands as a facilitator of bioenergetic change: The response of *in vivo* human hemoglobin. *International Journal of Psychoenergetic Systems*, 1, 121–129.

Lewin, K. (1964) *Field theory in the social sciences*. (D. Cartwright (Ed.) New York: Harper Torchbooks.

Madrid, M. and Winstead-Fry, P. (1986). Rogers' conceptual model. In P. Winstead-Fry (Ed.), *Case studies in nursing theory*. New York: National League for Nursing.

Malinski, V. (1986) *Explorations on Martha Rogers' science of unitary human beings.* Norwalk, CT: Appleton-Century-Crofts.

Meleis, A.I. (1988) Book reviews (Malinski, V.M. (1986) Explorations on Martha Rogers' science of unitary human beings). *Research in Nursing and Health*, 11, 59–63.

Moccia, P. (1985) A further investigation of dialectical thinking as a means of understanding systems-in-development: Relevance to Rogers' principles (Commentary). *Advances in Nursing Science*, 7(4), 33–38.

Newman, M.A. (1979) *Theory development in nursing*. Philadelphia: F.A. Davis.

Newman, M.A. (1986) *Health as expanding consciousness*. St. Louis: C.V. Mosby.

Phillips, J.R. (1989) Science of unitary human being: Changing research perspective. *Nursing Science Quarterly*, 2(2), 57–60.

Polanyi, M. (1958) *Personal knowledge*. Chicago: University of Chicago Press.

Porter, L.S. (1972) The impact of physical–physiological activity on infant growth and development. *Nursing Research*, 21(3), 210–219.

Quinn, J.F. (1989) Therapeutic touch as energy exchange: Replication and extension. *Nursing Science Quarterly*, 2(2), 74–78.

Rogers, M.E. (1970) *An introduction to the theoretical basis of nursing*. Philadelphia: F.A. Davis.

Rogers, M.E. (1980a) Nursing: A science of unitary man. In J.P. Riehl and C. Roy (Eds.), *Conceptual models for nursing practice* (2nd ed.). New York: Appleton-Century-Crofts.

Rogers, M.E. (1980b) The science of unitary man. (Audiotapes) New York: Media for Nursing.

Rogers, M.E. (1980c, December) Science of unitary man: A paradigm for nursing. Paper presented at the International Congress on Applied Systems Research and Cybernetics, Acapulco, Mexico.

Rogers, M.E. (1983a) Science of unitary human being: A paradigm for nursing. In I.W. Clements and F.B. Roberts (Eds.), *Family health: A theoretical approach to nursing care*. New York: John Wiley & Sons.

Rogers, M.E. (1983b, June). Nursing science: A science of unitary human beings. Paper presented at the First National Rogerian Conference, New York University.

Rogers, M.E. (1985) A paradigm for nursing. In R. Wood and J. Kekahbah (Eds.), *Examining the cultural implications of Martha E. Rogers' science of unitary human beings*. Lecampton, KS: Wood-Kekahbah Associates.

Rogers, M.E. (1986) Science of unitary human beings. In V. Malinski (Ed.), *Explorations on Martha Rogers' science of unitary human beings*. Norwalk, CT: Appleton-Century-Crofts.

Rogers, M.E. (1987) Rogers' science of unitary human beings. In R.R. Parse (Ed.), *Nursing science: Major paradigms, theories, and critiques*. Philadelphia: W.B. Saunders Company.

Rogers, M.E. (1988) Nursing science and art: A perspective. *Nursing Science Quarterly*, 1(3), 99–102.

Rossi, L. and Krekeler, K. (1982) Small-group reactions to the theoretical framework "Unitary man" (1980). In M.J. Kim and D.A. Moritz (Eds.), *Classification of nursing diagnosis: Proceedings of the third and fourth national conference*. New York: McGraw-Hill.

Schodt, C.M. (1989) Parental-fetal attachment and couvade: A study of patterns of human–environment integrality. *Nursing Science Quarterly*, 2(2), 88–97.

Smith, M.J. (1986) Human–environment process: A test of Rogers' principle of integrality. *Advances in Nursing Science*, 9(1), 21–28.

Smith, M.J. (1988) Testing propositions derived from Rogers' conceptual system. *Nursing Science Quarterly*, 1(2) 60–67.

Whelton, B.J. (1979) An operationalization of M. Rogers' theory throughout the nursing process. *International Journal of Nursing Studies*, 16, 7–20.

Winstead-Fry, P. (1984). Personal communication.

Chapter *15*

On Interactions

Several nurse theorists addressed nursing as a process of interaction. Some, such as Ida Orlando, developed the focus of the nursing process in nursing. I selected the following theorists to represent the central domain concepts related to interaction: Imogene King, Ida Orlando (Pelletier), Josephine G. Paterson and Loretta T. Zderad, Joyce Travelbee, and Ernestine Wiedenbach. Orlando's, Travelbee's, and Wiedenbach's theories may also be utilized as the frameworks to describe and explain significant questions related to the nursing process.

Imogene King—A Theory of Goal Attainment

THEORY DESCRIPTION

King's theory evolved in the mid-1960s with questions related to the role of theory in nursing. The development of her convictions and conceptualization progressed from recommending that nursing could be provided through a framework that contains a synthesis of ideas (a frame of reference that she entitled, in 1971, "Toward a Theory for Nursing") to the development of a theory that prompted the title to shift to "A Theory for Nursing" in 1981. In a curious way, the difference between the first tentative title and the second is analogous to nursing's tentativeness about theory in the 1970s and the determination to theorize in the 1980s. The difference between King's two books can be found in the last chapter of the second book, where she articulated her theory "for" nursing.

King provided nursing with four sets of concepts as part of her conceptual framework for nursing (King, 1988). These concepts are central to the field of nursing and provide the basis upon which she developed a theory of goal attainment, beginning with an assumption that nurses as human beings interact with patients as human beings, and both are open systems who also interact with the environment. Therefore, the personal systems (nurse and patient) interact with each other in an interpersonal system and with the environment that she called the social system (society). The relationships between these systems led to the development of the theory of goal attainment, with a distinct set of concepts, some of which were derived from the conceptual framework. Other theories may evolve from the conceptual framework. To understand the theory fully, it should be read in conjunction with the conceptual framework.

The theory deals with the central questions of interaction between nurses and clients. King considered questions related to the nature of the process of interaction that lead to the achievement of goals and the significance of mutual goal-setting in achieving nursing care goals. The theory evolved from several explicit assumptions (Table 15-1). These assumptions are congruent with the popular view held in nursing at this time. They speak to the significance of patient involvement in the care process as well as in the decision-making process, the importance of collaboration, and the humanity of the nurse–patient encounter.

It is important to note, too, that King's assumptions encompass the nurse's perceptions, goals, needs, and values, and these are expected to influence the interaction process and, indeed, the outcomes. Although King designated the nurse as a central concept in nursing theory, she did not go as far as Paterson and Zderad in focusing on the significance of the consideration of the continuous growth of the

Table 15-1
Assumptions—King

Explicit Assumptions

- The central focus of nursing is the interaction of human beings and environment, with the goal being health for human beings (King, 1982, p. 143).
- Individuals are social, sentient, rational, reacting, perceiving, controlling, purposeful, action-oriented, and time-oriented beings (King, 1981, p. 143).
- The interaction process is influenced by perceptions, goals, needs, and values of both the client and the nurse (1981)
- Human beings as patients have rights to obtain information, to participate in decisions that may influence their life, health, and community services, and to accept or reject care (1981).
- It is the responsibility of health care members to inform individuals of all aspects of health care to help them in making "informed decisions" (1981).
- Incongruities may exist between the goals of health care givers and recipients. Persons have the right to either accept or reject any aspect of health care (1981, pp. 143–144).

Implicit Assumptions

- Patients want to participate actively in the care process.
- Patients are conscious, active, and cognitively capable to participate in decision making (Austin & Champion, 1983, p. 56).

nurse in every interaction. The theory assumptions explicitly address the rationality of human beings and proceed to develop consistent concepts related to clients who can perceive, interpret, and solve problems. Austin and Champion (1983) argued that, as such, the theory is not useful to some situations in nursing, for example, when patients are comatose or psychotic.

There are inconsistencies in the different lists of concepts provided by King (Table 15-2). In one instance, she listed human being, environment, health, and society as the abstract concepts. She also identified personal, interpersonal, and social systems as the major concepts (1981, p. 142). She proceeded to define

Table 15-2
Concepts: A Conceptual Framework for Nursing—King

Personal Systems

Perception	Growth and development
Self	Time
Body Image	Space

Interpersonal Systems

Role	Transactions
Human interaction	Stress
Communication	Coping

Social Systems

Organization	Goal Attainment
Power, authority, status	Decision making
	Control

Concepts: A Theory of Goal Attainment

Interaction	Time
Perception	Space
Communication	Goal attainment
Transaction	Effective nursing care
Role	Appropriate information
Stress	Satisfaction
Growth and development	

Concepts: A Theory of Administration

Organization	Decision making
Power	Perception
Authority	Communication
Status	Interaction
Role	Transaction
Control	

interaction, perception, communication, transaction, role, stress, growth and development, time, and space as they represent the theory of goal attainment. Although King clarified the relationship between the latter set of concepts in the interpersonal system, it is not clear how these "major concepts in the theory" relate to human beings, environment, health, and society (King, 1988). Perception appears to be a central concept in her theory (Bunting, 1988).

King offered, in the conceptual framework, almost every concept that nurses may have historically used in nursing care (Table 15-2). It is not entirely clear how the goal attainment theory evolved from the myriad concepts that appear in the conceptual framework. In the goal attainment theory, she restricted concepts to the interaction system, central to the nursing act. Most of her concepts are derived, except for goal attainment, health, transaction, effective nursing, appropriate information, and satisfaction. Although the derived concepts are defined conceptually and have the potential for operational definition, they have not been delineated as central concepts, nor were they defined theoretically or operationally. However, the theory purports to have, as a goal, nurse–patient interactions.

Other concepts not defined are satisfaction and effective nursing care, and although these are seemingly central to patient outcomes, they are neither conceptually nor operationally defined. To attain goals, appropriate information should be given; what is "appropriate," what is considered "information," and who decides what is appropriate or information are only a few of the questions that point out the lack of theoretical definitions and lack of boundaries between concepts (Table 15-3), and incongruence between assumptions, concepts, and statements (Uys, 1987).

Table 15-3
Definition of Domain Concepts—King

Nursing	"A process of human interaction between nurse and client whereby each perceives the other in the situation and, through communication, they set goals, explore means, and agree on means to achieve goals" (King, 1981, p. 144), "and their actions indicate movement toward goal achievement" (1987, p. 113). "A process of action, reaction, interaction and transaction" (1971, p. 89 and 1981, p. 2). Nursing services are called upon when individuals cannot function in their roles.
Goal of nursing	"To help individuals to maintain their health so they can function in their roles" (1981, p.3). "To help individuals to attain and restore health or die in dignity" (1981, p.13). The goal of nursing is then to maintain, restore, and promote health.
Health	"A dynamic life experience of a human being, which implies continuous adjustment to stressors in the internal and external environment through optimum use of one's resources to achieve maximum potential for daily living" (1981, p. 5 and 1983, p. 186).

(*continued*)

Table 15-3 (Continued)

	Ability to function in social role. Process of growth and development.
Environment	The internal environment of human beings transforms energy to enable them to adjust to continuous external environmental changes (1981, p. 5). The external environment is the formal and informal organization. "A social system is defined as an organized boundary system of social roles, behaviors, an practices developed to maintain values and the mechanisms to regulate practice and rules" (1981, p. 115). The nurse is part of the patient's environment.
Human being	Rational, sentient, social being, perceiving, thinking, feeling, able to choose between alternative actions, able to set goals, to select means toward goals, to make decisions, and to have a symbolic way of communicating thoughts, actions, customs, and beliefs. Is time-oriented and reacting. Reactions are based on perceptions, expectations, and needs (1981, p. 19).
Nursing client	A unique, total, open system with perception, self, body image, time, space, growth, and development throughout the life span and with experiences of changes in structure and function of body influencing perception of self (1981, pp. 19–20). Person as open system exhibits permeable boundaries permitting an exchange of matter, energy, and information (1981, p. 69). A person who cannot perform daily activities and cannot carry the responsibilities of their roles (1976).
Nursing problem	Inability to meet needs for daily living (1981, p.5). Inability to function in their roles (1981, p.3). The central problem is nonmutual goal-setting and lack of agreement on goals and means leading to unattained goals (1981, p. 144) "Felt needs" as perceived by patient or real needs as perceived by nurse (1968, p. 29).
Nursing process	A focal concept in King's theory. The goal of nursing is to help patients attain their goals. The mechanism for that is the nursing process. Through this process, nurses interact purposefully with clients (1981, p. 176). The purpose is information sharing, setting of mutual goals, participation in decisions about goals and means, implementing plans and evaluations.
Nurse–patient relations	"A process of perception and communication between person and environment and between person and person, represented by verbal and nonverbal behaviors that are goal-oriented" (1981, p. 145). Variables affecting interactions are knowledge, needs, goals, past experiences, and perceptions of nurse and patient. The interaction process also includes reaction and transaction (1981, p. 145).
Nursing therapeutics	Transactions: informing, sharing, setting of mutual goals, participation in decisions about goals and means (1981, p. 176). Goal-oriented nursing record (1983, pp. 183–186).

There is incompleteness and inconsistency in how health is viewed by King. Health is defined in terms of ability to function in a social role, but as Magan (1987) indicated, ways by which the levels and quality of that functioning could be assessed are not described. Explication of health in terms of morbidity and mortality data and accidents is more congruent with a disease orientation than a role-functioning orientation.

King's views of health and illness are also problematic. As Magan puts it:

> The difficulty with a consistent understanding of health in King's framework is further complicated by her assertion that health and disease do not constitute polarities, while she also maintained that illness is an interference or disturbance in health. (Magan, 1987, p. 119)

The inconsistencies in King's definition of health are manifest in viewing health and illness as nonpolar and not dichotomies and illness as an interference or disturbance, and at the same time viewing health in terms of a dynamic life experience.

King offers examples of how her theory can be tested through a set of propositions that link perceptions, transactions, goal attainment, satisfaction, and effective nursing care. Propositions are relative and tend to be deterministic (Zetterberg, 1963). They are based on a cause-and-effect approach and are designed for prediction, not description. Propositions link some of the defined concepts (transactions, interactions, role performance), but they also link the undefined concepts.

THEORY ANALYSIS

The Theorist

Imogene King is well-known for more than her theory; she is one of the pioneers who promoted a theoretical base for nursing (King 1964; 1975; 1976). She is, like a number of other theorists, a graduate (Ed.D., 1961) of Teachers College of Columbia University. Prior to that, she had graduated from St. John's Hospital School of Nursing, St. Louis, in 1945 and received a bachelor's degree in nursing education in 1948 and a master of science in nursing in 1957. She completed a postdoctoral study in systems research, advanced statistics, research design, and computers (King, 1986a).

A clinician, an administrator, but primarily an educator, King is currently a professor at the College of Nursing, University of South Florida at Tampa. She has been dean of the School of Nursing at Ohio State University, Columbus, and professor of nursing at Loyola University in Chicago. Besides being an author, she is an effective speaker whose joy in presenting and describing her theory are readily apparent to her audiences.

Paradigmatic Origins

King used the language of system theory in the introduction of her ideas. Fawcett classified her as a system theorist (1989, p. 116) and George classified her as an adaptation theorist (1980, p. 186). Her conceptual framework evolves out of all paradigms that have been used in nursing, for example, the developmental paradigm (growth and development), systems (structural–functional view of role, open systems, social systems, energy), adaptation (continuous adjustment to stressors), psychoanalytical (self), and stress (energy response to environment). The theory of goal attainment derives a great deal from symbolic interactionism, and what King offers helps in understanding the nursing process and the process of interaction, and therefore prompts a classification of her theory as an interactionist theory.

Although King personally stated that she never used the symbolic interactionist school of thought (in Fawcett, 1989, p. 116), the influence of interactionism is marked. Several indications of parallelism between King's theory and symbolic interactionism are the descriptions of a person as a social being, actor, and reactor, who is constantly structuring and restructuring his perception of the world, thereby communicating through symbols. Nurse–patient interactions occur with the perceptual repertoire of both. Present meaning of any situation and perceptions of time of both nurse and patient are significant to the interaction (King, 1981, p. 148). In addition, King's use of roles (though more congruent with a structural–functional approach) and the personal element perception and interpretation are also indications of an interactionist approach. King recognized that a functionalist view of role is related to the study of social systems, but

> [t]he interactionist view of role is basic to understanding individuals in organizations when role is thought of as a relationship with another person or group of individuals, it is related to interpersonal systems. . . . The interactionist view relates to social interaction. (1981, p. 90)

Therefore, the entire focus of theory and the central question around process, interaction, and goal attainment make it more congruent with a symbolic interactionist approach. Refinement of theory could be enhanced if the backdrop is interaction rather than the inconsistent and mixed use of both system and interaction paradigms. Finally, both the paradigmatic origin and the theory suffer from the limitation of viewing a person as a social being rather than a bio-psycho-social being.

Internal Dimensions

The microtheory of goal attainment was developed from a field approach around concepts rather than propositions and is therefore concatenated in structure. It is a mental image, with a constructive beginning deduced from a conceptual framework whose concepts were also deduced from other paradigms. Its scope is limited to the process of interaction, focusing on perceptions of clients for the purpose of goal attainment. It deals with interactions of one nurse with one patient. Despite the fact that King extensively discusses the social system, her theory evolving from the interpersonal system is limited to nurse–patient interactions, as it ought to be. She later expanded it to incorporate the family and their perceptions (1983a; 1983b).

The microtheory of goal attainment purports to predict processes inherent in goal attainment and provides descriptions of the concepts and properties of the interpersonal system. The theory would be classified as providing a description of the nursing process; it mainly explains how and when to use transactions to achieve mutually agreed-upon goals. It is a single-domain theory with an average abstraction. King developed her theory using a logical method of development. The parts of the interactional system (interaction, transaction) lead to goal attainment.

THEORY CRITIQUE

The utility of King's theory for practice, research, education, and administration has been limited but promising. Theory development progressed from a conceptual framework—a variety of unrelated concepts—to a theory of nursing in the interpersonal system. King herself completed one research project and operationalized the theory for practice. Propositions emanating from the theory are presented in Table 15-4.

King's theory is parsimonious, with distinct concepts and limited relationships, but teleological because interaction is defined by interaction and transaction (King, 1981, p. 145). Goal attainment appears to be a process of transaction toward effective nursing care and is a product that is equated with effective nursing care and satisfaction (King, 1981, pp. 147 and 153).

Considering that interaction has emerged as one of the central concepts in nursing, King's contribution is substantial to nursing knowledge (King, 1987b). The theory clarity is enhanced when considered as a theory to describe and answer questions related to nurse–patient interactions for the purpose of setting goals. The nursing care process has been conceived as a process involving assessment, diagnosis, intervention, and evaluation (King, 1986a). The process depends on two significant clinical tools: observation and interaction.

King offers the nursing profession a description of the properties of interaction and one of its goals—attainment of mutually agreed-upon goals. King also offers a unique variation of the nursing process. The Goal-Oriented Nursing Record (GONR), developed as a tool analogous to the Problem-Oriented Medical Record developed by Weed (1969), includes both "process and outcomes in nursing situations" and a record of the goals, the means to achieve those agreed-upon goals, and the process used to achieve them. It consists of five components: a data base, a problem list, a goal list, a plan, and progress notes (King, 1981, pp. 164–165).

GONR is similar to the nursing process utilized by other theorists, but it offers a more dynamic dimension that addresses the process and not only the goals. GONR has the potential of offering organized nursing care, and it could facilitate nursing audits, enhance abilities in making nursing diagnoses, increase focus on patients'

Table 15-4
Propositions—King

---

1. If perceptual accuracy is present in nurse–patient interactions, transactions will occur.
2. If nurse and patient transact, goals will be attained.
3. If goals are attained, satisfactions will occur.
4. If goals are attained, effective nursing will occur.
5. If transactions are made in nurse–patient interactions, growth and development will be enhanced.
6. If role expectation and role performance, as perceived by nurse and patients, are congruent, transactions will occur.
7. If role conflict is experienced by nurse or patient or both, stress in nurse–patient interactions will occur.
8. If nurses with special knowledge and skills communicate appropriate information to patients, mutual goal-setting and goal attainment will occur.
9. Knowledge of oneself will bring about a helping relationship with patients.
10. Accurate perceptions of time and space in nurse–patient interactions lead to transactions.

From King, I. M. (1981) A theory for nursing: Systems, concepts, process. *New York: John Wiley & Sons, p. 149 and King I. M. (1986)* King's theory of goal attainment. *In P. Winstead-Fry (Ed.)* Case studies in nursing theory. *New York: National League for Nursing.*

---

participation, and validate perceptions of patients during the process (King, 1981, p. 172).

There are numerous examples of use of King's theory in clinical practice (Smith, 1988), including: the theory's use with an elderly patient with a cerebral vascular accident (King, 1983a), a patient with renal disease (King, 1984), in caring for families (King, 1983b), in providing community health nursing care (Asay and Ossler, 1984), in psychiatric care (Gonot, 1983), in caring for comatose patients (King, 1986a), and in caring for adults with diabetes (Husband, 1988).

Despite these examples of the clinical utility of the theory, the theory appears to be more useful for assessing active, autonomous, collaborative, and individual (rather than group or aggregate) relationships with nurses. It is more useful for long-term nurse–patient relationships in order to evaluate "satisfaction, goal attainment, and effective nursing care." The utility of GONR for care of infants, children, patients in coma, some psychiatric patients, or some mentally retarded patients is still in question (Stevens, 1984; Austin and Champion, 1983). King's theory is also limited in utilization to only some health care settings.

> The theory would have limited application in settings where clients are unable to interact competently. In addition, it is not clear how the theory could be utilized with groups. Utilizing transactions with groups of

individuals who had different goals is not addressed by King. (Austin and Champion, 1983, p. 60)

King expanded her theory to incorporate the family as a client in 1983 (Gonot, 1983; 1986).

There are a number of other limitations to clinical utility. The theory does not give guidelines to assessment, diagnosis, or intervention. The theoretical boundaries to help a practitioner in assessing problems and potential problems and in deciding on clinical therapeutics are not identified. It analyzes problems but does not offer guidelines for interventions. The specificity to other nursing phenomena is lacking. Interaction is a process in all helping relationships; its uniqueness to nursing stems from its relationship to other phenomena. This is lacking in King's theory.

Nursing administration could utilize the theory in developing a recording system for nursing care plans with refinement and modifications related to patient care outcomes. King promised that, if nurses use goal attainment theory and GONR to enhance accurate documentation and recording of goals identified and attained in interactions, effective nursing care could be measured (King, 1981, p. 155; King, 1989, pp. 42–45). King discussed the development of a theory of administration utilizing the same principles used in developing a theory of goal attainment. King believed that when such theory is communicated in the literature, it will be useful for both nursing science administration and nursing education administration. Elberson (1989) presented a description of the utility of King's theory in nursing administration.

King's theory is amenable to utilization in nursing education as a basis for learning, one significant phase and component of the nursing process. While utilization in practice and administration have not been documented, there is evidence that the theory provides both a conceptual framework for curricula (Daubenmire and King, 1973; King, 1978) and guides a curriculum in continuing education (Brown and Lee, 1980). King provided guidelines for implementation of her theory in an educational setting (1968, p. 30), and in 1986, she published a book on curriculum development in which she carefully demonstrated how her theory could be utilized as a framework for curricula (King, 1986b). She also summarized the potential utility of theory in curricula (King, 1988; Gulitz and King, 1988). King's theory has been used as a conceptual framework for a baccalaureate program at Ohio State University School of Nursing in Columbus (Daubenmire and King, 1973; King 1986b). Other schools also used her theory or components of it as a framework (Fawcett, 1989).

Diagrams depicting relationships between central concepts of the theory, central concepts in nursing, and major propositions would have enhanced the clarity of the theory and would have pointed out the gaps in linkages.

External Components of Theory

The theory is congruent with values and beliefs about nursing, humanity, autonomy, patient advocacy, self-reliance, and planning that are espoused by Western societies, especially the United States, pertaining to the conscious, self-directed patient. The focus of the theory on mutual goal-setting and attainment, on interacting with individuals, and on helping individuals become healthy enough to function in roles is congruent with Western philosophy and mores of pragmatism and usefulness of adult members of society. Many other societies that consider patients helpless, that espouse the sick role as abandonment of social roles and responsibilities, and that support the rights of patients to be sheltered from prognosis and health care goals (such as some Middle Eastern cultures) would consider this theory culturally limited (Meleis and Jones, 1983). Patients in these societies prefer to relinquish all decisions and goal-setting to the expertise of the health care professionals.

THEORY TESTING

King outlined hypotheses for testing her theoretical propositions (King, 1987a) and proposed future studies to test these hypotheses (King, 1986a; Uys, 1987). Fawcett (1989) reports that in February 1988 a conference held at the University of South Florida College of Nursing focused on research designed to test King's theory. As Fawcett indicates, this is a reflection of a growing body of knowledge related to King. King also developed a criterion-referenced instrument that was designed to assess physical and behavioral functional abilities, goal-setting with clients, and goal attainment (King, 1986a).

Several studies testing various properties derived from King's theory are reported in the literature. Brower (1981) described nurses' attitudes toward the elderly; Rosendahl and Ross (1982) described the relationship between attending behaviors on mental status; and Frey (1989) described the development and initial testing of parent support, child support, family health, and child health in families with insulin-dependent, diabetes mellitus. Frey used King's theory as the basis for defining concepts, selecting indicators, and developing propositions for testing. The finding lends support to the relationship between interaction and health as proposed by King. The researcher questions the availability of appropriate instruments to use in testing King's theory (Frey, 1989, p. 146). There are also indications of the international utility of King's theory in research (Roake and Norberg, 1988).

King also tested her theory and reported the results in her 1981 book. The study was designed to answer three questions:

1. What elements in nurse–patient interactions lead to transactions?
2. What are the relationships between the elements in the interactions that lead to transactions?
3. What are the essential variables in nurse–patient interactions that result in transactions? (King, 1981, p. 151)

The results of this descriptive study supported the components of the interpersonal system and lent construct validity. The study limitations are numerous, but the study could be considered a pilot for further research. The study was based on data generated by nonparticipant observations of verbal and nonverbal behaviors of nurses and patients. The sample consisted of 17 cases. The results of this descriptive study support the components of the interpersonal system and provide construct validity. Specifically, King's study indicated that interaction was verbal and nonverbal and that nurse–patient interactions lead to transactions, identification of problems, concerns, or disturbances in the patient's environment. Variables that helped in the achievement of goals were "accurate perceptions of the nurse and patient, adequate communication, and mutual goal setting" (King, 1981, p. 155). Despite several limitations of the study (sample size, biases of the researchers, limited analysis), it is a pilot study that indicates the potential testability of the theory.

Ida Orlando

THEORY DESCRIPTION

In the mid to late 1950s, the Yale School of Nursing shifted from undergraduate to graduate education and integrated psychiatric concepts into the entire curriculum. Orlando's theory grew out of processes inherent in these curricular changes and out of dissatisfaction with the possibility that nursing care was being prompted by organizational rules rather than by attention to patients' needs. Orlando's theory is based on the central questions: What prompts nursing actions? What are the properties of dynamic nurse–patient relationships that may lead to effective care?

When Orlando began formulating her conceptualization of nursing, the answer to the first question was that nurses were prompted in their actions by physician's prescriptions, organizational needs, and personal repertoire of experiences rather than by patient needs; in other words, for reasons other than the patients' immediate experiences and immediate needs (1961, p. 60). This answer did not satisfy Orlando and may have initiated the ideas for the development of her theory.

The focus of Orlando's theory is on identifying and clarifying problematic situations. To her, basically, nurses' reactions or responses to patients may be automatic, "discipline professional," "nursing process disciplined," (1972) or "deliberative" (1961). In each situation, the reaction is based on observation of the patient's verbal or nonverbal behavior and is influenced by perceptions, thoughts, and feelings related to the patient's action that prompted the nurse's reaction, or vice versa. The automatic response is guided by "secretiveness;" neither the meaning of the behavior nor the perceptions of the nurse or the patient are validated. The "disciplined professional response" is guided by "explicitness" of perceptions, of thoughts, and of feelings, indicating that the patient's needs are validated and ambivalence and distress is explored. The disciplined professional response also indicates the nurse has validated the effectiveness of nurses' actions in helping the patient.

The nursing disciplined process requires the following conditions:

- ○ What the nurse says to the individual in the contact must match (be consistent with) any or all of the items contained in the immediate reaction.
- ○ What the nurse does nonverbally must be verbally expressed, and the expression must match one or all of the items contained in the immediate reaction.
- ○ The nurse must clearly communicate to the individual that the item being expressed belongs to herself.
- ○ The nurse must ask the individual about the item expressed in order to obtain correction or verification from that same individual (1972, pp. 29–30).

On the other hand, not all interactions are based on a nursing process discipline. Nurses may give automatic nursing care, exemplified in routine care (1961, 1972). Automatic nursing care does not encompass perception, thoughts, and feelings. These deal less with finding out and meeting the patients' needs for help. There are two types of automatic responses. One is stimulated by the patient's needs and, insofar as nurses respond to needs that patients cannot take care of by themselves, automatic response is expected to be effective. This is deliberative, automatic response. The other automatic responses are those that result from reasons other than the patients' immediate needs for help. Automatic responses neither acknowledge nor consider patients' perceptions and thoughts of the problem.

A nurse's professional identity is exemplified by her offering disciplined professional actions that are stimulated by knowledge of patient needs and that are validated by patient responses. These actions involve a continuous process of reflection as the nurse attempts to explore the meaning of the behavior of the patient. The nurse perceives the behavior and its meaning, shares these perceptions, and explores and validates the meanings of these perceptions with the patient. By sharing, exploring, and validating perceptions, misinterpretations are minimized. Modeling for interpretation and validation would enhance further use of this process and would enhance understanding of our own and others' reactions and actions (Schmieding, 1987).

When nurses provide these actions, the result is a patient who experiences improvement in his behavior, who has needs met, who feels comfortable, who has a sense of adequacy, and who does not manifest helplessness or distress. Nurses deal with "immediate needs" in "immediate experiences" of a patient in an illness situation by engaging in "immediate exploration" of the patient's perceptions, thoughts, and feelings (Orlando, 1961, p. 65). If nurses provide effective nursing care, they will see immediate behavioral changes for the better, they will see increased ability and adequacy in better care of self and, eventually, they will see an increased sense of well-being. Need "is situationally defined as a requirement of the patient that, if supplied, relieves or diminishes his immediate distress or improves his immediate sense of adequacy or well-being" (Orlando, 1961, p. 5). Orlando based her conceptualization of nursing as dynamic interaction on several implicit assumptions (Table 15-5). It is also based on acknowledgement of feelings and emotions.

Table 15-5
Assumptions—Orlando

Implicit Assumptions

○ When patients cannot cope with their needs without help, they become distresssed with feelings of helplessness. (Orlando 1961, p. 11).

○ Nursing, in its professional character, does not add to the distress of the patient (1961, p.9).

○ Patients are unique and individual in their responses (1961, p. 59).

○ Nursing offers mothering and nursing analogous to an adult mothering and nurturing of a child (1961, p.4).

○ Nursing deals with people, environment, and health.

○ Patients need help in communicating needs; they are uncomfortable and ambivalent about dependency needs (1961, p. 24).

○ Human beings (nurses and patients) are able to be "secretive" or explicit about their needs. perceptions, thoughts, and feelings (1972, p. 26).

○ The nurse–patient situation is dynamic; actions and reactions are influenced by both nurse and patient (1961).

○ Human beings attach meanings to situations and actions that are not apparent to others.

○ Patient entry into nursing care is through medicine (1961, p. 5).

○ The patient cannot state the "nature and meaning of his distress for his need without the nurse's help or without her first having established a helpful relationship with him" (1961, p. 23).

○ "Any observation shared and explored with the patient is immediately useful in ascertaining and meeting his need or finding out that he is not in need at that time" (1961, p. 36).

○ Nurses are concerned with needs that patients cannot meet on their own (1961, p.5).

There are three problems with the assumptions. First, it is not clear how Orlando derived her assumptions; no documentation exists. Second, the nature of some of her assumptions limits nursing to administering only to patients who are under the care of medicine and who cannot meet their own needs comfortably. Neither of these assumptions are acceptable in nursing today; nurses may care for patients who are not under medical care and may help to more effectively meet the needs of patients who are able to meet their own needs. Third, the ratio of assumptions to propositions is high, necessitating too many conditions for the number of propositions and placing a severe limitation on the exploratory power of the theory.

Orlando's theory contains more primitive concepts (deliberative, automatic, disciplined professional, dynamic nurse–patient relationship) than derived concepts (needs, helplessness, environment), which would give the theory the neces-

Table 15-6
Concepts—Orlando

Need for help	Reaction
Distress	Perception
Immediate	Thought
Need	Feeling
Experience	Actions
Exploration	Secret
Behavioral changes	Automatic response
Sense of adequacy	Explicit
Helplessness	Personal response
Situational conflict	Improvement
Nursing process discipline	Reactions
Deliberative nursing process	Explicit
Disciplined professional response	Secret

sary content to enhance its power (Table 15-6). Many of the central concepts are not defined (environment, health) or, when defined (*e.g.*, interaction), they are non-variables (Hage, 1972). (See Table 15-7.) Because the concepts evolved out of her conceptual image of nursing's potential reality, they have empirical references and therefore have the potential to be operationalized (Andrews, 1983).

    Properties of action and reaction are well-explicated, but outcomes are not defined—such as improvement, distress, need for help, helplessness—making it difficult not only to ascertain conceptually the need for help but also to ascertain the consequences of either automatic or deliberate nursing actions. The most significant variable—effective nursing care—is equated with either the disciplined professional process or lack of helplessness, distress, and even, at times, meeting the needs of patients, making the theory both tautological and teleological.

Table 15-7
Definition of Domain Concepts—Orlando

Nursing	"Is responsive to individuals who suffer or anticipate a sense of helplessness." "Process of care in an immediate experience . . . for avoiding, relieving, diminishing, or curing the individual's sense of helplessness" (Orlando, 1972, p. 13). "Finding out and meeting the patient's immediate need for help" (1972, p. 20).
Goal of nursing	Increased sense of well-being; increase in ability, adequacy in better care of self and improvement in patient's behavior (1961).
Health	Sense of adequacy or well-being. Fullfilled needs. Sense of comfort (1961, p.9).

(continued)

Table 15-7 (Continued)

Environment	Not defined.
Human being	Developmental beings with needs.
Nursing client	Patients who are under medical care and who cannot deal with their needs or who cannot carry out medical treatment alone.
Nursing problem	Distress due to unmet needs due to "physical limitations," "adverse reactions to the setting," or "experiences which prevent the patient from communicating his needs (1961, p. 11). Ineffective nursing activities: acting in a way not helpful to patient or not achieving professional purpose (1961, p. 72). Ineffective patient behavior such as being uncooperative, unreasonable, demanding, or commanding behaviors that prevent the nurse from carrying out her care of maintaining a satisfactory relationship with the patient.
Nursing process	The interaction of "1) the behavior of the patient, 2) the reaction of the nurse, and 3) the nursing actions which are assigned for the patient's benefit" (1961, p. 36). Process by which a nurse acts (1972, p. 29).
Nurse–patient relations	Central in theory and not differentiated from nursing therapeutics or nursing process.
Nursing therapeutics	Direct function: "1) Initiates a process of helping the patient express the specific meaning of his behavior in order to ascertain his distress and 2) helps the patient explore the distress in order to ascertain the help he requires so that his distress may be relieved." Indirect function: Calling for the help of others (1961, p. 29). "Whatever help the patient may require for his need to be met" (*i.e.*, for his physical and mental comfort to be assured as far as possible while he is undergoing some form of medical treatment or supervision [1961, p. 5]). Automatic or deliberative instructing, suggesting, directing, explaining, informing, requesting, questioning, making decisions for the patient, handling the body of the patient, administering medications or treatments or changing the patient's immediate environment. Automatic activities: 1) routines of patient care such as serving food, evening care, 2) routines to protect the interests and safety of patient, such as locking doors, adjusting side rails, 3) routine practices of organization, such as signatures for consent forms, and releases (1961, p. 84). Automatic activities redefined in 1972: 1) perception by five senses, 2) automatic thoughts, 3) automatic feelings, 4) action (p. 25). Disciplined and professional activities: automatic activities plus matching of verbal and nonverbal responses, validation of perceptions, matching of thoughts and feelings with action (1972, pp. 25–32).

THEORY ANALYSIS

The Theorist

Ida Jean Orlando Pelletier was an associate professor and the director of the graduate program in mental health and psychiatric nursing (1958–1961) at Yale University School of Nursing when her 1961 book was published. The book was a product of a 1954–1959 National Institute of Mental Health Grant to integrate mental health concepts in nursing programs (Crane, 1980). Her second book, in 1972, was a result of another supported research project (by the National Institute of Mental Health, Public Health Service) and a general research grant. She was, at that time, a clinical nurse consultant at McLean Hospital, Belmont, Massachusetts (1962–1972).

Orlando has held numerous other positions, including consultant to nursing service administration and nursing education to schools, to health departments, and to the many students who called her from across the United States. She was appointed consultant to the New England Board of Higher Education and the board of the Harvard Community Health Plan. Orlando's most recent position was director of nursing at the Tri-City Unit of Metropolitan State Hospital in Waltham, Massachusetts.

According to Schmieding (1986), Orlando's 1961 book has been translated into five languages. Orlando worked closely with and was influenced by Wiedenbach; she, in turn, influenced Travelbee's theoretical notions of nursing.

Paradigmatic Origins

Although Orlando's theory evolved from extant practice through the analysis of some 2,000 nurse–patient interactions to discern what is good and bad practice, Orlando's writing appears to be influenced by Peplau's (1952) focus on interpersonal relationships in nursing. Peplau defined nursing in terms of relationships between a person in need of help and the nurse who is able to recognize such a need. Definitions by Orlando and Peplau have some common properties and, considering that Peplau's ideas were published in 1952 and Orlando began to formulate hers in 1954 (Yale received a grant for the purpose of developing an integrated program and, later, a faculty research development grant that facilitated testing some of Orlando's theoretical propositions), one can make an assumption of Peplau's influence on Orlando. Peplau acknowledged the influence of Harry Stack Sullivan on the development of her ideas; therefore, one may deduce that Orlando's theory has also utilized some of Sullivan's concepts and assumptions (dynamic relations, inadequate communication).

Perceptions, meaning, and evaluation of meaning are central concepts in the theory and are also central to symbolic interactionism. Considering that Orlando used a method of research that grew out of the Chicago school of symbolic interactionism in the 1950s, understanding her theory could be enhanced by studying the assumptions and major concepts of symbolic interactionism. Orlando used field methodology before it became a world view in research.

Schmieding (1987) suggested that by studying established theories in other disciplines, nursing theories could be better clarified and developed. She therefore proposed to analyze Orlando's theory by utilizing John Dewey's theory of inquiry. She described the similarities and the differences between Orlando's and Dewey's organizing principles around the meaning of experience, habit, and functions in acting and reacting. She demonstrated that Orlando used experiences, the meaning of experience, and the immediacy of nurse–patient situations as the basis for her theory and that these same principles are central to Dewey's theory.

Internal Dimensions

Orlando analyzed some 2,000 nurse–patient interactions to identify the properties, dimensions, and goals of interaction. The theory that evolved inductively from these analyses focused on the nature of interactions. All statements in the theory converge on interactions; therefore, it is a concatenated theory. She used a field approach in developing the theory. Orlando's background in psychiatric nursing (her academic objectives were to identify psychiatric content that should be integrated in nursing curricula) has most probably influenced the focus of the theory on describing the psychosocial aspects of the nurse–patient interactions.

As a single-domain theory that is also a microtheory of nurse–patient interactions around illness, it is limited to immediate exploration and immediate responses to a given situation. The nurse is an integral part of this theory; nurses' perceptions, thoughts, and feelings affect the nurses' actions and patients' reactions. The entire theory is built on nurse–patient encounters; therefore, using Stevens' (1984, pp. 29–52) classification method of theory development, Orlando used a mixture of operational and problematic methods—more of the former than of the latter.

Orlando identified a number of problems (helplessness, distress) and what nurses should do to handle these problems. The concepts in the problems are not operationally defined, and this limits the development of research hypotheses. Orlando's theory is focused on the delivery of nursing care through a disciplined nursing process. However, her focus is on how to deliver care and not on what care to give; therefore, it is an attempt to conceptualize knowledge of process. It is a nursing process theory of medium- to low-level abstraction, leaning more toward the low-level abstraction.

THEORY CRITIQUE

The early 1960s marked a milestone shift in the way the nursing perspective was viewed. The interaction theorists, epitomized by Orlando, marked a shift in the perspective of nursing from phenomena dealing with nurses, functions of nurses, and needs of patients to a focus on the process of interaction and the potential consequences for the patient. Orlando's theory—with its major proposition a deliberative nursing process, or the nursing process discipline, as it was relabeled in 1972—is a more effective process for identifying patient needs and evaluating patient care; therefore, providing effective care was the focus of many research projects. In fact, Orlando's theory provided the framework for numerous Yale studies (Diers, 1970).

Systematic explorations of relationships between each of the concepts in the theory and patient outcomes is possible when patient outcomes (improvement, met needs) are articulated, defined, and operationalized. Explorations could also focus on the effect of the "nursing process discipline" on the assessment process and on implementation of other clinical therapeutics (Orlando, 1972, p. 4). Examples of potential propositions are presented in Table 15-8.

Although Orlando considered the theory to be a theoretical framework for the practice of professional nursing (Orlando, 1972, p. 1), the theory is more congruent in guiding nurse–patient interactions for the purpose of assessing needs and in providing the nursing therapeutics that are deemed necessary to patient care. The process is in fact considered a universal process of interactions between patients and all health professionals (Marriner-Tomey, Mills, and Sauter, 1989). What may make it more unique to nursing is the addition of such dimensions as space (hospital) and length of encounters (number of hours nurses interact with patients).

The theory has several limitations, among them the seeming focus on ill people in hospitals, and the focus on individuals—particularly those who are aware and conscious—on immediate time and situations, on short-term rather than long-term care and planning, and on the virtual absence of reference group or family members. Other limitations are the lack of definition of environment, health, patient outcomes, physiological aspects of needs, and nonvariable nature of the central concepts of the theory (*e.g.*, improvement, immediacy, effectiveness). When we consider the theory goals to be limited only to describing the nurse–patient interaction for assessment of needs and for evaluation of care, then its limitations diminish.

Table 15-8
Propositions—Orlando

○ There will be greater improvement in patient behavior and more effective nursing care when nurses use the disciplined professional response than when they use automatic personal response.
○ The nursing situation includes perceptions, thoughts, feelings, and actions.
○ When a nurse assesses a patient's immediate needs, immediate experiences, and immediate resultant behaviors, nursing care is more effective in decreasing distress and helplessness and increasing comfort.
○ When nurse–patient dynamics and an "explicit" relationship are established, the patient is able to communicate his needs more clearly.

Nurses have used focused interactions and deliberative processes, whether they have been aware of it or not; even when they have been aware of this use, whether they credit Orlando or not remains debatable. Concepts and linkage from the theory, such as validation of observation and nurse–patient discussion of feelings, thoughts, perceptions, and reactions, are used in psychiatric settings and most probably in other settings. Further utilization would be enhanced by refinements, extensions, and proposition testing.

Orlando's theory evolved out of the need for curricular changes, and it is therefore logical that her first test of ideas occurred in an educational setting (Yale University). The first book (1961) identified teaching and learning strategies and some of the content that could be used in teaching students how to use the deliberative nursing process.

In her second book (1972), Orlando relayed the results of a training program over a three-month period. The training was for 28 staff nurses (as opposed to students in an educational system) in the use of the nursing process discipline. The purpose was to change their responsiveness from one that was "personal and automatic" to one that was "disciplined and professional" (Orlando, 1972, p. 4). Outcome variables were observed in nurses, and the study results indicated effective use of nursing process discipline in nurse–patient encounters by those nurses who were in the training program (Orlando, 1972).

Although there are limited indications of the use of Orlando's theory in practice, educational, or administrative settings, the concepts permeate our educational and practice settings. Schmieding (1986) provides the most comprehensive use of Orlando's theory in nursing practice and nursing administration. Each situation presented focused on problematic situations either with patients, nurses, physicians, or other colleagues. Nurses' immediate responses and deliberate process responses are then described illustrating Orlando's propositions. In each one of the vignettes offered, the deliberative process clarified assumptions, cleared misconceptions, checked judgmental thoughts, and enhanced expressions and interpretations.

External Components of Theory

The theory represents a shift from a view of nursing that was task-oriented and function-oriented, with goals that stemmed out of organizational needs and with therapeutics that were offered and that were based on physicians' prescriptions to nursing as an interaction process. Values of nursing shifted because of, or as a product of, interaction theories. These theories proposed that nursing is a process, patients are the focus, patients should be consulted in their own care, and patients should be spared the distress and discomfort associated with misconceptions, misinterpretations, and noninvolvement in their own care. Patients' behaviors and participation in interpreting meaning and validating perceptions should be significant factors in nurses' reactions. Although the patient was still viewed as helpless and the deliberative process appeared to be always initiated by the nurse, many of the assumptions of the theory are congruent with social and professional values of the 1980s and 1990s.

The theory is culturally bound. Patients in other parts of the world and from other subcultures may not want to participate in identifying their needs, nor do they feel free to engage in interpretations of meanings. They may prefer to rely on their significant others and the health care professionals to do that for them. They may misinterpret the continuous validation proposed in this theory as lack of knowledge, lack of expertise, or lack of accountability in the care process (Lipson and Meleis, 1983). The uniqueness of individuals assumed by the theory could counteract automatic responses of nurses because even a nursing process discipline or deliberative nursing process could turn into an automatic response if the nurse forgets the basic assumptions guiding the theory.

THEORY TESTING

The theory evolved from Orlando's observations of nurse–patient interactions. Although the findings were not reported in a research report, her 1961 book is based on that research. The research was done in various patient settings to explore the effect of the deliberative process, which includes perceptions, thoughts, and feelings of the patient and the nurse regarding patients' needs and the care given. Validation of perceptions, thoughts, and feelings is essential for enhancing the congruence between patients' needs and the care given. Results indicate unique nursing process is more effective than other approaches in dealing with pain (Barron, 1966; Bochnak, 1963), in reducing stress (Mertz, 1962), in understanding patients' needs (Cameron, 1963), in decreasing postoperative vomiting (Dumas and Leonard, 1963), in relieving distress experienced by patients during the process of admission to a hospital (Elms and Leonard, 1966), on the outcome of implicit and explicit verbal acceptance of a nursing procedure as well as on the degree of effectiveness of enemas and progress in labor (Tryon, 1963), and on the effectiveness of the enema, with the indicators being higher retention rate, more fecal return, and higher ratio of fluid intake and return (Tryon and Leonard, 1964).

A number of studies focused on explicating the properties and components of nurse–patient interactions (Diers, 1966; Gowan and Morris, 1964; Pienschke, 1973; Rhymes, 1964; Wolfer and Visintainer, 1975). Others explored the relationship between the nurses' social approval of patients and postoperative recovery behavior as an outcome, finding that there is a significant but weak inverse relationship between physical status (self-report) and social desirability (Eisler, Wolfer and Diers, 1972). These authors question the process and intent of validating experiences with patients (central to Orlando and Wiedenbach), suspecting that some patients may respond to validation on the basis of social expectation rather than "the patient's inner experience" (Eisler, Wolfer and Diers, 1972, p. 524).

A significant central concept in Orlando's theory—perceptions—was used as a framework to describe needs of grieving spouses. A study of the grieving spouses' perceptions of their own needs before and after the death event revealed high reliability in ability to identify needs and a consistency in the identified needs (Hampe, 1975). However, when identified needs were compared with met needs, a discrepancy became apparent. Implicitly, if the nurses had asked the grieving spouses to identify their own needs, perhaps the nurses would have more systematically and effectively planned to meet each of those needs. A deliberative interaction process can elicit perceptions of needs even when patients cannot communicate their needs (Gowan and Morris, 1964). When nurses used the previously identified needs of grieving spouses as specific targets in their nursing interventions, grieving spouses experienced more met needs (Dracup and Breu, 1978). In this latter study, the greater satisfaction in nursing care was attributed to the systematic approach in need identification.

Another study that supports Orlando's differentiation between presenting problems as perceived by nurses and those as perceived and validated by patients was by Gilliss (1976), who demonstrated that fewer patients suffering from sleeplessness required sleep medication in an experimental group in which Orlando's deliberative process was implemented. In this group, patients' specific needs were identified, defined, validated, and met.

Orlando's theory was used as a framework to research nursing administration. Schmieding (1988) demonstrated that nursing administrators did not explore the reaction of their staff to problematic situations, that the majority of them use an approach to handling problematic situations that did not involve the staff or they would tell the nurses what to do rather than solicit from nurses their thoughts or action plans.

The processes of interaction, action, and decision making in nursing administration are similar to these processes involved in nurse–patient interactions. Schmieding systematically explored the nature of interaction, decision making, and action processes in problematic situations in nursing administration and found out that Orlando's theory could provide the needed nursing focus in nursing service administration (1983). An instrument was developed to describe the action process of different members of nursing service personnel (Schmieding, 1987). Orlando's theory was also used in describing the responses of nursing students to distressed patients (Haggerty, 1987).

The findings lend support to consideration of the interaction process in achieving effective patient and nursing care outcomes. However, there are numerous methodological issues related to need identification and increasing patterns of interaction in the nursing process discipline. One such problem is the paucity of research tools to identify patient needs. Williamson (1978), in attempting to identify patient needs, questioned the existence of mutually exclusive variables such as physical and emotional needs and the contextuality of needs and socioeconomic cultural variables.

Josephine Paterson and Loretta Zderad

THEORY DESCRIPTION

The central questions for Paterson and Zderad (1988) were: How do nurses and patients interact? and How can nurses develop the knowledge base for the act of nursing? The humanistic practice nursing theory proposes that the nurse and the patient are significant components in the nurse–patient situation. The act of caring increases the humanness of both. They both approach the situation with experiences that influence the encounter. Nurses, therefore, should consider such encounters as existential experiences and should describe them from a phenomenological perspective. The sum total of all these experiences will enhance the development of the science of nursing.

In selecting existentialism and phenomenology as context and method for the development of nursing knowledge, Paterson and Zderad operate from several premises. The progress of nursing as a human science is hampered by the mechanistic, deterministic, cause-and-effect methods that have dominated it; in other words, they rejected the received view, the logical positivism view of theory development (Paterson, 1971, p. 143). Paterson and Zderad were a decade ahead of the literature in nursing that later advocated such a move. They have also developed their ideas on the premise that the experiences of nurses in practice supply the impetus for any useful theory for nurses. However, they also warned us that preconceived notions influence what is significant and determinately affect the development of knowledge.

Nursing is a lived dialogue that incorporates an intersubjective transaction in which a nurse and a patient meet, relate, and are totally present in the experience in an existential way that includes intimacy and mutuality (Paterson and Zderad, 1970–1971). Nursing brings a person together with a nurse because of the call of that person for help and the response of the nurse. The encounter is influenced by all other human beings in the patient's and nurse's lives and by other things, whether ordinary objects (such as utensils, clothes, furniture) or special objects (such as life-sustaining equipment). The dialogue during these encounters occurs in a time frame as experienced by both partners. When there is synchroneity in timing, the intersubjective dialogue is enhanced. Dialogue occurs in a certain space that is objective—the physical setting, or subjective—personal space.

Paterson and Zderad's theory is based on a number of implicit assumptions (Table 15-9). The theory has the potential for highly abstract propositions related to nurse–patient interactions (Table 15-10). The level of abstraction does not render propositions ready for testing. Concepts of the theory are well delineated (Table 15-11); however, some conceptual definitions are not complete in the theory (I/thou, I/it, we, all at once), and others provide useful conceptual definitions such as empathy (Zderad, 1969) and nursology (Paterson, 1971). The theorists did not offer operational definitions. Central nursing phenomena, such as environment or well-

Table 15-9
Assumptions—Paterson and Zderad

Implicit Assumptions

- ○ Nursing involves two human beings who are willing to enter into an existential relationship with each other.
- ○ Nurses and patients as human beings are unique and total bio-psycho-social beings with the potential for becoming through choice and intersubjectivity.
- ○ The present experiences are more than the sum total of the past, present, and the future, and are influenced by the past, present, and future. In their totality they are less than the future.
- ○ Every encounter with another human being is an open and profound one, with a great deal of intimacy that deeply and humanistically influences members in the encounter.
- ○ Human beings are free and are expected to be involved in their own care and in decisions involving them.
- ○ All nursing acts influence the quality of a person's living and dying.
- ○ Nurses and patients coexist; they are independent and interdependent.
- ○ A nurse has to "accept and believe in the chaos of existence as lived and experienced by each man despite the shadows he casts, interpreted as poise, control, order, and joy" (Paterson and Zderad, 1988, p. 56).
- ○ Human beings have an innate force that moves them to know their angular views and other's angular views of the world (Paterson and Zderad, 1976; Zderad, 1969).

From Paterson J. G. and Zderad, L. T. (1976) Humanistic nursing, New York: John Wiley & Sons; Zderad, L. T. (1969) Empathetic nursing: Realization of a human capacity. Nursing Clinics of North America, 4, 655–662; and Paterson, J. G. and Zderad, L. T. (1988) Humanistic Nursing. NLN Publication, March (41–2218).

Table 15-10
Propositions—Paterson and Zderad

- ○ Nursing's existential involvement in patient care is manifested in the active presence of the whole nurse in time and space as viewed by the patient.
- ○ Nursing's goal of more well-being is enhanced by both nurse and patient as they experience the process of making responsible choices.
- ○ Because nursing is involved with human beings, its phenomena are a person needing help and a person helping in his own situation.
- ○ Intimacy and mutuality in relationships enhance more well-being.

Table 15-11
Concepts—Paterson and Zderad

Between	Becoming
Nurturing	I/Thou
Comfort	I/it
Being and doing	We
Lived dialogue	All at once
Nurturing	Well-being
Intersubjective transaction	More-being
Meeting	Choices
Relating	Authenticity with one's self
Presence	Intellectual awareness
Intimacy	Community
Mutuality	Concepts for research
Call and response	Authenticity with self
Other human beings	Nursology
Things	
Time	
Synchronicity	
Space	

Table 15-12
Definition of Domain Concepts—Paterson and Zderad

Nursing	A human discipline involving one human being helping another in an interhuman and intersubjective transaction "containing all the human potentials and limitations of each unique participant" (Paterson and Zderad, 1988, p. 3). Incorporates all human responses of a person needing another. "The ability to struggle with other man through peak experiences related to health and suffering in which the participants in the nursing situation are and become in accordance with their human potential" (1988, p. 7).
Goals of nursing	1) Humanistic nursing itself is a goal. 2) Help patients and self to develop their human potential and to come toward, through choice and intersubjectivity, well-being or more well-being. To help patients and self to increase possibility of making responsible choices (1988, p. 14–17).
Health	More than absence of disease: equated with more well-being, as much as humanly possible (1988, p. 12).
Environment	Objective world as manifested in "other human beings" and things. The subjective meaning of the people and things. Refers to nurses' and patient's environment (1988, pp. 31–33, 37).
Human being	A unique and "incarnate being always becoming in relation with men and things in a world of time and space" (1988, p. 18). Has the capacity to reflect, value, experience to become more. One who asks for help and one who gives help.

(continued)

Table 15-12 (Continued)

Nursing client	Both nurse and patient are the nursing clients (incarnate men), who are unique, when they "meet in a goal-directed (nurturing well-being and more well-being) intersubjective transaction (being with and doing with) occurring in time and space (as measured and as lived by patient and nurse)" (1988, p. 21).
Nursing problem	Seeming discomfort that prompts a call for help. "A person with perceived needs related to the health/illness quality of living" (1988, p. 18).
Nursing process	"Deliberate, responsible, conscious, aware, nonjudgmental existence of the nurse in the nursing situation, followed by disciplined, authentic reflection and description" (1988, pp. 7–8). Based on awareness on the part of the nurse, continuous assessment (p. 16), and developing the human potential of the patient for responsible choosing between alternatives.
Nurse–patient relations	The human dialogue is the essence of nursing, interaction is nursing. Nurse–patient experience is an intersubjective transaction with empathy.
Nursing therapeutics	A human dialogue involves being and doing, nurturing, well-being or more well-being, and comforting. Existential involvement that is an active presence besides the doing, to provide nurturing and comfort and involves experiencing, reflecting, and conceptualizing (1988, p. 12–23). Nurses offer alternatives and support responsible choosing, share self, knowledge, and experience.
Focus of nursing	On the person's unique being and becoming (1988, p. 19).

being, are not defined, nor are central concepts of the theory, such as nurturance, comfort, empathy, and clinical process. Derived concepts, such as the nursing dialogue as meeting, relating, and presence are more comprehensively defined than any of the primitive concepts (Table 15-12).

THEORY ANALYSIS

The Theorists

Josephine G. Paterson, D.N.S. and Loretta T. Zderad, Ph.D. are nurse researchers at the Veterans Administration Hospital in Northport, New York. Paterson (diploma from Lenox Hill Hospital, B.S.N.E. from St. Johns University, M.P.H. from Johns Hopkins University) received her D.N.S. from the Boston University School of Nursing. Zderad (diploma from St. Bernard's Hospital, B.S.N.E. from Loyola University, M.S.N.E. from Catholic University) received her Ph.D. from Georgetown University. Their interest in public health and psychiatric nursing, respectively, is complementary and well-represented in their theory. Their ideas evolved in 1960 while collaboratively teaching graduate students. After completing their respective doctorates, they developed a course on humanistic nursing at the Veterans Administration Hospital in 1972. In the process of teaching the course, their theory evolved. Their 1976 collaborative book is a result of their teaching and observing clinicians in practice. Their book was republished by National League of Nursing in 1988, an indication of the contemporary nature of their ideas.

Paradigmatic Origins

It is quite easy to determine the paradigmatic origins of Paterson and Zderad's theory. The origins are explicitly identified as being existential philosophy for theory development and phenomenology for research. Existentialism considers a person as a unique being and the sum of all undertakings. It does not purport to find out the "why" of a human experience, but just describes the "is" of it. It views human existence as inexplicable and emphasizes the freedom of human choice and responsibility for one's acts. Existential philosophy projects that a person exists but lacks a fixed nature and is always in a state of becoming.

Phenomenology is the study of all aspects of a phenomenon in all its richness, in all its dimensions, in its entirety—without attempting to separate the human experiences of any partners in the study (Stevens, 1984, p. 239). The focus is on the here and now. Nursing deals with more than that; therefore, any limitations in the theory are limitations of the paradigmatic origins.

Paterson and Zderad relied heavily on such existentialist philosophers as Teilhard de Chardin, Martin Buber, Gabriel Marcel, and Frederick Nietzsche to develop their theory of nursing, and they also relied on such phenomenologists as James Agee. Both existentialism and phenomenology are compatible paradigms and allow the humanistic nursing theory to evolve. Stevens identified several advantages in the use of these paradigms to develop the nursing domain. A person could be considered in totality, experience could be viewed as a whole, and knowledge for nursing could be viewed as more than the sum total of diverse views from a variety of disciplines. Indeed, these paradigmatic origins give nursing its *raison d'etre* (Stevens, 1984, pp. 233–250). Existential nursing furthers a better understanding of the environment of one's self. To utilize the accepting nature of existentialism is antithetical to the advocacy needed to make changes in intolerable and oppressive situations that are mitigated by illness or by other social or political conditions. Existential nursing may provide the rationale for accepting an unhealthy and noneffective status quo.

Internal Dimensions

The purpose of the theory is to describe humanistic nursing and its components and the human method of *nursology*: the study of nursing aimed toward the development of nursing theory. Paterson and Zderad used a method to develop theory, and the theory is the method. They aimed to develop a theory, using methodology and proposing research, congruent with the nature of nursing as a human science (Kleiman, 1986). The theory evolved deductively from a philosophical view—

existentialism—but they used a phenomenological approach to inductively develop a theoretical conception of nursing. Because most of the concepts are derived from existentialism, one can deduce that the theory is more deductive than inductive.

This is a highly abstract theory developed around an interest in exploring interaction as a concept. The theory focuses on properties of the human encounter—the human situation that exists between nurses and patients; therefore, it is classified as a microtheory, with more derived than primitive concepts. Its scope is narrow, describing one aspect of nursing therapeutics or the nursing process—interaction—and one aspect of interaction—human encounter. Therefore, it is a single-domain theory. It deals with knowledge of process: How do people interact, particularly when one needs help and one is willing to give help?

Paterson and Zderad use a dialogue form for describing the "nursing dialogue." Therefore, McKeon (undated, cited in Stevens, 1984, p. 51) would consider their approach to theory development a dialectical one. They presented a whole, explaining the whole (humanistic nursing) through the parts (the various concepts) and the parts through the whole. The uniqueness of this theory lies in the lack of boundaries between the experience of the authors as nurses, theoreticians, methodologists, and writers. Concepts in the theory describe all that, and all experiences describe concepts.

THEORY CRITIQUE

The theorists, in proposing their humanistic theory of nursing, have also proposed a methodology congruent with the assumptions of the theory to develop nursing knowledge (Paterson, 1971). They use the logic of phenomenological methodology and call it *phenomenological nursology*. The method is aimed at the reality as experienced by the nurse and the patient subjectively and objectively. They propose the method for research and nursing practice. Existentialism is the context of nursing, and concepts are utilized to develop theory. Phenomenology is the process for clinical nursing and for research in nursing. Phenomenological nursology evolved out of nursing practice and is usable for nursing research.

The theorists proposed five phases of phenomenological nursology (Paterson, 1971, pp. 144-146):

1. "Preparation of the nurse knower for coming to know." This could be accomplished by total immersion in selected and related literary work. Immersion includes reflecting, contemplating, and discussing.
2. "Nurse knowing of the other intuitively" by seeing the world through the eyes of the subject or the patient, becoming an insider rather than an outsider.
3. "Nurse knowing the other scientifically" by replaying the subjective experiences, reflecting on them, and transcribing the amalgamated view. The nurse considers relationships and analyzes, synthesizes, and then conceptualizes.

4. "Nurse complementarity synthesizing known others" by comparing and contrasting the differences of like nursing situations to arrive at an expanded view.
5. "Succession within the nurse from the many to the paradoxical one," evolving from the multiple realities to an inclusive conception of the whole that incorporates the multiplicities and contradictions.

This is a method to find truths related to everyday practice in nursing or as evolving out of nursing research.

The theory depicts a way of life, an attitude toward humanity, a goal of actualization worth striving for on all levels of personal and professional lives. However, it is limited in the form of guidelines for nursing practice. The only indication of the use of this theory in practice has been offered by Paterson and Zderad as occurring in the Veterans Administration Hospital in Northport, New York.

The theory is a philosophy and a methodology that purports to improve not only the quality of care but also the quality of life for the nurse, the teacher, and the administrator. Objective criteria to measure outcomes are antithetical to the theory and the methodology proposed. Therefore, the subjective/objective assessment of each individual nurse is expected and accepted; there are no valid or reliable criteria to measure concepts, nor are they warranted within the philosophical view that guides the theory.

This is a tautological theory; the process of humanistic nursing is described by the goal of humanistic nursing, and the complexity of the phenomenon it addresses stems from abstractness and lack of boundaries between its concepts. It appears to focus on the nurse rather than the on patient as becoming and actualizing in the course of nursing care. Stevens (1984, p. 243) asked if what we need is really a holistic nurse, in which case the proper subject matter of existential nursing theory would appropriately be the nurse rather than the patient. If that is one of the focuses of nursing, and Donaldson would agree (1983), then Paterson and Zderad have offered a theory that appropriately describes one of the nursing phenomena.

External Components of Theory

The theory may be incongruent with some prevailing values of practice that address outcome over process, but it is congruent with values surrounding research and knowledge development in nursing that emerged in the mid-1980s in the United States. Humanistic theory proposes understanding of human beings and their experiences as they exist rather than how they ought to be or rather than changing them. The goals of humanistic nursing of understanding, supporting, and maintaining may be in direct conflict with other professional values and goals, such as intervention goals for changes in pain responses or for alleviation of suffering.

As illustrated by Stevens (1984, p. 229), it is a common existential position that suffering serves to bring about a state of heightened self-awareness, thereby creating an openness to authentic experience that the patient might not otherwise experience and express. Suffering creates a state in which the person is brought face to face with his own being. Most nurses, however, seek to remove (alleviate) suffering. It might be very difficult for a nurse who is adhering to this theory to justify nursing acts that remove a patient from the authentic experience of suffering. Neither Travelbee nor Paterson and Zderad would advocate the removal of suffering. Nursing to them is to help patients articulate their perceptions of the situation and the meaning of the suffering and to grow through this suffering.

According to this theory, a nurse–patient encounter involves an open human dialogue that incorporates a high degree of intimacy to enhance understanding of the subjective world of the patient (Stevens, 1984). How many such meetings can a nurse be involved in, in the course of her working day, and is there potential for emotional drainage leading to burnout? Do all patients seek and approve of such genuine encounters? Paterson and Zderad would argue that the higher levels of experience gleaned from each encounter indicate rejuvenation rather than burnout.

The theory is congruent with that segment of society that espouses subjectivity and being, but patients may want to experience and evolve their being in genuine encounters within their own circle rather than with the nursing staff.

When, in 1960, Paterson and Zderad were developing the seeds of their theory, they may or may not have anticipated the supportive literature of the 1980s that advocated phenomenology as the methodology most compatible with nursing. The 1980s witnessed an emerging world view in nursing, denouncing the empirical positivist view (see Chapter 4) and supporting a phenomenological view (Menke, 1978; Munhall, 1982; Oiler, 1982). Paterson and Zderad advocated respecting nursing experiences as sources of knowledge and, indeed, of wisdom, providing nursing with nonmechanistic and nonpositivistic strategies for theory development and research (Paterson, 1978; Zderad, 1978). Nursing would do well to adopt their views.

THEORY TESTING

Although no research is reported specifically using Paterson and Zderad's method, there are numerous research findings that have used grounded theory, modified phenomenological approaches, and qualitative approaches to nursing research. Researchers have used these concepts interchangeably to describe methodologies depicting part of each (Stern, 1980; Wilson, 1977). Paterson and Zderad have used the approach to articulate concepts of empathy (Zderad, 1968; 1969; 1970), and comfort (Paterson and Zderad, 1976), but these reports appear to be clinical insights as a prelude to systematic research findings.

Research to explore these theory propositions has potential after the concepts have been operationalized. For example, the concepts of authenticity, the "between," more well-being, and all-at-once are abstract and lack definition to render them researchable. The potential of the theory to generate research is exemplified in the use of the self (the nurse) and different patterns of presence in the patient's "time-space spheres."

Joyce Travelbee

THEORY DESCRIPTION

Nursing to Travelbee is an interpersonal process between two human beings, one of whom needs assistance because of an illness situation and the other who is able to give such assistance. The goal of the assistance is to help a human being cope with an illness situation, learn from the experience, find meaning in the experience, and grow due to the experience. For a nurse to be able to achieve that goal, she also has to find meaning in each encounter. Because illness is suffering and pain, the role of the nurse is to deal with suffering and pain. If the nurse experienced personal suffering, she would be far better able to understand the patient's suffering. Nurses should not shy away from becoming very involved with their patients because it is through such involvement that empathy, sympathy, and, eventually, rapport is established.

The central questions that Travelbee's theory answers are: How do nurse–patient, human-to-human relationships get established? For what purpose? Travelbee further asked: What is it that enables some individuals to cope with stress over a prolonged period of time? (Travelbee, 1970, personal communication.) In attempting to answer these questions, Travelbee theorized that suffering is a common life experience that every person encounters at some point, that particularly occurs around illness, and that is divided into phases.

Human relationships help people cope with suffering, and Travelbee conceptualized relationships as progressing in stages, beginning with the phase of original encounter and evolving to the phase of rapport. A person's attitude toward suffering ultimately determines how effectively he copes with illness. The nurse's role is focused on helping patients find different meanings for suffering, meanings that are of particular importance to them.

Travelbee provides us with an exhaustive conceptualization of sympathy, rapport, and suffering as fine examples of a factor-isolating theory. Suffering is defined as

> . . . a feeling of displeasure that ranges from simple transitory mental,
> physical, or spiritual discomfort to extreme anguish and to those phases
> beyond anguish; namely, the malignant phase of despair, the feeling of "not
> caring," and the terminal phase of apathetic indifference (Travelbee, 1966,
> p. 70).

It is an experience that is variable in its intensity, duration, and depth. Beyond the beginning feelings of suffering, and when suffering becomes very intense physically, mentally, and spiritually, suffering progresses to the malignant phase in which a person experiences anger, helplessness, and bitterness. If suffering persists, a person ceases to complain or express feelings related to anger and helplessness and instead displays apathetic indifference.

Although reactions to suffering are individualistic, there are some common responses. These are "nonacceptance, blaming self or others, bafflement, anger, self-pity, depression, anguish" during a "why me?" stage (Travelbee, 1966, p. 88). Or human beings may respond to suffering through no protest or even with an affirmative reaction, thereby accepting the suffering. Acceptance may occur because of personal philosophy, perception of the nature of humanity, or religious convictions. Pain and suffering are related. "To suffer is to be immersed in a black ocean of pain" (Travelbee, 1966, p. 89).

To deal with pain and suffering, a nurse has to establish nurse–patient interactions by getting to know the patient, by becoming involved, by ascertaining needs, and by fulfilling the purpose of nursing, which is to alleviate suffering and to help people find meaning in a situation. Communication is the key tool for the nurse. Nurses use various clinical therapeutics to keep channels of communication open, such as validating perceptions, reflecting by self or with patient, and using open-ended comments to solicit more information. Nurses can deliberately prevent communication breakdown by perceiving patients as human beings, recognizing levels of meaning when communicating, listening with reflection, and avoiding cliches, automatic responses, and undue interruptions (Travelbee, 1966, pp. 91–117).

Communication is the vehicle through which nurse–patient relationships are established. Such a relationship is defined as "an experience or series of experiences between a nurse and a patient . . . [or] a family member . . . in need of the service of the nurse." The relationship has two characteristics: it is a "mutually significant meaningful experience" and, through it, the nursing needs of the individual (or family member) are met (Travelbee, 1966, p. 125). Nurses and patients go through several stages to achieve the goal of established nurse–patient relationships. Each stage has certain tasks, and healthy development of the relationship is accomplished by mastering each task. The stages are as follows:

1. **Phase of the original encounter**: Emotional knowledge colors impressions and perceptions of both nurse and patient during initial encounters. The task to be accomplished is "to break the bond of categorization in order to perceive the human being in the patient" and vice versa (Travelbee, 1966, p. 133).
2. **Phase of emerging identities**: Both nurse and patient begin to transcend their respective roles and perceive uniqueness in each other. Tasks to be accomplished are separating oneself and one's experiences from others and avoiding "using oneself as a yardstick" by which to evaluate others. Barriers to such tasks may be due to role envy, lack of interest in others, inability to transcend the self, or refusal to initiate emotional investment.
3. **Phase of empathy**: This phase involves sharing another's psychological state but standing apart and not sharing feelings. It is characterized "by the ability to predict the behavior of another" (Travelbee, 1966, p. 143).
4. **Phase of sympathy**: Sharing, feeling, and experiencing what others are feeling and experiencing is accomplished. This phase

demonstrates emotional involvement and discredits objectivity as dehumanizing. The task of the nurse is to translate sympathy into helpful nursing actions (Travelbee, 1964).

5. **Phase of rapport**: All previous phases culminate into rapport, defined as all those experiences, thoughts, feelings, and attitudes that both nurse and patient undergo and are able to perceive, share, and communicate (Travelbee, 1963; 1966, pp. 133–162).

When relationships are established, the nurse can help patients to accept and find meaning in their experiences or to accept their humanness through either circuitous or indirect methods (avoiding direct confrontation by using parables or by the nurse opening herself and sharing similar personal experiences) or direct methods (asking pertinent questions or logically explaining the situation). Establishment of rapport in nurse–patient relationships and finding meaning in suffering eventually lead to the development of hope in patients (Travelbee, 1971).

Travelbee based her theory on numerous assumptions that are interspersed throughout her book. These assumptions are presented in Table 15-13. Travelbee's assumptions are explicit and congruent with selected concepts and theory propositions. The concepts are abstract and have face validity, but the boundaries are not clear or operationally defined (What is hope and how can it be measured?) (Table 15-14). Travelbee is consistent in her views of humanity, uniqueness, existential encounters, and nursing. The theorist's definitions of health, nursing, relationships, nursing problems, and nursing therapeutics are conceptually clear, with the integrity of the assumptions preserved throughout the definitions (Table 15-15). Rapport is a phase toward the nurse–patient relationship, but it also has the same properties as the nurse–patient relationship; the phases overlap. Further operationalization will help determine which behaviors belong in which phase of the process of establishing nurse–patient relationships. Travelbee often relied on dictionary definitions. Research relating to different concepts was not cited. The theory lends itself to numerous propositions that are central to the practice of nursing. Examples are offered in Table 15-16.

THEORY ANALYSIS

The Theorist

The late Joyce Travelbee was a faculty member at several schools of nursing. She worked as an assistant professor in the Department of Nursing, Louisiana State University, New Orleans; then as an instructor in psychiatric and mental health nursing in the Department of Nursing Education at New York University; then as a professor at the University of Mississippi School of Nursing in Jackson; and finally at Hotel Dieu School of Nursing in New Orleans. She received a diploma in nursing from Charity Hospital, New Orleans, a bachelor of science from Louisiana State University, and graduated from Yale with a master of science in nursing. She acknowledged Ida Orlando's influence on her work.

Table 15-13
Assumptions—Travelbee

- The nurse–patient relationship is the essence of the purpose of nursing (Travelbee, 1966, p. 13).
- Human beings are rational, social, and unique beings and are more different than alike (1966, p. 29).
- All human beings undergo certain experiences and will serach for meaning in them during the process of living. These experiences could be considered as coherent wholes and could be understood (*e.g.*, illness, anxiety, joy, harm). Therefore, likeness and similarities between human beings are in the nature of their experiences (1966, p. 30).
- Labels tend to evoke stereotypical categories. Nurses should remember that patients are human beings who differ from other human beings only in "requesting the assistance of other human beings believed capable of helping them solve health problems" (1966, p. 34).
- Relationships are established when both partners perceive each other's uniqueness. Then, such human relationships transcend roles and are true, meaningful, and effective relationships based on perceptions of uniqueness (1966, p. 36).
- Nurse–patient relationships are based on perceiving the patient as an illness or nursing as a task. Illness is only understood in the context of perceptions of the patient and the nurse
- Illness, suffering, and pain experiences could be self-actualizing if individuals find meaning in them.
- Human beings are motivated to search for and understand the meaning of all life experiences.
- Illness and suffering are not only physical encounters for human beings, they are emotional and spiritual encounters as well (1966, p. 69).
- Nurse–patient interaction, when purposeful, fulfills the goals of nursing (1966, p. 93).
- "Communication is a process that can enable the nurse to establish a nurse–patient relationship and thereby fulfill the purpose of nursing—namely to assist individuals and families, to prevent and cope with the experience of illness and suffering and, if necessary, to assist them to find meaning in these experiences." (1966, p. 94).
- Nurses are expected to ascertain the meaning of exchanged messages.

Paradigmatic Origins

Travelbee based her theoretical formulations on existentialist philosophy from which she drew many of the theory assumptions. A developmental approach is somewhat demonstrated in her writing as she utilized the concepts of stages of development of the nurse–patient relationship, stages of suffering, tasks to be mastered, constant change and development, and the becoming nature (Chin, 1974), after going through each of the stages. The continuous sense of becoming is both a developmental and an existential concept.

The incongruence perhaps lies in assumptions of developmental theory of an orderly progression and the lack of orderliness inherent in the existentialist philosophy. Despite this shortcoming, Travelbee has effectively and usefully synthesized assumptions and concepts of both developmental theory and existential philosophy

Table 15-14
Concepts—Travelbee

Perception	Finding meaning in illness and suffering
Pain	Circuitous
Suffering	Parable approach
Communication	Veiled
Therapeutic self	Personal experience
Hope	Direct
Self-actualization	Questioning
Transcend self	Explanation
Therapeutic self	Transitory discomfort
Nurse–patient relationship/human to human relationship	Anguish
Phase of original enocunter	Malignant despair
Phase of emerging identities	Not caring
Phase of empathy	Apathetic indifference
Phase of sympathy	Love
Phase of rapport	

Table 15-15
Definition of Domain Concepts—Travelbee

Nursing	An interpersonal process and service vitally concerned with change and influence of others. An interpersonal process whereby the professional nurse practitioner assists an individual or family to prevent or cope with the experience of illness and suffering and, if necessary, to assist the individual or family to find meaning in these experiences (Travelbee, 1966, pp. 5–6).
Goal of nursing	To assist an individual or family to prevent or cope with the experience or illness and suffering and, if necessary, to assist the individual or family to find meaning in these experiences (1966, pp. 10–12, 20), with the ultimate goal being the presence of hope (1971).
Health	World Health Organization (WHO) definition: "Health is a state of complete physical, mental, and social well-being and not merely the absence of disease or infirmity. The enjoyment of the highest attainable standard of health is one of the fundamental rights of every human bieng without distinction of race, religion, political, economic, or social condition." (1966, p.7).
Environment	Not defined.
Human being	A unique thinking, biological, amd social organism, an irreplaceable individual who is unlike any other person, who is influenced by heredity, environment, culture, and experiences. Always in the process of becoming and capable of choosing (1966, pp. 26–34).

(continued)

Table 15-15 (Continued)

	Understanding of a human being is through his perception of himself.
Nursing client	A patient is a human being who requests assistance from another human being who he believes is capable of helping and will help in solving his health problems.
Nursing problem	Communication breakdown and distortion: "1. Failure to perceive patient as a human being 2. Failure to recognize levels of meaning in communication 3. Failure to listen, using value statements without reflection 4. Cliches and automatic responses 5. Failure to interrupt" (1966, pp. 106–117)
Nursing process	Process to ascertain needs, validate inferences, decide who should meet needs, plan a course of action, and validate. "Disciplined intellectual approach," a logical method of approaching nursing problems, using knowledge and understanding of concepts from all other sciences and nursing in caring for patients (1966, p. 15).
Nurse–patient relations	An experience between an individual in need of the services of a nurse, and a nurse for the purpose of meeting the needs of the individual.
Nursing therapeutics	Therapeutic use of self (nurse). Disciplined intellectual approach to patient problems. Everything the nurse does for and with the patient is designed to help the individual or family in coping with or bearing the stress of illness and suffering in the event the individual or family encounters these experiences (1966, p. 8). Help patients find meaning in their experiences (1966, p. 10). Methods to find meaning are: 1) Circuitous (indirect) method, which includes (a) parable method (tell analogous story), (b) veiled problem approach (use indefinite pronouns), or (c) personal experience approach (shared experience); 2) Direct method, which includes questioning in jest and explaining (1966, pp. 16–19, 173–179). "Communication techniques: Use of open-ended comments or questions Use of reflecting technique Use of sharing perceptions Deliberate use of cliches" (1966, pp. 106–110).

by depicting the complexity of humanity through significant milestones (Sarlore, 1966). Her conception of empathy could be clearer if cast within the framework of role theory, particularly role-taking.

Travelbee herself credited Victor Frankel (1963) (with whom she corresponded and met) and Rollo May (1953) with the influence on her theories.

Table 15-16
Propositions—Travelbee

- To know and understand perceptions of time and life experiences increases the nurse's abilities to meet the needs of patients.
- "The nurse's perception of patients is a major factor in determining the quality and quantity of nursing care she will render each patient" (Travelbee, 1966, p. 34).
- If nurses perceive patients as illnesses, tasks, or sets of stereotype characteristics, their focus in care in (institutional) rather than person-centered (1966, p. 36–41).
- As patients become a "chore and a task, the nurse withdraws and directs her energy toward meeting institutional needs" and patients experience anger, irritability, tension, restlessness, sadness, depression, hopelessness, apathy, and transient somatic symptoms (1966, pp. 38–40).
- An individual's socioeconomic status affects the level of dehumanization a person is subjected to.
- "The quality of nursing care given any patient is determined by the nurses' beliefs about illness, suffering, and death" (1966, p. 55).
- "The spiritual values of the nurse or her philosophical beliefs about illness and suffering will determine the extent to which she will be able to help patients find meaning (or no meaning) in these situations" (1966, p. 55).
- Nurses are able to empathize with patients who are similar to themselves (1966, p. 142).
- Experience of illness affects, to a varying degree, all those associated with the patient, and subsequently affects the patient's perception of the experience (1966, p. 66).
- There is a direct relationship between caring and suffering; the more a person cares and is attached to an object or a person, the more the person suffers when that object or person is lost (1966, p. 72).
- Responses to pain are influenced by cultural background of the person, philosophical premises, spirituality, level of anxiety, and responses of others to the person in pain (1966, p. 81).
- What are the properties of hope, determinants of hope and hopelessness (1971)?
- There is a direct relationship between the extent to which the individual's need for cognitive clarity and security are met and the individual's anxiety level (1971, p. 190).

Internal Dimensions

Travelbee's theory is a hierarchical theory developed around the concepts of nurse–patient relationship, suffering, and pain to explore the relationship among them. It is both a concatenated theory, isolating and conceptualizing the central theory concepts, and a hierarchical one, as it interprets the relationship among these variables. Travelbee used the field approach in developing her theory, as is demonstrated in conceptualizing rapport in terms of other phases leading to and incorporating rapport. It is a descriptive and prescriptive microtheory that is also considered a single-domain theory.

The theory addresses one of the major concepts in nursing—interaction—but is limited to interaction surrounding illness. The theory focuses on the components of illness of concern to nursing: suffering and pain. It adds mainly to knowledge of process in nursing and provides significant existence propositions (nurse–patient interactions proceed through phases) and relational propositions (rapport increases patient's acceptance of illness).

Travelbee uses an operational method to develop highly abstract relationships. She incorporates the nurses' perceptions and acceptance with components of the nursing problem areas and nursing therapeutics. The nurse perceives, understands, and assigns meaning to behavior and is therefore part of the theory. The nurse's communication is one of the nursing problems, and the self could be used as the intervention through empathy and sympathy.

An operational method of theory development allows choices between alternate theories and actions. An example can be seen in the alternatives that Travelbee provides to dealing with suffering through using the direct method of confronting the patient with his suffering or the indirect method of sharing one's own experiences. Operational methods tend to be more acceptable to nurses because of their preferences for well-identified choices.

The theory's explanatory power is low (higher ratio of assumptions to explicitly-stated propositions) and is limited to knowledge of disorder (suffering) and knowledge of process (relationships).

Travelbee used a deductive approach to develop her theory (Duffey and Muhlenkamp, 1974). Although she explicitly stated the sources that influenced the theory deductively (existentialist philosophy), the inductive approach is more assumed than explicit. It is assumed that she observed nurse–patient relationships in acute and suffering incidents. Such observations are not an integral part of her theory, and it is not clear whether she developed her theory based on extant or ought-to-be practice. One can deduce that it was the former rather than the latter.

THEORY CRITIQUE

The theory is teleological. The process of establishing relationships is achieved after several stages in nurse–patient encounters, including rapport; however, rapport is the nurse–patient interaction. It is both goal and process; it is both process and product. The theory is tautological and parsimonious; assumptions and relationships could be presented without the numerous repetitions; and more attention needs to be given to the propositions. Finding meaning is analogous to coping but leads to coping, and vice versa.

The complexity of the theory is demonstrated in the abstractness of the concepts, limited operational definitions, and potential multiplicity of relationships. Therefore, its use in research, practice, education, and administration appears to be limited.

Although many of the central concepts in Travelbee's theory are derived from other theories (empathy, sympathy), she does not appear to have developed her propositions utilizing findings of other research. Some of Travelbee's ideas are common practice in nursing. The nursing process as we have come to teach it and use it involves several of the steps outlined by Travelbee. Observations are carried out to validate the needs of patients, to validate inferences made, to make decisions about personally taking action or not, and to then plan a course of action; then, the action is evaluated. The patient is the final authority.

Doona (1979), in preparing a second edition of an earlier Travelbee book (1969), used Travelbee's intervention theory as a guideline for the field of psychiatric nursing. Beyond this publication, no published evidence was found that directly develops, implements, or refines Travelbee's ideas. The theory has the potential for use in practice within the limitations of its scope and its microtheory nature, both of which refer only to individual patients who are ill and suffering, who are conscious, who are willing to invest in the development of rapport, and who participate in finding meaning in and making decisions about their care.

Cook (1989) demonstrated the utility of the theory in assessing suffering of nurses due to job distress at the height of the nursing shortage that forced their hospital to adopt a new system of patient care. The theory was used to define the nature and degree of suffering, the nature of each phase in the development of meaningful interactions between members of a group of nurses who met regularly to deal with their job stress. The rapport described by Travelbee was achieved prior to planning interventions. The intervention plan based on Travelbee (1971) included alleviating suffering, redefining the situation, and finding meaning in their experiences through disciplined and intellectual approaches and the use of the self (Cook, 1989, p. 205). The process of rapport development and the interventions helped the group members to feel less victimized and to gain control over their professional lives. The result was improved self-esteem, better problem solving, a more supportive environment, and rediscovery that a new system is providing them with greater autonomy and more challenging roles.

There is no other published material indicating the use of Travelbee's theory in education or administration, despite favorable review of her 1966 book (Sloane, 1966; Wolff, 1966). Travelbee indicated that the University of Mississippi School of Nursing in Jackson was beginning to modify its curriculum to use her theory (1970, personal communication). However, the limited scope of the theory restricts its utility for all aspects of nursing.

External Components of Theory

The focus of the theory on the uniqueness and dignity of the human being, on humanity, on autonomy, and on acceptance of others' values makes the assumptions of the theory congruent with Western values. The more recent emphasis on the role of hope—the ultimate goal of finding meaning in suffering—in healing and recovery tends to give more theoretical credence to Travelbee's propositions pertaining to the meaning of an illness and attitudes toward suffering. However, illness is viewed by society as an aberration, an abnormality, or a condition to be avoided and eliminated. This value is antithetical to Travelbee's basic assumption that illness is a part of life, and finding meaning in illness and suffering is a growing experience. Therefore, professional values could clash with the theory values (used here as an assumption). Many patients could consider the assumption of shared nurse–patient relationships to find meaning problematic and may even go as far as questioning the cost-effectiveness of such emphasis on relationships. The lack of a biological view of the patient and the limited positivistic orientation of the theory undoubtedly limit the utility and the acceptance of the theory by nurses.

Relationships are significant in the helping fields, they are an integral part of assessment for care, and they are focal in delivering care. Travelbee articulated for nursing how such relationships are formed and for what purpose. Hers is a theory to describe one of the central domain concepts in nursing.

THEORY TESTING

Central relationships in Travelbee's theory—nurse–patient relationship's effect on suffering and coping—have not been researched. However, the concept of empathy has been the center of numerous research studies. Various tools have been developed to measure degrees of empathy (Barrett-Leonard, 1962; Cartwright and Lerner, 1963; Truax and Carkhuff, 1967). Most of the studies of the 1960s and 1970s concluded that existing tools lacked construct and predictive validity and that their reliability was low (Chinsky and Rappaport, 1970; Kurtz and Grummon, 1972).

Other studies utilizing Travelbee's theory explore differences between perceptions of high and low empathizers in effective communication (Stetler, 1977) and properties of interaction surrounding pain (McBride, 1967). Results have been inconclusive. Freihofer and Felton (1976) explored the nature of nursing actions perceived to offer support, comfort, and ease the suffering of a terminally ill patient and significant others of terminally ill patients. More descriptive studies of this type will lend data to explore the construct validity of nurses' actions and options for suffering patients.

Ernestine Wiedenbach

THEORY DESCRIPTION

Ernestine Wiedenbach developed a concept of nursing that was congruent with the prevailing ideas at Yale in the late 1950s and early 1960s and that shifted nursing focus from the medical model to a patient model. In her early work (1963), she attempted to develop a concept that encompassed all nursing; this evolved into a prescriptive theory. The theory addresses the central question: How do nurses help patients meet their needs? Help, to Wiedenbach, is an integral part of nursing, and it is all actions that enable individuals to overcome whatever hampers their ability to function.

Needs and functions that dominated nursing at the time continue to do so with an added dimension. Needs can only be ascertained if the nurse validates her perceptions, feelings, and thoughts with those of the patient. Therefore, nurses' actions should abide by the following parameters: actions should be mutually understood and agreed upon with full knowledge of implications, and they should be either patient-directed or nurse-directed or both. When they are nurse-directed, they must be deliberate and based on patient needs. To Wiedenbach, nurses develop a helping prescription with the reality of the situation (physical, physiological, psychological, emotional, and spiritual) by exploring nurses' philosophies of nursing (central purpose and assessment of the situation). Throughout a continuous process of observation and validation, nurses' observations are focused on determining inconsistencies (deviations from normal) and perseverances in making the patients realize their needs. Nurses make plans for action to "minister help needed." The plan has to be validated by patients before implementation. Nurses use themselves, the patients, or others who are appropriate as therapeutic agents.

Wiedenbach (1970a) identified several assumptions that guided her theory, and there are other implicit assumptions (Table 15-17). There are some inconsistencies in the assumptions, such as uniqueness and orderliness, self-directed and dependent, but on the whole, Wiedenbach made a deliberate effort to identify the philosophical premises upon which she developed her theory. A student of her theory may be confused with the numerous premises appearing at different points throughout her work. Inconsistencies also exist in using principles, philosophy, and assumptions interchangeably, when, at times, any one of these also were used to mean propositions.

Assumptions and concepts are congruent (Table 15-18). Concepts in the theory are mostly derived (needs, interaction, perception), and because Orlando, Wiedenbach, Dickoff, and James all worked together closely in developing their ideas, despite some of their perceptions of differences (Wiedenbach, 1970b), it is not easy to discern which concepts are primitive and which are derived. All these theories are extensions of each other; while Wiedenbach developed the concept of validation, validation is an integral part of Orlando's nursing process discipline. For Wiedenbach, one of nursing's goals is to promote comfort; for Orlando, it is to alleviate distress. Wiedenbach focused on perceptions of people in need of help and Orlando focused on perceptions as a significant concept in interaction. Concepts in general are not operationally defined, perhaps by design, because whether a patient is comfortable or not depends on the patient's perception and the meaning he attributes to the event and situation (Table 15-19).

The major concepts in this theory tend to be concrete and nonvariable (comfort, validation, need for help). The definitions are contextual, and this has the advantage of allowing variable definitions (comfort is in the eye of the beholder), but it also decreases utility in practice and research. Health and environment are not defined; a nursing client is defined in terms of hospital care and is contingent upon awareness of needs. Relationships between concepts in Wiedenbach's early and later writing are not always clear (*i.e.*, prescription, validation). The explanatory power of the theory is hampered by a lack of clarity.

The theory lacks propositions and linkages between concepts, but one can derive propositions related to the process of assessment and intervention. The

Table 15-17
Assumptions—Wiedenbach

Explicit Assumptions

- "Each human being is endowed with a unique potential to develop within himself the resources that enable him to maintain and sustain himself" (Wiedenbach, 1970b, p. 1058).
- "The human being basically strives toward self-direction and relative independence and desires not only to make best use of his capabilities and potentialities, but desires to fulfill his responsibilities as well" (1970b, p. 1058).
- "The human being needs stimulation in order to make best use of his capabilities and realize his self-worth" (1970b, p. 1058).
- "Whatever the individual does represents his best judgment at the moment of doing it" (1970b, p. 1058).
- "The helping art of clinical nursing is a deliberate blending of thoughts, feelings, and overt actions" (1964, p. 11).
- "There are three more basic premises in nursing: "reverence for the gift of life," "respect for dignity, worth, autonomy, and individuality of each human being," and "resolution to act dynamically in relation to one's beliefs" (1964, p. 16).
- "Characteristics of professionalism: clarity of purpose, mastery of skills and knowledge, sustaining purposeful working relationships with others, interest in advancing knowledge and dedication to furthering the goal of mankind" (Dickoff, James, and Wiedenbach, 1968).

Implicit Assumptions

- Patients are dependent beings normaly willing to utilize help (Wiedenbach, 1970, p. 1060).
- Patients can use their sensitivities to frustrate health care givers and "thwart their efforts to obtain the results they desire" (1970b, p. 1060).
- Individuals like to live an orderly life, and life is an orderly process.
- Factors such as physical, physiological, psychological, and spiritual influence the nursing situation.
- Individuals want and have the resources to be healthy, comfortable, and capable (1964).
- Professional nursing respects dignity, worth, autonomy, and individuality of each human being.

Table 15-18
Concepts—Wiedenbach

Need for help	Ministeration
Help	Realities
Inconsistency/consistency	Central purpose
Purposeful perseverance	Prescription
Self-extension	Skills
Preconception	Procedural
Interpretation	Communication
Actions	
Rational	
Reactionary	
Deliberate	

Table 15-19
Definition of Domain Concepts—Wiedenbach

Nursing	A helping art with knowledge and theories. A goal-directed and deliberate blending of thoughts, feelings, perceptions, and actions to understand the patient and his condition, situation, and needs, to enhance his capability, improve his care, prevent recurrence of problem, and deal with anxiety, disability, or distress (Wiedenbach, 1964).
Goal of nursing	"To facilitate the efforts of the individual to overcome the obstacles which currently interfere (or maybe later interfere [1970b, p. 1058]) with his ability to respond capably to demands made of him by his condition, environment, situation, and time" (1963, p. 55). "To meet the need the individual is experiencing as a need for help" (1963, p. 55).
Health	Not defined.
Environment	Conglomerate of objects, policies, setting, atmosphere, time, human beings, happenings past, current, or anticipated that are dynamic, unpredictable, exhilarating, baffling, and disruptive (1970, p. 1061).
Human being	Possesses self-direction and relative independence, makes best use of capabilities, fulfills responsibilities, has resources to maintain self; in other words, is a functioning being (1964).
Nursing client	A person who is under care of some member of health care personnel, who is in a vulnerable position, with a perceived need for help.
Nursing problem	Inability or impaired ability of an individual to cope with situational demands due to interferences (1963, p. 56). Discomfort.
Nursing process	Deliberative, to identify need for help and interferences with ability to cope. Through observation, understanding, and clarification of the meaning of cues, determination of causes of discomfort (through inspection, palpation, temperature, etc.) and determination of whether or not patient is able to meet his own needs. Ministration of help needed and, the last step in the process, validation that help given was indeed help needed (1963, p. 56–57).
Nurse–patient relations	The deliberate use of nurses' perceptions, thoughts, feelings, and actions.
Nursing therapeutics	Deliberate action that is either nurse-directed, patient-directed, or mutually understood and agreed upon (1970b, p. 1059). (These are the nurse's options and the choice is hers.) It is designed to deal with a person who is in need of help by "any measure or action required and desired by the individual that has the potential for restoring or extending his ability to cope with the demands implicit in his situation" (1963, p. 56). Help, which is any measure or action that enables the individual to overcome whatever interferes with his ability to function capably in relation to his situation (1963, p. 56). Giving advice, information, referral, ministering or applying a comfort measure. Deliberate actions are mutually understood and agreed upon, patient-directed, and nurse-directed. Communication is an important tool. Helping is based on three principles: inconsistency or consistency, purposeful perseverance, and self-extension (1970).
Focus of nursing	Goal-directed activities focused on identifying "the patient's perception of his condition" and his need for help (1963, p. 55).

Table 15-20
Propositions—Wiedenbach*

○ When nurses observe inconsistencies in patients' actions, they use their perseverence in identifying the need for help and in offering help.
○ Exploration and validation of nurses' and patients' perceptions, thoughts, and feelings increase the effectiveness of help offered to patients in need of help.
○ Deliberate nursing action is an overt act consisting of several components: the need for help, validation, and ministration of help.
○ Congruent nurse and patient perceptions of the need for help and evaluation of help enhance effective care and decrease discomfort.
○ Mutually understood and agreed-upon nursing actions will have a positive effect on the patient.
○ Help give to individuals in need of help is categorized as: identification of variance from normal (principle of inconsistency/consistency); identification of an individual's need for help (principle of purposeful perseverence); utilizing self or others for help, advice, information, referral, or comfort (principle of self-extension).

* *Propositions delineated under Orlando could also be propositions derived from this theory.*

principles of help are amenable to the development of existence propositions and, subsequently, relational propositions (Table 15-20).

THEORY ANALYSIS

The Theorist

Ernestine Wiedenbach holds a bachelor of arts degree from Wellesley College, Wellesley, Massachusetts, and a diploma in nursing from Johns Hopkins School of Nursing, Baltimore, Maryland. She received her master's degree from Teachers College, Columbia University, in public health nursing. She practiced as a nurse midwife. At the time of theory development, she was an associate professor of maternity nursing at the School of Nursing, Yale University (she began working there around 1952) (Bennet and Foster, 1980). She worked closely with two philosophers, Patricia James and William Dickoff, who were teaching a course in philosophy for nurses. She also worked closely with Ida Orlando. Currently, Wiedenbach is retired and an associate professor emeritus.

Paradigmatic Origins

Basically, Wiedenbach's view of a human being and her view of a nurse are functional. She views patients in terms of their capabilities to function and carry out their responsibilities. Wiedenbach was influenced by Ida Orlando, James Dickoff, and Patricia James (and perhaps the reverse is also true). Such influence is seen in her explication of nurses' actions and reactions and the focus on interpretation and validation of perceptions, feelings, thoughts, and actions. Therefore, it would be useful for the reader to also review the discussion of paradigmatic origins found under Orlando.

Some of Wiedenbach's assumptions and concepts regarding the motivation of human beings and nurses' impulsive responses appear at times to reflect conditions or stimulus-response types of actions and reactions (Wiedenbach, 1968). Careful analysis of the theory may identify developmental themes or parallel themes with a psychoanalytical orientation, such as internal needs, frustrations, and motivations. However, the meaning of the situation or the event as perceived and expressed by an individual demonstrates a departure from psychoanalytical concepts to a phenomenological approach. These are speculations on paradigmatic origins. One origin is clear and documented; the theory evolved out of 40 years of clinical and teaching experiences (Wiedenbach, 1964, p. vii; 1968; 1969), and later developments supported the process nature of the theory (Wiedenbach and Falls, 1978).

Internal Dimensions

Wiedenbach's theory was developed around the need for help and validation of such need through patient perceptions and is therefore a concatenated theory that lends itself first and foremost to existence propositions. It is an inductive theory evolving from observations of clinical practice and patients' needs for help after many years of practice in the maternal and child nursing subspecialty. It is a microtheory explicating a component of the interaction process focused on validating perceptions, thoughts, and feelings before a deliberate action is planned. It is a theory with narrow scope—the deliberative nurse–patient interactive process in a clinical situation to identify needs and verify actions. It addresses one component of one of the central concepts in nursing: nurse–patient interaction. It deals with knowledge of process, describing a component of the process inherent in assessing and providing care.

Wiedenbach used a field approach in identifying dimensions of interaction and validation and used a combination of operational and problem approaches to theory development. She focused her conceptualization around problems of discomfort and the need for help and around the function of the nurse in observing, assessing, and exploring and validating feelings, thoughts, and fears. She used persuasion and personal beliefs to drive the concepts home to nurses.

Perhaps because of the concreteness of the theory, the circle of contagiousness of ideas was wide and reached diverse geographical locations and settings.

Although nurses may not articulate the concepts and linkages emanating from Wiedenbach, the central ideas of her theory are used widely. Her's is a good example of theory with tautology, lack of parsimoniousness in presenting ideas (presented in philosophical dialogue), and teleology (identifying the need for help is both a process and an outcome). The ratio of assumptions to existing propositions decreases its current power of explanation.

THEORY CRITIQUE

The patient's perspective has become an integral part of the lexicon of nursing since the 1980s. Whether these concepts infiltrated nursing thought as a result of Orlando and Wiedenbach can only be determined through extensive analysis of nursing literature and through comparison of writings the decades prior to 1960 and the decades following the publications of Orlando, Wiedenbach, Travelbee, Paterson, Zderad, and other interactionist theorists. An analysis of networking of ideas and people and the development of conceptual genealogical trees may enable us to ascertain the influence of the different theorists on the development of nursing knowledge.

It is apparent that the circle of contagiousness for research was limited to research in or surrounding Yale, but the circle of contagiousness for practice was much wider and engulfed the United States and foreign countries. Concepts such as patient-centered care, perceptions, validation, and exploration of thoughts, feelings, and actions are used in many practice settings. The theory gives guidelines for implementing the nursing process and has stimulated many attempts at conceptualizing the interaction process, but it is limited in its power for prescription (Rickleman, 1971). The scope of the theory remains limited to individuals who are conscious in a hospital setting, who are basically motivated to participate in their own care, who are inconsistent (in a state of disharmony with their surroundings, situation, or expectations) (Wiedenbach, 1965), and who are able to perceive their need for help. Patients who are consistent (do not deviate from normalcy), who are noncompliant, and who do not perceive a need for help are not nursing clients. Therefore, its use in practice is limited.

Administration literature in nursing may be considered an extension of Wiedenbach's theory; however, deliberate action, perceptual clarification, and validation could be claimed by any effective and efficient organizational theory.

External Components of Theory

The external components of Wiedenbach's theory are the same as those for Orlando's theory.

THEORY TESTING

As with Orlando's theory and perhaps in combination with it, numerous research studies were launched to test the what and how of a deliberative process and validation of interaction in assessing and intervening with patients in need of help. A review of the research and publications based on Wiedenbach's theory revealed two findings: first, both Orlando and Wiedenbach are cited in most research related to concepts of either theories, and second, Wiedenbach's ideas are still appearing in the literature as researchers continue to test propositions emanating from theory.

One type of research using Wiedenbach's theory focused more on the prescriptive propositions of effect of deliberate nursing process (validation) on several patient outcomes. Such research was hospital-oriented (preoperative preparation, admission procedures, obstetrical preparation, and patients in need of pain relief). (See discussion under Orlando.) Experimental groups usually received care that included identification of patient's needs focused on verbal and nonverbal behavior (Shields, 1978); nurses' perceptions compared and contrasted with patients' perceptions; and actions to provide help to restore the patient's functional ability based on a continuous process of validation.

On the other hand, nonexperimental care given to the control group was personal, automatic, technique-oriented, organizationally focused, and more authoritarian or friendly, but not deliberate and goal-oriented. Patient outcomes generally were significantly better in the first than in the second group. Outcomes considered included physiological measures, such as emesis during postoperative or postdelivery recovery, and degree of change in heart and respiration. Other outcomes were psychological and included subjective patient reports of alleviation of distress (Elms and Leonard, 1966; Leonard, Skipper and Woolridge, 1967; Wolfer and Visintainer, 1975).

Other research was related to the exploration of an implicit assumption that the client is truthful in validating the nurse's perception of his condition. Eisler, Wolfer, and Diers (1972) found that a slight correlation existed between social approval needs of patients (but not the patients' inner experience) and their reports of physical well-being, thereby casting doubt on previously unchallenged assumptions that validation indeed gets at patients' true perceptions of the situation.

Numerous other research reports could be related to the theory, providing further validation or invalidation of its concepts. For example, Larson (1977) found that a client's socioeconomic status and social desirability of the diagnosis affected the nurse's perceptions of the patient's characteristics. The "should" advice in Wiedenbach's theory is therefore expanded to include the "realities" of the nurse–patient situation. There is no indication that Wiedenbach made any substantial changes in her conceptualization based on the results of these research studies. A set of propositions for using change as an outcome variable is presented in Table 15-20.

REFERENCES

King

Asay, M.K. and Ossler, C.C. (Eds.) (1984) Conceptual models of nursing. Applications in community health nursing. Proceedings of the Eighth Annual Community Health Nursing Conference. Chapel Hill, NC: Department of Public Health Nursing, School of Public Health, University of North Carolina.

Austin, J.K. and Champion, V.L. (1983) King's theory for nursing: Explication and evaluation. In P. Chinn (Ed.), *Advances in nursing theory development*. Germantown, MD: Aspen.

Brower, H.T. (1981) Social organization and nurses' attitudes toward older persons. *Journal of Gerontological Nursing*, 7, 293–298.

Brown, S.T. and Lee, B.T. (1980) Imogene King's conceptual framework: A proposed model for continuing nursing education. *Journal of Advanced Nursing*, 5(5), 467–473.

Bunting, S. (1988) The concept of perception in selected nursing theories. *Nursing Science Quarterly*, 1(4), 168–174.

Daubenmire, M.J. and King, I.M. (1973) Nursing process models: A systems approach. *Nursing Outlook*, 2(8), 512–517.

Elberson, K. (1989) Applying King's model to nursing administration. In B. Henry, C. Arndt, M. Di Vincenti, and A. Marriner-Tomey (Eds.), *Dimensions of nursing administration*. London: Blackwell Scientific Publications.

Fawcett, J. (1989) *Analysis and evaluation of conceptual models of nursing* (2nd ed.). Philadelphia: F.A. Davis.

Frey, M. (1989) Social support and health: A theoretical formulation derived from King's conceptual framework. *Nursing Science Quarterly*, 2(3), 138–148.

George, J.B. (1980) Imogene King. In The Nursing Theories Conference Group, *Nursing theories: The base for professional nursing practice*. Englewood Cliffs, NJ: Prentice-Hall.

Gonot, P.J. (1983) Imogene M. King: A theory for nursing. In J.J. Fitzpatrick and A.L. Whall (Eds.), *Conceptual models of nursing: Analysis and application*. Bowie, MD: Brady.

Gonot, P.J. (1986) Family therapy as derived from King's conceptual model. In A.L. Whall (Ed.), *Family therapy for nursing: Four approaches*. Norwalk, CT: Appleton-Century-Crofts.

Gulitz, E.A. and King, I.M. (1988). King's general systems model: Application to curriculum development. *Nursing Science Quarterly*, 1(3), 128–132.

Husband, A. (1988) Application of King's theory of nursing to the care of the adult with diabetes. *Journal of Advanced Nursing*, 13, 484–488.

King, I.M. (1964, October) Nursing theory: Problems and prospects. *Nursing Science*, 2, 394–403.

King, I.M. (1968) A conceptual frame of reference for nursing. *Nursing Research*, 17(1), 27–31.

King, I.M. (1971) *Toward a theory for nursing*. New York: John Wiley & Sons.

King, I.M. (1975) A process for developing concepts for nursing through research. In P.J. Verhonick (Ed.), *Nursing Research* (Vol. 1). Boston: Little, Brown & Co.

King, I.M. (1976) The health care system: Nursing intervention subsystem. In W.H. Werley, et al. (Eds.), *Health research: The systems approach*. New York: Springer-Verlag.

King, I.M. (1978) USA: Loyola University of Chicago, School of Nursing. *Journal of Advanced Nursing*, 3, 390.

King, I.M. (1981) *A theory for nursing: Systems, concepts, process.* New York: John Wiley & Sons.

King, I.M. (1983a) The family coping with a medical illness. Analysis and application of King's theory of goal attainment. In I.W. Clements and F.B. Roberts (Eds.), *Family health: A theoretical approach to nursing.* New York: John Wiley & Sons.

King, I.M. (1983b) King's theory of nursing. In I.W. Clements and F.B. Roberts (Eds.), *Family health: A theoretical approach to nursing.* New York: John Wiley & Sons.

King, I.M. (1984) Effectiveness of nursing care: Use of a goal oriented nursing record in end stage renal disease. *American Association of Nephrology Nurses and Technicians Journal*, 11(2), 11–17, 60.

King, I.M. (1986a) King's theory of goal attainment. In P. Winstead-Fry (Ed.), *Case studies in nursing theory* (Chapter 7). New York: National League for Nursing.

King, I.M. (1986b) *Curriculum and instruction in nursing.* Norwalk, CT: Appleton-Century-Crofts.

King, I.M. (1987a) King's theory of goal attainment. In R. Parse (Ed.), *Nursing science: Major paradigms, theories, and critiques.* Philadelphia: W.B. Saunders.

King, I.M. (1987b) Translating research into practice. *Journal of Neuroscience Nursing*, 19(1), 44–48.

King, I.M. (1988) Concepts: Essential elements of theories. *Nursing Science Quarterly*, 1(1), 22–25.

King, I.M. (1989) King's systems framework for nursing administration. In B. Henry, C. Arndt, M. Di Vincenti, and A. Marriner-Tomey (Eds.), *Dimensions of nursing administration.* London: Blackwell Scientific Publications.

Magan, S. (1987) A critique of King's theory. In R. Parse (Ed.), *Nursing science: Major paradigms, theories, and critiques.* Philadelphia: W.B. Saunders.

Meleis, A.I. and Jones, A. (1983) Ethical crises and cultural differences. *Western Journal of Medicine*, 138(6), 889–893.

Roake, L. and Norberg, A. (1988) Problematic and meaningful situations in nursing interpreted by concepts from King's nursing theory and four additional concepts. *Scandinavian Journal of Caring Sciences*, 2(2), 80–87.

Rosendahl, P.B. and Ross, V. (1982) Does your behavior affect your patient's response? *Journal of Gerontological Nursing*, 8, 572–575.

Smith, M.C. (1988) King's theory in practice. *Nursing Science Quarterly*, 1(4), 145–146.

Stevens, B.J. (1984) *Nursing theory: Analysis, application, and evaluation* (2nd ed.). Boston: Little, Brown & Co.

Uys, L.R. (1987) Foundational studies in nursing. *Journal of Advanced Nursing*, 12(3), 275–280.

Weed, L.L. (1969) *Medical records, medical education, and patient care.* Cleveland: Case Western Reserve University Press.

Zetterberg, H.L. (1963) *On theory and verification in sociology*, rev'd ed. Totowa, NJ: Bedminster Press.

Orlando

Andrews, C.M. (1983) Ida Orlando's model for nursing. In J. Fitzpatrick and A. Whall (Eds.), *Conceptual models of nursing: Analysis and application.* Bowie, MD: Robert J. Brady Company.

Barron, M.A. (1966) The effects varied nursing approaches have on patients' complaints of pain (Abstract). *Nursing Research*, 15(1), 90–91.

Bochnak, M.A. (1963) The effect of an automatic and deliberative process of nursing activity on the relief of patients' pain: A clinical experiment. *Nursing Research*, 12(3), 191–192.

Cameron, J. (1963) An exploratory study of the verbal responses of the nurse–patient interactions. *Nursing Research*, 12(3), 192.

Crane, M.D. (1980) Ida Jean Orlando: In Nursing Theories Conference Group, *Nursing theories: The base for professional nursing practice*. Englewood Cliffs, NJ: Prentice-Hall.

Diers, D.K. (1966) The nurse orientation system: A method for analyzing the nurse–patient interactions (Abstract). *Nursing Research*, 15(1), 91.

Diers, D. (1970) Faculty research development at Yale. *Nursing Research*, 19(1), 64–71.

Dracup, K.A. and Breu, C.S. (1978) Using nursing research findings to meet the needs of grieving spouses. *Nursing Research*, 27(4), 212.

Dumas, R.G. and Leonard, R.C. (1963) The effect of nursing on the incidence of postoperative vomiting. *Nursing Research*, 12(1), 12–15.

Eisler, J., Wolfer, J., and Diers, D. (1972) Relationship between the need for social approval and postoperative recovery and welfare. *Nursing Research*, 21(5), 520–525.

Elms, R.R. and Leonard, R.C. (1966) The effects of nursing approaches during admission. *Nursing Research*, 15(1), 39–48.

Gilliss, L. (1976) Sleeplessness: Can you help? *The Canadian Nurse*, 72(7), 32–34.

Gowan, N.I. and Morris, M. (1964) Nurses' responses to expressed patient needs. *Nursing Research*, 13(1), 68–71.

Hage, J. (1972) *Techniques and problems of theory construction in sociology*. New York: John Wiley & Sons.

Haggerty, L.A. (1987) An analysis of senior nursing students' immediate responses to distressed patients. *Journal of Advanced Nursing*, 12, 451–461.

Hampe, S.O. (1975) Needs of grieving spouses in a hospital setting. *Nursing Research*, 24(2), 113.

Lipson, J. and Meleis, A.I. (1983, December) Issues in health care of Middle-Eastern patients. *The Western Journal of Medicine*, 139, 854–861.

Marriner-Tomey, A., Mills, D., and Sauter, M. (1989) Ida Jean Orlando (Pelletier): Nursing process theory. In A. Marriner-Tomey (Ed.), *Nursing theorists and their work*. St. Louis: C.V. Mosby.

Mertz, H. (1962) Nurse actions that reduce stress in patients. In *Emergency intervention by the nurse* (Monograph 1, pp. 10–14). New York: American Nurses' Association.

Orlando, I.J. (1961) *The dynamic nurse–patient relationship*. New York: G.P. Putnam's Sons.

Orlando, I.J. (1972) *The discipline and teaching of nursing process*. New York: G.P. Putnam's Sons.

Peplau, H.E. (1952) *Interpersonal relations in nursing*. New York: G.P. Putnam's Sons.

Pienschke, D. (1973) Guardedness or openness on the cancer unit. *Nursing Research*, 22(6), 484–490.

Rhymes, J. (1964) A description of nurse–patient interaction in effective nursing activity. *Nursing Research*, 13(4), 365.

Schmieding, N.J. (1983) An analysis of Orlando's theory based on Kuhn's theory of science. In P.L. Chinn (Ed.), *Advances in nursing theory development*. Rockville, MD: Aspen Systems.

Schmieding, N.J. (1986) Orlando's theory. In P. Winstead-Fry (Ed.), *Case studies in nursing theory*. New York: National League for Nursing.

Schmieding, N.J. (1987) Problematic situations in nursing: Analysis of Orlando's theory based on Dewey's theory of inquiry. *Journal of Advanced Nursing*, 12, 431–440.

Schmieding, N.J. (1988) Action process of nurse administrators to problematic situations based on Orlando's theory. *Journal of Advanced Nursing*, 13, 99–107.

Stevens, B.J. (1984) *Nursing theory: Analysis, application, and evaluation.* Boston: Little, Brown & Co.

Tryon, P.A. (1963) An experiment of the effect of patients' participation in planning the administration of a nursing procedure. *Nursing Research*, 12(4), 262–265.

Tryon, P.A. and Leonard, R.C. (1964) The effect of patients' participation on the outcome of a nursing procedure. *Nursing Forum*, 3(2), 79–89.

Williamson, Y. (1978) Methodologic dilemmas in tapping the concept of patient needs. *Nursing Research*, 27(3), 172.

Wolfer, J.A. and Visintainer, M.A. (1975) Pediatric surgical patients' and parents' stress responses and adjustment. *Nursing Research*, 24(4), 244–255.

Paterson and Zderad

Donaldson, S.K. (1983) Let us not abandon the humanities. *Nursing Outlook*, 31(1), 40–43.

Kleiman, S. (1986) Humanistic nursing: The phenomenological theory of Paterson and Zderad. In P. Winstead-Fry (Ed.), *Case studies in nursing theory.* New York: National League for Nursing.

McKeon, R. (undated) Philosophic semantics and philosophy inquiry. Cited in B.J. Stevens (1984), *Nursing theory: Analysis, application, and evaluation* (p. 51). Boston: Little, Brown & Co.

Menke, E.M. (1978) Theory development: A challenge for nursing. In N.L. Chaska (Ed.), *The nursing profession: Views through the mist.* New York: McGraw-Hill.

Munhall, P.L. (1982) Nursing philosophy and nursing research: In apposition or opposition? *Nursing Research*, 31(3), 776–786.

Oiler, C. (1982) The phenomenological approach in nursing research. *Nursing Research*, 31(3), 178–181.

Paterson, J.G. (1971) From a philosophy of clinical nursing to a method of nursology. *Nursing Research*, 20(2), 143–146.

Paterson, J.G. and Zderad, L.T. (1970–1971) All together through complementary syntheses are the worlds of the many. *Image* 4(3), 13–16.

Paterson, J.G. (1978) The tortuous way toward nursing theory. In *Theory development: What, why, how?* (NLN Publ. No. 15–1708, pp. 49–65.) New York: National League for Nursing.

Paterson, J.G. and Zderad, L.T. (1976) *Humanistic nursing.* New York: John Wiley & Sons.

Paterson, J.G. and Zderad, L.T. (1988) *Humanistic nursing* (2nd ed.). New York: National League of Nursing.

Stern, P.N. (1980) Grounded theory methodology: Its uses and processes. *Image*, 12, 20–23.

Stevens, B.J. (1984) *Nursing theory: Analysis, application, and evaluation.* Boston: Little, Brown & Co.

Wilson, H.S. (1977) Limiting intrusion: Social control of outsiders in a healing community. *Nursing Research*, 26(2), 103–111.

Zderad, L.T. (1968) A concept of empathy. Doctoral dissertation, Georgetown University.

Zderad, L.T. (1969) Empathetic nursing: Realization of a human capacity. *Nursing Clinics of North America*, 4, 655–662.

Zderad, L.T. (1970) Empathy: From cliche to construct. *Proceedings of the Third Nursing Theory Conference.* Lawrence, KS: University of Kansas Medical Center Department of Nursing.

Zderad, L.T. (1978) From here and now to theory: Reflections on "how." In *Theory development: What, why, how?* (NLN Publ. No. 15–1708, pp. 35–48.) New York: National League for Nursing.

Travelbee

Barrett-Leonard, G.T. (1962) Dimensions of therapist responses as causal factors in therapeutic change. *Psychological Monographs,* 76(43, Whole No. 562).

Cartwright, R.D. and Lerner, B. (1963) Empathy, need to change, and improvement with psychotherapy. *Journal of Consulting Psychology,* 27, 138–144.

Chin, R. (1974) The utility of system models and developmental models for practitioners. In J. Riehl and C. Roy (Eds.), *Conceptual models in nursing practice.* New York: Appleton-Century-Crofts.

Chinsky, J.M. and Rappaport, J. (1970) Brief critique of the meaning and reliability of "accurate empathy" ratings. *Psychological Bulletin,* 73, 379–382.

Cook, L. (1989) Nurses in crisis: A support group based on Travelbee's nursing theory. *Nursing and health care,* 10(4), 203–205.

Doona, M.E. (1979) *Travelbee's intervention in psychiatric nursing* (2nd ed.). Philadelphia: F.A. Davis.

Duffey, M. and Muhlenkamp, A.F. (1974) A framework for theory analysis. *Nursing Outlook,* 22(9), 570–574.

Frankel, V. (1963) *Man's search for meaning: An introduction to logotherapy.* New York: Washington Square Press.

Freihofer, P. and Felton, G. (1976) Nursing behaviors in bereavement: An exploratory study. *Nursing Research,* 25(5), 332–337.

Kurtz, R.R. and Grummon, D.L. (1972) Different approaches to the measurement of therapist empathy and their relationship to therapy outcomes. *Journal of Consulting and Clinical Psychology,* 30, 106–115.

May, R. (1953) *Man's search for himself.* New York: W.W. Norton.

McBride, M.A. (1967) Nursing approach, pain, and relief: An exploratory experiment. *Nursing Research,* 16(4), 337–341.

Sarlore, J.P. (1966) Existentialism. In W.V. Spanos (Ed.), *A casebook on existentialism.* New York: Thomas V. Crowell.

Sloane, A. (1966) Review of "Interpersonal aspects of nursing" by J. Travelbee. *American Journal of Nursing,* 66(6), 77.

Stetler, C. (1977) Relationship of perceived empathy of nurses' communication. *Nursing Research,* 26(6), 432–438.

Travelbee, J. (1963) What do we mean by rapport? *American Journal of Nursing,* 63(2), 70–72.

Travelbee, J. (1964) What's wrong with sympathy? *American Journal of Nursing,* 64(1), 68–71.

Travelbee, J. (1966) *Interpersonal aspects of nursing.* Philadelphia: F.A. Davis.

Travelbee, J. (1969) *Intervention in psychiatric nursing.* Philadelphia: F.A. Davis.

Travelbee, J. (1970) Personal communication.

Travelbee, J. (1971) *Interpersonal aspects of nursing* (2nd ed.). Philadelphia: F.A. Davis.

Truax, C. and Carkhuff, R.R. (1967) *Toward effective counseling and psychotherapy.* Chicago: Aldine.

Wolff, I.S. (1966) Review of "Interpersonal aspects of nursing" by J. Travelbee. *Am J Nurs*, 66(7), 1504–1506.

Wiedenbach

Bennett, A.M. and Foster, P.C. (1980) Ernestine Wiedenbach. In The Nursing Theories Conference Group, *Nursing theories: The base for professional nursing practice.* Englewood Cliffs, NJ: Prentice-Hall.

Eisler, J., Wolfer, J.A., and Diers, D. (1972) Relationship between the need for social approval and postoperative recovery welfare. *Nursing Research*, 21(5), 520–525.

Elms, R.R. and Leonard, R.C. (1966) Effects of nursing approaches during admission. *Nursing Research*, 15(1), 37–48.

Larson, P.A. (1977) Nurse perception of client illness. *Nursing Research*, 26(6), 416–421.

Leonard, R.C., Skipper, J.K., and Woolridge, P.J. (1967) Small sample field experiments for evaluating patient care. *Health Services Research*, 2(1), 47–50.

Rickleman, B.L. (1971) Bio-psycho-social linguistics: A conceptual approach to nurse–patient interaction. *Nursing Research*, 20(5), 398–403.

Shields, D. (1978) Nursing care in labor and patient satisfaction. A descriptive study. *Journal of Advances in Nursing*, 3, 535–550.

Wiedenbach, E. (1963) The helping art of nursing. *American Journal of Nursing*, 63(11), 54–57.

Wiedenbach, E. (1964) *Clinical nursing: A helping art.* New York: Springer-Verlag.

Wiedenbach, E. (1965) Family nurse practitioner for maternal and child care. *Nursing Outlook*, 13, 50–52.

Wiedenbach, E. (1968) Nurse's role in family planning: A conceptual base for practice. *Nursing Clinics of North America*, 3(2), 355–365.

Wiedenbach, E. (1969) *Meeting the realities in clinical teaching.* New York: Springer–Verlag.

Wiedenbach, E. (1970a) Comment on beliefs and values: Basis for curriculum design. *Nursing Research*, 19(5), 427.

Wiedenbach, E. (1970b) Nurses' wisdom in nursing theory. *American Journal of Nursing*, 70(5), 1057–1062.

Wiedenbach, E. and Falls, C.E. (1978) *Communication: Key to effective nursing.* New York: Tiresias Press.

Wolfer, J. and Visintainer, M. (1975) Pediatric surgical patients' and parents' stress responses and adjustment. *Nursing Research*, 24(4), 244–255.

Chapter *16*

On Nursing Therapeutics

The nursing activities and actions that are deliberately designed for caring for patients, potential patients, or people at risk (or families or communities) are grouped under nursing therapeutics. Theorists have described and discussed nursing therapeutics with various degrees of emphasis. Two images emerge when the concept "nursing therapeutics" is considered. One is Levine's proposed actions for conservation of energy and the second is Orem's proposed strategies to enhance self-care. Others may be delineated from the writings of different theorists (see Chapter 12, Tables 12-6, 12-12, and 12-18). Levine's and Orem's theories are evaluated in this chapter.

Myra Levine

THEORY DESCRIPTION

The central questions that Levine addressed are: What are the ways in which nursing care is delivered? What are the goals of nursing actions? and Why are nursing actions provided? To answer these questions, Levine conceptualized the methods of nursing as conservation of patient resources, as alteration of environment to fit the resources, and as an extension of the patient's perceptual system until his own system is healed. These questions address nursing therapeutics and, to a lesser degree, a perspective on health.

The impetus for Levine's conceptualization of nursing appears to be her attempt to separate the domains of medicine and nursing. Her very first published work focused on proposing "trophicognosis" as a new label for nursing assessment and "plan of action to substitute the concept of nursing diagnosis" (Levinc, 1966a, p. 57). Her rationale for the proposal was her desire to differentiate between diagnoses that have the connotation of medical diagnosis and disease orientation; the medical diagnosis tends to address and highlight the overlap between medicine and nursing rather than highlight the differences.

Simply put, *trophicognosis* is defined as "a nursing care judgment arrived at by the scientific method" (Levine, 1966a, p. 57). It denotes the knowledge of the art of nursing and is analogous to diagnosis and prognosis for the art of medicine. Labeling nursing assessment as a nursing diagnosis is only giving medical diagnosis a new label, but when trophicognosis is used, it emphasizes nursing care judgment based on the process of scientific method. Levine offered, then, a useful beginning for the use of the nursing process. Although the new label was not used in nursing, Levine's attempts in 1965 (published in 1966a) supported what other theorists had begun doing: delineating nursing's focus and differentiating between nursing and medicine. However, Levine later admonished nurses to simplify their language and not to invent language that confuses other health care providers (1989a).

Levine then put her energy into conceptualizing a human being as an adaptive being, in constant interaction with the environment, whose behaviors are integrated wholes in response to internal and external environmental stimuli. Nurses are interested in integrated responses of whole patients to noxious stimuli, particularly when the individual is not able to adapt behavior to environmental demands. Nursing is expected to create an atmosphere (therefore environment was beginning to emerge here as a central phenomenon in nursing) to encourage healing and to promote adaptation (1966b). Although this is classified as a theory that focused on nursing therapeutics, and some have used it as a framework for diagnosis and intervention (Taylor, 1989), Levine provided a detailed description of environment. She described environment dimensions as internal and external. Responses of human beings emanate from the internal environment. Both the internal and external environments influence each other, and the internal environment is constantly challenged to meet the external environment's demands. Throughout these challenges and changes, the body maintains its integrity through some control mechanisms that lead to autoregulation of the internal environment (Levine, 1973).

The external environment is perceptual, operational, and conceptual. The *perceptual environment* is that component "which an individual responds to with sense organs" (Levine, 1973, p. 12). The *operational environment* includes all that affects an individual physically, such as microorganisms and pollutants. The *conceptual environment* includes symbols, values, culture, language, thinking, and personal styles, among others (Levine, 1973; 1989b). The interaction between the internal and the external environments is where a person's adaptation resides; it is where the fit between person and environment occurs (Levine, 1989b).

Levine (1973) identified nine models to guide assessment (the relationship between each major theory concept and every model is not entirely explicit):

1. Vital signs;
2. Body movement and positioning;
3. Ministration of personal hygiene needs;
4. Pressure gradient systems in nursing intervention (fluids);
5. Nursing determinants in provision for nutritional needs;
6. Pressure gradient system in nursing (gases);
7. Local application of heat and cold;

8. Administration of medication; and

9. Establishing an aseptic environment

Assessment would include organismic and environmental systems. The first allows for description of all physiological and biological adaptive integrative systems, such as response to fear (fight or flight), response to inflammation, and response to stress. The other systems of response are to the environment, which is more than one's immediate surroundings (Levine, 1969). It is the perceptual environment "depending on the ability of a person to receive sensory stimuli via his sense organs," the operational environment, including all those physical entities that do not need to be recorded by senses (radiation, microorganisms), and the conceptual environment "determined by the dependence of human beings on the symbolic exchange of language and ideas." It also includes cultural determinants (Levine, 1971a, p. 262).

The "holistic nursing challenge" is to nurse whole patients at the interface of organism and environment to promote adaptation. Adaptation could be accomplished through conservation. Conservation of energy is important to the disease process and begins with regulation of metabolism in response to noxious forces that have instigated the disease process. It does not only mean limitation of activity, it also means "proper disbursement of energy expense, allowing for activity within the range of the individual's capability, safety, and comfort" (Levine, 1971a, p. 259). Conservation of structural integrity is accomplished through tasks that support the physiological and anatomical positioning. Conservation of integrity is related to environmental processes. It includes conservation of personal integrity through preservation of sense of worth and integrity and conservation of social integrity through the recognition of cultural, ethnic, religious, and family relationships (Levine, 1967).

Maintenance of system integrity depends on perceptual systems (basic orienting, visual, auditory, hepatic, and taste and smell). When perceptual systems are deficient, the organismic responses are altered, and the nurse uses her perceptual system in an attempt to maintain wholeness in the individual. This is how healing can proceed (Levine, 1969).

Levine's conceptualization is based on numerous implicit and explicit assumptions that were dispersed throughout her writings between 1966 and 1989. They are presented in Table 16-1. Basic to her theory are her beliefs in wholeness of patients (not clients, because clients come from a Latin root that means a follower) (Levine, 1989c, p. 126). Patients are partners in the care process and nurses should help in developing a trusting dialogue.

All major concepts are derived from other paradigms except for the concepts of trophicognosis and conservation, which are primitive to this theory (Table 16-2). Both are theoretically defined; the first was also operationally defined, but because of its esoteric nature, nurses preferred "nursing diagnosis" over trophicognosis. The derived concepts are not operationally defined and have unclear boundaries. Concepts such as wholeness, social well-being, integrity, and adaptation are used interchangeably and are not well-differentiated (Table 16-3).

Table 16–1.
Assumptions—Levine

Implicit Assumptions

○ The nurse creates an environment in which healing could occur (Levine, 1966a).
○ A human being is more than the sum of parts.
○ Human beings respond in a predictable way (1966a).
○ Human beings are unique in their responses (1966a).
○ Human beings know and appraise objects, conditions, and situations (1985).
○ Human beings sense, reflect, reason, and understand (1985).
○ Human beings' actions are self-determined even when emotional (1985).
○ Human beings are capable of prolonging reflection through such strategies as raising questions or redirecting attention.
○ Human beings make decisions through prioritizing courses of actions.
○ Human beings must be aware and able to contemplate objects, conditions, and situations in order to act purposively.
○ Human beings are agents who act deliberately to attain goals (1985, pp. 12–13).
○ Adaptive changes involve the whole individual (1967).
○ A human being has unity in his response to the environment. He responds in an integrated way (1966a).
○ Every person possesses a unique adaptive ability based on one's life experience, which creates a unique message (1967).
○ There is an order and continuity to life (1966a).
○ Change is not random.
○ A human being (as a whole) responds organismically in an everchanging manner (1967).
○ A theory of nursing must recognize the importance of detail of care for a single patient within an empiric framework that successfully describes the requirements of all patients (1966a).
○ A human being is a social animal.
○ A human being is in constant interaction with an everchanging society.
○ Change is inevitable in life (1973, p. 10).
○ Nursing meets existing and emerging demands of self-care and dependent care (1985).
○ Nursing is associated with conditions of regulation of exercise or development of capabilities of providing care (1985).

Levine's theory offers existence propositions that are based on conceptualizing assessment of levels of responses, internal and external environments, and focus of nursing as conservation of energy and integrity through therapy or support. It offers concepts that appear on the surface to be linked together; however, relationships between each set of these concepts are not clear (*e.g.*, well-being and adaptation, conservation and responses). Therefore, as it stands now, this is a theory with existence propositions and no relational ones. Levine's propositions are summarized in Table 16-4.

Table 16–2.
Concepts—Levine

Wholeness	Intervention
Holism	Supportive
Noxious stimuli	Therapeutic
Organismic response	Perceptual systems
Fight or flight	Basic orienting
Inflammatory response	Visual
Stress	Auditory
Perceptual awareness	Hepatic
Homeostasis	Taste, smell
Homeorhesis	Environment
Adaptation	Perceptual
Equilibrium	Operational
Environmental exchange	Conceptual
Orderly synchronization = Health	Perceptual systems
Desynchronization = Disease	Basic orienting
Conservation	Anatomical
Energy	Visual
Integrity	Dynamic exchange
Structural	Trophicognosis
Personal	
Social	

Table 16–3.
Definition of Domain Concepts—Levine

Nursing	Has a unique body of knowledge and is a human interaction. Its goal is to conserve energies and integrities through changes in the environment.
Goal of nursing	Restoration of individual's wholeness, integrity, well-being, and independent activity. Conservation of energy, social, personal, and structural (Levine, 1967). When necessary, maintenance of appropriate balance between patient abilities, involvement in the care, and nurses' actions. Maintenance of individuality.
Health	"Health and illness are patterns of adaptive change" (1966a, p. 2452). Is equated with successful adaptation; in fact, one criterion of successful adaptation is the attainment of social well-being (1966a, p. 2452).
Environment	Is both internal and external. It is a setting, a background, and the dynamic exchange that involves both the individual organism and the setting and background. Environment is perceptual, operational, and conceptual. Perceptual environment is based on

(continued)

Table 16–3. (Continued)

	a person's sense organs' interpretation. Operational environment includes the things that affect an individual physically, such as virus, and the conceptual environment evolves out of an individual's cultural patterns, values, and spirituality and is mediated by symbols of language and thought (1969, p. 94; 1973, p. 12).
Person	An everchanging organism who is in constant interaction with his environment and who is constantly striving to maintain his integrity. Responses of a human being are a unified whole.
Nursing client	A total, whole person, a system of systems, in a state of dyssynchronization and in need of assistance to conserve energy, structural, personal, and social integrity (1969; 1973) An ill client maintains his integrity through four levels of physiologically predetermined protective responses. These are fear, inflammatory process, stress, and perceptual awareness as mediated through sense organs.
Nursing problem	The internal or external environment as it threatens the total integrity of a whole person. Organism responses to threat coexist in a single individual: 1) Response to fear by fight or flight, an instantaneous reaction, a most primitive reaction; 2) Inflammatory response, a second-level response, a response of entire resources of an individual, a systematized energy directed as exclusion and removal of intruding irritant or pathogen; 3) Response to stress produces defensive response in the form of changes that are nonspecific in a human being. Structural changes and gradual loss of adaptation energy occurs, until exhaustion is reached; 4) Sensory response producing perceptual awareness, the information and experience in life are only meaningful when perceived in an integrated whole by the individual. All are energy exchange transmissions from individual to environment and back. The result is a physiological or behavioral activity.
Nursing process	Assessment, diagnosis, and intervention, using steps of the scientific method, with great emphasis on observation as a central tool (1973, pp. 23–29).
Nurse–patient relations	"Depend on perceptual system of both persons" (1969, p. 97). The nursing process and action are for conservation.
Nursing therapeutics	The nurse acts in a therapeutic way when the intervention changes the course of adaptation toward a renewed social well-being. The nurse acts in a supportive way when the intervention maintains or fails to maintain the status quo and when there is no alteration in the course of adaptation (1966; 1967). Focus is on creating an atmosphere where healing could occur; therefore, the target is the environment. Based on appreciation of the patient's responses. To conserve patient's resources, alter the environment to fit the resources and act as the patient's perceptual system when his own is impaired.

(*continued*)

Table 16–3. (Continued)

Adaptation	The process of change whereby the individual retains his integrity, his wholeness within the realities of his environment (1969, p. 95).
Focus of nursing	Organism responses that are singular but integrated, maintenance of wholeness. Nurse–patient interaction.
Consequences	Adaptation process of change within which an individual maintains his integrity and his wholeness.
Illness	Dyssynchronization with outer events Loss of a portion of well-being Loss of wholeness; "Health and illness are patterns of adaptive response (Levine, 1966a, p. 2452)."

Although Levine described the conservation principles in what may be construed as assumptions, her principles could formulate the major propositions. She proposed that the goal and the process of nursing action is the conservation of energy and integrity. Such propositions are supported by assumptions emanating from other paradigms about the significance of energy and integrity for a human being.

Levine in a personal communication (cited in Fawcett, 1989, p. 157) provided further support for the classification of her theory as a theory for nursing therapeutics. She proposed a theory she called "therapeutic intervention" in which she described seven areas of therapeutic interventions that are still in the process of being developed. These are therapeutic regimens to support the healing process of the body, to substitute for failure of autoregulation, to focus on restoring integrity and well-being of individuals, to promote comfort and human concern, to decrease the threat of disease, to create functional changes, and to correct metabolic imbalances.

Table 16–4.
Propositions—Levine

Awareness of an environment influenced behavior at all times.

Conservation of patients' energy is a consequence of nursing intervention.

Components of nursing interventions are conservation of individual patient's structural integrity, personal integrity, and social integrity.

Nurses are participants in every patient's environment and influence patient's adaptation.

THEORY ANALYSIS

The Theorist

Myra Levine is a graduate of the Cook County diploma program, and she has a non-nursing bachelor degree from the University of Chicago and a master of science in nursing from Wayne State University, Detroit. She is currently retired and a professor emeritus in the medical-surgical nursing graduate program at the University of Illinois, Chicago, where she taught and collaborated in teaching the theory seminars. Her writings evolved while she was a predoctoral and postgraduate student at the University of Chicago. She has an extensive clinical (private duty nurse, staff nurse), administrative (director of nursing), and teaching background (preclinical instructor in Cook County; a faculty member at Loyola University, at Rush University, and at the University of Illinois) (Esposito and Leonard, 1980).

Paradigmatic Origins

In introducing holism in the mid-1960s, Levine was quite critical of the scientific approach that advocated experimentation, deductive thinking, and analysis of experiences that only led to more mechanistic and dualistic approaches to patient care. The ultimate result was compartmentalization of human beings. She recommended an inductive approach that evolved from experience and clinical practice and incorporated the wisdom of the person. To her, there was a paradox between holism and humanism on the one hand and dualism and scientific thought on the other hand. Despite these admonitions, Levine used a deductive approach to develop her theory and recommended the scientific method for collecting data about nursing care.

Levine's clinical background in medical-surgical nursing and the close association of this background with medical, biological, and pathophysiological sciences have influenced the development of her theory. The theory draws on concepts and assumptions from systems theory (Bertalanffy, 1968), adaptation theories (Dubos, 1966; Selye, 1956; and Cannon, 1939), developmental theory (surprisingly, Erik Erikson (1968) was cited for the definition of wholeness, totality, and system [Levine, 1969, p. 94]), existentialism (Buber, 1967; Tillich, 1961), and nursing theorists (Nightingale, 1969; Rogers, 1961; Abdellah and Levine, 1986).

Levine also drew her ideas from several concepts that, in her view, had a major impact on nursing. These are the natural healing concept, the germ theory, theory of multiple factors, and the unified theory of health and disease. Although she promoted the scientific method for nursing in both the development of nursing science (Levine, 1966b) and in the development of nursing process (Levine, 1966a), she encouraged us to consider life processes holistically by transcending the duality of mind and body. She also warned against the apparent dissociation between environment and individual as evidenced in the nature/nurture arguments. Cause-and-effect mechanistic views are dehumanizing and antiholistic. Organism responses, purposeful life, integrative approach, and adaptation are concepts that guided her view of nursing. She advocated a return to nursing as it used to be.

Nursing has always been characterized by an intensely humanistic purpose, an expression at once of the selfless giving, selfish rewards that accompany human interaction. (Levine, 1971a, p. 263)

It is, after all, in the role of patient advocate that the nurse has historically fulfilled her responsibility to bring compassion, protection, and commitment to the bedside. (Levine, 1971b, p. 43)

Internal Dimensions

Levine's is a concatenated theory developed around concepts of adaptation, conservation, responses, and environment and therefore has an appropriate set of existence propositions. It is a microtheory with limited scope, addressing conservation of energy and integrity. It evolved deductively out of hypothetical beginnings, a view of what nursing ought to be. It is a descriptive theory that attempts to describe strategies of nursing care and of the nursing client. It addresses mainly phenomena of disorder, fight or flight, stress responses, inflammation responses, and perceptual awareness responses.

Levine used a problematic method approach in her theory (Barnum, 1990, pp. 48–51). Responses of people are holistic but are differentiated into four different problems; conservation is offered separately in four different types. Whereas a person is not reduced to components, responses are limited to four problematic responses. Nurses' actions are limited to conservation. It could be argued, therefore, that there is a certain element of reductionism in Levine's theory.

THEORY CRITIQUE

Levine developed her notions in the mid-1960s when nurses were struggling with increasing mechanization, when they were beset with fragmentation due to specialization, and when they were trying to differentiate between different types of nursing and also between nursing and medicine. She began by differentiating between medical and nursing judgment, by offering trophicognosis to replace nursing diagnosis. She saw the process of clinical judgment—the nursing process —as a means of focusing on nursing issues in patient care. Holism and humanism, person–environment interactions, are abstract concepts attached to the nursing act and not clearly defined, but Levine was among the first to redraw our attention to them. The essence of the nursing act is conservation. It is what all human beings strive for and, when not able to adapt to noxious stimuli, the nurse becomes their conservator.

Fortunately, or unfortunately, the theory drew heavily from pathophysiology and was therefore perceived as a theory oriented to acute care of ill individuals. However, Hirschfeld (1976) discussed the cognitively impaired older adult and demonstrated how Levine's four principles of conservation could be applied to give direction to nursing interventions when impairments are present. This appears to be the only published indication of Levine's utility in the practice arena, and it does provide support for the notion that the theory can be clinically utilized.

Levine is inconsistent in her use of holism, humanism, and integrative approaches to understanding response and in nursing care. The inconsistency arises from the view of human beings through a pathophysiological approach and reduction of responses to those responses that are biologically bound. The inclusion of perceptual awareness amidst the focus on biological responses to fear, stress, and inflammation almost seems an additive thought and not an integrative one. The major concepts of the theory adaptation and energy are not well-defined.

The complexity of the theory is perhaps due to the lack of clarity and disconnectedness of its concepts. It is a teleological theory, adding to the lack of clarity of the boundaries of the concepts (Levine, 1971a, p. 258). Conservation is a goal and an intervention process in different parts of the theory, but an organismic and environmental response overlap when Levine discusses perceptual awareness. It could be argued that three responses—fear, stress, and inflammation—are simply syndromes in response to stress as defined by Selye. Complete definitions and development of propositions connecting responses, environment, and conservation would render this theory testable.

There are other functional limitations in the theory that may have deterred others from using it. Holistic nursing appears to be limited to integrating social and personal aspects of care in acute care individuals who are dependent on the health care professional. It does not lend itself readily without extensive interpretation to long-term care and care of families or communities. The theory offers guidelines for assessment of responses and environment and guidelines for goals of nursing therapeutics, but it is limited in conceptualizing the means by which the nurse can achieve these goals. The theory does not lend itself readily to preventive and health promotion care, but the potential for extensions exists.

Some have used the theory in curricula development for educational settings. (Hall, 1979; Riehl, 1980). Others have used it in administration settings as a framework for identification of outcome criteria for nursing care of patients on a neurology unit (Taylor, 1974). Taylor's account of her use also substantiates the utility of the theory for the use of the nursing process in assessment and diagnosis.

As evidenced previously, the circle of contagiousness of the theory is limited. The use of theory for research, education, and administration has suffered from the problematic approach in articulating the theory, the lack of interpretation of holistic and total human being, the limited operationalization of integrative responses, the overlap between concepts (*e.g.*, personal and social integrity), and, most of all, the theory's lack of propositions. That is not to say that the potential is not there; it only means that the existing literature by Levine focuses on assumptions, concepts, and definitions. Each of the conservation principles lends itself to existence propositions and each of the nine descriptive models can generate research questions.

External Components of Theory

The theory is congruent with general professional and societal views of health and patient care. Levine espoused holistic care before holism became an accepted lexicon in both nursing and societal language. The total individual has a parallel in

Rogers' unitary human being (1970). Two other of Levine's ideas are widely accepted now in nursing thought: the focus of nursing on life processes and the significance of the environment (Donaldson and Crowley, 1978; Flaskerud and Halloran, 1980).

To use an individual's natural resources, to conserve energy, and to preserve the integrity of the individual are values of the future. Their social significance would make the theory appealing to the general public, but the challenge remains. How do we achieve these goals of nursing care? What are the outcome criteria by which we nurses know when we have and when we have not achieved these goals? Are they or are they not cost-effective in prevention and intervention?

While nursing is attempting to devise ways to measure energy and study unitary human beings and the meaning of healing, Levine demonstrates inconsistencies in ideas and displayed impatience with the lack of use of scientific data in studying therapeutic touch. In response to an article by Krieger, she wrote a scathing letter to the editor, admonishing nurses to stick to science in developing nursing (Levine, 1979). In this letter she warned:

> The professional implications of nurses engaging in "healing" based on the spurious notion that "excess of energy" in the human body can be transmitted to the "ill person who can be thought of as being in less than an optimal energy state" are frightening. The science is spurious, as is the explanation that this "appears to be done physiologically by a kind of electron transfer resonance." (p. 1379)

Levine charges that this type of thinking will take nursing on to a "hocus pocus" " faith healing" path and that nursing cannot afford to indulge in this kind of "charlatanism." (p. 1380).

Levine is an advocate of theoretical formulations that are based on coherence, but calls for corroboration of truth in nursing. She offered nursing in the mid-1960s a forward view of environment, holistic nursing, the total person, potential significance of perceptual apparatus in nursing, and nursing action as conservation.

THEORY TESTING

One research study tested a proposition that could be viewed as an extension of Levine's theory. The proposition states that mediation of stimuli through the perceptual system of the nurse could be enhanced if the nurse and the patient share the same subjective time. To explore this proposition, which is closely related to Levine's notion of hepatic perceptual system (which mediates touch, thought, muscles, joints, and skeletal system), Tompkins (1980) explored the effect of restricted mobility on perceived duration. She found that "decreased perceived duration . . . may be a mechanism for preserving system integrity in those whose mobility is restricted" (p. 333). This is the only published study that has tested the relationship between system integrity and perceptual systems.

Hirschfeld (1976) applied Levine's theory to the care of the cognitively impaired elderly patients and found the theory useful in determining priorities. Newport (1984) used Levine's theory as a framework for a study designed to contrast temperatures of newborns who were put in warmers with those who were placed in a skin-to-skin contact with mothers. Other research could evolve from the propositions described earlier in Table 16-4.

Dorothea Orem

THEORY DESCRIPTION

Orem's theory has been one of the most discussed and utilized theories in nursing. The impetus of Orem's ideas, as is the case for a number of other theorists, was to define content for nursing curricula. The seeds of her theory were first published in 1959 in a guide for developing a curriculum for practical nurses (Orem, 1959). As a member of a curriculum subcommittee at Catholic University (1965–1968), Orem recognized that work needed to continue in developing a conceptualization of nursing. Five of the subcommittee members continued to work with another six colleagues for about a decade (1968–1979) to formalize a theory of the process of nursing. In the process, Orem published the first formal articulation of her ideas (1971), and the group articulated the process of nursing theory development and identified universal elements in nursing that are congruent with Orem (Nursing Development Conference Group, 1973, 1979). The second edition of her book appeared in 1980, when she refined and extended the theory that appeared in the first edition.

Orem proposed three theories that are interrelated and have come to be considered as one by many of the utilizers. Central to all three theories is that people function and maintain life, health, and well-being by caring for themselves. The first theory, "self-care deficits," is the most comprehensive and is the core of her ideas. It is a conceptual image of the recipients of care as people who are incapable of continuous self-care or independent care due to health-related or health-derived limitations (Orem, 1985, p. 34). The second theory, "theory of self-care," is based on the central idea that a relationship exists between deliberate self-care actions and the development and functioning of individuals and groups. The third theory, "theory of nursing system(s)," describes therapeutic self-care requisites and the actions or systems involved in self-care.

The focus of the three theories is on *self-care*, defined as "the practice of activities that individuals initiate and perform on their own behalf in maintaining life, health, and well-being" (Orem, 1985, p. 84). Self-care is not limited to a person providing care for himself; it includes care offered by others on behalf of the person. Care may be offered by members of the family or outsiders until a person is able to perform self-care. Self-care is purposeful and contributes to human structural integrity, functioning, and development (Orem, 1985, p. 86). The purposes to be attained are universal, developmental, and health-deviation self-care requisites (see Table 16-5).

The focus of nursing is on the identification of self-care requisites, the designing of methods and actions to meet the requisites, and "the totality of the demands for self-care action" (Orem, 1985, p. 88).

Table 16–5.
Self-Care Requisites—Orem

Universal Self-Care Requisites

○ The maintenance of a sufficient intake of air
○ The maintenance of a sufficient intake of water
○ The maintenance of a sufficient intake of food
○ The provision of care associated with elimination processes and excrements
○ The maintenance of a balance between activity and rest
○ The maintenance of a balance between solitude and social interaction
○ The prevention of hazards to human life, human functioning, and human well-being
○ The promotion of human functioning and development within social groups in accord with human potential, known human limitations, and the human desire to be normal (Orem, 1985, pp. 90–91)

Developmental Self-Care Requisites

○ The bringing about and maintenance of living conditions that support life processes and promote the processes of development; that is, human progress toward higher levels of the organization of human structures and toward maturation
○ Provision of care either to prevent the occurrence of deleterious effects of conditions that can affect human development or so as to mitigate or overcome these effects from various conditions (1985, p. 96)

Health-Deviation Self-Care Requisites

○ Seeking and securing appropriate medical assistance in the event of exposure to specific physical or biological agents or environmental conditions associated with human pathological events and states, or when there is evidence of genetic, physiological, or psychological conditions known to produce or be associated with human pathology
○ Being aware of and attending to the effects and results of pathological conditions and states
○ Effectively carrying out medically prescribed diagnostic, therapeutic, and rehabilitative measures directed to the prevention of specific types of pathology, to the pathology itself, to the resolution of human integrated functioning, to the correction of deformities or abnormalities, or to compensation for disabilities
○ Being aware of and attending to or regulating the discomforting or deleterious effects of medical care measures performed or prescribed by the physician
○ Modifying the self-concept (and self-image) in accepting oneself as being in a particular state of health and in need of specific forms of health care
○ Learning to live with the effects of pathological conditions and states and the effects of medical diagnostic and treatment measures in a life-style that promotes continued personal development (1985, pp. 99–100)

The totality of self-care actions to be performed for some duration in order to meet human self-care requisites by using valid methods and related sets of operations or actions is termed the therapeutic self-care demand. (1985, p. 88)

The provider of self-care, whether self or other, is considered a *self-care agent*. It is an entity to be described in terms of development and operability, which is influenced by such variables as genetics, cultural or experiential backgrounds, and in terms of adequacy. The latter could be evaluated by considering self-care capabilities and self-care demand (Orem, 1987).

Nursing care is therapeutic self-care designed to supplement self-care requisites in the absence of capabilities to do so. Nursing actions, called "the theory of nursing systems," are:

- **Wholly compensatory:** The nurse is expected to accomplish all the patient's therapeutic self-care or to compensate for the patient's inability to engage in self-care, or when the patient needs continuous guidance in self-care;
- **Partly compensatory:** Both nurse and patient engage in meeting self-care needs;
- **Supportive educative system:** The system requires assistance in decision making, behavior control, and acquisition of knowledge and skills. Under this system, patients are able to perform self-care with assistance (Orem, 1985, pp. 152–156).

Orem's theory is based on explicit and implicit premises (Orem, 1983; 1987) (Table 16-6) that "do not express a singular belief in a clear way at either the philosophical or more general level of discourse" (Smith, 1987, p. 93).

Orem provides nursing with a number of primitive concepts that are defined theoretically and operationally, the esoteric nature of the terminology being one of the obstacles that may have influenced the initial slow use of the theory in practice (Anna, Christensen, Hohn, Ord and Wells, 1978). The theory includes both abstract (health, self-care agency) and concrete (universal self-care needs) variables (Table 16-7).

When concepts are defined, their relationships are not entirely clear as, for example, with health and self-care or illness and self-care deficit. The primitiveness, the overlap, and the undefined boundaries between concepts create multiple interpretations, particularly for those who are new to operationalizing the theory. The self-care agency is an example of an undefined concept or a primitive concept with multiple meanings. When should an agent be identified? What is the extent of self-care performed by an agent to make it self-care by self or by others? How do you determine the agent? By whose perception? (Anna, *et al*, 1978; Smith, 1979) These are examples of what an adequate theoretical and operational definition could do to decrease ambiguity and enhance clarity. Some of the variables are nonvariables (*e.g.*, self-care), thereby limiting their propositional power (Table 16-8).

Table 16–6.
Assumptions—Orem

Explicit Assumptions

- ○ Nursing is a deliberate, purposeful helping service performed by nurses for the sake of others over a period of time.
- ○ Persons (human agency) are capable and willing to perform self-care for self or for dependent members of the family.
- ○ Self-care is part of life that is necessary for health, human development, and well-being.
- ○ Education and culture influence individuals.
- ○ Self-care is learned through human interaction and communication.
- ○ Self-care includes deliberate and systematic actions performed to meet known needs for care (Orem, 1980, pp. 34–38).
- ○ "Human agency is exercised in discovering, developing and transmitting to others ways and means to identify needs for and make inputs to self and others" (1987, p. 73).

Implicit Assumptions

- ○ People should be self-reliant and responsible for their own care needs as well as for others in the family who are not able to care for themselves.
- ○ People are individuals with entities that are distinct from others and from their environment.

Orem proposed three specific theories: theory of self-care deficit (or dependent care deficit), theory of self-care, and theory of nursing systems. The theory of self-care deficit describes the needs of individuals who are incapable of self-care due to health-related limitations (Orem, 1985, p. 34). The theory of self-care describes self-care behaviors that regulate human structural integrity, functioning, and human development (Orem, 1985, p. 36). The theory of nursing systems—a

Table 16–7.
Concepts—Orem

Self-care	Self-care requisites
Deficits	Universal self-care
Capabilities	Developmental self-care
Demands	Health-deviation self-care
Dependent care	Therapeutic self-care
Dependent care deficit	demands
Nursing systems	Self-care agency
Wholly compensatory	Dependent care agency
Partly compensatory	Theory of self-care
Supportive educative	Theory of self-care deficits
	Theory of nursing systems

Table 16–8.
Definition of Domain Concepts—Orem

Nursing	Nursing is art, a helping service, and a technology (Orem, 1985, pp. 144–146).
	Actions deliberately selected and performed by nurses to help individuals or groups under their care to maintain or change conditions in themselves or their environments (p. 5).
	Encompasses the patient's perspective of health condition, the physician's perspective, and the nursing perspective. Universal, developmental, and health deviation self-care requisites.
Goal of nursing	To render the patient or members of his family capable of meeting the patient's self-care needs (1985, p. 54).
	"1. To maintain a state of health; 2. To regain normal or near normal state of health in the event of disease or injury; 3. To stabilize, control, or minimize the effects of chronic poor health or disability" (1980, p. 124).
Health	"Health and healthy are terms used to describe living things . . . [it is when] they are structurally and functionally whole or sound . . . wholeness or integrity . . . includes that which makes a person human, . . . operating in conjunction with physiological and psychophysiological mechanisms and a material structure (biologic life) and in relation to and interacting with other human beings (interpersonal and social life)" (1980, pp. 118–119).
	"A state of being whole and sound" (1985, p. 176).
	Well-being is a perception of contentment, happiness and pleasure, by spiritual experiences and through a sense of personalization (1985, p. 179).
Environment	Environment components are environmental factors, environmental elements, environmental conditions, and developmental environment (1985, pp. 140–141).
	Limited view of environment to its usefulness as a helping method. Therefore defined under Nursing Therapeutics. Though environment is mentioned in a diagram (1985, p. 85) and in the definition of nursing , (1985, p. 53), it is not defined.
Human being	Has the capacity to reflect, symbolize, and use symbols (1985, p. 174).
	Conceptualized as a total being with universal, developmental needs and capable of continuous self-care (1985).
	A unity that can function biologically, symbolically, and socially (1985, p. 175).
Nursing client	A human being who has "health-related or health-derived limitations that render him incapable of continuous self-care or dependent care or limitations that result in ineffective or incomplete care" (1985, pp. 34–35). A person who is deficient in universal, developmental, or health-related self-care requisites. . . . A human being is the focus of nursing only when a self-care requisite exceeds self-care capabilities (1985, p. 35).
Nursing problem	Deficits in universal, developmental, and health-derived or health-related conditions.

(continued)

Table 16–8. (Continued)

Nursing process	A system to determine 1) why a person is under care, 2) a plan for care, 3) the implementation of care.
Nurse–patient relations	Not defined.
Nursing therapeutics	Deliberate, systematic, and purposeful action. Total compensatory, partly compensatory, or educative supportive care in universal, developmental, and health-deviation self-care deficits, using several helping methods; acting or doing for others, guiding, supporting, providing a developmental environment, teaching (1985, pp. 88–90).
Focus	"The special concern of nursing is the individual's need for self-care action and the provision and management of it on a continuous basis in order to sustain life and health, recover from disease or injury, and cope with their effects." (1985, p. 54) Dependency or incapacities due to health/illness situation (1983, p. 208).

general theory of nursing—describes and explains nursing actions and products within the context of their contractual and interpersonal relations with human beings with self-care deficits (Orem and Taylor, 1986, p. 44).

Orem offers propositions that are summarized in Table 16-9. Propositions developed by Orem (1985) correspond to her three proposed themes and their central ideas. Propositions address the nursing client and nursing therapeutics. No propositions could be derived for the other major nursing phenomena. Propositions are limited to linking nursing therapeutics and human beings, but do not link all the theory's central concepts. Self-care requisites, demands, and needs are at times used interchangeably, decreasing the clarity of the theory. Propositions are mainly existence propositions, attesting to the stage of development of the theory. Despite these limitations and the complexity of the construct of self-care, Orem's theory has become part of the lexicon of health care and is beginning to be adopted by patients and health care professionals alike.

THEORY ANALYSIS

The Theorist

Dorothea Orem earned her diploma and bachelor of science in the 1930s and master of science in 1945 from the Catholic University of America, Washington, D.C. and honorary doctorates in 1976 from Georgetown University, Washington, D.C. and in 1980 from Incarnate Word College, San Antonio, Texas. She has established a private consulting company, Orem and Shields, Inc., in Chevy Chase, Maryland, perhaps to accommodate the diverse practice arenas that are using her theory and that need her consultation. She has been involved in nursing practice, nursing

Table 16-9.
Propositions—Orem

Person and Nursing Client

○ Human beings have capabilities to provide their own self-care or care for dependents to meet universal, developmental, and health-deviation self-care requisites. These capabilities are learned and recalled.

○ Self-care abilities are influenced by age, developmental state, experiences, sociocultural background as well as other variables.

○ Self-care deficits are to balance between self-care demands and self-care capabilities and an indication of a state of social dependency.

○ Self-care or dependent care is mediated by age, developmental stage, life experience, sociocultural orientation, health, and available resources.

Nursing Therapeutics

○ Therapeutic self-care includes actions of nurses, patients, and others that regulate self-care capabilities and meet self-care needs.

○ Nurses assess the abilities of patients to meet their self-care needs and their potential for refraining from performing their self-care.

○ Nurses engage in selecting valid and reliable processes or technologies or actions for meeting self-care demands.

○ Components of therapeutic self-care are wholly compensatory, partly compensatory, and supportive–educative.

Based on Orem (1985) and Orem & Taylor (1986).

---

service, and nursing education at different levels of education (practical, diploma, baccalaureate, and masters). She taught at two schools of nursing: the Catholic University of America and the Medical College of Virginia, Richmond (Foster and Janssens, 1980).

The impetus of Orem's theory was an attempt to conceptualize a curriculum for a diploma program by isolating and specifying nursing actions. She continued her theory development activities as a member of two overlapping crucial groups, the Nursing Model Committee of the Catholic University nursing faculty and the Nursing Development Conference Group.

Paradigmatic Origins

Orem's theory has been classified as a systems theory by Riehl and Roy (1980), as an interaction model by Riehl-Sisca (1989), and as developmental by Fawcett (1989). Orem used concepts from these three paradigms that may lead to the conclusion that the theory evolved from them. Her definition of health as a state of wholeness, her conception of the integrity of the person, and the use of systems of nursing all evolved from systems theory. These, however, are isolated concepts, more like terms, not derived conceptually or defined in terms of the original paradigm. A system model implies a feedback mechanism between nurse and patient, and such bidirectional movement is not congruent with this theory in which the nurse–patient relationship is predicated by the one-way transfer of agency (Melnyk, 1983, p. 173).

Similarly, Orem views a person with self-care deficits as socially dependent; the capability to engage in self-care and to meet universal self-care needs appears to characterize a more integrated development. These are concepts reflecting a developmental view of humanity, yet their lack of centrality in the theory, lack of definition, and absence of developmental stages and deliberate progression to more complex entities deny the theory a developmental origin. In fact, classifying the theory as either a system or a developmental theory would highlight gaps in defining concepts and propositions central to the two paradigms but quite tangential to Orem's theory.

The paradigmatic origin of the theory is more appropriately the needs theory of Henderson (1966) or the functional theory of Abdellah, Beland, Martin, and Matheney (1961). Henderson (1966, pp. 16–17) identified 14 needs. Universal self-care needs are similar to the needs identified by Henderson, although the uniqueness of Orem's theory lies more in the expectation of that person's capability to engage in his own self-care. Health-deviation requisites are an extension and not a refinement of Henderson's concept of nursing. Orem offers a fine example of the process inherent in theory development based on other theories in which new concepts evolve and others are derived. It is an example to be emulated as nurses refine and extend other theories.

Internal Dimensions

Orem's theories are interrelated and centered around self-care. Their level of development and interrelationship suggest that they are concepts and part of one theory, a nursing therapeutic theory of self-care. Orem's theory of self-care is a descriptive theory developed around an attempt to clarify the components of care offered by nurses and a conceptualization of the nursing client. It is a deductive theory with a hypothetical constructive beginning (Orem, 1985). It is a concatenated theory with more potential for existence propositions to describe the properties of the various concepts and to delineate the elements of such complex constructs as the exercise of self-care. It uses a field approach to theory construction. The units are understood in terms of other mini-units.

The theory is focused on and limited to dealing with individual self-care deficits rather than with the biopsychological being. It deals essentially with one of the domain concepts—clinical therapeutics—and offers one modality for care—the development of self-care abilities. It focuses on actions and deals with knowledge of control. It is a theory developed using an operational method; alternative methods of action are dependent on the nurse's discrimination and decision about the needs and the action (Barnum, 1990, p. 51). It is the agent's perspective that decides on alternative action.

THEORY CRITIQUE

Orem's theory has been operationalized and implemented in research, practice, and administration. It lends itself to research for a number of reasons. Orem herself has developed propositions linking the theory concepts and addressing at least two of the central concepts in nursing. However, the theory is a nursing therapeutic theory and appeals to the "relevance to nursing criteria" and is therefore used more to guide practice than research. It is about practice and for practice. When used to guide evaluation, it has lent itself to evaluation of the clinical efficacy of the theory (Backscheider, 1974).

The theory demonstrates a great but limited utility for nursing practice. Despite this limitation, there are several reasons for the rather speedy adoption of the theory by nursing practice. The language of the theory extends concepts advanced by Henderson, Abdellah and, to some extent, Nightingale. Nurses, when shifting from a medical model, have utilized a needs and functional approach to nursing care; therefore, the shift becomes more gentle and gradual, both of which are integral to Orem's theory. Orem also delineated the technical and professional aspects of nursing practice in both the Nursing Development Conference publications (1973, 1979) and in her first book (Orem, 1971).

Orem's theory also incorporates the medical perspective rather than rejects it (Johnston, 1983) and purports to build nursing practice on it. Furthermore, it uses medical science language, with which most nurses are familiar and many prefer. The theory is developed around the ill person and conveys the centrality of individual and institutional care, perhaps the most appealing feature for the majority of nurses who care for the sick. Orem extended the use of the theory to the care of families (Orem, 1983). It also appeals to those who wish to model Kinlein (1977) who "hung her own shingle" when she went into private practice. It is perhaps due to all these reasons, and the operational method in theory development, that we see more documentation in the literature of the utility of this theory for practice than is true of other theories.

The wide appeal of theory in practice is demonstrated in utilizing the theory to care for chronically ill patients, particularly the diabetic patient (Allison, 1973; Backscheider, 1971, 1974; Fitzgerald, 1980), in caring for amyotrophic lateral sclerosis patients (Taylor, 1988), in psychiatry (Buckwalter and Kerfoot, 1982; Caley, Dirksen, Engalla and Hennrich, 1980; Underwood, 1980), in acute care settings (Mullin, 1980), in preoperative and postoperative care (Bromley, 1980; Campuzano, 1982; Dropkin, 1981), in hospice care (Murphy, 1981; Walborn, 1980), and with adolescents (Michael and Sewall, 1980) and adult and geriatric patients (Anna *et al.*, 1978). The theory was used to individualize care for cancer patients (Morse and Werner, 1988), for patients with end stage renal disease (Greenfield and Pace, 1985), and for patients with drug problems (Compton, 1989). The theory was also used for caring for gerontological patients in community health nursing settings (Clark, 1986).

Limitations of the theory to practice are demonstrated in the analysis of the definitions and the central propositions in the theory. It appears that the theory is illness-oriented, both acute and chronic, with no indication of its use in wellness settings. Although some extended its use to the care of patients other than adults (Michael and Sewall, 1980), the theory itself addresses adults more than any other group (Melnyk, 1983). It presumes a list of needs that evolve out of a pathophysiological or medical focus, explaining its utility to hospital care. It establishes a relationship between a sick person and a nurse and not enough of a relationship between a well person and a nurse. The clarity of the theory is questionable when Orem's ideas are critiqued, but the diversity of its utility is demonstrated in a variety of subspecialties. It provides nurses with collegial visibility (Bennett, 1980).

Nurse administrators have found the theory amenable to implementation in a number of institutions. Orem (1989) herself proposed a framework for nursing administration. Miller (1980) challenged nursing administrators to create a climate to enhance the use of theory, although she did not give much guidance or exemplars for implementation on a large scale involving nursing administrators. She offered a model for nursing practice based on Orem's theory, demonstrating its utility for care in acute illness, convalescence, and restored health. The model was based more on a developmental, health/illness continuum than on Orem's theory. Others have described the utility of the theory as "a guide for the nursing activities within a hospital nursing service" (Coleman, 1980, p. 323) in organizing nursing care in independent practice (Backscheider, 1974), in psychiatric units (Underwood, 1980), particularly, in nurse-run clinics (Allison, 1973), and in five pilot units at the Toronto General Hospital (Reid, Allen, Gauthier and Campbell, 1989).

The theory evolved out of interest in curricula for diploma and baccalaureate programs and the need to differentiate between technical and professional education. Therefore, its utility to nursing education is enhanced by the theorist's interest. The curriculum subcommittee of the School of Nursing, Georgetown University in Washington, D.C. in which Orem, Backscheider, and Kinlein were members, developed a curriculum based on ideas of theory (or theory ideas evolved out of curriculum). Not surprisingly, the theory has been used as a conceptual framework in associate degree programs (Fenner, 1979). The framework is also used in the schools of nursing at the University of Southern Mississippi in Hattiesburg and the University of Missouri at Columbia (Fawcett, 1989, pp. 236–237).

The theory's circle of contagiousness in research, education, and administration is limited, but it has the widest circle of all theories in practice.

External Components of Theory

Orem's theory is congruent with the era of nursing practice that prevailed and focused on the ill and the institutionalized. As we shift focus to the well individuals and to the community, extensions and refinements will need to be made. The focus on health deficits due to illness creating self-care deficits will need to be supplemented with focus on health deficits versus self-care deficits (Melnyk, 1983), thereby allowing prevention and health promotion care. Its congruence with the social values is paradoxical; while the theory promotes the patient as being responsible for his own self-care and a partner in all decisions pertaining to his care (a prevailing value in nursing, specifically, and in Western society, in general), the theory gives the impression that the patient is dependent, expecting goals to be set for him, goals that involve him in developing the highest potential for self-care. Furthermore, what if a patient prefers that others take care of him?

The theory seemingly needs adaptation for use with other cultures; for example, values of patients in Japan include group care and the inseparability of the environment and the individual. On the other hand, it is usable in some societies where, though hospital patients are not expected to be self-care agents, family members are expected to and actually do become the self-care agents, as in many Middle Eastern countries. The nurse's role in these countries is to educate and support family members who assume the care. When these patients come to the United States alone, without their families or other self-care agents, they are unreceptive to nurses' attempts to promote self-care skills.

Orem's proposed theory may indeed make a substantial and valued difference in the lives of people whose self-care abilities are curtailed due to acute or chronic conditions, but it may not make the same difference in enhancing prevention and promoting health and well-being.

THEORY TESTING

Orem's theory has been utilized as the basis for the development of research instruments to assist researchers in utilizing the theory (Clinton, Denyes, Goodwin and Koto, 1977; Denyes, 1982; Kearney and Fleischer, 1979; Kuriansky, Gurland, Fleiss, and Cowan, 1976). Kearney and Fleischer (1979) described the development of a valid and reliable instrument to measure the exercise of self-care agency (McBride, 1987). The instrument can be used to measure the level of involvement of patients in self-care, and eventually measurements could be developed to determine outcomes of the increase in patients' abilities of self-care. Hanson and Bickel (1985) and Weaver (1987) developed, described, and critiqued an instrument to measure patients' perceptions of self-care agency. The Danger Assessment Instrument (Campbell, 1986) was developed to measure the danger level of homicide for battered women. Along the same lines, the Performance Test of Activities of Daily Living (PADL) is another tool developed to measure the self-care agency (Kuriansky *et al.*, 1976).

The focus of these studies lends support to the need for a process of operationalizing complex theory constructs and for the development of valid and reliable instruments based on these constructs. These studies represent effective steps in the further testing of central theory propositions that now exist, but with the potential for relational ones. The lack of clarity of concepts and tautology in ideas may have limited applications, but they have prompted the present line of investigation.

Fawcett reported that there are numerous unpublished ongoing or completed studies that have been presented in the annual conferences based on theory that are held at Georgetown University School of Nursing and Wichita (Kansas) State

University. Fawcett also reported on dissertations that used Orem as a theoretical framework for the research (Fawcett, 1989, p. 233). While published literature is limited, the potential for research is available.

Several descriptive studies focused on self-care practices. Allan (1988) examined the use and interpretation of health information in the practice of self-care activities of women as related to their weight. She found that women in her study were more concerned about their self-image than risk factors, and she was able to describe the self-care activities that they used to protect that image in the face of the reality of failure to maintain their weight. Miller (1982) used the theory to identify categories of self-care needs for diabetic patients, and Storm and Baumgartner (1987) illustrated through a research case study method the use of self-care theory in the successful discharge of ventilator-dependent patients. Kubricht (1984) described self-care needs of radiation patients, and Sandman, Norberg, Adolfsson, Axelsson, and Hedly (1986) described Alzheimer-type dementia patients and nurses' needs and actions. Maunz and Woods (1988) described self-care actions by women.

Other studies tested relationships between propositions. One example is Denyes (1988) who provided partial support for the relationship between self-care agency and self-care in determining health outcomes. Hartley (1988) tested the relationship between nursing system and self-care behavior by examining the congruence between teaching strategies and learning styles of women and their effect on accuracy and frequency of performance of breast self-examination. The study demonstrated that self-care agency could evolve through the recall of observations or actions of others: "Knowledge of self-care breast self-examination developed through the use of supportive-educative nursing system, a system through which efficient and effective learning occurred" (Hartley, 1988, p. 166).

Other tests of interventions lend further support to the utility of Orem's theories. The relationship between self-care as a nursing therapeutic and nursing outcome was examined in a number of studies. For example, Toth (1980) examined the relationship of a structured transfer-preparation on patients' anxiety; Rothlis (1984) explored the effect of self-help groups on perceptions of hopelessness and helplessness; and Moore (1987) described the effects of various learning strategies on the development of autonomy and self-care agency among school-aged children. Dashiff (1988) reviewed research and clinical literature in psychiatric nursing that is based on Orem's self-care deficit theory. She compared the contributions of this literature to the development of theory for use in psychiatric nursing with other nursing specialties and concluded that psychiatric nurses are utilizing Orem's theory; however, there were limited indications of research productivity.

An indirect effect of focusing on a nursing theory was reported by Denyes, O'Connor, Oakley, and Ferguson (1989). A collaborative research project was initiated between nursing service and nursing education, focusing on contraceptive nursing care and self-care of women using primary care facilities. The results of the research—that women are their own self-care agents—gave impetus "for revising the clinic's family planning standards so that they would more fully operationalize the concepts" (Denyes *et al.*, 1989, p. 144).

As with all other theories, Orem's could be used more broadly as a schematic to analyze the focus of research conducted in nursing and to set a direction for future research in nursing (Smith, 1979). On the whole, although the potential is there, the theory is utilized more as a guide for practice, with few having used it to evaluate the outcome of care (Chang, 1980; Roberts, 1982).

REFERENCES

Levine

Abdellah, F.G. and Levine, E. (1986) *Better patient care through nursing research* (3rd ed.). New York: Macmillan.

Barnum, B.J. (1990) *Nursing theory: Analysis, application, and evaluation* (3rd ed.). Boston: Little, Brown & Co.

Bertalanffy, L. (1968) *General system theory*. New York: George Braziller.

Buber, M. (1967) *Between man and man*. New York: Macmillan.

Cannon, W.B. (1939) *The wisdom of the body*. New York: W.W. Norton.

Donaldson, S.K. and Crowley, D.M. (1978) The discipline of nursing. *Nursing Outlook*, 26(2), 113–120.

Dubos, R. (1966) *Man adapting*. New Haven, CT: Yale University Press.

Erikson, E. (1968) *Identity, youth and crisis*. New York: W.W. Norton.

Esposito, C.H. and Leonard, M.K. (1980). Myra Estrin Levine: In Nursing Theories: The Base for Professional Practice. The Nursing Conference Group. Englewood Cliffs, NJ: Prentice-Hall.

Fawcett, J. (1989) *Analysis and evaluation of conceptual models of nursing* (2nd ed.). Philadelphia: F.A. Davis.

Flaskerud, J.H. and Halloran, E.J. (1980) Areas of agreement in nursing theory development. *Advances in Nursing Science*, 3(1), 1–7.

Hall, K.V. (1979) Current trends in the use of conceptual frameworks in nursing education. *Journal of Nursing Education*, 18(4), 26–29.

Hirschfeld, M.J. (1976) The cognitively impaired older adult. *American Journal of Nursing*, 76(12), 1981–1984.

Levine, M.E. (1966a) Trophicognosis: An alternative to nursing diagnosis. In *Exploring progress in medical-surgical nursing practice*. New York: American Nurses' Association.

Levine, M.E. (1966b) Adaptation and assessment: A rationale for nursing intervention. *American Journal of Nursing*, 66(11), 2450–2453.

Levine, M.E. (1967) The four conservation principles of nursing. *Nursing Forum*, 6(1), 45–59.

Levine, M.E. (1969) The pursuit of wholeness. *American Journal of Nursing*, 69(1), 93–98.

Levine, M.E. (1971a) Holistic nursing. *Nursing Clinics of North America*, 6(2), 253–264.

Levine, M.E. (1971b, June) Time has come to speak of health care. *AORN Journal*, 13, 37–43.

Levine, M.E. (1973) *Introduction to clinical nursing* (2nd ed.). Philadelphia: F.A. Davis.

Levine, M.E. (1979) The science is spurious (letter to the editor). *American Journal of Nursing*, 79(8), 1379–1383.

Levine, M.E. (1989a) The ethics of nursing rhetoric. *Image: Journal of Nursing Scholarship*, 21(1), 4–6.

Levine, M.E. (1989b) The four conservation principles: Twenty years later. In J.P. Riehl, *Conceptional models for nursing practice* (3rd ed.). Norwalk, CT: Appleton & Lange.

Levine, M.E. (1989c) Ethical issues in cancer care: Beyond dilemma. *Seminars in Oncology Nursing*, 5(2), 124–128.

Newport, M.A. (1984) Conserving thermal energy and social integrity in the newborn. *Western Journal of Nursing Research*, 6, 176–197.

Nightingale, F. (1969) *Notes on nursing. What it is and what it is not.* New York: Dover.

Riehl, J.P. (1980) Nursing models in current use. In J.P. Riehl and C. Roy (Eds.), *Conceptual models for nursing practice* (2nd ed.). New York: Appleton-Century-Crofts.

Rogers, C.R. (1961) *On becoming a person.* Boston: Houghton-Mifflin.

Rogers, M.E. (1970) *An introduction to the theoretical basis of nursing.* Philadelphia: F.A. Davis.

Selye, H. (1956) *The stress of life.* New York: McGraw-Hill.

Taylor, J.W. (1974) Measuring the outcomes of nursing care. *Nursing Clinics of North America*, 9(2), 337–348.

Taylor, J.W. (1989) Levine's conservation principles: Using the model for nursing diagnosis in a neurological setting. In J. Riehl-Sisca (Ed.), *Conceptual models for nursing practice* (3rd ed.). Norwalk, CT: Appleton & Lange.

Tillich, P. (1961) The meaning of health. *Perspectives in Biology and Medicine*, 5, 92–100.

Tompkins, E.S. (1980) Effect of restricted mobility and dominance on perceived duration. *Nursing Research*, 29(6), 333–338.

Orem

Abdellah, G.F., Beland, I.L., Martin, A., and Matheney, R.V. (1961) *Patient-centered approaches to nursing.* New York: Macmillan.

Allan, J.D. (1988) Knowing what to weigh: Woman self-care activities related to weight. *Advances in Nursing Science*, 11(1), 47–60.

Allison, S.E. (1973, July–August) A framework for nursing action in a nurse-conducted diabetic management clinic. *Journal of Nursing Administration*, 3(4), 53–60.

Anna, D.J., Christensen, D.G., Hohn, S.A., Ord, L., and Wells, S.R. (1978) Implementing Orem's conceptual framework. *Journal of Nursing Administration*, 8(11), 8–11.

Backscheider, J.E. (1971) The use of self as the essence of clinical supervision in ambulatory patient care. *Nursing Clinics of North America*, 6(4), 785–794.

Backscheider, J.E. (1974) Self-care requirements, self-care capabilities, and nursing systems in the diabetic nurse management clinic. *American Journal of Public Health*, 64(12), 1138–1146.

Bennett, J.G. (1980) Forward to the Symposium on the Self-care Concept in Nursing. *Nursing Clinics of North America*, 15(1), 129–130.

Bromley, B. (1980, February) Applying Orem's self-care theory in enterostomal therapy. *American Journal of Nursing*, 80(2), 245–249.

Buckwalter, K.C. and Kerfoot, K.M. (1982) Teaching patients self-care: A critical aspect of psychiatric discharge planning. *Journal of Psychiatric Nursing and Mental Health Services*, 20(5), 15–20.

Caley, J.M., Dirksen, M., Engalla, M., and Hennrich, M. (1980) The Orem self-care nursing model. In J.P. Riehl and C. Roy (Eds.), *Conceptual models for nursing practice* (2nd ed.). New York: Appleton-Century-Crofts.

Campbell, J.C. (1986) Nursing assessment for risk of homicide with battered women. *Advances in Nursing Science*, 8(4), 36–51.

Campuzano, M. (1982, April/May) Self-care following coronary artery bypass surgery. *Focus*, 55–56.

Chang, B.L. (1980) Evaluation of health care professionals in facilitating self-care: Review of the literature and a conceptual model. *Advances in Nursing Science*, 3(1), 43–58.

Clark, M.D. (1986) Application of Orem's theory of self-care: A case study. *Journal of Community Health Nursing*, 3(3), 127–135.

Clinton, J.F., Denyes, M.J., Goodwin, J.O., and Koto, E.M. (1977) Developing criterion measures of nursing care: Case study of a process. *Journal of Nursing Administration*, 7(7), 41–45.

Coleman, L.J. (1980) Orem's self-care concept of nursing. In J.P. Riehl and C. Roy (Eds.), *Conceptual models for nursing practice* (2nd ed.). New York: Appleton-Century-Crofts.

Compton, P. (1989) Drug abuse, a self-care deficit. *Journal of Psychosocial Nursing*, 27(3), 22–26.

Dashiff, C.J. (1988) Theory development in psychiatric-mental health nursing: An analysis of Orem's theory. *Archives of Psychiatric Nursing*, 2(6), 366–372.

Denyes, M.J., O'Connor, N.A., Oakley, D., and Ferguson, S. (1989) Integrating nursing theory, *Research*, 31(1), 63.

Denyes, M.J., O'Connor, N.A., Oakley, D., and Ferguson, S. (1989) Integrating nursing theory, practice and research through collaborative research. *Journal of Advanced Nursing*, 14, 141–145.

Dropkin, M.J. (1981, April) Development of a self-care teaching program for postoperative head and neck patients. *Cancer Nursing*, 103–106.

Fawcett, J. (1989) *Analysis and evaluation of conceptual models of nursing* (2nd ed.). Philadelphia: F.A. Davis.

Fenner, K. (1979) Developing a conceptual framework. *Nursing Outlook*, 27, 122–126.

Fitzgerald, S. (1980) Utilizing Orem's self-care nursing model in designing an educational program for the diabetic. *Topics in Clinical Nursing*, 2(2), 57–65.

Foster, P.C. and Janssens, N.P. (1980) Dorothea E. Orem. In The Nursing Theories Conference Group (Eds.), *Nursing theories: The base for professional nursing practice*. Englewood Cliffs, NJ: Prentice-Hall.

Greenfield, E. and Pace, J. (1985) Orem's self-care theory of nursing: Practical application to the end stage renal disease (ESRD) patient. *Journal of Nephrology Nursing*, 2(4), 187–193.

Hanson, B.R. and Bickel, L. (1985) Development and testing of the questionnaire on perception of self-care agency. In J. Riehl-Sisca, *The science and art of self-care*. Norwalk, CT: Appleton-Century-Crofts.

Hartley, L.A. (1988) Congruence between teaching and learning self-care: A pilot study. *Nursing Science Quarterly*, 1(4), 161–167.

Henderson, V. (1966) *The nature of nursing*. New York: Macmillan.

Johnston, R.L. (1983) Orem self-care model of nursing. In J. Fitzpatrick and A. Whall (Eds.), *Conceptual models of nursing: Analysis and application*. Bowie, MD: Robert J. Brady Company.

Kearney, B.Y. and Fleischer, B.J. (1979) Development of an instrument to measure exercise of self-care agency. *Research in Nursing and Health*, 2(1), 25–34.

Kinlein, M.L. (1977) Self-care concept. *American Journal of Nursing*, 77, 598–601.

Kubricht, D. (1984) Therapeutic self-care demands expressed by outpatients receiving external radiation therapy. *Cancer Nursing*, 7, 43–52.

Kuriansky, J., Gurland, B., Fleiss, J., and Cowan, D. (1976) The assessment of self-care capacity in geriatric psychiatric patients by objective and subjective methods. *Journal of Clinical Psychology, 32,* 95–102.

Maunz, E.R. and Woods, N.F. (1988) Self-care practices among young adult women: Influence of symptoms, employment, and sex-role orientation. *Health Care for Women International, 9,* 29–41.

McBride, S. (1987) Validation of an instrument to measure exercise of self-care agency. *Research in Nursing and Health, 10,* 311–316.

Melnyk, K.A.M. (1983) The process of theory analysis: An examination of the nursing theory of Dorothea E. Orem. *Nursing Research, 32*(3), 170–174.

Michael, M.M. and Sewall, K.S. (1980) Use of the adolescent peer group to increase the self-care agency of adolescent alcohol abusers. *Nursing Clinics of North America, 15,* 157–176.

Miller, J.F. (1980) The dynamic focus of nursing: A challenge to nursing administration. *The Journal of Nursing Administration, 10*(1), 13–18.

Miller, J.F. (1982) Categories of self-care needs of ambulatory patients with diabetes. *Journal of Advanced Nursing, 7,* 25–31.

Moore, J.B. (1987) Effects of assertion training and first aid instruction on children's autonomy and self-care agency. *Research in Nursing and Health, 10,* 101–109.

Morse, W. and Werner, J.S. (1988) Individualization of patient care using Orem's theory. *Cancer Nursing, 11*(3), 195–202.

Mullin, V.I. (1980) Implementing the self-care concept in the acute care setting. *Nursing Clinics of North America, 15*(4), 177–190.

Murphy, P.P. (1981) A hospice model and self-care theory. *Oncology Nursing Forum, 8*(2), 19–21.

Nursing Development Conference Group. (1973) *Concept formalization in nursing: process and product.* Boston: Little, Brown & Co.

Nursing Development Conference Group. (1979) *Concept formalization in nursing: process and product* (2nd ed.). Boston: Little, Brown & Co.

Orem, D.E. (1959) *Guides for developing curriculae for the education of practical nurses.* Washington, D.C.: U.S. Department of Health, Education, & Welfare, Office of Education.

Orem, D.E. (1971) *Nursing: Concepts of practice.* New York: McGraw-Hill.

Orem, D.E. (1980) *Nursing concepts of practice* (2nd ed.). New York: McGraw Hill.

Orem, D.E. (1983) The self-care deficit theory of nursing: A general theory. In I.W. Clements and F.B. Roberts (Eds.), *Family health: A theoretical approach to nursing care.* New York: John Wiley & Sons.

Orem, D.E. (1985) *Nursing: Concepts of practice* (3rd ed.). New York: McGraw-Hill.

Orem, D.E. (1987) Orem's general theory of nursing. In R. Parse, *Nursing science: Major paradigms, theories, and critiques.* Philadelphia: W.B. Saunders.

Orem, D.E. (1989) Theories and hypotheses for nursing administration. In B. Henry, M. Di Vincenti, C. Arndt, and A. Marriner (Eds.), *Dimensions of nursing administration. Theory, research, education, and practice.* Boston: Blackwell Scientific Publications.

Orem, D.E. and Taylor, S.G. (1986) Orem's general theory of nursing. In P. Winstead-Fry (Ed.), *Case studies in nursing theory.* New York: National League for Nursing.

Reid, B., Allen, A., Gauthier, T., and Campbell, H. (1989) Solving the Orem mystery: An educational strategy. *Journal of Continuing Education in Nursing, 20*(3), 108–110.

Riehl, J.P. and Roy, C. (Eds.). (1980) *Conceptual models for nursing practice* (2nd ed.). New York: Appleton-Century-Crofts.

Riehl-Sisca, J.P. (1989) *Conceptual models for nursing practice* Norwalk, CT: Appleton-Lange.

Roberts, C.S. (1982) Identifying the real patient problems. *Nursing Clinics of North America,* 17(3), 481–489.

Rothlis, J. (1984) The effect of a self-help group on feelings of hopelessness and helplessness. *Western Journal of Nursing Research,* 6, 157–173.

Sandman, P.O., Norberg, A., Adolfsson, R., Axelsson, K., and Hedly, V. (1986) Morning care of patients with Alzheimer-type dementia. A theoretical model based on direct observations. *Journal of Advanced Nursing,* 11, 369–378.

Smith, M.C. (1979) Proposed metaparadigm for nursing research and theory development. *Image,* 11(3), 75–79.

Smith, M.C. (1987) A critique of Orem's theory. In R.R. Parse, *Nursing science. Major paradigms, theories, and critiques.* Philadelphia: W.B. Saunders.

Stevens, B.J. (1984) *Nursing theory: Analysis, application, and evaluation.* Boston: Little, Brown & Co.

Storm, D.S. and Baumgartner, R.G. (1987) Achieving self-care in the ventilator-dependent patient: A critical analysis of a case study. *International Journal of Nursing Studies,* 24, 95–106.

Taylor, S.G. (1988) Nursing theory and nursing process: Orem's theory in practice. *Nursing Science Quarterly,* 1(3), 111–119.

Toth, J.C. (1980) Effect of structured preparation for transfer on patient anxiety on leaving coronary care unit. *Nursing Research,* 29(1), 28–34.

Underwood, P.R. (1980) Facilitating self-care. In P. Pothier (Ed.), *Psychiatric nursing.* Boston: Little, Brown & Co.

Walborn, K.A. (1980) A nursing model for hospice: Primary and self-care. *Nursing Clinics of North America,* 15(1), 205–217.

Weaver, M.T. (1987) Perceived self-care agency: A LISREL, factor analysis of Bickel and Hanson's questionnaire. *Nursing Research,* 36, 381–387.

Part **6**

Our Theoretical Future (A Holograph of Past and Present)

*P*art Six views the future of theoretical nursing as it is evolving from its past and present. It considers future stages and milestones as they relate to the stages and milestones articulated and discussed in Part One. Further progress is explored under some of the premises also presented in Part One. The view presented in this part is not linear but holographic, that is to say, it sees past, present, and future through the same glasses and at the same instant. The view is not static either, but is limited to forces that exist today. As new paradigms that are evolving gain support in societies (paradigms that combine the empiricism of the West with the mysticism of the East) and as new trends influence nurses and their clients as human beings, the view may take different shapes and different forms.

This part closes with a short summary of salient future recommendations representing the perspective taken in this book.

Chapter 17

On Practical Wisdom

Most of the popular theories that exist to describe, explain, and predict human health and well-being have emerged from a biomedical perspective. The biomedical model as a framework for health care has been challenged due to its limited effectiveness (Engel, 1977) and challenged by nurses as inappropriate for the mission of nursing (Shaver, 1985; Allan and Hall, 1988). Others have described the differences in perspectives between nursing and other health fields and the uniqueness of the nursing perspective despite its dependent and interdependent functions (Visintainer, 1986).

Nursing theorists are among those nurses who not only challenged the biomedical model, but who also proactively conceptualized different aspects of the territory of nursing. Their conceptualizations provide the bases for identifying nursing perspectives and for defining our nursing domain. It is because of their pioneering work that I became interested in exploring theoretical nursing in its various dimensions.

This concluding chapter has three purposes. Its first purpose is to discuss the relationship between theory and nursing diagnoses, nursing education, and nursing administration. Its second purpose is to identify the next stages and milestones in the development and progress of theoretical nursing. Its third purpose is to provide the reader with some recommendations and guidelines related to the continuous progress of theoretical nursing. The ultimate purpose of this chapter is to maintain an open and an ongoing dialogue about theoretical nursing.

The relationships among theoretical nursing, nursing practice, and nursing research have been discussed throughout this text with the premise that no discussion of any part is complete without discussion of the whole. The relationships between theoretical nursing and nursing diagnosis, nursing education, and nursing administration deserve a pause in this concluding chapter.

THEORETICAL NURSING
AND NURSING DIAGNOSIS

The work on defining and identifying nursing diagnosis began in nursing in 1950 (McManus, 1950; Gordon, 1979) and was seriously considered after the pioneering efforts of Gebbie and Lavin, who initiated the first national conference on classification of nursing diagnosis in St. Louis in 1971 (Gebbie and Lavin, 1975). The results of seven such conferences have been the identification of 50 to 70 labels for nursing diagnosis and an increasing number of research projects in which the authors designed studies to validate nursing diagnosis and other studies to identify nursing diagnosis in diverse groups (Gordon, 1985; Kim, 1989). The result also has been an acceptance of nursing diagnosis as a significant step in clinical judgment and as a concept with great utility in nursing practice, as evidenced in the number of clinical writings about the concept, its appearance on agendas, for nursing conferences and its inclusion in the definition of nursing in the Social Policy Statement (American Nurses' Association, 1980).

The extent to which nursing diagnosis has influenced the development and progress of nursing theory has not been carefully explored. There are two ways to consider the relationship between nursing theory and nursing diagnosis: first, one can consider how nursing theory has influenced the development of nursing diagnosis; and second, one can consider how nursing diagnosis has contributed to the development of nursing theory.

The impetus for the development of nursing diagnosis has some theoretical characteristics when viewed from the perspective of identifying and defining labels for judgments that nurses make in their daily practice. As Kritek (1978) indicated, these judgments about assessments are examples of factor-isolating theories, which were defined by Dickoff, James, and Wiedenbach in 1968. This type of theory specifies, describes, defines, and classifies concepts.

The process of identifying what nurses assess and what judgments they make is also characterized by some features that later nursing philosophers and theorists advocated. Nurses were asked to look at their own practice, to trust their assessments, to uncover their judgments, and to collaborate in a long process of specifying, defining, and identifying. The processes that organizers of the nursing diagnosis conferences, the attendees, and all others who participated in the nursing diagnosis movement have utilized are processes of theoretical thinking geared toward the goal of the theoretical development of the discipline.

Nursing diagnoses, however, did not emerge from a coherent philosophical approach nor from a theoretically defined domain. While they represent the realities of those nurses who participated in developing the diagnoses, they do not represent the majority of nurses who have been caring for clients and for communities for years and whose levels of expertise range from the novice to the expert, nor could they do that. Assumptions held by nurses and shared assumptions of the domain have not been adequately, carefully, or systematically discussed, nor have they reflected on the nursing diagnosis literature. Therefore, to summarize comments on ways by which nursing theory has influenced nursing diagnosis, I would say that the quest for theoretical development of the discipline may have guided the *process* of attempting to classify labels used in judging the condition of nursing clients, but it did not guide the *content* of these labels. The content of the classification process was predicated on diverse values, assumptions, and visions of the mission of nursing that remain to be identified and defined; they were also predicated on a problem orientation to care rather than an asset approach to care. A theoretical approach based on assets, health maintenance, and health promotion is a more congruent approach to the mission of nursing. This approach is lacking in the current framework for nursing diagnosis.

Attempts at relating existing nursing theories to the accepted diagnoses and to the development of useful, coherent, and supported nursing theories that may create new diagnoses should be of interest to theory students. One approach to theory development may be more useful than the other; however, with the current level of enthusiasm in the nursing diagnosis movement, I propose that we carefully chart mechanisms to ensure that the former approach (accepted diagnosis) does not overshadow the latter (the development of theory leading to new diagnosis).

A second way by which the relationship between nursing theory and nursing diagnosis could be considered is to analyze the contributions of nursing diagnoses to the development of nursing theory. There are at least three consequences of the nursing diagnosis movement to theoretical nursing.

First, nursing diagnosis created a theoretical discourse in the literature that is useful in analyzing philosophical bases and values and potentially useful in the further development and progress of theoretical nursing. Examples are the Shamansky and Yanni (1983) and Kritek (1985) debates about assumptions regarding the development of nursing diagnosis, the role of nursing diagnosis in knowledge development in the discipline, and the implicit limitations of the concept of nursing diagnosis. Other examples are the analysis of implicit values inherent in nursing diagnosis and in the dependent and independent roles of nurses (Kritek, 1979; Kim, 1985; Jacoby, 1985).

Second, the publication and use of nursing diagnoses have prompted a reevaluation of some of the labels and their meanings, a theoretical process that is defined as concept classification (Dennison and Keeling, 1989; Jenny, 1987).

Third, the nursing diagnosis movement has stimulated nursing researchers to initiate studies to identify nursing diagnoses and to validate existing ones (Kim, 1989; Gordon, 1985). A next step beyond the analysis of research findings is the initiation of further dialogue to interpret the theoretical and philosophical implications of these findings.

A taxonomy of nursing diagnoses does not represent a theory; it is just a classification system. Each of the diagnostic labels represents a concept that may be a building block for a potential nursing theory related to that concept, if and when the concept is defined within a context of assumptions, values, nursing mission, and other concepts representing the domain of nursing; and when it is related to health and well-being as the goals of nursing. Two types of theories could be developed: descriptive/explanatory and prescriptive theories. The nursing diagnosis label of "comfort (alterations in)," for example, is only meaningful within a theory that describes comfort and its relationship to the health of clients as viewed from the perspective of the domain of nursing, with its focus on person–environment interaction and responses to health and illness.

THEORETICAL NURSING AND NURSING EDUCATION

Theoretical nursing includes a discourse about the structure of nursing knowledge, the philosophical bases of nursing science, theory development, the history of nursing knowledge, and nursing theories. Aspects of these components have been included in doctoral nursing programs in the United States (Jacobs-Kramer and Huether, 1988) and internationally. A more limited version has been included in master programs with more emphasis on presentations and critique of existing nursing theories (Jacobson, 1987). Although nursing theories have been used as frameworks for nursing curricula in undergraduate programs during the 1970s and 1980s, only a limited number have included opportunities to discuss theoretical nursing and approaches to theory development (Meleis and Price, 1988; Jacobs-Kramer and Huether, 1988).

Theoretical thinking, the pride a member of a discipline has in the theoretical threads in one's discipline, a belief in the self as a proactive developer of knowledge, and an identity that incorporates the ability to structure nursing knowledge are values, the seeds for which could and should be planted as early as possible in nursing education. It is not enough to promote these values in doctoral programs, or in master's programs.

> If nursing expects seriously to impact through development and use of
> theory, content related to the purpose, generation, and use of theory must be
> introduced into the curricula much earlier than it currently is (Jacobs-Kramer
> and Huether, 1988, p. 376).

Introducing theoretical nursing to students at the undergraduate level is not too early (Batra, 1987). However, when content related to theory and knowledge development is introduced as a separate component of a nursing curriculum, students and faculty experience difficulties in relating this content to other curricular components. While this practice may have been necessary in the decades when the primacy of theoretical nursing was still debated, faculty members and students may now be ready to integrate that content with clinical and research components of the curriculum.

Theoretical nursing provides nursing curricula with a perspective that is uniquely nursing; it provides nursing students with frameworks that help them define their values, concepts in their work, significant problems in their fields, and approaches to structuring and developing knowledge. More importantly, a theoretical nursing perspective promotes the primacy of discovering, developing, and structuring nursing knowledge.

The relationship between theory and nursing curricula is similar to the relationship that research had to nursing curricula. Educators asked whether or not research courses should be in the curriculum, at what level they should be introduced, and what should be included (Wilson, 1985). The questions related to theory, theoretical nursing, and philosophy are no longer whether theory should be a component of nursing programs, or at what level it should be introduced; rather the questions educators will grapple with in the 1990s are what aspects of theory should be introduced at every educational level and what are the most effective and meaningful ways by which it should be included.

NURSING THEORY AND NURSING ADMINISTRATION

> Nursing administrators can directly influence efforts to generate nursing's knowledge by providing access to a virtually untapped theory building resource—the non-university service setting (DeGroot, Ferketich, and Larson, 1987, p. 38).

This sentiment of the close connection between nursing administration and nursing knowledge and of the potential of nursing theory construction by or as promoted by nursing administrators has been expressed repeatedly in the late 1980s (an example is the volume edited by Henry, Arndt, Di Vincenti and Marriner-Tomey, 1989). Until the late 1980s, there was a limited dialogue about the relationship of nursing theory and nursing administration (Christmyer, Catanzariti, Langford, and Reiz, 1988). Some addressed the shortcomings of that limited dialogue, indicating that specialty nursing cannot afford to be distanced from mainstream nursing by claiming that nursing theories do not represent them (Dashiff, 1988).

Viewing nursing administration from a domain perspective and investigating theoretical and clinical questions from that perspective could lead to a more coherent approach to structuring knowledge that is as useful to clinicians as it may be to administrators. Theoretical aspects of the domain of nursing may provide clinicians and administrators with a unifying framework that could further contribute to the development of coherent theories to guide nursing care (Meleis and Jennings, 1989; Jennings and Meleis, 1988).

NEW STAGES . . . NEW MILESTONES

Stages

In Chapter 3, the development of theoretical nursing was described in terms of five stages. These were:

Stage of Practice;
Stage of Education and Administration;

Stage of Research;
Stage of Nursing Theory; and
Stage of Philosophy.

In Chapter 7, nursing was described as a scholarly discipline. The next stages in the development of nursing knowledge are projected as the stage of structure and integration and the stage of reaching out.

Stage of Structure and Integration

A first characteristic of this stage is substantive dialogues and discussions focused on identifying coherent structures of the discipline of nursing at large and of the specific areas of specialization (Schlotfeldt, 1988). The structures include nursing scientific, theoretical, philosophical, and clinical knowledge that is focused on the nursing domain and its phenomena. These dialogues take place in conferences, think tanks, and theme journal editions devoted to the development of middle-range and single-domain theories focused on an aspect of the domain of nursing.

A second characteristic of this stage is the development of educational programs that are organized around substantive areas through the integration of theory, research, and practice. It is also manifested in the ease by which nursing administrators, clinicians, and educators use theoretical nursing and in the increasing dialogue among members of the discipline regarding matters related to knowledge, discovery, and development that is focused on and emanates from the domain of nursing.

A third characteristic of this stage is the evaluation of different aspects of theoretical nursing by members of the discipline representing nursing clinicians, teachers, administrators, researchers, and theoreticians. Evaluation is not limited to theory testing; it includes description, analysis, and critiques as well. Each of these processes is important in the development and progress of our discipline because of its diverse philosophical bases.

A fourth characteristic of this stage is the attention that members of the discipline give to the strategies of knowledge development that are congruent with the discipline's shared assumptions and that take the conditions of holism, patterning, experience, and meaning into consideration.

A fifth characteristic is the involvement of members of specialty fields in developing theories that are pertinent to the phenomenon of that particular field. This involvement does not preclude similar attention to theories related to phenomena of the domain of nursing at large.

A final characteristic is the systematic reappraisal of philosophical and theoretical underpinnings that has guided the definitions and the conceptualizations of the central concepts of the domain of nursing. An example of such discourse is the reappraisal of the definition of client in the nursing literature and the congruency of these definitions with domain assumptions (Allen, 1987).

Stage of Reaching Out

Reaching out is defined as going beyond the confines of the discipline and beyond the usual mainstream nursing clients. Reaching out includes but is not limited to reaching out to develop theories that are useful in understanding and caring for clients from different socioeconomic and cultural backgrounds. It also includes having a voice and marketing nursing discoveries, ideas, and goals to members of other disciplines and the public.

Characteristics of this stage are the description and development of phenomena that are of interest to minorities and vulnerable, underserved, and underrepresented populations. Theories allow for understanding of phenomena from diverse perspectives. Communicating with the public through the media to describe and report nurses' goals and actions is another characteristic of this stage. An example of the gap in this information is nurses' claims of health and well-being as a domain focus and the apparent lack of recognition of such a focus by members of the other disciplines as well as the public.

Another significant characteristic of reaching out is manifested in the promotion of collaboration with international colleagues and the increase in published dialogues about phenomena that represent the nursing domain and represent diverse explanations.

MILESTONES

The following eight milestones were identified in Chapter 3:

Prior to 1955—From Florence Nightingale to nursing research;
1955–1960—The birth of nursing theory: The Columbia University Teachers College approach;
1961–1965—Theory: A national goal in nursing;
1966–1970—Theory development: A tangible goal for academics;
1971–1975—Theory syntax;
1976–1980—A time to reflect;
1981–1985—Nursing theories' revival: Emergence of the domain concepts; and
1986–1990—From metatheory to single domain theory.

These milestones represent the development of theoretical nursing up to 1990. During the period from 1981 to 1990, aspects of the domain of nursing became more accessible to nurses in many special clinical and functional fields and were utilized as the organizing framework for education, clinical practice, and research. There was less need for advocacy and synthesis of theory, the milestones that characterized the preceding periods. Nursing programs discussed and utilized nursing theories with the same ease as theories from other disciplines were discussed and utilized. Graduates of programs where nursing theories were utilized became aware of the strengths and limitations in utility of nursing theory and the strengths and limitations of theories that were developed to answer questions characteristic of other disciplines.

The syntactical debates (theory *vs.* conceptual framework, nursing theory *vs.* borrowed theory) faded and gave way to substantive debates (different views of health, environment, and client). Those who were engaged in refining and extending theories through research–practice–theory produced the milestone of this period. Indications of refinement/extension were already beginning in 1984. Relationships between domain concepts were being explored using existing nursing theories and other pertinent theories, such as interpersonal relations and the delivery of nursing care (nursing therapeutics), resulting in theoretical exemplars that could guide nursing research (Kasch, 1984).

Although philosophical discussions and theoretical exchanges are useful, their utility is limited without considering related research as an integral part of these discussions. This view is congruent with the more contemporary view of science (Laudan, 1981). Theorists, researchers, clinicians, and educators began to explicitly state the theoretical underpinnings of their work and to engage in dialogues with self and others to help in identifying relationships or lack of them with the nursing domain. Such discussions helped to refine both the domain and the work being done.

Because our scholarly work centers around and emanates from the domain, special interest groups emerged as (what Merton calls) a "community of scholars" who, in turn, helped in the refinement and extension processes (Merton, 1973). These communities of scholars were organized around substantive nursing areas, such as mobility, rest, and nursing therapeutics.

While striving for an approach in care and in research that is congruent with holism and nonreductionism, we accepted that our limited tools and methodologies have not limited serious work that may mix reductionism with holism, objectivity with subjectivity, stability with change, and empiricism with historicism. To hold up theoretical and research investigation until all our premises, concepts, propositions, and research are congruent would be to hold up progress. Inconsistencies, paradoxes, and oppositions, if viewed as functions of the time, may still contribute to the goal of total congruence or collaboration. Neither end of the pole (that is, total congruence or total incongruence) is conducive to solving problems in a field. A healthy presence of multiple perspectives, even though sometimes inconsistent, is bound to help us understand the richness of the multiple realities of nursing.

Nursing theories of the past, present, or the future do not answer all the questions that nurses may ask; neither do sociological, psychological, physiological, or engineering theories. Different theories in each of these disciplines answer different questions, and yet there are still some questions that have not been answered satisfactorily. Other questions that appeared to be answered satisfactorily were being challenged by new data and new competing explanations, for example Margaret Mead's cultural determinism and Sigmund Freud's seduction theories. These we have learned were not reasons to condescendingly brush away nursing theory or nurses' abilities to develop theories. The next milestones demonstrated a new maturity in the discipline.

1990–1995: The Development of Prescriptive Theories

Descriptive theories are followed by the development of prescriptive theories designed to provide nurses with frameworks for action that includes maintenance, restoration, or change. The relevance of theories to nursing practice becomes more prominent when theories are developed to provide nurses with guidelines for action.

1995–2000: Second and Third Generation Theorists

Theorists who focus on the development of middle range and single domain theories substitute current theorists. The focus shifts from theorists to theories.

THE END FOR NOW!
ON PRACTICAL WISDOM

The major goals of this book are to make a contribution to raising our consciousness about the theoretical development and progress of our discipline, to acknowledge our theoretical history, to place the present in the context of our history, and to develop an awareness of the potential inherent in members of the discipline, men or women. To paraphrase McBride (1986): We must consider the future neither with apologies nor with our inadequacies waving, but with a sense that (theoretical nursing) has contributed mightily to the present maturity of the (discipline) (p. 31).

Within these goals, the following points were made in this book:

1. Nurses have a fine and useful theoretical heritage that is worthy of analysis. By understanding how and why our heritage evolved as it did, we may be in a better position to have control of a future of theory development.

2. Nurses have the resources by which they can conceptualize different aspects of their universe for the purpose of facilitating understanding, increasing autonomy in their actions, and enhancing control over their domain for the ultimate objective of providing the kind of quality care they aspire to. The resources and the tools differ, based on education and experience; however, it was proposed here that the clinicians are as valuable as the theoreticians because they articulate their practical wisdom into exemplars that may help to solve other clinical problems.

3. The scientific development of the discipline of nursing has followed a unique path that was charted by nursing to suit its unique features and its nursing care complexities. Sociology of nursing science and philosophy of nursing science are legitimate and significant areas of investigation to discern the progress and development of the discipline. As nurses question the empiricist's view of science and begin to embrace the historicist's conception of science, the behavior of scientists and theoreticians, the processes of selection of research and theories, the historical environment, and the sociocultural context for the development and utility of the discipline's theories become legitimate and central questions.

4. Our theoretical history, our epistemology, and our domain are the bases for our theoretical future. The novice should be acquainted with them, the advanced should explore and question the relationships between the parts and, together with the experienced, they should shape and reshape nursing knowledge. More specifically, I propose three avenues to pursue to begin a pattern of practical wisdom. These are not exhaustive, but should be considered as a beginning for others the reader may identify:

   ○ Analytical and critical consideration of nursing theories should be a cornerstone of curricula in nursing, from community college to doctoral programs, with different goals at each educational level. For example, a choice of discussion of human beings as nursing clients may be organized around nursing theories that discuss human beings and the different goals of the different perspectives.
   ○ Consideration of research and clinical exemplars that are related to different domain concepts and questions and beginning attempts at a thorough review may help in creating some coherence and may delineate further avenues of investigation.
   ○ The advanced clinicians and clinical specialists can be coached to develop and share their wisdom gleaned from their clinical practice in the form of exemplars. Exemplars identify, model, and direct problems of concern to nursing and ways of solving these problems.

Out of all that, we return to what Johnson referred to as "practical wisdom" (1959, p. 294), and the age of wisdom will then emerge. It encompasses all the properties of the other stages nursing has gone through, not in a cumulative way but rather synthetically and developmentally, with experience and practice as its hallmark. There will be more acceptance of the complexity and fluidity of nursing concepts and the significance of the temporal dimension in our research and theory development. Natural turns and detours will be made with ease and comfort, just as Newton made a natural turn to astronomy because, at that time, finding one's way in the sea had been a preoccupation of the time, or just as Kepler turned to astrology and used it during the Thirty Years War.

Using theories and developing new theories will benefit from temporal experiences. From such use and further development comes wisdom. Although we must not forget Bacon's reasoning for empirical testing or Kant's insistence on *a priori* conceptual schemata independent of experience, a practice discipline such as nursing cannot exist if it forgets Kaplan's advice that the pursuit of wisdom expresses a deep concern with the good that can be achieved in human life. Those benefits resulting from nursing practice have to be conveyed to the public, to whom nursing is ultimately accountable. It is such public awareness and accountability that are the main pillars upon which the discipline of nursing will rest.

This book presents our domain as we see it today, and such are the consequences we must nurture in the 1990s. At any particular time, the recognized domain will include many phenomena that are not entirely clear or apparently consequential, or they might create genuine and inquisitive stances. This does not reflect the lack of maturity of a discipline but rather indicates its continuing growth. During the age of wisdom, the bond between scientific endeavors and reflection will become stronger, adaptation and demand will be the key forces of progress instead of structure and inflexibility. We will accept limitations in the discipline of nursing as limitations of the time rather than as the discipline's shortcomings.

Wisdom is the "capacity to take account of all important factors in a problem and to attach to each its due weight" and to know which ends to pursue (Russell, 1957, p. 29). It combines knowledge, feelings, morals, and practice. Wisdom is a sense of proportion. Knowledge can give us nursing therapeutics to enhance self-care, increase mother–infant attachment, increase social support or networks, ease effects of transition, or maintain integrity of the individual. Only wisdom and understanding can ensure their appropriate use for our clients without imposing our own values. Wisdom is a total perspective, seeing an object, event, or idea in all its pertinent relationships. Spinoza defined wisdom as seeing things "*sub specie aeternitatis,*" in view of eternity (Copleston, 1963, p. 253); Durant (1957) suggested defining it as seeing things "*sub specie totuis,*" in view of the whole. Considering the stages of development of knowledge in nursing and considering nursing as a whole leads to the proposition that nursing is currently encountering a scholarly evolution.

Emerson once said, "To the philosopher, all things are friendly and sacred, all events profitable, all days whole, all men (or women) divine." To nursing, all stages were essential to bring us to the stage of scholarliness, and from all stages will emerge the age of wisdom. "Knowledge is power, but only wisdom is liberty" (Durant, 1957, p. 9). Once there was a there. Now "there" is here. Let us acknowledge and enjoy our accomplishments; but we must also remember, there is no end to what lies ahead because it is the process that is the future.

REFERENCES

Allan, J. and Hall, B. (1988) Challenging the focus on technology: A critique of the medical model in a changing health care system. *Advances in Nursing Science*, 10(3), 22–34.

Allen, D.G. (1987) The social policy statement: A reappraisal. *Advances in Nursing Science*, 10(1), 39–48.

American Nurses Association. (1980) *Nursing: A social policy statement.* Kansas City, MO: ANA.

Batra, C. (1987) Nursing theory for undergraduates. *Nursing Outlook*, 35(4), 189–192.

Christmyer, C.S., Catanzariti, P.M., Langford, A.M., and Reiz, J.A. (1988, August) Bridging the gap: Theory to practice—Part I, clinical applications. *Nursing Management*, 19(9), 42–50.

Copleston, S.J. (1963) *A history of philosophy. Volume 4, Modern philosophy: Descartes to Leibniz.* Garden City, NY: Image Books. (Baruch Spinoza, pp. 211–269.)

Dashiff, C. (1988, December) Theory development in psychiatric mental health nursing: An analysis of Orem's theory. *Archives of Psychiatric Nursing*, 2(6), 366–372.

DeGroot, H.A., Ferketich, S.L., and Larson, P.J. (1987) Theory development in a non-university service setting. *Journal of Nursing Administration*, 17(4), 38–4.

Dennison, P.D., and Keeling, A.W. (1989) Clinical support for eliminating the nursing diagnosis of knowledge deficit. *Image: Journal of Nursing Scholarship*, 21(3), 142–144.

Dickoff, J., James, P., and Wiedenbach, E. (1968) Theory in a practice discipline: Part 1. Practice oriented theory. *Nursing Research,* 17, 415–435.

Durant, W. (1957) What is wisdom? *Wisdom: The Magazine for Knowledge for All America,* 20(8), 25.

Engel, G.L. (1977, April) The need for a new medical model: A challenge for biomedicine. *Science,* 196, 129–137.

Gebbie, K.M. and Lavin, M.A. (1975) *Proceedings of the first national conference on classification of nursing diagnosis.* St. Louis: C.V. Mosby.

Gordon, M. (1979) The concept of nursing diagnosis. *Nursing Clinics of North America,* 14(3), 487–496.

Gordon, M. (1985) Nursing diagnosis. *Annual Review of Nursing Research,* 3, 127–146.

Henry, B., Arndt, C., Di Vincenti, M., and Marriner-Tomey, A. (Eds.) (1989) *Dimensions of nursing administration: Theory, research, education, practice.* Boston: Blackwell Scientific Publications.

Jacobs-Kramer, M. and Huether, S.E. (1988) Curricular considerations for teaching nursing theory. *Journal of Professional Nursing,* 4(5), 373–380.

Jacobson, S. (1987) Studying and using conceptual models of nursing. *Image: Journal of Nursing Scholarship,* 19(2), 78–82.

Jacoby, M.K. (1985) Eliminating the double standard. *American Journal of Nursing,* 85(3), 281, 285.

Jennings, B.M. and Meleis, A.I. (1988) Nursing theory and administration practice: Agenda for the 1990s. *Advances in Nursing Science,* 10(3), 56–69.

Jenny, J.L. (1987) Knowledge deficit: Not a nursing diagnosis. *Image: Journal of Nursing Scholarship,* 19(4), 184–185.

Johnson, D.E. (1959) The nature of a science of nursing. *Nursing Outlook,* 7(5), 291–294.

Kasch, C. (1984) Interpersonal competence and communication in the delivery of nursing care. *Advances in Nursing Science,* 6(2), 71–88.

Kim, M.J. (1985, March) Without collaboration, what's left? *American Journal of Nursing,* 85(3), 281–284.

Kim, M.J. (1989) Nursing diagnosis. *Annual Review of Nursing Research,* 7, 117–142.

Kritek, P.B. (1978) The generation and classification of nursing diagnoses: Toward a theory of nursing. *Image: Journal of Nursing Scholarship,* 10(2), 33–40.

Kritek, P.B. (1979) Commentary: The development of nursing diagnosis and theory. *Advances in Nursing Science,* 2(1), 73–79.

Kritek, P.B. (1985) Nursing diagnosis in perspective: Response to a critique. *Image: Journal of Nursing Scholarship,* 17(1), 3–8.

Laudan, L. (1981) A problem solving approach to scientific growth. In I. Hacking (Ed.), *Scientific revolutions.* Oxford, UK: Oxford University Press.

McBride, A.B. (1986, September) Theory and research. *Journal of Psychosocial Nursing,* 24(9), 27–32.

McManus, R.L. (1950) Assumptions of functions of nursing. In *Regional planning for nurses and nursing education.* New York: Bureau of Publications. Teachers College, Columbia University.

Meleis, A.I. and Jennings, B.M. (1989) Theoretical nursing administration: Today's challenges, tomorrow's bridges. In B. Henry, C. Arndt, M. Di Vincenti and A. Marriner-Tomey (Eds.), *Dimensions of nursing administration: Theory, research, education, practice.* Boston: Blackwell Scientific Publications.

Meleis, A.I. and Price, M.J. (1988) Strategies and conditions for teaching theoretical nursing: An international perspective. *Journal of Advanced Nursing,* 13, 592–604.

Merton, R.K. (1973) *The sociology of science: Theoretical and empirical investigations.* Chicago: University of Chicago Press.

Russell, B. (1957) The world's need for wisdom. *Wisdom: The Magazine for Knowledge for all America*, 14, 29.

Schlotfeldt, R.M. (1988) Structuring nursing knowledge: A priority for creating nursing's future. *Nursing Science Quarterly*, 1(1), 35–38.

Shamansky, S.L. and Yanni, C.R. (1983) In opposition to nursing diagnosis: A minority opinion. *Image: Journal of Nursing Scholarship*, 15(2), 47–50.

Shaver, J. (1985) A biopsychosocial view of human health. *Nursing Outlook*, 33(4), 186–1101.

Visintainer, M. (1988) The nature of knowledge and theory in nursing. *Image: Journal of Nursing Scholarship*, 18(2), 32–38.

Wilson, H.S. (1985) *Research in nursing.* Menlo Park, CA: Addison-Wesley.

Part 7

Our Theoretical Literature

*L*iterature in nursing is rich with writings in theory, of theory, and on theory. Some of the writings provided significant milestones in the shaping of the theoretical progress in nursing. The last two chapters in this book are organized around these writings. They provide an analytical review of the central literature in metatheory and theory up to the beginning of the 1980s as well as a comprehensive bibliography up to the beginning of the 1990s.

These chapters are offered for students, faculty, clinicians, and researchers. The serious theory student needs analytical familiarity with the significant writing that shaped the progress in the discipline of nursing. The cursory theory student can find these chapters helpful as an overview of the writing related to nursing theory. Everyone concerned with the discipline of nursing will find that the literature relates, in some way, to their specific area of expertise. This literature is a significant component of our heritage without which our practice, teaching, and research are limited.

Chapter *18*

Analysis of Theoretical Writing in Nursing

To develop, analyze, or critique theories, a theory student, utilizer, or developer needs a background that includes all the significant writings related to theoretical nursing. This chapter provides the reader with a critical assessment of the central writing contained in the nursing literature of the 1980s. With the publication of *Advances in Nursing Science*, as well as other theoretically oriented journals and books, theory literature has developed and proliferated exponentially, and it is therefore no longer possible to include a comprehensive critical assessment of writings in theory. As many as possible of the writings up to the early 1980s that are considered classic in theory are included in this chapter.

The chapter is divided into two sections. **Section I** includes analysis and critique of the metatheory literature. **Section II** includes analysis and critique of the literature on nursing theory, written by the nurse theorists or by others who have used the nursing theory in research, practice, education, and administration. All analytical abstracts are listed alphabetically within the two sections.

There are many ways a reader could use this chapter: *first*, the reader can use it in conjunction with the contents of various chapters in the book; *second*, when studying a particular theorist's work, the reader can identify citations related to the theorist and can pull out those that have been abstracted for review; *third*, Section I could be read in its entirety as a way to prepare for a general overview of nursing theory; *fourth*, the reader can divide the writings in Section II into those relating to a particular theorist in order to read the abstracts related to each theorist separately; and *fifth*, readers interested in the development of theoretical nursing may wish to have a temporal perspective by reading abstracts according to year of citation.

The intent of the abstracts is to challenge readers to different interpretations and not to critique the writing. *Readers are encouraged to read original writings and to use these analytical abstracts only to provide them with one perspective of the writings.* Finally, the reader should remember that the analyses here include the interpretation of the authors who abstracted them, which may or may not agree with others' interpretations.

Section I
ABSTRACTS OF WRITINGS
IN METATHEORY, 1960–1984

Ellen Mahoney and Afaf Meleis

Abdellah, F.G. (1969) The nature of nursing science. *Nursing Research*, 18(5), 390–393.

This article seeks to move toward the "identification of a nursing science." History is reviewed, and nursing scientists are exhorted to build on the work of nurse pioneers who were mainly theorists. Nursing science is defined as a body of cumulative scientific knowledge (drawn from the physical, biological, and behavioral sciences) that is uniquely nursing. Emphasis is on an evolving science. The more that nursing research is directed by scientific theory, the more likely its results will contribute to the development of a nursing science. There are too few nursing scientists (should be 1%), but the numbers are growing. "It is the inescapable role of the nurse-scientist to point the way for change in nursing."

This is a short overview article, but it contains details of nursing history and random observations of interest.

Andreoli, K.G. and Thompson, C.E. (1977) The nature of science in nursing. *Image*, 9(2), 32–37.

The theoretical basis of practice is the science of nursing, and it defines nursing's uniqueness. Science is defined as a system of knowledge based on scientific principles. It's ultimate goal is the discovery of new knowledge, the expansion of existing knowledge, and the reaffirmation of previously held knowledge. Nursing is defined by abstracting the major elements from the conceptions of several nursing theorists. Science in nursing (the body of verified knowledge found within the discipline of nursing) is distinguished from the science of nursing (that body of verifiable knowledge that will be derived from nursing practice, the unique way in which nursing utilizes borrowed knowledge). Nursing will attain the status of a science once it has clearly identified a verifiable knowledge base that can be contested and corroborated. This knowledge base will come from practice. Specific attention is given to the scientific methodologies of nursing research, conceptual models in nursing, the nursing process, and nursing diagnosis as a means of developing a knowledge base.

The fact that the article offers more than the others in the category is an interesting argument for the integration of basic and applied science and the sections on scientific methodologies in nursing that stress the theory–practice–research link. One might argue that the "unique" elements of nursing presented are really not so unique. The definition of "science" comes from the dictionary; the conceptions of nursing science presented (especially by Johnson and Rogers) should be read in the original.

Batey, M.V. (1972) Values relative to research and to science in nursing as influenced by a sociological perspective. *Nursing Research*, 21(6), 504–508.

Central to the development of a science of nursing is the continuing issue of the function of values in research and in science. This article is a response to the question: How does preparation in one of the disciplines related to nursing bear upon the identification and conceptualization of nursing research problems and approaches used to design and carry through an investigation? Batey's response is organized in three topics: (1) an overview of her conceptual and methodological orientation in sociology; (2) illustrations of the research in her work; and (3) contrasting perspectives of science with thought geared toward nursing science. It is to the third topic that the abstract is addressed.

Research is a tool of science; the goal of science is the continuing advancement of an objective body of knowledge. Batey contrasts two perspectives of science: (1) as a social system with values (expressed) as the desired goal toward which science strives (*i.e.*, an advancing and objectively verified body of knowledge), *norms* (expected standards of behavior, including disinterest, organized skepticism, and communality) and *parteined relations* (the expectation of a competent response to one's creative effort); versus (2) as a means (knowledge for use). An investigator's perspective will influence types of research problems identified as well as the selection of knowledge brought to bear for their conceptualization and research methodologies. In nursing, where knowledge is valued for its use, (perspective 2) it is hypothesized that there is a greater emphasis on descriptive studies than on the subsequent stages of the discovery process toward an objectively verified body of knowledge. Until we alter our normative system in nursing relative to science, we can expect little movement toward nursing science.

Whereas a major thrust of the article focuses on the dilemma of conflicting values for nurses educated in other fields, the section "Perspectives of Science" (pp. 507–508) is provocative and well worth reading, particularly after exposure to explications of nursing science and arguments for practice theory. Does the reader agree with Batey's hypothesis that a discipline emphasizing knowledge for use will emphasize descriptive research?

Batey, M.V. (1977) Conceptualization: Knowledge and logic guiding empirical research. *Nursing Research*, 26(5), 324–329.

This is an excellent article analyzing functions and processes of research conceptualization. Analyzing a systematic sample of articles published in *Nursing Research*, Batey identified "limiting features" representing problems of: (1) the *conceptual phase* ("fallacies of reasoning, specification of meaning, and use of knowledge in conveying the problem, conceptual framework, and/or purpose"); (2) the *empirical phase* ("technical processes related to the methods and procedures of data production and reduction"); and (3) the *interpretative phase* ("analytical processes related to deriving meanings of findings"). Batey judged that the vast majority of problems are due to limitations of the conceptual phase, particularly the lack of clear definition and inadequate development or utilization of a conceptual framework. Factors contributing to conceptual limitations are identified, as are their consequences.

The remainder of the paper is an explication of the conceptual phase of research in order to achieve a reduction of the limitations noted. Components of the conceptual phase are as follows: (1) The *problem* determines the context of the study by setting the major parameters of the phenomenon of concern; it includes what, how, why, or under what conditions phenomena occur, and a normative statement; (2) the *conceptual framework* involves background knowledge that delineates the present knowledge state about the problem and that yields the theoretical statement through which the investigator attempts to construct an accurate image of the phenomenon of study; it includes background (review of literature) and rationale (theoretical framework); and (3) the *purpose* is derived from the rationale; the research purpose is the hypothesis to be tested.

The article also includes brief but helpful sections on purposes and methods for literature review, scientific versus common sense meanings of concepts, tips on critical reading, and guidelines for the interpretative phase and its dynamic relation to conceptualization.

There is some overlap and lack of clarity in defining the three components of the conceptual phase, and it would have been appropriate to explicate more on the theoretical background of a study. This article should be read in the context of other articles that address conceptualization and conceptual frameworks. Besides tying these phases together, this article provides useful criteria for the design and evaluation of research.

Becker, C.H. (1983) A conceptualization of concept. *Nursing papers: Perspectives in Nursing,* 15(2), 51–58.

The first part of this article is a series of lists. The first list has to do with characteristics of concepts: ambiguity, conventional meaning, dependent on context, neither false nor true, and either significant or nonsignificant. The author inserts an observation: "Concepts arise in the mind of an individual as a result of attempts to make order out of what is observed."

The next list describes modes of concept analysis (from Edel, 1979): Socratic (general and essential), element analysis, genetic (how evolved), functional, systems, pragmatic, logical, operational, phenomenological. A summary list gives the requirements for an appropriate use of concepts in theory development: "(1) concepts have intention; (2) concepts are seen as models of some aspect of reality; (3) the concepts selected are significant; (4) the mode of concept analysis dictates the method of investigation of the concept; (5) the value bias and semantic overtones are inherently present in the concepts selected for study; and (6) concepts are subject to continual analysis and refinement."

Then, micro-concepts are endorsed: "micro-concepts rather than general macro-concepts may have the potential to contribute more to the structuring of nursing knowledge." An example is given: self-esteem (micro) versus personality (macro). The author presents the following reasoning: "Macro-concepts, because of their generalness, have a loose flexibility of meaning. Micro-concepts would not allow this looseness." There are also fewer variables in micro-level concepts: (1) the intention of the author is easily understood; (2) meaning is not so easily distorted; (3) the most appropriate mode of analysis is easily identified; and (4) there is not polarity.

Beckstrand, J. (1978) The notion of a practice theory and the relationship of scientific and ethical knowledge to practice. *Research in Nursing and Health*, 1(3), 131–136.

Beckstrand critiques several authors who have supported a "practice theory" (Dickoff and James, Jacox, etc.). For such notions to be meaningful, practice knowledge must be shown to be different from scientific knowledge or ethical knowledge, or else "no need for a separate practice theory would exist." Two primary aspects of practice knowledge, the knowledge of how to make changes and the knowledge of what is "good" are examined. First *science*, "the knowledge of lawlike empirical relationships," is studied to determine if it includes the knowledge used to control phenomena in practice. Beckstrand provides an extended summary discussion of the nature of scientific knowledge, relating it to the notion of "control." "The potential for controlling a phenomenon is synonymous with lawlike relationships and the potential for prediction that they provide . . . . Science seeks to establish the knowledge that allows for this kind of control." To make changes one must have some control. Although practice often seeks this control through invalid argument, "functional argument," and empirical generalization, these are "based on the knowledge of scientific laws and lawlike relationships." The controls possible in scientific experimentation are impossible in the practice situation, but despite uncertainty of outcome, practice methodology nonetheless proceeds by valid deduction from scientific laws.

Next is a review of the field of ethics. Ethics is concerned with the knowledge of what is right, good, or obligatory. Both normative ethics and metaethics have relevance to practice. But theories of the moral obligations of practitioners "are identical in form" to other theories of moral obligation; theories of moral value in practice do not represent unique forms of theory. The goals defined in practice are not moral values that may be determined by the methods of ethical philosophy and no others. In short, "it would appear that there is no need for a practice theory distinct from a scientific or ethical theory."

The bulk of the article is Beckstrand's reading in the philosophy of science and ethical theory. Her more abbreviated attempts to apply these readings to Dickoff and colleagues are dependent on crucial unargued and unevidenced assertions. For example, (1) the relation of "practice knowledge," (Beckstrand's term) to "practice theory," which is the focus of the authors she surveys), after all, to have a theory of teaching is not to have the knowledge to teach a course in Russian history; (2) the assertion that practice knowledge can be broken down into two generalizations— "how to make changes" and "what is good"—without oversimplification or distortion; and (3) the assertion that unscientific reasoning and procedures are "based" on scientific reasoning and procedures. Although Beckstrand argues that the knowledge on which practice is based is science-knowledge, she admits outright that the reasoning process in practice is often unscientific, and she ignores experience, tradition, or even nonscientific logic as bases.

Beckstrand emphasizes what might be called "content" with regard to science and practice theory (*i.e.*, concern only for the knowledge in science and practice and not the reasoning processes, and concern only for just what information, basically, is used in it and not for the descriptive shape of the activity, its form, nor its outline-definition). Beckstrand reverses herself when discussing ethics, saying that although there may be specific ethical obligations or directives especially and uniquely applicable to a practice, the form of the theory is that of an ethical theory. Might one not ask her then, why a theory of practice (although the information used in it may well be the same as ethics and science) cannot remain unique because its shape and its form is that of a practice theory?

Beckstrand, J. (1978) The need for a practice theory as indicated by the knowledge used in the conduct of practice. *Research in Nursing and Health*, 1(4), 175–179.

Beckstrand's aim is to extend her previous argument. Her first article said that "much of the knowledge required for practice is the knowledge of science and ethics." Here, she "examines" practice to see if "the theoretical knowledge used in practice is completely defined by science, ethics, and logic." To determine this, she turns to the definition of the purpose of practice: "Practice attempts to *change* an entity or phenomenon in such a way that a greater good is realized." Accomplishing change in practice necessitates the knowledge of both change and action. This knowledge can be reduced to limited categorization, but Beckstrand broadens the base of necessary knowledge here to include "the domain of logic in general."

Following this is the logical analysis of the conduct of practice. First, she discusses conditions. She asserts that "[t]o say that an interaction is meaningful is to say that the interaction has logical implications in relation to existing scientific or ethical knowledge." She argues that although the combination of conditions in each situation can draw on infinite numbers for infinite variance, and that because the "human potential" to perceive or the "personal knowledge" of the practitioner are limited, only a finite number of conditions are attended to or identified, and they are identified in a way "most dependent on the practitioner's scientific and ethical knowledge."

Next under the rubric of "description" of the conduct of practice, Beckstrand discusses values and goals. She restates that the goal of practice is change toward the greater good. Determination of this greater good depends on the values of the practice discipline, values that "reflect normative ethical theories." A practitioner sometimes accepts a hierarchy of values "implicitly and uncritically, but these hierarchies and their implementation represent ethical decisions." She concludes that the knowledge of practice "depends not on some special aspects of practice, but on science and ethics alone."

Immediately in her introduction, Beckstrand, without calling attention to it, puts forward two new factors missing from her first article: "theoretical knowledge" presumably now will bridge her pass from "theory" to "knowledge" (whereas this formulation does not appear at all in her first essay, it is seen three times in this introduction to her second), and "logic" is added (again, without comment) to science and ethics, to subsume practice theory. One might hypothesize that these additions reflect a reaction to criticism (her own or that of others) of the first piece, and therefore that problems are to be addressed. The body of the article never again mentions "theoretical knowledge" but instead substitutes "knowledge" alone, as in the first essay. What is more, as she freely interchanges "theoretical knowledge used in practice" with "knowledge used in practice" one may deduce a confusion in the use of the concept "theoretical." What of the goal to maintain health *against* changes?

In addition, it would have been helpful if Beckstrand had considered, even as an error to be refuted, that a theory of nursing might be as relevant to "nursing ethics" as a theory of ethics. Finally, her conclusion forgets her introduction and its specificities of "theoretical" and "logic." "Thus, the knowledge of practice depends not on some special aspects of practice, but on science and ethics alone." Both articles are thought to be provoking and central readings in metatheory.

Beckstrand, J. (1980) A critique of several conceptions of practice theory in nursing. *Research in Nursing and Health*, 3, 69–79.

Although the title and summary suggest a survey of ideas about "practice theory," half of this article (roughly five pages) is devoted to what Beckstrand characterizes as the "set of rules" conception of practice theory, which she attributes to Ada Jacox. Other writers, most notably Dickoff, James, and Wiedenbach, who provide the opening focus of the essay, are given remarkably short shrift. The initial section, "The notion of Dickoff *et al.*," attempts to explain their notion, mixing restatement of their formulations with a series of asserted exemplifications of what they mean: "the articulation of the conceptual frameworks . . . practitioners actually use"; "in changing a flat tire a practice theory is being employed"; an identity between their notions and "technology" (*i.e.*, "the totality of a plan of action used to bring about a goal that is presumed desirable").

The big interest for Beckstrand is Jacox (1974). Jacox's is presented as an incorrect interpretation of Dickoff *et al.*—incorrect because Beckstrand appears to interpret Dickoff and James' position in terms of each practitioner having her own practice theory formula. Jacox, according to Beckstrand, suggests a rigid, compulsion-carrying deck of directives, which one shuffles on each occasion to find the right rules of procedure. Nurses are "compelled to conform . . . to a set of rules imposed by an external authority." Under this conception, "prescriptive practice theory becomes a set of universally prescribed rules for practice."

Following this is the longest section of the essay (by far)—an attack on the Jacox position so characterized. Beckstrand produces a discussion of ethics intended to demonstrate that you cannot prescribe a goal without making an unjustifiable value judgment. Then she makes a series of "practical arguments." Prescriptions cannot take into account all the variables in a given situation. Sometimes, two prescriptions will come into conflict. The practitioner will be forced to make an "arbitrary" decision between them. She takes time to "demonstrate" that you could not have a prescription specific to every situation. She responds to objections by saying that, even under such a theory, scientific and ethical judgment would still be required. Granted this, Beckstrand asserts that the change would be nil. She argues that such a theory will not be valuable in the education of practitioners because she has already shown it is not valuable in practice. Nursing-education does not involve prescriptions of this kind, because those in education "are not imperatives carrying sanctions for their adoption or violation." Sets of rules for practice are no aid in research because "as prescriptions, they imply no deductively derivable empirically true or false consequences (predictions)."

Other notions of practice theory are briefly examined. Conceptual frameworks of nursing, such as Roy's or Jones' "are not scientific theories but ideologies" because they are "legitimately alterable on the sole basis of personal or public discretion." Beckstrand also differs with those (like Peterson) who wish to try to delineate the bounds of nursing inquiry. In theory development and in research, you do not know *a priori* what is relevant, rather, you let the characterizations and categorizations emerge and evolve from the situation.

In this article, Beckstrand provides a unique interpretation of Dickoff and colleagues and of Jacox. Although the problem with Dickoff *et al.* inevitably represents some difficulties with their exposition, most attempts like this at reduction can be problematic (as they dismiss and refute such approaches in their 1975 article) simply because they fail to include all the elements Dickoff, James, and Wiedenbach insist on (*i.e.*, a conceptual framework with built-in goal orientation, prescriptions, and a survey list). The set of rules theory attributed to Jacox also has some flaws. We would assume that Jacox would argue that her proposed system is not intended to be a straightjacket and that provisions for "breaking" rules are made. Beckstrand's arguments against Jacox would seem to apply to any attempts to teach practice, or to any potential contributions from research. She sees the possibility of this objection: "one might argue that if a prescriptive practice theory of the set-of-rules type cannot be justified, then no decision can be made about what to do in practice."

As to her paragraph on metatheory, first, under Carnap's definition, all theories of nursing are metatheories. Second, after all these attempts to discredit practice theory, she says that if you will call it metatheory, it is okay, and Dickoff and colleagues' may be considered a beginning (and worthy) metatheory of nursing practice. Beckstrand notes that because Dickoff and colleagues "did not fully explicate or formalize their theory," they have only offered "undeveloped ideas." Dickoff *et al.*, of course, do not have a theory. (That is to say, they do not have a "practice theory.") These appear to be unfortunate mix-ups. Despite our analytical arguments, we consider Beckstrand's writing stimulating, challenging, and an absolute must for a theory student.

Benoliel, J.Q. (1977) The interaction between theory and research. *Nursing Outlook,* 25(2), 108–113.

This essay explores relationships between theory and research as reciprocal elements in an ongoing process through which scientific knowledge relevant to nursing is created, expanded, tested, and refined. Practice can serve as a stimulus to research and can therefore form part of the cyclical process. There is also a brief section on sources of knowledge in nursing.

This is a simple account of the "constantly flowing interchange between the realities of practice, theory development, and scientific investigation." The inductive/deductive cycle is demonstrated, as is an example of building a body of knowledge by the "application of different philosophical approaches to the study of a particular human phenomenon." Better "sources of knowledge" include Rogers, Carper, and Beckstrand.

Berthold, J.S. (1968) Prologue: Symposium on theory development in nursing. *Nursing Research*, 17(3), 196–197.

According to the author, no substantive definition of "theory" can be applied with any generality due to the ambiguity and complexity of the concept "theory." Differential use of terms necessitates clear understanding of their use to avoid semantic confusion and to allow for attention to the substance of various positions.

In this introduction to the Symposium, Berthold states: "The questions . . . involve a discussion of various positions about and approaches to developing a conceptual structure of knowledge useful and necessary to attain the goals established by nurses." In elaborating on this statement, the author stresses: thought processes that result in theoretical constructs, ordered in a systematic way; knowledge that is verified; theory that is useful in stimulating new observations and insights and in generating propositions concerning relevant events; and goals that are established and controlled by nurses for nursing.

This is a brief overview that succinctly captures the major issues, questions, and debates about nursing theory development addressed in the Symposium. (See articles by Schrag, Crowley, Folta, and Brown, as well as Panel Discussion).

Brown, M.I. (1964) Research on the development of nursing theory: The importance of a theoretical framework in nursing research. *Nursing Research*, 13(2), 109–112.

Two major questions are addressed: (1) How far have we progressed through research toward the development of an integrated body of nursing theory? and (2) How can we determine if a research project has a theoretical framework that will make possible a contribution to scientific knowledge? Sections of the paper include: the need for nursing theory, concept validation through research, and assessing the theoretical framework of a research project. A research project that contributes to nursing theory can be identified by certain characteristics, such as: an aim to pursue knowledge for its own sake, the statement of the relationship of the problem to research and nursing literature, the use of established meaningful terms, the association of findings to the work of others, and the logical but creative exposition of implications and further hypotheses for testing.

This early, easy-to-read article is a brief reminder of the theory/research symbiosis. The article emphasizes rationale rather than criteria for selecting theoretical frameworks. Would Brown's conclusions be different if this article was written in the 1980s?

Brown, M.I. (1968) Theory development in nursing: Social theory in geriatric nursing research. *Nursing Research*, 17(3), 213–217.

This is an exemplification of Brown's theme—the nature of nursing research and its relation to theory formation. The article is a descriptive account of the use of the concept of socialization in a gerontological research project.

Although Brown asks how theories of the basic and other applied sciences relate to nursing research, her response stresses problems intrinsic to the theories. Other authors (see especially Klein, Crawford, and Johnson *et al.*) emphasize the implications of "borrowing" theories formulated in other disciplines. The article is part of the 1968 Symposium on Theory Development in Nursing.

Brown, M.L. (1983) Research questions and answers: The use of theory and conceptual frameworks in nursing research and practice. *Oncology Nursing Forum*, 10(2), 111–112.

The author presents an initial distinction: "A theory explains the nature of phenomena and a conceptual framework identifies what variables are important." Both are important to "identify, categorize, and expand nursing knowledge in an organized and thoughtful way. A catalog of notions of theory is then offered. The author summarizes: "Theory, then, helps identify the research problem, defines . . . appropriate evidence . . . and determines methods to obtain, organize, and integrate information."

In dealing with conceptual frameworks, on the other hand, the author simply presents a definition: "A conceptual framework is an organized grouping of ideas or concepts that assists in providing overall structure to the research project and the nursing process."

The author follows Derdiarian's delineation of the need for order and systematization in nursing research, education, and practice. Finally, she cites Marino's conceptual framework for cancer nursing.

This article is actually a columnist's response to a question by readers about the terms "theory" and "conceptual framework." More elaborate and somewhat different presentations are available elsewhere in the literature.

Burgess, G. (1978) The personal development of the nursing student as a conceptual framework. *Nursing Forum*, 17(1), 96–102.

Burgess proposes "personal development" of the student nurse as a conceptual framework in professional nursing education. Rationales are presented (enhanced potential for professional effectiveness; improved quality of care; criteria for retention of students) as well as means of operationalizing personal development (ability to articulate goals and philosophy and to evaluate accomplishments and needs; change in attitudes; increased sensitivity to others).

A conceptual framework is defined, by analogy, as a unifying central theme that provides the mechanism for articulating and relating all parts of the curriculum. Course objectives are the means of providing attachment to the central theme, and the courses themselves (content plus learning experiences) are "free to respond to currents of movement and creative expression," while maintaining their attachment to the central theme.

The proposed conceptual framework provides a provocative, if controversial, alternative to more common subject or process-oriented curricula. The major value of this article however, is its simple, yet creative and very helpful explanation of the characteristics and purposes of the conceptual framework and its emphasis on the need to operationalize concepts.

Bush, H.A. (1979) Models for nursing. *Advances in Nursing Science.* 1(2), 13–21.

This article examines types of models, the relationship between models and theories, and the use of models in nursing research, education, and practice.

Models provide a means for ordering, clarifying, and analyzing concepts and their relationships; they provide analogs to reality and stimulate the scientific process by identifying new possibilities. A model primarily expresses structure, whereas a theory provides substance. Models used in nursing must represent the ordered reality of focus on human beings, their environment, their health, and nursing itself (*i.e.*, isomorphic). Models are used: (1) in research, to conceptualize the research process itself and to facilitate thinking about concepts and their relationships; (2) in education, to guide curricula planning; and (3) in practice, to guide assessment, intervention, and evaluation.

This article provides a good summary of types of models and their purposes in nursing. More pragmatic information on the development of models may be found in Jacox and McKay.

Carper, B.A. (1978) Fundamental patterns of knowing in nursing. *Advances in Nursing Science*, 1(1), 13–23.

A classification of the patterns of knowledge in nursing is presented here. The article addresses the question: "What kinds of knowledge are most valuable to the discipline of nursing?" Answers are meant to provide: (1) perspective and significance to the discipline; (2) awareness of the complexity and diversity of nursing knowledge; and (3) an operational definition of nursing.

Four patterns of knowing are identified:

1. *Empirical* (the science of nursing). The science of nursing is in a healthy but embryonic stage; theoretical models are presenting new perspectives.
2. *Aesthetics* (the art of nursing). Aesthetics is achieved by empathy, "dynamic integration" of parts into the whole, and the recognition of particulars versus universals.
3. *Personal Knowledge.* Personal knowledge is concerned with the quality of interpersonal contacts, promoting therapeutic relationships, and individualized care.
4. *Ethics* (the moral component) "What ought to be done." Each individual pattern of knowing is necessary, but not sufficient, for achieving the goals of nursing. It is their interrelationship that defines the whole. These patterns provide structure and boundaries, dictate subject matter for nursing education, and,

together, represent a complete approach to the problems and
questions of the discipline of nursing.

The reader of this article should consider several points. The "Aesthetics of
Nursing" section appears to confuse knowledge with action ("a science teaches us
to know, and an art to do") and blurs distinctions between intuition, perception,
instinct, and what we more ordinarily call knowledge. Perhaps most important, the
identification of aesthetic with *empathy* loses any sense of clear distinction between this and her third category, described as "acceptance." In this case, Carper is
rejecting an approach to the client as an "object," and is rejecting establishing
"authentic personal relationships."

In addition, the "Ethics of Nursing" obscures a major oversight of this paper
(something emphasized by Donaldson and Crowley)—that nursing involves history
and philosophy as well as science and art. The delineation of goals, principles, and
values and of the hierarchies among these that are specific to nursing are the
continuing products of nursing experience and of thought in nursing that is broadly
theoretical. The value of this article lies in its provision of a broader perspective of
nursing knowledge than has been previously presented in the literature.

Chapman, C.M. (1976) The use of sociological theories and models in nursing. *Journal of Advanced Nursing*, 1, 111–127.

Theory development has not kept pace with expanding roles in nursing and does
not support nursing actions. Nursing and sociology are similarly defined as interactive processes between individuals, and the author therefore suggests the potential
contribution of sociological theories and models to the development of nursing
theory.

Social exchange theory is proposed to explain how patients and nurses satisfy
their own needs and goals, and organizational theories are considered in the context
of their effect on goal achievement, communication, and compliance. Concluding
remarks stress that: (1) borrowed theories must be validated in the new situation,
and (2) theories in the behavioral sciences can describe and explain more accurately than they can predict due to the variability in human behavior.

The bulk of this article focuses on the effects of organizational structure on
nurse roles and behaviors in the United Kingdom. The reader might question
comparisons between nursing and sociology and assumptions about nurses and
patients. The article emphasizes theories related to the delivery of care and the
development of nursing theory that would support clinical practice. Whereas the
ideas presented in the conclusions are important, their development is somewhat
limited.

Chinn, P.L. and Jacobs, M.K. (1978) A model of theory development in nursing. *Advances in Nursing Science*, 1(1), 1–11.

The process of theory development is a means of facilitating the evolution of
nursing science, and is the most critical task facing the nursing profession. Theory is
defined as "an internally consistent body of relational statements about phenomena

which is useful for prediction and control." Conceptual frameworks are presented as less-developed theoretical statements allowing description and explanation.

The model of theory development contains four separate but interrelated components: (1) examination and analysis of concepts; (2) formulation and testing of relational statements; (3) theory construction; and (4) practical application of theory. These components may be differentiated by the nature of the operations involved: cognitive (1 and 3); empirical (2 and 4); and by their functions: description and explanation (1 and 2); prediction and control (3 and 4). As a whole, the model demonstrates, "how different types of research yield varying types of products, each contributing to the total development of the science." Also included in the model are boundaries that delimit areas of nursing concern, while allowing free exchange of content and processes among sciences, and a central core denoting the influence of history on theory development in nursing. The importance of the theory–practice linkage and the dynamic and contextual nature of the process of theory development are emphasized.

Two major arguments are developed: (1) "The process of theory development has greater value for nursing than the product"; and (2) the emphasis in theory development should be prediction and control. These positions should be contrasted with authors who emphasize the preliminary importance of descriptive and explanatory theories, the importance of the "product" for building a science of nursing, and the guiding influence of a clear conception of nursing.

Clark, J. (1982) Development of models and theories on the concept of nursing. *Journal of Advanced Nursing*, 7(2), 129–134.

This article aims to show that models and theories in nursing have "practical value for the ordinary clinical nurse." One must relate theoretical work to what nurses actually do, built around concepts that can be operationalized. The failure to do this explains "the relative lack of impact on nursing practice . . . of the work in theory development undertaken in recent years."

Clark presents a "simple model of nursing." The model is a "gross simplification," but deliberately so, as more elaborate models are less universal. Often, models do not easily fit all fields of nursing.

How can such a model help the ordinary practicing nurse? (1) It purports explicitly that there is something called "nursing" that has an identity of its own ("versus those who still see nursing merely as a collection of tasks undertaken on the initiative of . . . doctors"), (2) it stresses the reciprocity of the nurse–patient relationship and the significance of environment, and (3) it stresses cause and effect relationships; "considerably more attention must be paid than in the past to outcomes of nursing care."

The remainder of the article is an application to her own situation. Clark demonstrates by considering her own nursing care in light of the model.

More popularizing than theory or scholarship, the article provides a role model of informal, thoughtful, and conscious practice, and does a good job of presenting serious ideas in attractive and readily understandable ways. It is a well-written example of what it argues—relating scholarship in nursing to practice, making it available to "consumers." It is a soft-sell for theory-based practice and is quite effective.

Cleland, V.S. (1967) The use of existing theories. *Nursing Research,* 16(2), 118–121.

Theory serves two major functions: as a tool, it gives direction to empirical investigation; as a goal, it tends to abstract, summarize, and order research findings. The goal function of theory, which is the basis for progression of science, has been less adequately used in nursing. The functional method of research, which begins with a significant problem or question and then searches for relevant theoretical formulations, enables the nurse researcher to take advantage of advances made in other disciplines, while ensuring nursing relevance. It permits the researcher to work inductively from existing empirical data and deductively from other theoretical formulations. An example of this is given to illustrate the inherent limitation of research that has no theoretical framework (and, of course, the superiority of one that does).

This rationale for conceptual frameworks is similar to others on the subject, and may be contrasted with the "grounded" approach (see Quint). Although the authors in this group of articles agree on the values of a framework, consider the integral relationship of this section and the one on theory critique.

Collaizzi, J. (1975) The proper object of nursing science. *International Journal of Nursing Studies,* 12(4), 197–200.

The beginning of a science should be a philosophical inquiry into its appropriate domain. In initiating a science of nursing, considerable theoretical ambiguity has resulted from the assumption that nursing science is synthetic. Although we have amassed a body of scientific findings (that can be properly called health technology), what we have failed to do is circumscribe that which is uniquely nursing. Although nursing takes place within both technical and existential dimensions, the proper object of nursing science is the human experience of health and illness. Therefore, the research methods of human science, rather than those of natural science, must be used to investigate the questions that arise within this (existential) dimension.

This article offers an intelligent support of prevalent and influential conceptions of nursing science that emerged in the 1980s.

Collins, R.J. and Fielder, J.H. (1981) Beckstrand's concept of practice theory: A critique. *Research in Nursing and Health,* 4(3), 317–321.

The authors find two major flaws in Beckstrand's analysis. First, they attack her claim that "the knowledge nurses need to effect changes is scientific knowledge." Specifically, they follow Toulmin's suggestion that there is a "plurality of different types of medical knowledge," and they quickly collapse it into two "modes." Beckstrand has overlooked or ignored the subjective, the knowledge of the particular, "knowing the client as a particular human being." Several of the authors' statements on this issue are memorable: "The role of the nurse and the biographer are similar; both must turn their attention to knowing individuals in all of the uniqueness and particularity. . . . The nurse's role is perhaps closer to that of the priest, intimate friend, or therapist—seeking not only knowledge of the individual but also the person's well-being. Understanding is not the primary goal, but a way of becoming an effective adviser and advocate for the person's interest."

Second, there are moral issues in nursing that will not be resolved by appeal to ethics but are specific to nursing. The authors point to activities or goals that are not obligatory but that are praiseworthy; these are characterized as, "[M]oral ideal. . . . The questions of which, if any, moral ideals an individual pursues is not answered by an ethical theory. The theory may be used to justify an ideal as a moral ideal, but the choice of which ones to pursue must flow from an individual's concept of what kind of life the person wishes to lead. . . . The profession of nursing has only recently emerged from the role of being the physician's handmaiden and is now in the process of defining itself as a profession in its own right, embodying certain moral ideals. Just what those ideals should be is one of the major elements of a practice theory."

This is an interesting, analytical article. It nicely adjusts and fills out Beckstrand's work, without any excessive negativity. It is a good example of the sense of a shared enterprise: Beckstrand is a colleague whose work is to be built on.

Crawford, G., Dufault, S.K., and Rudy, E. (1979) Evolving issues in theory development. *Nursing Outlook*, 27(5), 346–351.

This review of nursing theory literature addresses issues in historical perspective: Is nursing theory borrowed or unique? Is nursing a basic or applied science? Should there be theories *of* nursing or *for* practice? What are the approaches to theory development? The purpose of the article is to redefine these issues in light of Donaldson and Crowley's article.

A strong bias for unique, practice-oriented, "situation-producing" theories is presented. Problems of borrowing are presented (*e.g.*, lack of isomorphism). Authors agree with Johnson that the nature of knowledge required for nursing will foster theory development that is unique to nursing.

As defined in the 1968 nursing science conference, basic science supports knowledge for its own sake, whereas applied science demonstrates knowledge with practical aims and applications. Donaldson and Crowley present the need to increase understanding of phenomena (basic), demonstrate applicability of basic knowledge in real situations (applied), and explain how to utilize knowledge to achieve goals in practice (prescriptive theory). Together, these comprise nursing science.

Regarding the issue of theory *of nursing* (delineation of definition and scope of or about nursing and the nursing process) versus *for practice* (conceptualizations guiding nursing action to achieve desired goals), these authors address the question of unified versus diverse theories, supporting Jacox's "middle-range theories." It is possible that they confuse "unified theory" with the values of a theoretical framework. The complexities of the arguments for and against unified and diverse theories are not addressed.

This approach to theory development lends support to inductive, deductive, historical, and philosophical methods. Theories should be developed to generate new knowledge and to organize knowledge about the discipline of nursing (supporting Donaldson and Crowley). The author states McKay's questions about which methods are most appropriate and what are criteria for acceptance of findings. She also supports Stevens' advice to ask the significant questions and only then to seek appropriate research methodologies.

This article provides a good overview of critical issues in nursing theory development from a historical perspective. While one is attempting to resolve these issues, the complexities of the arguments and contrasting positions are not always fully addressed, precluding comprehensive, definitive resolution. Nevertheless, this article is a good synthesis of supporting positions and contains an excellent bibliography on theory development in nursing.

Dickoff, J. and James, P. (1968) Researching research's role in theory development. *Nursing Research*, 17(3), 204–205.

Research is for the sake of theory and theory is for practice. However, research alone will not produce theory, and theory produced without research has little hope of viability. Research is a tool to be used in conjunction with adequate conceptualization and with a level of precision that, although scientifically sound, does not preclude practical usefulness. The purpose of research (creating or testing theory) should determine the methodology employed.

This excellent, humorous, and atypically brief article by Dickoff and James is one of the best articles on the research–theory–practice link available in the literature.

Dickoff, J. and James, P. (1968) A theory of theories: A position paper. *Nursing Research*, 17(3), 197–203.

Dickoff and James begin by defining theory as: a conceptual system or framework invented for some purpose. (There are other kinds of theory besides "predictive theory.") Because a profession shapes reality, nursing theory must provide conceptualizations to guide the shaping of reality to nursing's professional purpose. Therefore, nursing theory is at the fourth or highest level—situation-producing theory—because the nursing aim is practice. Nursing has an advantage to offsetting the difficulty of producing so complex a theory, namely, "the privileged and habitual intercourse with empirical reality carried on in a practice discipline," together with the practical wisdom passed on in apprenticeship. (There follows a summary of "Theory in a Practice Discipline"—see abstract of that article for this information.) Natural and social science theories will be offered by contributors, but one should realize that conceptualization at a very sophisticated level constitutes the integration of these into nursing theory. The authors' summary indicates that definition and types of theory delineated are the crucial points made. They suggest valuation of their theory or theories to rest on "whether or not the proposed position constitutes a fruitful view of theory."

This is a stimulating introduction to the ideas of Dickoff and James, and contains some knowing asides (*e.g.*, the authors encourage nurses to persist in theory building despite "the smoother sailing and quicker payoff in status and funds to be found in repetition or imitation of inquiry" in other disciplines). Nevertheless, the article is simply an overview, and depends on the more elaborate articulations ("Theory in a Practice Discipline," etc.) for substantive support.

Dickoff, J., James, P., and Wiedenbach, E. (1968) Theory in a practice discipline: Part I—Practice oriented theory. *Nursing Research*, 17(5), 415–435.

This is the first of two articles on the nature and development of theory in a practice discipline. A major thesis is made explicit at the outset: theory is relevant to practice, practice to theory, and both are relevant to research. The movement is delineated from felt discomfort/criticism to articulation of a problem, and then to speculative and eventual practical resolution. This "epitomizes that theory is born in practice and must return to practice." What is theory? Theory is a "conceptual framework to some purpose." There is some discussion of the nature of theory and misconceptions about theory.

The four levels of theory are: (1) factor-isolating theories; (2) factor-relating theories (descriptive); (3) situation-relating theories (predictive, etc.); and (4) situation-producing theories (prescriptive). Each of these is then described: (1) involves naming, classifying; (2) is depicting or "natural-history-stage" theory; (3) extends from predictive theory into "promoting and inhibiting" theories; (4) is the primary subject of the article, situation-producing theory. The three essential ingredients of a situation-producing theory are: (1) goal content specified as an aim for activity; (2) prescriptions for activity; and (3) a survey list to serve as a supplement.

Each of these ingredients is discussed, the first two briefly, the survey list at some length. As to the first, "No more feeling of reverence to some shadowy high ideal can substitute in theory for the conception of goal as goal." As to prescriptions, they are commands giving a directive, aimed at a specified end, and directed toward some specified agent. The survey list accounts for the agent's judgment, experience, and practical insight. It bridges the gap between particular activity and the goal content and prescriptions. Such activity has six salient aspects: agency, patiency, framework, terminus, procedure, and dynamics.

What is nursing theory? It must be a theory at the most sophisticated level, a situation-producing theory. This article seeks to suggest what might be expected in a nursing theory. Again, the discussion is structured on the tripartite division—goal, prescription, and survey-list ingredients. The discussion of goal content identifies the goals as "beforehand specifications of situations the theorist deems worthy to produce," as well as, "explicit conceptualizations subject to revision." The treatment of the prescription ingredient merely expands with examples of what has been said already. Furthermore, "Appropriate specificity of goal content and prescription is an important consideration in any practice theory."

The survey list ingredients are explained and illustrated at some length. Under *agency*, the question is asked, "Who might be agents of activity that realizes the nursing goal?" The conclusion is that there is no theoretical reason that all nursing agents must be nurses or even persons. *Patiency*, similarly, is mainly the extension of that term to cover "[a]ny person or thing that receives the activity of a registered nurse." *Framework* asks: What in the context of activity, practically speaking, is relevant? *Terminus* is activity in terms of outcomes. This and *procedure* are fairly obvious discussions of viewing activity in terms of means and ends. *Dynamics* introduces interesting questions about the motivations of nurses and how these may be influenced. The question is of the "power sources" for successful nursing activity.

The article closes with a brief look at existing nursing theory. Actually, this is mainly a look at nursing literature. Beginning with the observation that there is no existing nursing theory to meet their paradigm, the authors argue nonetheless that extant nursing literature constitutes a contribution to, or preparation for, such a theory. They discuss the difficulties of "would-be" nursing theorists, they observe that there may be more than one good nursing theory, and then they propose to consider types of nursing literature (other than research studies): the "inspirational" literature of nursing, treatises and textbooks, and procedure and policy books. These constitute "a rich mine, if we know how to exploit the veins." The existence of something concrete to be examined critically—written materials and existing practice—is a necessary stepping stone. "In other words, even now, practice is guided in some incipient way by embryonic theory."

Dickoff and colleagues have much to offer: "As Einstein's theory of relativity is . . . so is our theory of theories." In fact, it is this very insistence that they are introducing a *new kind* of theory, substantively different, that provides the major ground for doubt or dispute. Whereas some parts of this article are dense and full of ideas, whole sections seem diffuse, rambling, simplistic, and often unnecessary. There is no bibliography. However, their pretensions to metatheory are the main objectionable elements (except for an occasional condescension to nurses and "would-be" nurse theorists). This is the major substantive article by these authors, and it is a "must read" because of the contagion and impact of their ideas. Critical reading of this article should be followed by reading of the article by Jacox and the series by Beckstrand.

Dickoff, J., James, P., and Wiedenbach, E. (1968) Theory in a practice discipline: Part II—Practice oriented research. *Nursing Research*, 17(6), 545–554.

To have a nursing theory, three sources must be tapped: awareness of practice theory, interest in developing it, and "openness to relevant empirical reality." The authors see the first two of these as covered in Part I of this article, which is briefly reviewed. Research and practice are the constituents of the required "openness." The essential aspect of practice as opposed to "mere" research lies in the accomplishment of something in the here-and-now. Research has as its goal "[i]nput to knowledge beyond the immediate particular." Possible research objectives are: to stimulate conception and to validate a conception already formed. "We can say that research has two objectives or that research has theory as its immediate objective but in two different ways." Simply put, though, research tests theory or stimulates theory.

There are two ways to stimulate theory: the researcher "encounters again and again, and with as many variations as possible, empirical reality." This is called planned "staring." A second way is to test theory at the just-preceding level. As for testing, only fourth-level theory testing is considered; it is "fairly well-accepted" that the others can be tested. The purpose of situation-producing theory is three-fold: (1) to achieve its goal; (2) that these results be desirable when achieved; and (3) that guiding action by the theory is feasible in terms of cost, etc. Testing means testing all three dimensions: the theory's *coherency* must be tested; its *palatability* must be assessed; and the *feasibility* claim must be evaluated. Research methodology is not absolute and can be expected to vary with the level of theory tested, and with its being strictly "test" *or* stimulation. The conditional nature of methodology is stressed in order to approach creatively the kind of research needed or to stimulate practice theory for nursing. Summary and conclusions follow. Noteworthy among these observations are the following:

"Research is for theory, theory for practice, so that practice fittingly
   has first place and theory has the mediating role."
"There is a thorough-going, mutual interdependence as among the
   three activities of practice, theorizing, and research."
"In short, to supply nursing image is to venture a nursing theory."

The authors are mostly to be commended for certain emphases, certain stressed elements, especially concerning the place and importance of theory in nursing. As with their other productions, this article fails to provide any bibliography. This article is not so controversial and seems not so valuable as their other contributions.

Donaldson, S.K. and Crowley, D. (1978) The discipline of nursing. *Nursing Outlook*, 26(2), 113–120.
This article poses a series of significant questions. It begins by noting the question of the nature of nursing, but addresses this through a subquestion: What are the recurrent themes in nursing inquiry? These could suggest "boundaries" for systematic study of the discipline of nursing. There follows a long discussion of the nature of classification of disciplines. Nursing is seen as a "professional" discipline. It is noted as a discipline different from nursing science (doctoral training for nursing historians as well as for nursing scientists is endorsed) and different from nursing practice (the discipline should be governing practice instead of vice versa). Finally, the structure of the discipline of nursing is considered, a generalization is offered ("Nursing studies the wholeness or health of humans"), and some "major conceptualizations in nursing" are presented.
   The article is somewhat ill-organized. The opening ideas are not developed and are unrelated to what follows (except for the assertion, not discussed, that they provide "boundaries"). On the second page, the authors state that what is truly important is to define the discipline of nursing. Having discussed the nature and relations of disciplines, one expected the next section to be entitled "The Discipline of Nursing." Instead, the authors launch into a discussion of nursing-as-practice

versus the discipline of nursing. The structure (as opposed to the nature or definition?) and nursing's "perspective" are not clearly delineated or related. Definition is never mentioned, and what is given is somewhat vague, broad, and unspecific to nursing, such as "Major conceptualizations in nursing: 1. Distinctions between human and nonhuman beings; 2. Distinctions between living and non-living. . . . 7. Human characteristics . . . such as consciousness, abstraction . . . aging, dying, reproducing."

Nevertheless, this seminal work is challenging, and it has had a wide and significant impact on the theory development literature because of the importance of the topic and its timeliness. It makes the point successfully that nursing is a discipline and gives support to its focus.

Ellis, R. (1968) Characteristics of significant theories. *Nursing Research,* 17(3), 217–222.

Significant theories for nursing are those that (1) improve practice by addressing the goal of nursing (represented by Henderson's definition) and (2) include the patient as a component. The purposes of theory development are (1) to distinguish fact from pseudo-fact, (2) to structure and synthesize facts from other fields, (3) to give direction to practice, and (4) to provide a framework for retrieval and use of generated and stored knowledge.

Seven characteristics of significant theories are enumerated: (1) *Scope* (the number of concepts related). Scope provides framework for ordering observations about a variety of phenomena, and it must include psychological and biological variables; the broader the scope, the greater the significance. (2) *Complexity* (the notion that theory should treat multiple variables or relationships of a single variable in its full complexity). The strength of this argument is Ellis' admonition that "incomplete conceptualizations lead to hazards of illusory comprehension." (3) *Testability* (focuses chiefly on the importance of recognizing theories as hypothetical constructs, amenable to change). (4) *Usefulness* (the ultimate criterion is that theories help develop and guide clinical practice). (5) *Implicit value* must be recognized and made explicit. (6) *Capability* of generating new information, new ideas, and practices must be there. (7) *Terminology* can be used meaningfully with, or applied to, phenomena observed in nursing.

These "characteristics of significant theories" speak directly or indirectly to evaluative methodologies and criteria for internal and external validity presented elsewhere, providing a succinct presentation of major considerations. Ellis' positions on scope and complexity should be compared with those of Jacox, Hardy, Stevens, Duffey and Muhlenkamp, and Hage. The major area of disagreement between Ellis and other authors is related to the characteristic of testability, which, she states, can be sacrificed in favor of scope, complexity, and clinical usefulness. Ellis she argues that "elegance and complexity of structure are to be preferred to precision in the meaning of concepts in the present state of knowledge." This view should be contrasted with the more prevalent argument for testability as the ultimate determinant of significance.

Fawcett, J. (1980) A framework for analysis and evaluation of conceptual models of nursing. *Nurse Educator*, 5(6), 10–14.

The purpose of this article is to provide a clear definition of conceptual models, to delineate the confused distinction between conceptual models and theories, and to develop a framework for analysis and evaluation of conceptual models.

A conceptual model is defined as a set of abstract concepts and the assumptions that integrate them into a meaningful configuration. By identifying relevant phenomena, (person, environment, health, and nursing), a conceptual model provides a perspective for scientists; by describing these phenomena and their interrelationships in general and abstract terms, the model represents the first step in developing the theoretical formulations needed for scientific activities.

A theory is a set of interrelated concepts, definitions, and propositions that present a systematic view of phenomena by specifying relations among variables (Kerlinger). It postulates specific relations among concepts and takes the form of a description, explanation, prediction, or prescription for action. Any theory presupposes a more general abstract conceptual system. The crucial distinction between a conceptual model and a theory is the level of abstraction; a theory is both more precise and more limited in scope than its parent conceptual scheme.

Based on this distinction between conceptual models and theories, different frameworks are required for analysis and evaluation. The remainder of the article is devoted to the presentation of a framework for analysis (philosophical base, context, scope) and evaluation (internal validity, etc.) of conceptual models of nursing.

This is an excellent, substantive article that is of value both in its articulation of differences between conceptual models and theories and its eclectic framework.

Gebbie, K. and Lavin, M.A. (1974) Classifying nursing diagnoses. *American Journal of Nursing*, 74(2), 250–253.

Report of the First National Conference on the Classification of Nursing Diagnoses. This article describes the process of developing a classification system and a list of tentative nursing diagnoses.

It is an example of what Dickoff and James call a factor-isolating theory. The relationship of nursing diagnoses to theory development, while observed in the article, is made explicit and developed in detail by Kritek (1978).

Gortner, S.R. (1983) The history and philosophy of nursing science and research. *Advances in Nursing Science*, 5(2), 1–8.

Only in the past few years have philosophy of science issues attracted serious attention in nursing research, as the research tradition moves into a new phase of development. Questions regarding method, discovery (as opposed to justification or proof), ethics, politics, and so forth are now prompting comment. This article presents an overview of this philosophical component of emerging nursing science and research, and does so in part through a historical perspective.

In the early years, practice was the source of knowledge. Efforts to generate a knowledge base for nursing through research have been much more prominent in the past two decades. Early research approaches included development of critical resources, surveys, conferences, studies of procedure, case analyses, and alliance with other disciplines. More recent times have seen the enlargement of critical resources (especially in doctoral education) and public support and new development of colleagueship, communication, and research designs and methods.

On this last subject, Gortner addresses a major point of discussion: "To assume that the choice of research methods used in nursing was influenced by a particular philosophy of science (*e.g.*, logical positivism) is to attribute too much deliberation or rationality to what was the result of social, political, and economic events." With doctoral training in other fields than nursing, nursing scientists brought with them methods that had served them well in other fields. They also had to face the pragmatics of funding. "Granting agencies prefer controlled studies in which variables are well-specified and instrumentation is precise." Finally, generalizability has become a critical element because "the capacity to affect practice depends heavily on this factor."

Consensus has emerged about the definition and subject matter of nursing and the research paradigms of its science. However, the philosophical orientation of the science remains chiefly empirical and naturalistic. Attempts to incorporate theoretical propositions are now being made, and the search is on to discover relationships. "Science (empirics), art (esthetics), morality (ethics), and intuition (personal or subjective) all represent sources of knowledge. . . . The profession surely can accommodate multiple paradigms (analytic, humanistic) and modes of inquiry (naturalistic, experimental, historical). In the formation of research questions and the choice of areas of inquiry, it can be expected that inquiry will be of a more fundamental nature in the future than was true in the past. Examples of phenomena that have relevance for nursing include self-care, social support, family functioning, and stress. Two other important areas are clinical therapeutics and investigation of environments.

Gortner concludes that "nursing science will make a major contribution, as science, in the interface of the biological and social sciences concerned with illness and health."

This article is significant because of its comprehensiveness and currency; it points forward to the shape of nursing's future.

Green, J.A. (1979) Science, nursing and nursing science: A conceptual analysis. *Advances in Nursing Science*, 2(1), 57–64.

This article examines the term "science" historically, linguistically, and contextually. The scientific method is considered ("science includes both methodology and knowledge"), and the functions of science are indicated. Various definitions are cited (Conant, Nagel, Fischer), and a synthetic definition is offered. The usefulness of this definition of science for nursing is said to be its potential for evaluating the status of nursing science: "It provides a standard to determine whether or not a designated body of knowledge constitutes a science." A distinction is established between science and technology.

A series of definitions of nursing are considered, with attention given to chronological development of the nurse's role (Henderson, Wiedenbach, Yura and Walsh, King, Travelbee). Following Travelbee, an analytical course is set. Nursing is seen as involving content and process. A comparison of nursing and medicine is made. Knowledge drawn from natural, behavioral, social, and medical sciences constitute the science in nursing. This is then transformed through application in clinical practice. So, a definition of nursing becomes "a service discipline that provides care, concern, and comfort to recipients experiencing a broad range of health-illness phenomena through the synergetic combination of its art and science." This definition precludes separate classification of technical and professional nursing.

The main value of this article is that it collects and presents good basic materials on the questions "What is science?" and "What is nursing?" Green's only argument for "nursing science" is a reference to Gortner and colleagues, who, she says, document its existence. Also, her synthetic definitions seem to be inferior to her citations from other sources.

Hall, B.A. (1981) The change paradigm in nursing: Growth versus persistence. *Advances in Nursing Science*, 3(4), 1–6.

Questions of emerging and competing paradigms in nursing theory development are addressed as they relate to shaping the values of the professional. The "change paradigm," which postulates continuous flux, has been pervasive in nursing theory (*e.g.*, adaptation, development). It is argued that: (1) a paradigm based on change may not be the most productive departure for the study of humans and health; (2) a focus on change leads to the illusion that things are changing when they are actually staying the same; and (3) nursing's attention may have been drawn to the phenomena of changes at the expense of increasing our understanding of the capacity for stability and persistence.

Hall's attention to the heuristic value of a paradigm is an interesting example of the sociology of science, and her admonitions about the acceptance of unverified assumptions underlying theory are provocative and important. Several interesting questions are raised that are based on Kuhn and have generalizability beyond the specific example; for example: What is the process by which a paradigm is accepted?; Why and when does a paradigm's shift occur?; What is the relationship between theory and value?; Can competing paradigms exist simultaneously, and with what implications?

The presentation of change and stability as competing theoretical notions may be somewhat oversimplified. Although Hall explicitly refrains from dropping models of change, her presentation is strongly biased in the direction of stability (albeit perhaps for the sake of balance). Perhaps change and stability are better viewed as which/when versus either/or phenomena. Kuhn's paradigm, espoused by Hall, would seem to preempt the possibility of dialectical theory development. This article should be read by the student with some background in theory development.

Hardy, M.E. (1978) Perspectives on nursing theory. *Advances in Nursing Science*, 1(1), 37–48.

Nursing theory development and evaluation are viewed within the context of stages of scientific development. Applying Kuhn's thesis on the development of scientific knowledge, Hardy argues that nursing is in a "preparadigmatic" stage of theory development, "characterized by divergent schools of thought which, although addressing the same range of phenomena, usually describe and interpret these phenomena in different ways." Nursing needs to struggle through and beyond the preparadigmatic stage of scientific development because confusion, wasted energy, and poorly focused, systematic research result from this lack of a well-defined perspective.

A "metaparadigm," or prevailing paradigm, on the other hand, presents a general orientation that holds the commitment and consensus of the scientists in a particular discipline. It determines the general parameters of the field, it provides focus to scientific endeavor, and it may subsume several "exemplar" paradigms, which are more concrete and specific in directing the activities of scientists. The existence of a prevailing paradigm facilitates the "normal work of science." Research is purposeful, orderly, and raises few unanswerable questions. Whereas the adoption of a metaparadigm cannot be decreed but rather will be based on its scientific credence and its potential for advancing scientific knowledge, nursing scientists can facilitate this process by being well-informed in a substantive area and participating actively in theory construction and research.

Subsequent sections of this article address the nature of theory, the relationship between theory and practice, criteria for "borrowing" theory from other disciplines, types (levels) of theory, and criteria for theory evaluation, including logical adequacy, empirical adequacy, usefulness, and significance. Each of these criteria is clearly elaborated.

Whereas Hardy's "perspectives" are not clearly interrelated, they are well worth reading. Before reflecting on the implications of nursing's "preparadigmatic" stage of theory development, consider: (1) the applicability of Kuhn's thesis to nursing; and (2) evidence for other conclusions on the status of nursing science. The sections on development and evaluation of theory are excellent. Hardy's criteria should be compared with other taxonomies.

Jacobs, M.K. and Huether, S.E. (1978) Nursing science: The theory-practice linkage. *Advances in Nursing Science*, 1(1), 63–73.

Nursing science is defined as both process and product: "the process of nursing science requires that concepts be defined, operationalized, linked into relationships, and verified. From verified conceptual linkages accrue the product, which is theory; and the theory explains and predicts nursing phenomena." The goal of nursing science is to define goals and guide practice; it is prerequisite to professional autonomy and impact.

The complementary and mutually dependent interrelationship of theory and practice are emphasized and demonstrated. Concepts, the building blocks of theory, must be empirically derived and operationalized in a clear and useful manner. They are then linked in theoretical formulations that are subject to empirical verification. Theory without practice is vacuous; practice without theory is intuitive rather than scientific. The contributions of both researchers and practitioners are crucial.

These authors present nursing as an evolving science. The current status of nursing science is illuminated by historical perspective; education and "cohesiveness will facilitate the advancement of nursing science." The article includes brief sections on the nature of science, the structure and function of science, and the process of concept selection and definition. The theory–practice linkage is clearly articulated and appropriately emphasized.

Jacox, A. (1974) Theory construction in nursing: An overview. *Nursing Research*, 23(1), 4–13.

Three levels or stages of theory development are discussed: (1) a period of specifying, defining, and classifying the concepts used in describing the phenomena of the field; (2) developing statements or propositions that propose how two or more concepts are related; and (3) specifying how all the propositions are related to each other in a systematic way.

Concepts are abstract representations of reality that indicate the subject matter of a theory. They may vary both in complexity (concepts, "higher-level" concepts, constructs), and in the degree to which they are observable versus symbolic (empirical–theoretical continuum). Precise operational definitions are emphasized.

Propositions are statements of constant relationships between two or more concepts or facts. All scientific propositions are based on empirical generalizations that may be proved false in the future. Types of relational statements include laws, axioms, theorems, hypotheses and principles—differentiated on the basis of degree of tentativeness. Although nursing has made wide use of principles on which to base nursing action, Jacox observes little attempt to relate these principles to one another systematically.

Scientific theory is defined as "a systematically related set of statements, including some law-like generalizations, that is empirically testable." The purpose of theory "to describe, explain, and predict a selected aspect of empirical reality" requires the use of both inductive and deductive reasoning and a close relationship between theory, practice, and research.

Jacox espouses nursing practice theory as that which guides the nurse's actions in attaining nursing goals in patient care. While presupposing and building upon theory that explains, describes, and predicts, nursing practice theory must allow the investigator to go beyond these levels in order to prescribe and control. She describes nursing as a discipline "in which the major concern is *use* of knowledge."

Other topics discussed in this article include: (1) definition and use of models to guide research; (2) arguments for "middle-range theories" in nursing (versus "grand theory" or abstracted empiricism"); and (3) a discussion of the nature and source of knowledge and theory in (of, for) nursing and the proper use of nursing resources in theory development.

This article is a good overview of theory construction, emphasizing the relationships between various elements of theories and emphasizing issues in the development of nursing theory. Jacox's nursing practice theory should be compared with Dickoff and James and the contrasting position of Beckstrand. Comparisons should also be made with Hardy, Donaldson and Crowley, and Green. Reflection on Jacox's description of the "state of the art" of theory construction in nursing is recommended.

Johnson, D.E. (1959) The nature of a science of nursing. *Nursing Outlook*, 7(5), 291–294.

The basis for the concepts set forth in this article is found in the earlier article by this author on the philosophy of nursing. Here, the focus is on exploring the nature of nursing as a science and as a discipline. Johnson identifies professional disciplines as representing applied sciences. One might be interested in comparing her thoughts on this with a more recent article by Donaldson and Crowley, noting that Johnson and Crowley were colleagues at the University of California, Los Angeles in the mid-1960s and that Crowley was influenced by Johnson (1978).

Johnson believes that the goals of nursing must be established in precise terms to give direction to the search for a body of knowledge. Although nursing shares the ultimate goal held by all health workers, its specific and unique goal is not as clearly understood or as widely accepted as that of medicine. It is through a discussion of nursing's professional goal that Johnson elaborates on her conceptions as a way of illustrating how the development of science can be given direction. Her conception of nursing care is borrowed from general systems theory, and the primary purpose of nursing care is expressed in terms such as tension, equilibrium, and dynamic state.

For nursing to achieve its goals, it is hypothesized that two kinds of knowledge are needed: the knowledge of people, which is shared; knowledge common to all health workers; and knowledge of the science of nursing. Furthermore, it is this author's thesis that "the science of nursing is developed through the reformulation of concepts drawn from the basic sciences to yield a body of knowledge fundamental to the development of theories of nursing diagnosis and nursing intervention."

Borrowing theory is a controversial approach to the development of nursing knowledge but is nonetheless a useful one, as demonstrated by a number of other nursing theorists as well as Johnson. Herein Johnson develops a rationale for that approach. We will later see how she herself does this using systems theory as a prototype to develop her behavioral systems model.

This article makes an important contribution to the early thinking about a science of nursing, in addition to showing us Johnson's early thinking about the behavioral systems model. The writing is clear, and the presentation is logically developed and expressed. This article should be read by those who are interested in Johnson's model, especially by those who wish to see how the model unfolded, and by all who are interested in the development and organization of nursing knowledge. Responses and patterns, part of the lexicon in nursing in the 1980s, were introduced as early as 1959, as is evident in this publication.

Johnson, D.E. (1968) Theory in nursing: Borrowed and unique. *Nursing Research*, 17(3), 206–209.

Differentiation of "borrowed" and "unique" theory in nursing may help clarify nursing's appropriate place and focus in theory development. Borrowed theory is defined as that knowledge that is developed in the main by other disciplines and that is drawn upon by nurses. Unique theory is defined as that knowledge derived from the observation of phenomena and the asking of questions unlike those that characterize other disciplines.

The question of borrowed and unique is analyzed first in respect to the nature of knowledge required for nursing practice and the availability of the knowledge. This knowledge may be divided into: (1) knowledge of order, that which describes and explains the "normal" state of people and the "normal" scheme of things (this kind of knowledge has been the focus of the basic sciences); (2) knowledge of disorder, that which helps us understand events that pose a threat to the well-being or survival of the individual or society; and (3) knowledge of control, that which allows prescription of a course of action that, when executed, changes the sequence of events in desired ways predicated on the knowledge of disorder and geared toward specified outcomes. Although knowledge of all these types is basic to nursing practice, it is in the area of disorder that efforts at nursing theory development should be concentrated.

A second perspective for analysis of the borrowed/unique issue considers the problem of nursing's objects in scientific investigation. Nursing is ill-defined as a field of practice and as a field of inquiry. The lack of definition constitutes a serious obstacle to professional and scientific development. If there is an area for study and theory development unique to nursing, it will evolve only through the study of phenomena and through asking questions in a way that is not characteristic of any other discipline. Behavioral system disorders represent such a focus.

Part of the 1968 Symposium on Theory Development in Nursing. This article is a "must read" because: (1) it is a cogent and effective analysis of one of the major issues in theory development; (2) Johnson's framework of order, disorder, and control is one of the major typologies in the literature; and (3) it serves as an introduction and rationale for Johnson's Behavioral Systems Model.

Johnson, D.E. (1978) Development of theory: A requisite for nursing as a primary health profession. In Chaska, N. (Ed.), *The nursing profession: Views through the mist.* New York: McGraw-Hill.

The development of a theoretical body of nursing knowledge is a means of acquiring professional status. Impediments to the development of nursing science are surveyed, and two questions are presented as means of providing direction: For what purpose is a theoretical body of knowledge intended? and What phenomena must be studied and what kinds of questions must be asked to develop the needed knowledge?

In response to these questions, Johnson discusses the evaluation of scientific disciplines and the professions as sciences. Sciences become differentiated on the basis of the distinctive perspective for observation and interpretation of selected phenomena. The focus of any profession's scientific concern is interdependent with its service (social function). Johnson discusses the implication of different conceptual models and alternative routes to theory development and presents three social criteria for evaluating models: congruence (Do nursing decisions and actions that are based on the model fulfill social expectations?); significance (Do nursing decisions and actions based on the model lead to outcomes for patients that make an important difference in their lives or well-being?); and utility (Is the conceptual system on which the model is based sufficiently well-developed to provide clear direction for nursing practice, education, and research?).

This is a good theoretical treatise on problems in nursing theory development and the evaluation of solutions to these problems. Direct responses to Johnson's guiding questions, however, must be supplemented from other sources (see sections on philosophy, practice, research, guidelines). Johnson's theory evaluation criteria, based on factors extrinsic to the substance of the model, represent an often neglected yet important dimension.

Kramer, S. (1969) Behavioral science and human biology in medicine. *The New Physician,* 18(11), 965–978.

The question is raised whether information in the biological, behavioral, and medical sciences can be used to develop a comprehensive theory of the human organism. Kramer presents the thesis that "in human development, the social environment, through its influence on genetically determined patterns of behavior together with the normal process of growth, is capable of modifying the development of every individual in characteristic ways." Examples of the interrelated nature of bio-psycho-social variables are given, using growth and development as a frame of reference. One major concept—"character structure"—is developed to define psychic, somatic, and social unity of the individual to explain the empirical finding that alterations of behavior in one realm are capable of influencing all other realms (as in stress reactions).

The proposed "medical-ecological model" of the human organism represents an attempt to develop an eclectic "grand theory." The rationale is presented intelligently, and recognition is given to some major obstacles, for example, the fact that individual disciplines use words in different ways and use different units of analysis, ranging from the molecular (physiology) to the molar (behavioral sciences). Implications for conceptualization or viable theory development are left to the reader.

Kritek, P.B. (1978) The generation and classification of nursing diagnosis: Toward a theory of nursing. *Image,* 10(2), 33–40.

In building nursing theory, we have skipped the first stage of specifying, defining, and classifying our concepts, and this has led to problems. To the degree that first-level theory (descriptive) is dissonant with or unclear when related to "what is" in nursing, the eventual level-four theory (prescriptive) will be dissonant or unclear. Returning to the level-one theory, building and doing first things first, may be a worthwhile place toward which we could redirect our energies. This is being done through the generation and classification of nursing diagnoses (see Gebbie and Lavin, 1974). This level-one theory is evaluated in terms of Ellis' criteria of a significant theory.

Read this article after Dickoff, James, and Wiedenbach (1968a, 1968b), Ellis (1968), and Gebbie and Lavin (1974). It is most insightful in the application and implications of Dickoff, James, and Wiedenbach's framework. Would you call nursing diagnoses theory?

Leininger, M.M. (1969) Introduction: Nature of science in nursing. *Nursing Research*, 18(5), 388–389.

This is a statement of conference goals to explore approaches and methods that will support a scientific discipline and a body of nursing knowledge. There is a core of nurses eager to develop both a scientific and a humanistic discipline of nursing within institutions of higher education. Though "a theory" of nursing is spoken of, it is healthy and desirable that there be multiple theories, models, and conceptual frameworks. An attitude of constructive skepticism and critique of colleagues is urged.

In addition to induction and deduction, an ethnoscientific approach is suggested: a systematic and descriptive documentary study of phenomena through the eyes of people in their situations. Nursing lacks systematic ethnological studies of concrete nurse–patient–other situations.

There is a need to be tolerant of one another's failures and frustrations. Finally, change must be accommodated. Students should be encouraged to explore problems and test ideas that seem "exotic, highly radical, or out-of-this-world."

This is a brief overview of concerns facing the conference.

McCarthy, R.T. (1972) A practice theory of nursing care. *Nursing Research*, 21(5), 406–410.

Can the format (of Dickoff, James, and Wiedenbach), applied to a real-life situation, produce useful theories of nursing (practice)?

The purpose of this article is to illustrate how a practice theory can be developed on four levels. McCarthy presents data from her survey of postoperative patterns of voiding in patients with spinal anesthesia to demonstrate the four levels of theory as described by Dickoff *et al.* (1968). Under first-level theory (factor-isolating), she categorizes patients according to type of surgery. Second-level theory (factor-relating) involves analyzing the relationships between need for catheterization, duration of surgery, fluid intake, and so on. So far so good. When we get to the third level we find that "a statement that 'patients who have not voided within 14 hours may have to be catheterized' could be said to constitute predictive theory." The highest level of theory—situation-producing or prescriptive—is a nursing care plan (*e.g.*, "note time of last voiding," note when patient expresses desire to void, offer assistance, etc.).

The article also includes an example of a survey list in operation. Is the reader's response to the opening question affirmative or negative? Does your response reflect comment on McCarthy or on Dickoff, James, and Wiedenbach?

McKay, R. (1969) Theories, and models, and systems for nursing. *Nursing Research*, 18(5), 393–400.

Theory is the cornerstone of all scientific work because the understanding, which is the goal of science, is expressed in terms of theoretical formulations. The article proceeds to give a lot of space to defining various senses of the term "theory." Nursing, at present, should use the word in a modest sense. "Models" are defined and analyzed. Models vary in two ways: level of abstraction and metaphor used. Two metaphors have been dominant—the machine and the organism. The organism is currently the dominant model in many fields, and, for both philosophic and practical reasons, it is dominant in nursing.

The concept of "systems" is the ultimate central focus of the article. Various definitions of systems are offered. Open and closed systems are discussed. Properties of open systems are articulated, and the suggestion is made that nursing could be represented by such a systems approach. Theorems or propositions based on general systems theory developed by James Miller are endorsed as particularly appropriate for nursing. Finally, a systems approach to the study of nursing education is proposed for the study of students and of curricula.

This is a valuable treatment of the subjects considered. Its value is due in great part to the many clear and careful definitions and to its detailed application of systems theory to nursing. There is a crucial question about models and metaphor: Is the model merely a restatement in other terms or does it accomplish extension or clarification? The late Dr. McKay was a central figure in metatheory. This represents a fine example of her writing.

McKay, R.C. (1977) What is the relationship between the development and utilization of a taxonomy and nursing theory? *Nursing Research*, 26(3), 222–224.

This essay is a brief description of the purposes and principles of classification schemes. The definition and arrangement of concepts in a taxonomy, presuming it reflects the natural system, is a descriptive model of reality and can be considered a theoretical design (factor-isolating or naming). The value of taxonomies for clinicians and educators are briefly listed.

It is another example of first-level theory; how it relates to the second level is not discussed. This article is really McKay's response to a reader's question.

Menke, E.M. (1978) Theory development: A challenge for nursing. In N.L. Chaska (Ed.), *The nursing profession: Views through the mist.* New York: McGraw-Hill.

Menke considers three issues related to theory development in nursing: the importance of theory development, the present status of theory development, and strategies to facilitate theory development in nursing.

Theory development is important for any discipline because it prescribes the conceptual framework for describing, explaining, and predicting phenomena. It serves as a means to isolate and classify facts, and it points to gaps in the available knowledge. Definitions and components of theories are discussed, as well as levels (Dickoff and James) or stages (Jacox) of theory development. The importance of lower-level theory development as a sound basis is emphasized, and consideration of theories about nursing rather than of nursing is proposed. Lack of theory development may have been caused by the lack of systematic direction and collaboration among theory developers. An eclectic approach to theory development is advocated.

This is an excellent, well-written, and substantive review of major issues in theory development.

Moore, M.A. (1968) Nursing: A scientific discipline? *Nursing Forum*, 7(4), 340–348.

Moore argues that, in our eagerness to break away from the apprenticeship tradition, nurses are trying to develop a scientific discipline without setting the foundation that is characteristic of every well-structured discipline. The fallacies and shortcomings of such practices as searching for a theory of nursing; borrowing concepts, tools, methods, and even questions from other disciplines; and allowing values to interfere with science are discussed, along with their ramifications. The only sensible basis for the development of a content area to be labeled "nursing" involves empirical generalizations regarding the effects on the patient of the activities we carry out as nurses.

This short, easy-to-read article should be read early in a nursing theorist's career because it provides an excellent overview of major issues and pitfalls in the development of nursing theory and nursing science. Moore's emphasis on clear, precise definition of terms is refreshing. While you can, now or later, argue about "the only sensible basis. . . ," Moore is obviously interested in the theory–practice–research linkage.

Murphy, S.A. and Hoeffer, B. (1983) Role of the specialties in nursing science. *Advances in Nursing Science*, 5(4), 31–39.

There is some conceptual movement away from specialization in nursing. Three trends have impact in this regard: (1) defining nursing as a discipline separate from medicine, (2) educating entry-level generalists, and (3) developing conceptual frameworks.

As to the first, perspectives of the two professions—medicine and nursing—are now clearly different. Medicine has become more specialized in an attempt to keep abreast of technological changes and increased knowledge, whereas nursing has become more generalized and holistic in its approach to health care.

Second, medical-surgical nursing was disease-based, psychiatric nursing was patient-based, and community health nursing was locus-based. Many schools determined that using specialty departments as organizing components of the curriculum was no longer efficient; many now offer a series of concepts basic to nursing, along with the nursing process, and they loosely refer to these as an integrated curriculum. One of the outcomes is that the specialties are no longer clearly distinguishable. Also, movement from the hospital setting to the university, as well as changing patterns of illness, have reinforced this direction.

Third, the new conceptual system in nursing provides direction for practice and education. However, none have delineated the role of the specialties. The role of nursing specialties is supported, nonetheless. The authors bring to their aid the social policy statement on nursing by the ANA: "The effectiveness of the profession is increased when specialists are available to focus their efforts on a particular aspect of clinical nursing, to test application of newly available theory to conditions germane to that clinical aspect, and to translate those theory applications into nursing approaches considered more useful than prevailing ones."

It appears that nursing specialties can best contribute to nursing science by generating and testing middle-range or limited-size theories. This type of theory is more directly relevant for addressing practice concerns. As practice-relevant theory was developed and refined in each specialty from its particular vantage point, the specialty would contribute to nursing science through both cumulative and didactic processes.

The article concludes with a brief discussion of the theory development process (inductive, deductive, adapted) and a sustained example drawn from mental health nursing, where a concept from nursing, "mutual withdrawal," is identified and traced through its history.

This article is especially important for its focus on a perhaps as yet unassimilated consequence of recent developments in nursing: the de-emphasis of the specialties.

Newman M. A. (1972) Nursing's theoretical evolution. *Nursing Outlook,* 20(7), 449–453.

Following a brief discussion of the evolution of nursing science, Newman elaborates on three main approaches to the discovery of nursing knowledge that emerged during the 1960s: (1) the borrowing of theory from other disciplines with an intent to integrate it into a science of nursing; (2) an analysis of nursing practice situations in search of the theoretical underpinnings; and (3) the creation of a conceptual system from which theories could be derived. While limitations and difficulties in the first two approaches are discussed, Rogers is credited with initiating the third phase. The clear-cut delineation of the individual as the focus of nursing gave direction to the development of theory that is basic to nursing.

Newman cites Hempel to evidence the value of the Rogerian approach and, by comparing Rogers with other nurse theorists, concludes that a conceptual system of nursing is evolving and does provide meaningful direction for research. Whether the theory evolves inductively from ideas conceived in clinical practice or deductively from broad generalizations within the theoretical framework does not seem particularly important. What is important is that the nursing investigator should determine the relationship of her study question to the overall conceptual system in nursing and should therefore expand and elaborate the system by the testing of theories that have derived from it. Nursing is coming of age.

Newman's article should be contrasted with that of Hardy, who sees nursing in a "preparadigmatic" stage (from Kuhn). She cites the problem of the past as a dearth of nursing knowledge while "the problem of the future will be an acceleration of that knowledge." Has this prediction been realized in the 20 years since this article was written? How does your answer attest to the veracity of Newman's characterization?

Notter, L.E. (1975) The case for nursing research. *Nursing Outlook,* 23(12), 70–763.

Slow progress in nursing research is attributed to views of nursing and women, too little cumulative effort, and the relatively new idea of nursing as an intellectual profession. The following are areas for concentrated effort: the need for more research based on theories consonant with nursing's domain of responsibility; the need for replication; the need for postdoctoral research and for individual researchers who select a problem area and continue to study it over time; and the need for more service agencies to develop clinical research programs that encourage staff participation in research.

Payne, G. (1973) Comparative sociology: Some problems of theory and method. *British Journal of Sociology*, 24(1), 13–29.

Comparative sociology is a method of inquiry that allows "explicit testing of sociological theories with data from various sources" and that examines "the nature of society as revealed by . . . the operation and interrelation of key processes in different societies, or areas of societies (historical, geographical, social)" (p. 13). The interrelationship of theory and method in the generation of social theory is examined, with emphasis on methodological issues in comparative analysis.

Societies that are similar in regard to a specific variable (*e.g.*, form, function, or structure) are studied to generate laws that explain that one type of society only. Problems inherent in this approach are categorization (defining categories and determining an acceptable level of similarity) and generalization (producing theories that have more than specific application). The purpose of comparing dissimilar societies is to yield universal laws. Defining and determining the appropriate scope of variables, as well as developing specific, meaningful hypotheses, are major difficulties. In both approaches, problems develop in selecting study variables and studying them outside of their cultural context. Nevertheless, the comparative method provides not only understanding and insight but also a means of verifying theory and developing a science of sociology.

This is an excellent, substantive article on a particular methodology for development of theory and science. Issues and problems of comparative study are addressed, and insight is given on the relationship of theory and methodology. What is missing in clarity of expression in this article is more than counterbalanced by the salience of ideas and the potential for applicability to nursing science development.

Payne, L. (1983) Health: A basic concept in nursing theory. *Journal of Advanced Nursing*, 8(5), 393–395.

The article traces the historical evolution of the concept of health. For centuries, disease has been the central focus for the examination of the phenomenon of health. Only one major formulation (Sigerist's in 1941) preceded the critical turning point statements in the constitution of the World Health Organization (1958): "Health is a state of complete physical, mental, and social well-being and not merely the absence of disease and infirmity."

Various paradigms have subsequently been developed: the ecological model, based on the relationship of people to the total environment (Blum, 1974; Rogers, 1960), and the equilibrium model, based on the body's self-regulatory powers to maintain constancy of the internal milieu (Dubos, 1965). Psychosocial models came later: sociocultural, philosophical, or relating health to notions or normality. A new emphasis on quality of life and high-level wellness emerged (Dunn, 1959) due to people's dissatisfaction with life despite their affluence; the idea of holism, originating in Gestalt theory, grew to a multidimensional approach, emphasizing self-responsibility, the whole person, and the process of care-giving; and the "salutogenic" model of health (Antonovsky, 1979) originated, in which "the origin of health lies in a 'sense of coherence,' that is, the way in which one sees life as meaningful, manageable, and comprehensible."

Assumptions based on traditional paradigms have bound nursing curricula and practice to the negative view of health in terms of absence of disease. "The concept of health constitutes a basic building block for nursing theory . . . . If the goal of nursing is the promotion of health, making this concept operational is essential for nursing practice." Finally, a definition of health is offered (a nursing concept of health): "Health is the effective functioning of self-care resources that ensures the operation and adequacy of self-care actions."

The article combines some history, some popularization, some commonplace information, and perhaps some helpful reminders.

Peterson, C.J. (1977) Questions frequently asked about the development of a conceptual framework. *Journal of Nursing Education*, 16(4), 22–32.

The relationship between theory and conceptual frameworks in nursing is examined. A conceptual framework is defined as "a loosely organized set or complex of ideas . . . that provides the overall structure of a curriculum (p. 25)." A theory is defined as a group of systematically interrelated propositions that provides organization to a body of content and, by allowing explanation and prediction, provides a guide for practice. A conceptual framework is an earlier evolutionary step that may be developed into theory, generating testable hypotheses.

Essential elements of a conceptual framework include: the nature of the service provided (nursing/nursing process), goal or outcome (health), rationale for services (nonhealth or illness), characteristics of the care-giver (nursing practitioner), characteristics of the recipient (patient/client), and context for service (care setting or environment). Explanations of the relationships of these concepts provide the framework.

The relationship of the conceptual framework to borrowed theories, program philosophy and objectives, and curricular threads, as well as its role in the development of a nursing curriculum, are also addressed.

This is an excellent article that demystifies the conceptual framework in a thorough, organized, and articulate manner. While emphasizing the use of conceptual frameworks in nursing curricula, the article provides much useful material on theory components (including simple but excellent definitions) and theory development. Excellent figures summarize major points. Peterson's selection of concepts may be compared with those of Dickoff and James, and her presentation of the conceptual framework should be contrasted with that of Torres and Yura.

Phillips, J.R. (1977) Nursing systems and nursing models. *Image*, 9(1), 4–7.

Because the primary goal of nursing theory is the generation of knowledge specific to nursing, the process of theory building must be couched in a nursing frame of reference. Otherwise, the obtained knowledge will not be nursing knowledge that can be used to build or expand nursing science or that can be used for nursing education, practice, or research. Models that nursing has borrowed (medical, psychological, ecological, social) are criticized on the grounds that not one of them views the person as a totality in interaction with the environment. Models of Rogers and Johnson are proposed as frameworks for nursing theory construction.

There are many agreements between the arguments of this article and one by Newman (1972). Although some good points are made about the shortcomings (*e.g.*, of the medical model), many of the arguments could be further developed. Are there any legitimate prototypes outside of nursing?

Putnam, P. (1965) A Conceptual approach to nursing theory. *Nursing Science*, 3, 430–442.

A theoretical framework is valuable as a stimulus in the development of nursing science. In the absence of adequate theory, nursing is limited by the concrete here and now; nursing then becomes restricted to immediate impressions and is unable to explain the past, evaluate the present, or predict the future. Despite the clear necessity of a generalized theory, development has been slow and piecemeal; contributing factors include complexity of the subject matter, the proximity (and therefore influence) of the scientist to the empirical data, and the necessity of delimiting a knowledge base that will encompass changing objects in changing environmental fields.

A key to the conceptual maze is the identification of the unique domain of nursing. The knowledge base of the nursing process, nursing science, is at least a four-dimensional synthesis of knowledge relating to biological function, psychological function, social function, and variations in organization of these factors. The operational identification of the intermixture of components in the synthesis, defined and tested through nursing research, would be a genuine contribution to science. Nurses make it possible for patients to accomplish their own energy exchanges with the external environment. The abstraction of the idea of how nursing makes these exchanges possible is an essential step in theory construction. The constant interplay between theory, practice, and research is stressed.

Although other articles provide more cogent arguments for the value of nursing theory, more enlightened definitions of nursing, or more pragmatic suggestions for theory development, Putnam is particularly eloquent on the problems of lack of adequate theory, the characteristics of conceptual difficulties in nursing theory, and the need to identify the unique domain of nursing.

Quint, J.C. (1967) The case for theories generated from empirical data. *Nursing Research*, 16(2), 109–114.

This work discusses a research approach in which a given problem area is studied for the purpose of developing a conceptual framework. Sections are devoted to the research problem and its overall design, the collection and analysis of data, and the reporting and interpretation of the findings.

This article is the precursor of an approach that has gained increased interest and credibility in the ensuing years.

Rogers, M.E. (1963) Some comments on the theoretical basis of nursing practice. *Nursing Science*, 1, 11–13, 60–61.

This substantive article contains many of the elements that are later to be incorporated into Rogers' *Introduction to the theoretical basis of nursing* (1970). It is recommended that this be read prior to reading the book, but it is not a requisite to understanding the theory.

There is a mix of philosophy, definitions, concepts, and goals—all about life, human beings, nursing, and nursing science. Elements of the prototype theory—systems theory—are also present. These are presented not as a theoretical basis of the nursing process but rather "to stimulate logical and creative thinking concerning its identification and development." Despite Rogers' intent, however, a rudimentary structure of the future theory appears to be taking shape here.

First, the philosophical statements and beliefs are presented, along with assumptions about human beings. Nursing is defined as a process and the goal of nursing is also stated. The concept-building process is discussed, with one concept—the life process—presented. Principles rest on the definitions of the concepts, and principles are integral to nursing science. As an example of a basic principle in nursing science, the adaptive mechanism in human beings is identified. Rogers states, "The human organism has an amazing, innate capacity to adapt: physically, biologically, socially." (An assumption!) What is the purpose of a principle is not discussed in detail.

Finally, Rogers says that the theoretical basis of nursing practice must include a philosophy and a concept of death as well as life. However, she does not undertake that task. Furthermore, though the term "health" was used, it was not defined. Nor does Rogers discuss the role of nursing as it relates to or interfaces with other health care givers. These, then, are a few limitations of this article.

The purpose of this article is to stimulate thinking concerning the identification and development of nursing science—the theoretical basis of nursing practice. Nursing science is a body of scientific knowledge characterized by descriptive, explanatory, and predictive principles about the life process of human beings. These principles rest on the review of the person as a unified "biophysicalpsychosocial" phenomenon in constant interaction with all parts of the environment. The body of knowledge develops through synthesis and resynthesis of selected information from the humanities and the biological, physical, and social sciences in order to form new concepts and understanding about the person and environment. It assumes its own "unique scientific mix" through selection and patterning of this information. The focus of nursing science is central to the formation and understanding of its theories. This focus is elaborated in the remainder of the article.

This is one of the original and most influential articles by one of nursing's true sages. This article, along with that of Johnson (1959), ushered in the era of nursing theory and nursing science. Rogers' characterization of nursing science has been a source of challenge and inspiration, and sometimes of conflict, to all subsequent nurse philosophers and theorists.

For its historical importance and strength of argument, this article should definitely be read. An introduction to Rogers' theory is an added bonus.

Rubin, R. (1968) A theory of clinical nursing. *Nursing Research,* 17(13), 210–212.

This article is part of the 1968 Symposium on Theory Development in Nursing. It is a brief and simple example of development of a model and its use in research.

Silva, M.C. (1977) Philosophy, science, theory: Interrelationships and implications for nursing research. *Image*, 9(3), 59–63.

This is an overview of the relationships among philosophy, science, and theory, with implications for the conduct of nursing research. Science developed into specializations; philosophy "unifies scientific findings so that man as a holistic being might emerge." Science aims to describe, understand, predict, control, or explain phenomena. Theory refers to a set of related statements that have been derived from scientific data and from which plausible hypotheses can be deduced, tested, and verified.

Implications for nursing research: (1) all nursing theory and research is derived from or leads to philosophy, (2) philosophical introspection and intuition are legitimate methods of scientific inquiry, and (3) nursing knowledge arrived at by the scientific method too often sacrifices meaningfulness for rigor.

The author argues that no real distinctions are made between different kinds of knowledge until the Industrial Revolution; Darwin and Freud set off a proliferation of knowledge. This appears to ignore much great work, including the obvious contributions of Francis Bacon. Silva's comparisons of the realms of philosophy, science, and theory are good beginnings in nursing. Her pleas for the recognition of nonscientific ways of knowing deserve attention.

Silva, M.C. and Rothbart, D. (1984) An analysis of changing trends in philosophies of science on nursing theory development and testing. *Advances in Nursing Science*, 6(2), 1–13.

Philosophy of science and nursing theory are in states of transition. Has nursing theory kept pace with new trends in the philosophy of science?

Two competing schools in the philosophy of science are traced and examined: logical empiricism (1940s–1960s) and historicism (1960s–present). The schools are compared in terms of their views of science: (1) its components, (2) its characterization, and (3) its outcomes.

Components: For logical empiricism—deductive system, theories linked to and tested through empirically observable properties; for historicism—research tradition that includes many theories, ontological commitments, and methodological commitments.

Characterization: For logical empiricism—product, scientific knowledge, theory validation; for historicism—the human activity of working scientists, theory discovery.

Outcome: For logical empiricism—verification leading to a body of truth; for historicism—problem-solving effectiveness.

There follows a review of the literature in nursing theory. Three time periods are examined: 1964–1969, 1970–1975, and 1976-present.

> 1964–69: Logical empiricist position everywhere (*e.g.*, Dickoff and
> James, Abdellah. The exception—Leininger offered an
> ethnoscience research methodology.
> 1970–75: Culmination of logical empiricism in Jacox and Hardy;
> conceptual frameworks; "The irony is that . . . the logical

empiricist viewpoints espoused were being strongly repudiated by a growing number of philosophers of science. . . . [N]ursing's theoretical link to philosophy of science was . . . about a decade behind the times."

1976–present: Continued commitment to logical empiricism; a beginning trend toward historicism (*e.g.*, in Newman, Hardy); revisions of conceptual frameworks and introduction of new ones, moving more explicitly toward logical empiricism; questioning of strictly quantitative methods.

Implications: (1) There should not be a single conceptual framework for nursing; (2) there will never emerge a static set of eternal truths; (3) historicism strongly encourages a careful study of actual practices, belief systems, and external factors; (4) the assessment of progress will be more practical (*i.e.*, problem solving).

Important recommendations: (1) Cooperation among nursing theorists, researchers, clinicians, and scholars; (2) exploration of innovative qualitative methods.

Because this article presents itself as expository rather than argumentative, the major questions are: Should one, after all, be trendy and in line with the latest fashion in the philosophy of science? In what ways do the ultimate recommendations differ from what Dickoff and James would suggest?

Stainton, M.C. (1982) The birth of nursing science. *The Canadian Nurse*, 78(10), 24–28.

"The birth of nursing science" celebrates the coming-to-terms of the new science by reviewing its history and describing the conditions necessary for its development. The history is detailed despite its brevity and is told in a lively style, with the added perspective of the author's Canadian nationality and focus.

The list of developmental requirements includes: a perception of nursing as a developing science in the minds and hearts of all nurses; a sense of the significance of each nurse's contribution; a cadre of nursing scientists; the conceptualization of nursing as a science; nursing research teams; monies; the introduction of nursing science to science in general; research and facilities in major centers of nursing; collaboration and international networks; replication of studies; nursing education at all levels of career development; an individual goal of professionalism; and an expectation that one day a nurse will be the recipient of the Nobel Prize for excellence in contributing to science.

The significance of this article should be considered in terms of its effects on the intended readership.

Tinkle, M.B. and Beaton, J.L. (1983) Toward a new view of science: Implications for nursing research. *Advances in Nursing Science*, 5(2), 27–36.

This article begins by pointing to two oppositions: the "hard" versus the "soft" science debate and the opposition between traditional historians of science and the "historicist" revisionists, such as Kuhn and Laudan. These oppositions are associated and identified in Sampson's formulation as Paradigm I versus Paradigm II.

"Context-free generalizations" comprise the object of Paradigm I; research guided by the view of Paradigm II is "often conducted in naturalistic settings, using observational methods."

The authors further contend that the dominance of Paradigm I science is a result of "nourishment it has received from a male-dominant, Protestant-ethic-oriented, middle-class, liberal, and capitalistic society." The implications for nursing are multiple. If scientific truth is acontextual, then little attention is likely to be paid to the values and biases underlying research endeavors, so methodological biases or determinations of proper research subjects may go unexamined.

Further, nursing is, at its most basic level, a relational profession. However, acontextual study is not likely to focus on interpersonal or person–situation interactions. Such studies are apt to lack "ecological validity" and to be removed from the "real world."

The overarching conceptualization of nursing that can be abstracted from nursing theory is centered around the view of a human being as a holistic being. Nursing involves each person's unique bio-psycho-social context. The impact of the environment is a recurrent theme. Sociocultural context is stressed. However, the experimental method is also held in the highest regard.

"What is proposed is a blending of both methodologies to produce a science that retains a critical concern for objectivity while ensuring that the research it produces has validity in the real world and the influence of contextual variables is acknowledged."

This article suffers from the very problems it indicts. It is too abstract and general (*i.e.*, it rarely provides *examples* of the kinds of studies it talks about), and when, as in two references to women's studies in psychology, it moves toward some specificity, the work is simply alluded to. It is also too far from real life; the proposal for blending the two methodologies in a future state moves toward the mystical: "This new synthesis will not consist of the use of Paradigm II methods in the context of discovery and the use of Paradigm I in matters of verification. Rather, a convergence will involve the higher organization of the opposites in both paradigms."

Nevertheless, the point of the article, that we must have an explicit awareness of the assumptions and biases underlying our methods (particularly, in this case, sexist ones), commands our assent.

Tucker, R.W. (1979) The value decisions we know as science. *Advances in Nursing Science*, 1(2), 1–12.

Tucker argues that the processes of science necessarily involve the making of value judgments (versus the ubiquitous image of science as "value-free"). After classifying value judgments along the dimensions: rationale (personal versus objective), subscribership (individual versus "market") and explicitness (formal versus contextual), he discusses the "value decision-making contexts in research." Tucker's position is that each step of the research process—from selection of a problem, theoretical framework, and methodology to analyzing and reporting data—involves value judgments. The principal activity of science is to make well-supported value judgments.

Tucker encourages an explicit awareness of "the value decisions we know as science." There are some valuable insights in this article—if you can avoid getting hung up on the PVJs, CVJs, and VDMCRs.

Wald, F.S. and Leonard, R.C. (1964) Toward development of a nursing practice theory. *Nursing Research*, 13(4), 309–313.

Nursing practice theory—based on the empirical approach of building knowledge directly from systematic study of nursing—is proposed as an alternative to "making borrowed concepts fit." In developing its own theories, nursing would become an independent discipline in its own right. In freeing themselves from the burden of looking only for applications of the basic sciences in their practice, nurses would at the same time take on the responsibility of developing their own science. This calls for the development of nursing practice theory.

Major sections of this article deal with: (1) the fallacy of nursing as an applied science ("accepted" principles may be invalid or inappropriate to nursing, nursing problems are being rephrased as social science cues rather than cues of practice); (2) characteristics of research methods for practice versus descriptive science (the difference lies in the selection of variables and the kind of hypotheses that are entertained); (3) characteristics of practice versus descriptive theory (practice must contain causal hypotheses); and (4) barriers to the development of research of practice theory in nursing (related to research attitudes, need to generalize, and skill in research methods).

This is the first article written on practice theory in nursing and should definitely be read. Those interested in nursing theory should certainly contrast "the fallacy of nursing as an applied science" with the more prevalent view of how nursing science is developed. In addition, consider the process of development of practice theory presented by Wald and Leonard (p. 311) that is clearly a precursor to the influential work of Dickoff, James, and Wiedenbach.

Weatherston, L. (1979) Theory of nursing: Creating effective care. *Journal of Advanced Nursing*, 4(7), 365–375.

Effective nursing care requires a *theory of nursing*—a phrase that connotes the interdependence of the two concepts. Conceptual analysis of "nursing," using Wilson's "model case" method is presented as a way to determine the "essence of nursing," and provides a basis for deciding what nursing theory is. The purpose of theory is to explain, predict, or control phenomena. In order to be a theory of nursing "the theory must be created and used with reference to the unique functions and intentions of nursing and the nature of nursing activity." The relationship of "microtheory" and "paradigmatic theory" are described. A model is developed to demonstrate the relationship of theory, practice, and education.

This article addresses several key issues, including the "essence" of nursing; the relationships among theory, practice, and education; and the rationale for and process of theory building in nursing. However, more sophisticated treatments of each of these subjects are available elsewhere, and should be read first. Many of the article's shortcomings are related to the nonevaluative use of several frameworks and definitions: Wilson's Model Case method, Peter's criteria for education, and conceptions of nursing that do not stress its scientific aspects.

Section II
ABSTRACTS OF WRITINGS IN NURSING THEORY, 1960–1984
Afaf Meleis and Sandra Scheetz

The citations abstracted in this section pertain to selected central writings related to only six of the nurse theorists presented in this text (Johnson, Levine, Orem, Rogers, Roy, and Travelbee). Only selected writings related to each of the theorists, and other's writings (based on theories) were described and analyzed below. The abstracts presented in this section are organized alphabetically according to theorist and author. This section is best used in conjunction with Chapter 3 and with the corresponding chapters in the text that focus on the analysis of the particular theory (Chapters 12, 13, 14, 15, and 16).

Dorothy Johnson

Auger, J.R. and Dee, V. (1983) A patient classification system based on the behavioral system model of nursing: Part 1. *Journal of Nursing Administration,* 13, 38–43.

This first article of a two-part series focused on the development of a patient classification system based on a nursing model and was presented from the combined perspectives of administration and clinical practice. Part 2 (Dee and Auger), to follow, focused on the implementation of the classification system in the clinical setting. The nursing model used was Johnson's behavioral system model and the clinical setting was psychiatric.

The specific intent of such a classification system was for use "as a clinical measure of patient progress in addition to the administrative determination of staffing levels" (p. 38). The importance of a framework common to both was stressed. The rationale for such a classification system versus the use of an existing classification system was discussed.

The rationale for using the Johnson behavioral systems model as the theoretical framework for the classification system in this psychiatric setting was threefold: (1) it could be used with the existing programs based on social learning theory; (2) it could be applied to all clinical settings because of the emphasis on bio-psycho-sociocultural factors; and (3) it identified universal patterns of behavior applicable to all individuals. The model addresses the eight subsystems outlined by Johnson that include ingestive, eliminative, sexual, dependency, affiliative, achievement, aggressive-protective, and restorative. These subsystems of behavior are "assumed to be universal and of primary significance to all persons" (p. 39).

Integrated with the nursing process, the model provided a focus for the assessment phase and is intended to link specific patient behaviors with the corresponding nursing interventions. Furthermore, the model allows for use in clinical settings other than psychiatry.

The development of the classification tool began by certain people addressing the nursing care requirements for patients admitted to either the adult or child psychiatric units of the agency where it was developed. Therefore, the tool had to be both comprehensive and flexible enough to describe behaviors reflective of a wide variety of diagnoses and age groups. To meet this challenge, a group of expert clinicians and nursing administrators was organized to develop the tool.

The criteria for item inclusion reflected several dimensions. First, each of the eight subsystems of the Johnson behavioral system model were operationalized in terms of both adaptive and maladaptive behaviors. The behavioral statements had to meet four criteria: "measurable, relevant to the clinical setting, observable, and specific to the subsystem" (p. 39). A panel of experts then evaluated the statements to make certain that they met the four criteria. The behaviors were also ranked in one of three categories according to their level of adaptiveness, with one being the most adaptive and three being the least adaptive, or maladaptive. Nursing interventions were also ranked according to requirements for intensity and frequency of nursing contact. A fourth level was included to reflect the intensity of one-to-one nursing care required for extremely maladaptive behavior.

After the initial set of critical behaviors were formulated, they were tested by letting a sample of 28 registered nurses, in pairs, serve as observers on seven inpatient units. "Each pair of observers was asked to rate each subsystem of behavior for all patients present on the unit during the shift. In addition, the observers rated the overall level of behavior for each patient" (pp. 39–40). Several exhibits were included to illustrate some components of the process thus far: first, the eight subsystems, definitions of behaviors, and critical behavior characteristics; second, characteristic patient behaviors and the requisite nursing intervention; and third, samples of level three (maladaptive) patient behaviors and nursing interventions for the eliminative and affiliative subsystems.

The implementation of the system was described briefly, with mention of the steps taken. The description did not provide adequate information if someone had been trying to duplicate the process. However, more depth was included in Part 2.

Preliminary testing of the tool revealed that there were several problem areas associated with patient assessment. There were disagreements among staff about ratings of patient behaviors, although it was recognized that these reflected difficulties inherent in defining and measuring behaviors. Observer bias was also an uncontrolled variable associated with measurement of patient behaviors. The two subsystems with the highest level of agreement were eliminative and sexual, probably because these required the least inference on the part of the observers. The subsystems of affiliative, dependency, and achievement—requiring a higher level of observer inference—were found to have lower levels of observer agreement in this preliminary testing.

The importance of minimizing the influence of observer interpretation was recognized, but only one suggestion about how to accomplish this was made, other than through the use of a model to structure the observed behaviors. The suggestion was for staff to "consistently identify and discuss their observations of patient behavior to develop a common frame of reference and achieve a higher degree of agreement (p. 43)." Instrument testing, (specifically, measures of content validity), reliability, and improving interrater reliability would also be important contributions to theory validation. In the long run, these would do more to contribute to the overall theory development and concept measurement. This is the next important step to be taken with the work done this far on the classification tool.

A number of administrative benefits of the classification tool were listed. They all reflected factors influencing decisions that considered cost-effectiveness and quality of care issues.

Broncatello, K.F. (1980) Auger in action: Application of the model. *Advances in Nursing Science*, 2(2), 13–23.

It has long been a given that continued development of conceptual models is an important part of the development of nursing as a science; it is also a given that a part of the continued development of models is application of the models in a variety of practices. However, what has become increasingly apparent in the 1980s is that application of the model to practice is insufficient for refinement of theory. This article is a good example; although it demonstrates application to practice, it does not offer extension or refinement, neither of which are possible in single-case application.

There are several other limitations. After giving a fairly extensive review (summary) of Auger's application of the Johnson behavioral system model to the chronically ill hemodialysis patient, the author attempts to apply the model using new concepts that are not central to either Johnson's or the extension offered by Auger. The section about applying the model begins with a discussion of self-concept and body image. A reader could rightfully question the fit of these concepts with the behavioral systems model.

Stressors are identified that could be extrapolated from the model, including: diet, which affects the eliminative subsystem, and dependence on a machine, which sounds as if it were related to the aggressive-protective subsystem, though logically, it is more directly a problem of the dependence subsystem. Careful analysis of relationships with Auger were better provided in the next section on the model in practice. Here, the author proposes to examine the consequences of hemodialysis on the eight subsystems outlined by Auger. The reader may continue to remain at a loss as to where body image and self-concept fit in the analysis.

This article provides labeling of nursing problems experienced by the chronically ill hemodialysis patient. The author also discusses interventions within the Johnson–Auger subsystems.

Dee, V. and Auger, J.R. (1983) A patient classification system based on the behavioral system model of nursing: Part 2. *Journal of Nursing Administration*, 13(May), 18–23.

The patient categorization tool (see Auger and Dee, Part 1), a major component of the classification system outlined in Part 1, provided a basis for the clinical application in terms of the nursing process in a child psychiatry inpatient setting. It was designed to be both comprehensive and flexible enough to allow for use with clients with a variety of diagnoses as well as a wide age range. (How this was implemented was the subject of Part 1.) What was required by way of inpatient unit revisions has been the focus of this second part.

The plan for development of materials and teaching strategies required revision of nursing assessment forms, teaching materials, staff seminars, and orientation of new employees. First of all, inpatient unit nursing assessment forms had to be revised to reflect the model. What had previously been two six-page assessment forms were replaced by four-page forms designed to assess patient factors or behaviors based on the Johnson model. Whereas the earlier forms had been specific to the patient populations, the new assessment form was specific to the Johnson model and was therefore useful in all clinical settings. In view of the fact that nurses vary in levels of education, clinical experience, and abilities, an interview guide was constructed to assist the nurses in eliciting information from the patient and family. The questions included reflected content from the eight subsystems of the Johnson Behavior System Model (JBSM) as they related to the specific psychiatric setting and patient population.

The clinical nurse specialists (CNS) and the nursing coordinators (NC) of each unit developed a package of the teaching materials to illustrate the clinical application of the model. "The materials consisted of samples of completed nursing assessment forms, nursing care plans, and a list of recommended readings pertinent to the behavioral systems model and each subsystem" (Dee and Auger, 1983, p. 19).

Two exhibits contribute to the overall presentation of the teaching materials developed and stand alone, not needing additional narrative to describe them to the reader. Exhibit 1 illustrates two pages of the nursing assessment form (with sample data) developed for one of the specific inpatient units; Exhibit 2 shows portions of a sample nursing care plan based on the assessment.

Staff seminars conducted totaled four hours and were required for all nursing staff on each unit. These were followed up by actual application on the units. All newly admitted patients were assessed, and care plans were developed based on the model using the new materials. Integration and follow-up of the nursing process was provided by the CNS through weekly nursing care plan meetings or individual clinical supervision.

The orientation of new employees consisted of didactic presentations of purpose and theory, audiovisual materials of examples of different levels of patient behaviors and the corresponding nursing intervention, and unit orientation. Subsequently, the orientee was required to complete a nursing assessment and care plan with supervision from an experienced R.N.

While theoretical advantages of using the model were anticipated, the practical advantages were realized only with continued use. There were many practical advantages. Some of the clinical advantages included: more systematic patient behavioral assessment resulting in a comprehensive baseline of behavior at time of hospitalization, more specific and expedited nursing care plans, a focus on patient strengths versus pathology, and improved monitoring of patient behavior over the course of hospitalization. These factors consequently provided more objective means for evaluating the quality of nursing care.

Administrative advantages included improved ability to determine required levels of staffing based on more accurate assessment of patient behaviors, and also a more appropriate assignment of new admissions to a unit based on the level of patient need and level of staffing available; thus achieving a better match of patient needs with staff resources. The corollary would then be that as the overall identified need rose and fell, staffing levels could be raised or lowered accordingly; affecting (conversely influencing) scheduling, budgeting, and nursing hours. Overall efficiency in the integration and balance of scheduling, budgeting, and nursing hours would be improved, resulting in more cost-effective management.

Although the work was written primarily for administrators and clinicians, this scholarly approach to applying theory to practice demonstrates the utility of the JBSM for practice in various inpatient psychiatric units and gives direction to research. It also provides a working model of the "how to" in implementing theory in a practice setting and provides a blueprint for those who might choose to implement this or another theoretical model.

Derdiarian, A.K. (1983) An instrument for theory and research development using the behavioral systems model for nursing: The cancer patient, Part I. *Nursing Research*, 32(4), 196–201.

Clearly stated by the author in the introduction are both the main purposes of the research carried out and the scope and content of each of a two-part series. The purpose was to develop a valid and reliable research tool to describe the behavioral changes of cancer patients as perceived by them. The research was conceptualized from the behavioral system perspective, and therefore much of the content of Part I is a synopsis of the Johnson behavioral systems model for nursing. For a reader who is unfamiliar with the model, this is an excellent review. The author's concise writing style makes the theoretical overview quite understandable, and the author remains true to Johnson's original work. Each of the seven subsystems (achievement, affiliation, aggressive-protective, dependence, eliminative, ingestive, and sexual) and the eighth subsystem that was added later (restorative) are reviewed, terms are defined, and relationships between concepts are spelled out. The goal of nursing is also stated.

In the rest of the article, the author reviews the support from the literature for the existence of each subsystem, both from work by Johnson and Auger as well as from others writing on the same topic. The author then identifies the major dimensions extrapolated for each of the subsystems. The impact of cancer on each subsystem is then described using previously reported research. The Johnson model provides a conceptual reservoir within which research findings find a coherent existence.

This is a fine example of how theory can be used to guide research findings. The author then presents a table containing each subsystem, the determinants of behavior, and behavioral manifestations. It is upon these that the variables of interest for measurement were based. These then comprised the items of the instrument developed by the author. The development of the items and the frequencies in the table are not clear to the reader and are incongruent with the theoretical discussion. The table fits in with Part II of the article, published in the next issue, where it is discussed and described.

Derdiarian, A.K. and Forsythe, A.B. (1983) An instrument for theory and research development using the behavioral systems model for nursing: The cancer patient, Part II. *Nursing Research*, 32, 260–267.

The focus and scope of Part II of this two-article series is on the process of establishing validity and reliability for an instrument that will test perceived behavioral changes of cancer patients, based on Johnson's Behavioral Systems Model. One hundred twenty-one change items, based on each subsystem, were delineated from previous research and were given to a homogeneous sample of 163 cancer patients. The criteria for inclusion and exclusion of subjects are listed. The authors' rationale for the "limitation of selection criteria was to maximize the homogeneity of the sample in terms of salient intervening variables such as visible, extensive body disfigurement, level of awareness, comprehension, absence of additional stress caused by a new treatment or procedure, and variables of adult life cycle (p. 261)." What is not clear is why there are such broad parameters for inclusion of subjects. The extreme age variation (20–70), various cancer diagnoses, and range of treatments do not logically suggest a homogeneous sample to achieve the desired results.

Patients were asked to identify changes they perceived happening due to or since they became ill and to add or subtract changes. They were also asked to indicate quantitatively and qualitatively the extent of the changes and, finally, their perceptions of the consequences of the changes. Figure 1 in Part I presents frequency distribution of responses. The authors did not discuss what decisions they made based on these frequency distributions.

Several approaches were used to estimate content validity and reliability of the instrument. What appears to be the first step was to use an expert panel of six members, divided into two groups. "The first group evaluated the comprehensiveness of the theoretical framework and its consistency with known theories, and the consistency of the operational definitions with the theoretical framework. The second group evaluated the consistency of the operational definitions with the categories and the times. The panel judged independently" (p. 262). A supplemental assessment of empirical validity was done using the theta coefficient estimation, which was derived from a factor analysis.

Described later in the "method" section are two other methods of evaluation of comprehensiveness. Here, a panel of three clinical nurse specialists in oncology independently judged the "other" changes added by the patients (p. 262). Because of these various methods used to evaluate comprehensiveness, some confusion is generated about the sequential timing of these evaluations as well as about when the pilot testing and the reliability testing were completed.

The Derdiarian behavioral system model (DBSM) instrument was pilot tested after construction and estimation of content validity, using three male and three female subjects. Test-retest reliability was assessed by administering the instrument to, apparently, all 163 subjects. The instrument did not have identifying information on it, and "a randomized permutation schedule always places a subsystem questionnaire designed for retesting for reliability in the third place in the sequence of the subsystem questionnaires" (p. 262). Time to complete the instrument as reported by subjects was approximately 1.75 hours. After a 15-minute respite, the patient was asked to complete the retest subsystem questionnaire.

Also evaluated in the overall process was the performance of each of the eight trained research assistants. Interviewer reliability was an ongoing concern as manifested by regular review of the tapes and rating of the interviewer behavior by two independent raters who were not involved in the data-gathering process.

Grubbs, J. (1980) An interpretation of the Johnson behavioral system model for nursing practice. In J.P. Riehl and C. Roy (Eds.), *Conceptual models for nursing practice.* **New York: Appleton-Century-Crofts.**

The purpose of this article is an attempt to operationalize the model so that it could be used as a systematic guide to nursing practice. The author indicates that this is her own interpretation of the Johnson behavioral system model.

The most obvious difference between Grubbs' interpretation and the original model is the addition of the restorative subsystem, with its goal being "to relieve fatigue and/or achieve a state of equilibrium by reestablishing or replenishing the energy distribution among the other subsystems" (p. 228). The additional subsystem was articulated by faculty members at the University of California, Los Angeles after long discussions and debates. Johnson continued to remind the faculty that restoration is a requirement for each subsystem, and its addition may therefore be teleological and tautological. Also described are the functional requirements, which are better defined in Auger (1976).

An important contribution this article makes to the reader is the use of this model in the prospective development of tools (*e.g.*, sample flow sheet and work sheet, which illustrate use of the model to guide the nursing process). There is even an appendix describing items, by systems, that should be included in the assessment. Furthermore, the language and terminology used in the examples are consistent both with systems theory in general and with the behavioral system model more specifically.

Overall, this article is a contribution to the understanding of the behavioral system theory and, if read with Johnson's own account of her theory in the same book, will help to clarify the theory components. The process demonstrated here shows thought and solid construction based on the model.

Holaday, B. (1980) Implementing the Johnson model for nursing practice. In J.P. Riehl and C. Roy (Eds.), *Conceptual models for nursing practice* **(2nd ed.). New York: Appleton-Century-Crofts.**

The focus of this article, which follows the Grubbs article, is the operationalization of the model and application of the nursing process to care of the individual patient, using Johnson's model. The author designed a new assessment tool and synthesized Piaget's definition of cognition with Johnson's view of a human being as a system of behavior.

This author devotes the entire article to cognition—not even one of the behavioral subsystems—and to the eliminative system, which was defined by Johnson to include the excretion of physiological wastes and which was expanded by Grubbs (and the faculty of UCLA) to include the expulsion of one's feelings, beliefs, and emotions.

Had the author developed a rationale for incorporating Piaget's theory and refined the integration of it within either a subsystem or a cultural or psychological variable, the argument would have been more defensible.

Overall, the article is limited because of the narrow focus on the redefined eliminative subsystem, even though the author does follow through with each phase of the nursing process in accord with the purpose of the article. The article offers some clarification of the use of the behavioral systems model in practice. Refinement and extension were not provided.

Johnson, D.E. (1959) A philosophy of nursing. *Nursing Outlook,* 7(4), 198–200.

At the time this article was written, the author had identified factors impinging on nursing that resulted in a confusion of goals and the division of nursing into two camps. The camps were divided into those who believed the professional nurse of the future would have largely supervisory and managerial responsibilities and, on the other side, those who believed that nursing could and would take its place as a professional discipline in relation to direct service to people who are "in need of nursing care."

Johnson belonged to the latter camp: the science of nursing and the art of nursing. The first of these—the discussion of the science of nursing, centered around the patient, the recipient of care—is phenomenal in that it is as relevant today as it was in the late 1950s. In fact, the discussion might almost be considered prophetic because three decades later, the client was identified as one of the nursing phenomenon. Nursing process, nursing diagnosis, and nursing science are no longer as esoteric as they seemed in 1959 when Johnson's article was published. Nursing art, to Johnson, represented ministration of the basic unmet needs of the patient. Also identified are those activities that are delegated and controlled by the physician.

A sociological analysis of the nursing role is used as a vehicle for understanding the division of labor between nurses and physicians. We will also see, much later in time, just how much of an impact this sociological analysis has had on Johnson's own theory.

Johnson, D.E. (1961) The significance of nursing care. *Nursing Outlook,* 61(11), 63–66.

This is a very significant, indeed, classic work in nursing knowledge. Here, Johnson introduces the notion of stability rather than change as the goal of nursing. Meeting the needs of the patient helps bring about that stability.

Because of pressures from the medical and hospital management on nursing to take on non-nursing tasks, Johnson believes that the view of nursing as a direct and individualized service has become less goal-oriented and more blurred. Three major components or types of nursing services were identified: (1) nursing care, (2) delegated medical care, and (3) health care. Of the three, only one—nursing care—has "no well-delineated theoretical framework or conceptual basis to give it meaning or direction (p. 64)."

The purpose of this article, then, is to delineate such a framework within the context of nursing's distinctive contribution to patient welfare and the specific purpose of nursing care.

Using concepts of physiological homeostasis borrowed from Cannon and stability in patterns of social interaction from Parsons, Johnson synthesized them and related them to individuals who are ill. Instability causes tension; if tension is intense, an individual experiences discomfort and displeasure.

Speculating from these, Johnson attempted to evolve a basis for nursing care, using concepts of equilibrium, stress, and tension. Each of these is defined in general terms and then as it applies to an individual patient (or group) or how the nurse might identify or assess stress, tension, or equilibrium. The conceptualization of equilibrium, stress, and tension presents a way of viewing the nature of disturbances that a patient might have as well as the purpose of nursing care, or what might be considered nursing's specific responsibility in nursing care.

Two nursing interventions within this framework are also suggested. First, reduction of the stressful stimuli through the management of the physical and psychological environment, and second, support of the patient's "natural defenses and adaptive processes" through "protective and sustaining measures." The focus of nursing is on immediate situations, universal needs, and patterns that belong to the patient and are gratifying to him. The seeds for Johnson's theory were planted in this writing.

Johnson, D.E. (1980) The behavioral system model for nursing. In J.P. Riehl and C. Roy (Eds.), *Conceptual models for nursing practice* **(2nd ed.). New York: Appleton-Century-Crofts.**

Dorothy Johnson, for the first time in writing, clearly presents the whole of her theory. Much of her unpublished work had been alluded to by her protegees and, though available in manuscript form, it suffered from limited distribution. This was the first time the original behavioral systems theory for nursing was published in its entirety.

According to its author, the behavioral systems model has its origins in a philosophical perspective and has been supported by an expanding empirical and theoretical base (*i.e.*, systems theory). (It would be helpful to read three of the author's early publications, two in 1959 and one in 1961, in conjunction with this one.) It is Johnson's perspective that both nurses and physicians theoretically have viewed a human being as a system. However, nurses view the patient as a behavioral system, whereas physicians view him as a biological system. It is the nursing view of the human being as a behavioral system that underlies this model. A review of this article shows that the underlying assumptions of the model are explicit. The concepts are embedded in the context and are not specifically defined. The system is identified as having seven subsystems, which are briefly defined. The four structural elements of each subsystem are listed and discussed.

The basic elements of the model that are briefly touched upon and that are implicit rather than explicit include values, goal of action, patiency, and source of difficulty. The latter is discussed only minimally; noticeably missing is a discussion of intervention.

In summarizing, the author indicated that the behavioral systems model "seems defensible and promising by three criteria." The criteria were named in the 1974 article and are social congruence, social significance, and social utility. She also said that the model has "proved its utility in providing clear direction for practice, education, and research." Although the present work does not provide any evidence to support this, some available documentation exists and is discussed in the section on Johnson in this book.

Despite these limitations of the model—that is, underdevelopment of some of the elements and lack of supportive evidence for the model's utility—this theoretical model for nursing is one of the major contributions to nursing theory development in the past two decades. Furthermore, Johnson's thinking has impacted on a great number of graduate students in nursing who have since gone on to develop other theoretical models. Johnson's stimulus for progress should not be underestimated; it has resulted in the advancement of nursing as a science.

Lovejoy, N.C. (1983) The leukemic child's perceptions of family behaviors. *Oncology Nursing Forum,* 10(4), 20–25.
Contributing to theory development and testing through the development of instruments to measure concepts is of utmost importance to the advancement of nursing science.

The author states that the Johnson model was selected as the theoretical framework "because of its basic premise that human behavior in health and illness is the independent domain of nursing" (Lovejoy, 1983, p. 20). In table form as part of the background materials, the author presented a comparison of the Johnson behavioral system model (JBSM) goals by subsystem and by theorist, showing differences between theorists. The theorists compared are Johnson, Grubbs, Auger, and Lovejoy; all of whom have elaborated upon and used the model. This provides a helpful summary and review of the subsystems for the reader familiar with the model. It is assumed, however, that the reader has some knowledge of the model. The author notes the disparity among the theorists regarding the scope of the goal-directed behaviors of the subsystems, but concludes that "the goals used in this research appeared to parsimoniously and discretely define special domains of behavior (Lovejoy, 1983, p. 21)." The reader is left wondering where the support for such a conclusion is. Little additional elaboration of or support for "discretely defined domains of behavior" was given.

The Family Relations (FR) test, the instrument upon which the family assessment instrument was modeled, was then described. The FR test situation was designed as a play situation in which the child was to decide what feelings fit what members of the family. The family assessment instrument (Lovejoy) consists of 47 items apparently designed to reflect the eight subsystems of the JBSM. The number of questions ranges from four to eight for each subsystem. No explanation is provided for having a variable number of items per subsystem. The items are shown in Table 2 and stand alone without additional explanation. Items for the assessment tool were generated and formulated based on a review of major growth and development theorists and a review of chronic illness research. Statements reflecting functional and dysfunctional family member behaviors were formulated from this review. The statements describing these behaviors were then placed on individual cards for later test administration. Noticeably missing was reference to how items were formulated to reflect the eight subsystems of the JBSM. This is an important omission given that the author purported that the instrument was "based on the Johnson Model for nursing (1983, p. 20)."

There are several major limitations with this instrument. First, there is little or no evidence of content validity and face validity within the context of either growth and development theory or the Johnson model. No evidence is presented indicating that the items were subjected to a review by experts either in growth and development or the Johnson model. This was also true of the review of the scoring guide, as discussed previously. Although it is a time-consuming and arduous task, some attempt to develop content validity is crucial, even for initial instrument development, and was overlooked in the development of this instrument.

Second, the scoring guide and the method of scoring described suggest that the rating of 0 to 2 is a scale, with equal distances between each measure. In application, these appear to be discrete categories and therefore not conducive to the summation-scoring method used.

It may be more appropriate to standardize the instrument by developing norms for each age group.

Rawls, A.C. (1980) Evaluation of the Johnson behavioral model in clinical practice: Report of a test and evaluation of the Johnson theory. *Image,* 12, 13–16.

In the introduction, the author clearly identifies the importance of model testing for the future of nursing in general and, specifically, her rationale for choosing to evaluate the application of the Johnson theory. The purpose and scope of the report are also identified. The title might suggest that the "test" was research when, actually, it was an exercise in whether or not the theory was clinically useful.

As background for the study, a brief history and an overview of other authors' contributions to the model is presented. Johnson's model is briefly reviewed to provide readers with an outline of how the model was used as a framework by the author. The subsystems and their components and the structure and function of the theory are all defined. For purposes of discussion only, the structure, function, and functional requirements of the subsystems are discussed in detail. After clarification of a few other components of the model, the use of the Johnson model (JM) as a guide for the nursing process is illustrated.

Each stage of the nursing process—assessment through evaluation—is described within the context of the JM subsystems using the Grubbs assessment tool and nursing process worksheet. These process and description are similar to those described by Janelli (1980) with Roy's model. Prior to the beginning of the "study," variables that may have influenced the outcome were explored. Four were identified: "limited knowledge of Johnson's theory," "lack of experience in utilizing Grubbs' assessment tool and nursing process worksheet," and patient's response to the researcher, to the assessment tool, and to the plan of care developed. Time available for the study and the size of the study group were also identified. The author chose to limit the sample size to one "due to the variables cited previously (Rawls, 1980, p. 13)."

The study focused on a case presentation of one subject, beginning with patient background, followed by first- and second-level assessment. The patient selected for the study was a white male who had been hospitalized for evaluation of an accidental injury, resulting in painful amputation of the left hand and distal phalanges approximately six months earlier. The first level assessment appeared to be more in keeping with the medical model in that information about past and present history of the problem, psychological assessment, family, and social, environmental, and development history were reviewed.

From the perspective of the JM, no examples of assessments of subsystems were presented. An exception was a statement indicating that because no problems were noted in the review to that point, a complete review of the behavior subsystems was conducted using Grubbs' assessment tool. Two problem areas in the achievement subsystem were identified. Because there were problem areas in only this one subsystem, the discussion was limited to that one. Second-level assessment proceeded from there. One concept—the concept of body image—was explored in depth.

The assessment phase was followed by a plan for care, again focusing on intervention for the two problems in the achievement subsystem only. The plan focused on how the patient's loss of his left hand and its function prevented him from meeting the conceptual goal of the achievement subsystem (*i.e.*, to achieve or master). Variables that might have influenced the patient's care were explored and identified. "The developmental, psychological, sociological, and level-of-wellness variables were all viewed as influencing variables that could be manipulated to benefit the patient" (Rawls, 1980, p. 16).

The next step was the identification of nursing problems. This step may be confusing in that problems were identified earlier in the assessment phases of the nursing process. Furthermore, the author did not clarify why this additional step of problem identification was necessary. Further reading led me to conclude that these additional problems were refinements of previously identified problems in the achievement subsystem. The nursing interventions for these problems were detailed, with numerous examples used for illustration. Both long-term and short-term goals of nursing intervention were formulated. The plan of care was evaluated and found to be appropriate, as measured by changes consistent with the short-term goals. The plan of care, with minor revisions, was also found to be appropriate to the patient's postoperative course.

The author's "evaluation of the Johnson Model" was more of an evaluation of the usefulness of the model for clinical practice than a critical review of the model itself. The author recommended that the model be tested further in a variety of settings with clients who have a variety of complex problems in each of the subsystems. To have stated this limitation is to the author's credit. Disadvantages of the model as perceived by the author included complex and unique terminology and the requirement of knowledge of systems theory in order to use the model more effectively. The author concluded that the advantages of the model for practice, in essence, outweighed the disadvantages; she believed that the Johnson model "offers the nurse a tool which will allow her to accurately predict the results of nursing interventions prior to care," and "formulate standards for care" (1980, p. 16).

The nursing educator who is interested in teaching the JM or in demonstrating the application of theory to practice (as well as the nursing theorist concerned about the utility of the model for practice) would find this article of some interest. The beginnings of the elaboration of the concept of body image as it relates to the achievement subsystem are present in this author's assessment phase.

Small, B. (1980) Nursing visually impaired children with Johnson's model as a conceptual framework. In J.P. Riehl and C. Roy (Eds.), *Conceptual models for nursing practice* (2nd ed.). (pp. 264–273). New York: Appleton-Century-Crofts.

Although nursing research that tests hypotheses of nursing theories is critical for the advancement of a particular theory, this study does not test hypotheses evolving from Johnson's theory, but it demonstrates that the theory could be utilized in working with visually impaired children.

The report of a research study is the first of two parts of this chapter. The second includes implications for nursing. The major assumptions underlying the theoretical framework of the study were derived from Piaget and cognitive developmental psychology. Two null hypotheses were tested and rejected. The first stated that "there would be no significant difference between the perceived body image of visually impaired and normally sighted preschool children." The second stated that there would be no significant difference between the spatial awareness of visually impaired preschoolers and those who were normally sighted.

The author explains results of the study using Johnson's theory. Vision plays an important role in the development of object permanence and the relation of objects in space. These two concepts are necessary for the development of a child's body image and for his awareness of his body in space. Therefore, if a child is visually handicapped, the implications are that nurses can intervene to meet his needs and to facilitate the development of his self-concept.

Once this line of reasoning was developed, and once a brief description of Johnson's model was presented, the author tended to focus more on interventions with the parents than with the child, therefore supporting Johnson's recommendations for intervention: manipulation of the environment to reduce tension.

Myra Levine

Esposito, C.H. and Leonard, M.K. (1980) Myra Estrin Levine. In the Nursing Theories Conference Group, *Nursing theories: A base for professional practice* (pp. 150-163). Englewood Cliffs, NJ: Prentice-Hall.

The content of this article is organized to include a summary of the components of Levine's theory, its application to the nursing process, and the relationship of the theory to five major concepts (humanity, society, health, learning, and nursing). In addition, a brief case study is included to demonstrate application to practice (*i.e.*, the utility of the theory for clinical practice).

One of the major contributions of this chapter is the identification of the explicit assumptions underlying Levine's theory. This is helpful because the assumptions are implicit in Levine's writing.

There is one important omission in this discussion of Levine's theory: the major theoretical underpinnings, namely systems theory, is not identified. Given that systems theory is not acknowledged, it becomes clearer why Levine's theory is identified as having a close kinship to Maslow's hierarchy of needs. One might agree that parallels could be drawn between the conservation principles and Maslow's levels of needs, but Maslow's theory must not be construed as the prototype for Levine's principles. Nowhere in Levine's writing is there any reference to Maslow's needs hierarchy.

Two potential problems in this chapter are the lack of identification of what is Levine's and what are Esposito's and Leonard's additions and that the parallels between Maslow's hierarchy of needs and conservation principles (tenuous at best) may be accidental and therefore do not justify this as a prototype paradigm. More support could be given to system or adaptations as guiding paradigms.

Hirschfeld, M.J. (1976) The cognitively impaired older adult. *American Journal of Nursing*, 76(12), 1981–1984.

In a very straightforward discussion of the possible cognitive impairments of older adults, and in the only published work on utilization of Levine's theory in practice, Hirschfeld demonstrates how Levine's four principles of conservation can be applied to give direction to nursing interventions when impairments are present. The goal of the interventions is specified as trying to keep remaining cognitive capacities intact and in use.

Each conservation principle, and examples demonstrating problems in the area it covered, were discussed separately. For example, a variety of problems are described wherein the balance of activity and rest were disturbed. Focusing on conservation of energy in this case gave the nurse direction for intervention.

Levine, M.E. (1966) Adaptation and assessment: A rationale of nursing intervention. *American Journal of Nursing*, 66(11), 2450–2453.

Levine introduced "trophicognosis" as an alternative concept to replace "nursing diagnosis" (Levine, M.E. (1966) Trophicognosis: An alternative to nursing diagnosis. In *Exploring progress in medical surgical nursing practice.* (pp. 55–70). New York: American Nurses Association. A series of papers presented at the 1965 Regional Clinical Conferences, November 3–5, 1965, Washington, D.C.). The latter conjures up medicine and disease orientation, whereas the former focuses attention on judgments related to nursing care utilizing the scientific method. In that earlier writing, it becomes apparent that Levine is interested in delineating nursing goals and differentiating them from medical goals.

In this second of four articles that precede the publishing of her book, *Introduction to Clinical Nursing,* Levine further demonstrates her conceptualization of nursing as utilizing the scientific method and as a coherent theory in guiding its actions. She argues that nursing practice and education have long been influenced by the prevailing beliefs about health and disease. As a result of a carry-over or a carry-through of earlier theories, nursing care has become "an unsynthesized "total," a sum of many disparate parts" (p. 2451). Thus there is an urgent need, as Levine sees it, for a restatement of the theoretical basis for nursing practice. This is what she attempted to do in this article.

Drawing from a variety of sources—philosophy, physiology, and sociology—a few basic ideas about human beings become implicit assumptions of the theory. Central ideas are (1) a human being's life is multidimensional, (2) a human being is in constant interaction with the environment, (3) a human being's internal environment is integrated and is dynamically balanced, (4) a human being responds to forces in the environment in a unique but integrated manner, (5) health and disease are patterns of adaptive change, and (6) the nurse is part of every patient's environment. One sees here the influence of systems theory: wholeness of human being, dynamic equilibrium, human being–environment interactions, and adaptation.

The author revived Nightingale's ideas of multicausality of illness, disease as a "reparative process," and nursing's goal as establishing a health environment that would enhance healing and reparative processes. Levine refocused nursing's attention on the wholeness of human beings, the uniqueness of each human being, and on the fact that a broad knowledge base is required by the nurse in order to give nursing care.

Levine's discussion of adaptation raises some questions. Adaptation is introduced but not really defined per se. For example, "all the processes of living are processes of adaptation," "diseases represent patterned responses or adaptations," "health and disease are patterns of adaptive change" (p. 2452). But what is adaptation? Levine indicates that a criterion of successful adaptation is the attainment of social well-being, which is neither defined nor related to the preceding physiological discussion.

The major ideas expressed about nursing are that the nurse is an agent who intervenes between a patient and his environment to facilitate adaptation and that the interventions are based on coherent and systematic knowledge and a scientific process in collecting data about the patient.

Levine, M.E. (1967) The four conservation principles of nursing. *Nursing Forum,* 6(1), 45–59.

This article is the third that this author wrote in an attempt to lay down a framework for nursing intervention. It is helpful to read this after reading the first two on trophicognosis and on adaptation and assessment in order to fully understand the process that Levine used in theory development: redefining central concepts, reconceptualization of nursing goals, and then nursing actions. She identified central concepts, stated assumptions, and proposed four central propositions.

The concept of adaptation as developed by Levine in her earlier article remains undefined. In the introduction alone, adaptation may be conceived or interpreted in three different ways. First, one can infer that it "can be manifested in patterns" and "has a course." One could also infer that adaptation is an outcome because it can be measured by "renewed social well-being." Third, in another context, one can infer that adaptation can be a capability or a characteristic of a person.

Aside from adaptation, the major focus of this article and Levine's major contribution to theory is the introduction of four conservation principles that are central to the mission of nursing. Levine identifies nursing principles as "fundamental assumptions which provide a unifying structure for understanding a wide variety of nursing activities" (p. 45). Here, each principle (labeled assumptions, but they may be the theory's propositions) is listed separately along with a statement about nursing intervention and is then followed by a discussion that supports the principle and the rationale for it. Clinical examples are included as supportive evidence. The four principles are all conservation principles. Conservation is defined as "keeping together," but the author emphasizes that this "should not imply minimal activity," especially on the part of the nurse.

The four principles are: "(1) The Principle of the Conservation of Patient Energy, (2) The Principle of the Conservation of Structural Integrity, (3) The Principle of Conservation of Personal Integrity, (4) The Principle of Conservation of Social Integrity." For each of these, nursing intervention is based on the conservation of the particular patient's need in focus. The four principles evolved from an assumption of the unity and integrity of the individual; they are well-developed and supported with clinical examples; and they are, in part, consistent with some assumptions from the systems theory.

Three critical questions are raised: (1) How did the author come to the point of identifying four and only four principles? (2) In principle 2, given the complex interrelationships of human structure and function (which Levine does discuss), why is the principle not stated in terms of both structural and functional integrity, or why weren't two separate principles for these developed? What is the rationale for focusing on structural integrity versus both structure and function? (3) Why aren't personal integrity and social integrity specifically defined?

Considering the dearth of theoretical frameworks for nursing available in the late 1960s, this framework made a substantial contribution to the science of nursing. Levine proved herself to be an insightful, forward-looking theorist.

Levine, M.E. (1969) The pursuit of wholeness. *American Journal of Nursing,* 69(1), 93–98.

Consistent with the first three articles and with systems theory, Levine views a human being as a system in constant interaction with the environment: "patients are complete persons, not groups of parts."

This article provides a view of the human being from a nursing perspective, as a system in a constant dynamic interchange with the environment and as part of a larger ecosystem. Information is exchanged between the human system and the larger ecosystem—by way of the perceptual subsystem. Disturbances in the perceptual subsystem, as well as the levels of organismic response used to protect the organism as it responds to the environment, give direction to nursing.

When the environment changes, the human being must change. Levine makes a fairly succinct theoretical statement here about what adaptation is. This process of change "whereby the individual retains his integrity—his wholeness—within the realities of his environment" is labeled adaptation (p. 95). The goal of the individual is to defend his wholeness.

There are at least four levels of organismic response, each physiologically predetermined. (This is an implicit assumption on Levine's part.) The responses are used to protect the organism so that it can make a viable adaptation to the environment. The four levels include: response to fear, inflammatory response, response to stress, and sensory response. These four levels are fairly well-documented.

Alone, this article does not contribute substantially to our understanding of Levine's theory; it must not be read in isolation. In the context of earlier articles and ones that come later, the perspective of this one becomes clearer.

Levine, M.E. (1971) Holistic nursing. *Nursing Clinics of North America*, 6(2), 253–264.

No new material is presented here. This is more of a synthesis of previously published material, which contributes to a better general understanding of the theory. The author brings together all the ideas, the separate parts, of the earlier four articles into a whole. The parts of Levine's theory—the assumptions, central concepts, definitions of person (who is the nursing client), goals of nursing, and nursing intervention—are put together, and the interrelationships between parts are then described.

Levine views holistic nursing as the challenge before nurses. This approach to nursing takes place at the interface between the organism (human being) and the environment. In other words, nursing is an interaction, and the nurse, in a sense, mediates between the organism and his environment, whether the environment in question is the organism's internal environment or external environment.

For the person desiring an overview of the theory, or some help in piecing together the earlier parts of the theory, this article could be most helpful and should then be read before the first four articles.

Levine, M.E. (1971) Time has come to speak of. . . health care. *AORN Journal*, 13, 37–43.

In a speech to the annual congress of the Association of Operating Room Nurses (AORN), focusing on the concerns of that group for viability, Levine indirectly presents arguments in support of her theoretical framework for nursing. Ostensibly, the focus of the speech is the threat of increased technological change and innovation to the roles of nurses, especially with the concomitant requirement for technicians to manage the machinery. The health care field has responded to the technological advances by increasing the number of technicians. Although operating room nurses were the first to be threatened by the influx, their area is not the only one inundated by technicians. For example, there are now ICUs, CCUs, trauma, dialysis, burn, coma, respiratory, and hyperbaric units.

Nevertheless, Levine argues that in all these settings there are both technical and professional roles to be filled. She further argues that situations continue to arise in which there are new threats of new technicians; however, her real concern is for the quality of care to patients. What will happen if the new physician assistants, for example, go into underserved areas and provide a second-class kind of medical care? If this is a trend, then nursing must make itself heard to prevent these inadequacies from occurring. Those in society who are now already underserved, already suffering, would be most affected by these inadequacies of health care.

Confusion in the roles of workers, both professional and technical, has been a result of all the changes in health care. However, there still remains one need that nurses can recognize and sustain: self-respect and humanity of the patient. The nurse traditionally has been and must remain the patient's advocate. Unless the effort is made to reach out and establish human contact, the patient will just become another part of the elaborate machinery of the technology. The technical role in this situation is supportive and essential, but it is the professional nurse who must be the patient's advocate, the humanizing agent, the one who brings "compassion, protection, and commitment to the bedside."

Given the changes in health care, the education of nurses must change too. In order to be the professional nurse, as described previously, Levine believes that the achievement of the education of a patient's advocate requires knowledge and skills of a global kind. Furthermore, there needs to be a conceptualization of nursing. She presents her formulations as valid forms of nursing intervention. She also suggests that the concepts inherent in the generalizations can be readily applied to all kinds of nursing intervention. It is here that we see Levine's support for her theoretical framework for nursing as one way to counter the threat of technological advances to nursing, to patients, and to health care.

Dorothea Orem

Allison, S.E. (1973) A framework for nursing action in a nurse-conducted diabetic management clinic. *Journal of Nursing Administration*, 3(4), 53–60.

This article is based on and follows the 1974 Backscheider article, although this one was published first. The author provides a comprehensive picture of the health care system, using the self-care model as a basis for the nurse-conducted diabetic management clinic. The author synthesizes some of Orem's and Backscheider's concepts: universal self-care, health deviation self-care (Orem), and mental, physical, motivational, emotional, and orientational capacities to follow a therapeutic regimen (Backscheider). The article provides a highly useful example of the use of Orem's ideas in a nurse-run diabetic clinic. Three models—self-care, health status, and environment—are offered as a framework for assessment and intervention. The author provides a very useful discussion of areas of responsibility and differentiates between traditional nursing roles (administrative) and practitioner roles (clinically oriented) as shared and as delineated for nursing, medicine, and other health services. Although this is an ideal setting for theory testing, the focus of the article is on application.

Anna, D.J., Christensen, D.G., Hohn, S.A., Ord, L., and Wells, S.R. (1978) Implementing Orem's conceptual framework. *Journal of Nursing Administration*, 8(11), 8–11.

The authors present a descriptive account of the implementation of Orem's model by a group of graduate students in a nursing home setting for adult patients (geriatric setting). In doing so, the authors provide a short summary of the theory, the use of the nursing process according to Orem, the strategies the students used in implementing the theory in the setting, and the obstacles preventing implementation by students, patients, and nursing staff. Difficulties experienced by the students in shifting to Orem's conceptualization (terminology, concept definitions, mechanization) are those that could be universal and could apply to all initial attempts at implementing any nursing theory. The conceptualization of a patient's role as that of a significant decision maker and eventually a performer of self-care activities presented another obstacle. Patients felt more comfortable as recipients of care. As expected, the nursing staff was resistant to change initiated by a group of temporary students. Evaluation of the implementation process was done by review of students' personal diaries. Themes were an increase in patient participation, motivation, and cooperation.

Backscheider, J.E. (1974) Self-care requirements, self-care capabilities, and nursing systems in the diabetic nurse management clinic. *American Journal of Public Health*, 64(12), 1138–1146.

This author provides a conceptualization of the diabetic-related component of therapeutic self-care, encompassing a set of patient responsibilities (related to the patient's own condition and therapy and to the effects of his condition and therapy) and a set of action capabilities (physical, mental, motivational, emotional, and orientational). Nursing care is needed when a patient has limited capability to meet the therapeutic self-care (self-care deficit). Nursing is a mediating system and is divided into four types. Nursing care (nursing system) is focused on the patient as a one-time guidance or teaching, on long-term assistance that is oriented toward maintenance and support, on more permanent compensatory care oriented toward some changes in the patient, or on compensatory care using changes in the environment.

When a given health care deviation occurs, the capabilities essential to meet that portion of the therapeutic self-care are determined first and foremost. Criteria can then be established. The nurse can assess the patient's capabilities against the established criteria to determine whether or not the patient can meet the self-care demands. This is a more positive approach, a more scientific one to establishing nursing interventions than by estimating the patient's abilities or limitations.

This is an important article to read in relation to the theory of self-care. It demonstrates the interaction between practice and theory development and shows potential for researchable questions.

Bromley, B. (1980) Applying Orem's self-care theory in enterostomal therapy. *American Journal of Nursing*, 80(2), 245–249.

The author, an enterostomal therapist, begins with a discussion of her own personal philosophy of nursing practice, with the most useful tool being the nurse. Her choice of Orem's theory was made because of the apparent congruency between hers and Orem's philosophies. The usefulness of this article lies in the author's synthesis of her perceptions of Orem's theory and the use of an exemplar to demonstrate the theory–practice fit, particularly around nursing interventions. The author writes clearly and does a particularly nice job of showing how the nursing systems of self-care are implemented in an inpatient (hospital) setting. Using an example, she shows how she has moved from a wholly compensatory system, through the partly compensatory system, to the supportive–educative system with a client.

For those interested in the appropriateness of Orem's model for inpatient practice in a surgical setting, this is a good example because the author followed the theory closely throughout.

Buckwalter, K.C. and Kerfoot, K.M. (1982) Teaching patients self-care: A critical aspect of psychiatric discharge planning. *Journal of Psychiatric Nursing and Mental Health Services*, 20(5), 15–20.

While ostensibly presenting clinical applications under the umbrella of Orem's self-care framework, this article is about discharge planning and teaching; it appears that the notion of self-care has been added after the fact. The abstract clues us in to the fact that self-care is not an integral part of the conceptualization of the discharge planning.

The content includes the following topics: understanding the diagnosis, stressors, signs and symptoms, resocializing issues, community support, and medication compliance. Each topic is briefly described and illustrated with clinical examples. A sample standardized protocol for depressives and their families is included.

The only references to Orem are the use of her definition of self-care and two references to kinds of nursing assistance, namely teaching and self-care guidance. Self-care concepts are not applied to the content. To be consistent with the theoretical framework, the content must also follow. For example, the summary of the five areas to be covered with patient and family in the discharge planning interview (p. 16) lend themselves to the six health deviation self-care requisites as elaborated by Orem (1980, pp. 48–51).

This article covers an important topic of present concern for all mental health practitioners—not just nurses—regarding maintaining the mentally ill in the community. Overall, the article is written in a straightforward and understandable style and presents important clinical content. What is of concern is that the authors state that they are using Orem's perspective. Although they do include topics under the rubric of self-care, Orem's framework in fact does not guide the conceptualization of the teaching and guidance plan.

Caley, J.M., Dirkensen, M., Engally, M., and Hennrich, M.L. (1980) The Orem self-care nursing model. In J.P. Riehl and C. Roy (Eds.), *Conceptual models for nursing practice* (2nd ed.). (pp. 302–314). New York: Appleton-Century-Crofts.

The intent of the chapter is to offer an example of the use of Orem's theory in a psychiatric setting, using a suicidal patient as the case study. The discussion of the model, brief and limited, is organized around the goal of action, patiency, actor's role, source of difficulty, intervention focus/mode, and consequences, both intended and otherwise.

It would be helpful for a theory novice who is focused on a theory-psychiatric practice link to read this chapter in conjunction with Orem's work, with the understanding that it is a limited expose and does not do complete justice to Orem's theories. The authors freely used concepts from Backscheider (1971; 1974) and the Nursing Development Conference Group (1973) in addition to Orem (1971).

Chang, B.L. (1980) Evaluation of health care professionals in facilitating self-care: Review of the literature and a conceptual model. *Advances in Nursing Science*, 3(1), 43–58.

The purpose of this article is stated in terms of needs. "A need exists for the evaluation of health professionals in facilitating self-care. Such an evaluation must take into account lay persons' judgments regarding the health care received. A conceptual framework is needed for the evaluation of the role of health professionals in facilitating self-care" (p. 44). The "why" of this, the importance, is not spelled out.

The author states that the derivation of her framework for the evaluation of health professionals is in part from Orem's work and in part from other literature related to the evaluation of quality of care. The dimensions of the framework are listed as "(1) patient or layperson characteristics, (2) health care professional characteristics, and (3) patient outcomes" (p. 44). A diagram illustrates the relationship of these dimensions and serves to introduce the components of these dimensions. The diagram contains all the dimensions and their components and the direction of the linkages. The third and last dimension, influenced by the preceding two, is the focus of the review of literature. Why only the third dimension—evaluation of outcomes of self-care—is reviewed in detail is not stated.

Although the author has presented a broad definition of self-care, a strong statement about the overall importance of the topic and why this particular definition of self-care was chosen over others commonly used in the literature has thus far not been presented.

There are numerous opportunities to use Orem's framework to guide the conceptualization of the model proposed, and they are not taken advantage of. In the review of the literature on evaluation of outcomes of self-care, specifically the three components, the author appears to have neglected to use important articles relevant to the framework presented. Examples of this include writings by Allison (1973), who addresses nurses and other health team members and their role in assisting patients to perform self-care regarding diabetic management, and by Backscheider (1974), who also addresses the role of nurses in assisting with the self-care practices of diabetics and the self-care competencies required by ambulatory diabetics.

Although the author may have accomplished her overall goals of presenting a conceptual model and reviewing some literature related to evaluation of health care professionals, conceptual linkages between the different dimensions, are missing.

Coleman, L.J. (1980) Orem's self-care concept of nursing. In J.P. Riehl and C. Roy (Eds.), *Conceptual models for nursing practice* (2nd ed.). (pp. 315–328). New York: Appleton-Century-Crofts.

The primary purpose of this article is to describe the implementation of Orem's theory in one nursing service department of a large metropolitan hospital. Therefore, Orem's model is first summarized by the author, with particular emphasis on those concepts and ideas that would be most useful for the nursing service department of a hospital (*e.g.*, nursing assistance, nursing process). The language of the chapter, to be sure, is the language of nursing administration, such as classification of patients, techniques essential for nursing practice, utilization of nursing personnel, and operational documents. The author then described what was involved in revising operational documents of a nursing service, including departmental philosophy and goals, departmental policies, divisional philosophy and objectives, position descriptions, nursing tools, and nursing care evaluation instruments in the process of operationalizing Orem's model. Also briefly described was the preparation of the nursing personnel for understanding and using Orem's concepts.

This chapter offers a "how to" contribution to the nursing administrator who wishes to implement the theory in practice.

Dickson, G.L. and Lee-Villasenor, H. (1982) Nursing theory and practice: A self-care approach. *Advances in Nursing Science*, 5, 29–40.

The stated purpose of this article is "to bridge the gaps between theory and practice through the research of the application of an evolving theory" (p. 29). The authors also present a "new nursing model in which to "think nursing" " (p. 30). The findings described were from a field study carried out by the authors in their own independent practice settings using their own clients.

The framework of self-care developed by Orem and modified by Kinlein was chosen as the theoretical model for practice and research because the beliefs underlying the model were in keeping with the authors' philosophy. The authors adequately describe and document these background materials sufficiently for those familiar with the model. For those unfamiliar with the model, the review is not adequate.

A nonexperimental, descriptive design was used. The source of data was the written recording of nurse–patient interactions from 35 time periods of four clients. Although the authors describe the four female subjects, they do not tell us why eight other prospective subjects were not included.

The research process proceeded as follows: during the clients' appointments and during the process of providing nursing care, the nursing researchers recorded their clients' words. At the time that a "need" was expressed, the nurse then identified self-care assets, the self-care demands, and the self-care measures with the client. The next step was a period of introspection for reflection on the nursing phenomena observed. Operational definitions were established, and four research questions were generated.

The data analysis yielded four categories of care: (1) the client's expression of need, (2) self-care asset, (3) self-care demand, and (4) self-care measures. These were analyzed using content analysis from the grounded field theory methodology. Further analysis, in keeping with the inductive method of research being used (Glaser and Strauss), focused on the integration of categories and their properties. Specifically, data were analyzed to determine properties of expressions of need and self-care assets. The latter were found to be similar to the indicators of self-care agency as identified by Kearney and Fleischer (1979).

In summary, the authors reflect on the limitations of the research, namely sample size and bias, implications for practice and research, and directions for future research. The authors demonstrate clarity in describing both the procedures and the process of their experiences in relating theory to practice and research. The complex helical relationship of the three is clearly illustrated and the scholarliness of their approach and writing adds to the overall readability. The model was their guide for practice and research and, with the model in mind, it helped to maintain their focus on their goals. For these reasons, this study would be of interest to theorists, researchers, and clinicians alike who espouse the self-care framework. More important, the article provides an exemplar for theory development using the practice–theory strategy.

Karl, C.A. (1982) The effect of an exercise program on self-care activities for the institutionalized elderly. *Journal of Gerontological Nursing*, 8, 282–285.

Although the title of this short report of a research study includes the concept of self-care, and although Orem is mentioned in the section, "Program Background," the self-care framework does not seem to guide the conceptualization of the study. The review of the research literature focuses on general topics of feelings of well-being and physiological benefits of exercise rather than on self-care. Furthermore, liberties are taken with Orem's framework when the author states that "the theoretical defense for a study of the positive effects an exercise program can have on the institutionalized elderly and their ability to care for themselves has been formulated by Orem in her theory of self-care" (p. 283). Also misstated were the "assumptions"; in fact, these are really the hypotheses tested by the study.

Miller, J.F. (1980) The dynamic focus of nursing: A challenge to nursing administration. *Journal of Nursing Administration*, 10(1), 13–18.

Although the title of this article suggests that the focus will be on nursing administration, and despite the introductory statement that "nursing administrators are challenged to establish a climate that facilitates the use of appropriate frameworks to guide nursing" (p. 13), this article is really about the application of a nursing framework—Orem's—to acute care. However, there is very little evidence of the self-care theory, which the author purports to use. What the author did, in fact, was to pull out the idea of changes in the health/illness continuum, suggesting that nurses focus on changes in the patient's health status as a model to guide intervention. The author presents three conceptual phases for acute care patients (acute illness, convalescence, and restored health), problems and nursing care strategies related to each, and a patient case study to demonstrate application. Only phases 2 and 3 are linked to patient development of self-care skills.

Although it takes into account where the person is on the health/illness continuum (which phase), the proposed "model for dynamic nursing practice" essentially ignores Orem's nursing systems, which give direction for nursing intervention based on the person's health self-care needs or self-care deficits regardless of where he is on the health/illness continuum. Therefore, this article offers a very limited application of Orem's theory.

Miller, J.F. (1982) Categories of self-care needs of ambulatory patients with diabetes. *Journal of Advanced Nursing,* 7, 25–31.

The stated purpose of this paper is to report a study of the identification of need categories of ambulatory diabetic patients within the context of the self-care nursing framework. The title of the article reflects this purpose. The method used to discover the categories of self-care needs was that of participant observation. The need for the research was identified, but why the self-care framework is "especially appropriate" (p. 25) was not explained.

The sample of 65 men and women, ranging in age from 22 to 83, came from different socioeconomic classes and were from various cultural backgrounds. No rationale for sample selection was presented. The clinic where the subjects were treated used the self-care concept for nursing practice. Data collection initially involved an assessment of the patient's self-care agency using an instrument designed by the researcher and published elsewhere.

Additional self-care evaluation was completed during later patient contacts, with all patients in the study having a minimum of three contacts. "The evaluation consisted of four parts: an interview, physical assessment, interpretation of findings, and mutually determined goals." (p. 26) During this process, nursing care was provided during the contact. "Data gathered were recorded on a care plan and collection continued until no new categories were discovered and each category had been saturated with examples" (p. 27). Ten categories of needs were identified: "acquire skills for self-care management, receive feedback regarding self-care management, become aware of own resources, have feelings of self-esteem enhanced, grieve over losses, work towards acceptance of chronic disease, have new or continuing health concerns evaluated, obtain services from various support agencies, alleviate physical and mental discomforts, identify positive role of the health care agency and feel like a full participant in determining care goals, and maintain family solidarity and support or assist ill member" (p. 27).

These findings reveal an interesting contrast to the findings of Dickson and Lee-Villasenor (1982), who similarly used the method of participant observation. The latter also made observations in a clinical setting with a quite different sample and gleaned their need categories from statements of needs as expressed by their subjects.

In the discussion and conclusions, there is a certain eagerness to apply the findings to the practice setting as the next step. Here, that application is premature. More appropriate to the present stage of theory development of Orem is the phase of reanalysis and refinement of the self-care need categories for this subpopulation.

This study makes an important contribution to nursing science by using the theoretical formulations of Orem to guide the organization of the observations made of 65 ambulatory diabetic clients into the need categories. These data and categories contribute important information for continued theory development, for the inductive approach, and, more specifically, for the development of the concept of self-care needs.

Murphy, P.P. (1981) A hospice model and self-care theory. *Oncology Nursing Forum*, 8(2), 19–21.

This brief article describes how Orem's self-care framework was used as a guide for nursing practice in a hospice setting. The focus of the article is on the role of nursing in this setting, using the three basic systems of nursing care described by Orem: (1) supportive–educative, (2) partially compensatory, and (3) wholly compensatory. Examples of level of interaction between the nurse and the patient for each system and a diagram illustrate how the hospice team operates using the self-care framework.

Although this article is not based on research but rather on clinical application, and although it does not provide any new insights or interpretations of Orem's work, it does demonstrate that the self-care framework is a useful guide for practitioners in a setting with terminally-ill patients.

Petrlik, J.C. (1976) Diabetic peripheral neuropathy. *American Journal of Nursing*, 76, 1794–1797.

While this article does not mention Orem's theory as a basis for the discussion of self-care, it is based on the earlier article by Backscheider on self-care requirements and self-care abilities and should be read in conjunction with it. In this case, the author focused on assessment of the self-care abilities of patients who have peripheral neuropathy and the concomitant long-term problems. The theory–practice analysis is useful in helping the reader delineate some research propositions.

Porter, D., and Shamian, J. (1983) Self care in theory and practice. *Canadian Nurse*, 79(8), 21–23.

Self-care as theory originated in the early 1950s. Orem was perceived as visionary, and the theory was labeled as revolutionary by the authors. Self-care was defined, and the assumptions of the theory and the goal of nursing were identified; the scope of practice—the role of nurse in relation to the client—was also discussed. How nurses might achieve the goal of nursing according to Orem was also explored in this article.

The basic needs of clients, which nurses assist in meeting, are classified by Orem as universal, developmental, and health deviational. While these are consistent with Orem's theory, only brief listings suggest what makes up each of these categories of needs. Citing Orem, the authors suggested that nursing interventions corresponding to the first two categories of needs could be considered primary prevention. Secondary and tertiary prevention would be those interventions related to health deviation self-care needs.

Within the context of Orem's theory, nursing care planning is facilitated by the development of nursing systems. Nursing system was defined, and the hierarchical components of the nursing system were outlined. These included wholly compensatory, partly compensatory, and supportive–educative; all of which were defined indirectly within the context of examples. Patients were to be categorized into one of these three systems through the nursing process when the nurse planned care.

The nursing process within the context of self-care theory included the identification of a number of factors influencing a person's ability to perform self-care. Some were listed. This concluded the brief description of the assessment phase. Likewise, the intervention phase was only briefly described.

Intervention is required when self-care abilities are inadequate to meet self-care demands. Nursing measures that help the client to achieve the goal of self-care as defined by Orem include: (1) acting or doing for; (2) guiding; (3) teaching; (4) supporting; and (5) providing a developmental environment. None of these was discussed by the authors. The meanings of major terms and concepts were illustrated within the context of a clinical situation and were offset for emphasis. This clinical example was titled "Self-care theory in practice at the JGH" (Jewish General Hospital).

Overall, the authors' description was in keeping with the theory, and the few omissions of concepts were not significant in terms of the model. The article provides a clear distillation or synopsis of the theory presented in an easy reading style, and although it is merely informative, it might be of interest to the newcomer to Orem's model. It might also be of interest to clinicians wishing a quick overview of the model and its potential utility in the practice setting.

Smith, M.C. (1979) Proposed metaparadigm for nursing research and theory development: An analysis of Orem's self-care theory. *Image*, 11(3), 75–79.

The purpose of this article is to "propose a classification scheme to structure the analysis of existing research and the design of future research in nursing." The author uses Orem's theory to illustrate the proposed scheme. The ultimate purpose using the proposed scheme is to "formulate a cohesive, organized body of knowledge for theory building and development in nursing" (p. 75) as well as to organize existing research and design future research studies from a nursing framework.

Having developed a scheme and labeled a metaparadigm, the author illustrated how the premises and propositions of this particular nursing theorist are or can be classified. The author acknowledges and makes explicit her personally biased assumptions regarding the *sine qua non* of professional nursing practice.

This article is relevant to discussions of central phenomena in nursing and to the relationship between nursing research, theory development, and nursing practice.

Sullivan, T.J. (1980) Self-care model for nursing. In *New directions for nursing in the '80s.* Kansas City MO: American Nurses' Association.

The introduction to this article is very broad, discussing the issues for nursing and society for the 1980s. This leads the reader to the present focus of self-care, the appropriateness of it for clients and for the nursing profession, specifically because of the values it embraces and their similarity to those embedded in our American sociocultural value system. Nowhere in the introduction is the reader made aware that the author has taken what she perceived to be a broad, abstract, and otherwise static grand-level theory and operationalized the concept of self-care to make it more usable. She undertook to organize a body of knowledge for nursing the aged, which resulted in a self-care model for nursing the aged.

More than one-half of the article focuses on a review of Orem's self-care model. This review includes a fairly comprehensive picture of the model and description of its components. The nature, philosophy (including four underlying assumptions), and conceptual framework of the self-care model are all presented. The conceptual framework includes definitions of the three major conceptual constructs: therapeutic self-care demand, self-care agency, and nursing agency. The relationships between these parts of the framework are also explicated. Nursing agency is defined, and the hierarchical systems and their hierarchical subsystems— technological, interpersonal, and social—of nursing care are further described and linkages noted.

In the author's discussion of the philosophy of self-care—more specifically within the discussion of the nurse–patient relationship—the author has taken what she described as a "lawlike generalization" and restated it as a proposition. Another statement of a corollary could also have been restated as a propositional statement. These statements were almost incidental to the purpose of this paper, yet they are what are critically needed to move this theory to the point of being tested by research. Elaboration of the concepts, development of propositional statements, and subsequent hypothesis generation are basic requirements for validation of the self-care model. This author's brief discussion provides an important step in this direction.

The development of the self-care model for the aged was accomplished following "analysis and review of nursing literature on the aged and self-care." The outcome was a self-care model for nursing the aged. The four levels of the self-care system that emerged were listed and discussed. Conclusions that were reached following identification of these four self-care systems were also listed. The author also addressed the reality that clients might be functioning partly on one level and partly on another and that the four levels of the self-care system are therefore fluid; they represent a continuum. The model also allows for movement over time, indicating that clients may move vertically from one level of self-care to another as well, in several identifiable directions.

The technological and interpersonal subsystems of the nursing systems overlap in the process of accomplishing the goals of self-care. These were discussed, and approaches for applying methods of assistance to the aged emerged as a result of the study. These approaches were listed from the highest level to the lowest level of client capability for self-care. Also listed from the highest level of client capability to the lowest were four interpersonal subsystems. The social subsystem dimension of the nursing subsystem was also briefly discussed. Horizontal linkages with the model were also discussed. The author noted that, while it was not within the scope of the paper to present the concrete referents identified in the model, they had been identified.

Implications for use of the self-care theory in general, and the self-care model for nursing the aged more specifically, were succinctly summarized. Implications for model development for nursing groups other than the aged, for nursing practice with an emphasis on health versus illness, for hypothesis generation leading to research, for nursing leadership roles in health care, and for issues in nursing such as accountability, legal and ethical, were all presented.

This article would be of interest to practitioners, educators, and researchers who desire to use the self-care model for any of those areas—and is recommended reading. For the student of the self-care model, it would be helpful reading as a succinct summary of the model, with examples of statements of propositions. It would also be of interest to those working with the elderly and those who are interested in the self-care model. Furthermore, for students of epistemology, it illustrates the process of model development through the operationalization of a grand-level theory. The article is clearly written and logically developed; overall, it is a scholarly work.

Martha Rogers

This article suggests that the model can be used as a curriculum model for gerontological nursing.

Egbert, E. (1980, January) Concept of wellness. *JPN and Mental Health Services*, 18(1), 9–12.

Based on the opening sentence in this article, it appears that Rogers' use of the term *health* (not wellness) in a statement about what nursing is was the stimulus for developing the concept of wellness. At no other time is there any reference to Rogers' work, nor is the concept of wellness, as it is developed, related back to her theory.

The concept of wellness as developed here was, in essence, distilled from a variety of definitions as a result of a review of the literature. Based on the review, the author determined that wellness could not be clearly defined. Instead, she delineated a list of characteristics of wellness from the conceptions described by several authors and institutions that attempted to define health, such as Freud, Maslow, Jourard, Perls, Jahoda, Wu, and the World Health Organization. The author suggested that although health and wellness could not be clearly defined, the list, a synthesis of many definitions, could provide guidelines for nursing intervention and prevention.

This article does not contribute to our understanding of Rogers' theory but provides us with a summary of some of the definitions of health.

Falco, S.M. and Lobo, M.L. (1980) Martha E. Rogers. In the Nursing Theories Confer-ence Group, *Nursing theories: The base for professional nursing practice.* Englewood Cliffs, NJ: Prentice-Hall.

Consistent with the other chapters in this edited volume, there is a brief history about the theoretician whose theory is presented. This summary of Rogers' *Theoretical basis of nursing* by Falco and Lobo is generally written clearly and concisely.

The authors present Rogers' definition of nursing and the five major assumptions about human beings that underlie the nursing science explicated by Rogers. What are not listed by these authors are the more general, broader assumptions underlying the four principles of homeodynamics, which are explicitly stated by Rogers. The second set of assumptions, similar to those about human beings, are grounded in systems theory. The four principles of homeodynamics are identified and elaborated on by the authors.

In the remainder of the article, the authors compare Rogers' theory with other theories, present clinical examples, and demonstrate the principles of homeodynamics, and then show how the principles might be used in the nursing process. This illustration shows the potential application of the model to clinical practice. Examples include series of questions to be used in the assessment phase to reflect each of the principles of homeodynamics. There are also examples of nursing diagnoses, planning, and implementation within the framework. Tables illustrate the relationship of the principles of homeodynamics to the nursing process. This use of Rogers' principles in the nursing process is only one of two known uses that are published (see also Whelton, 1979) and is an important contribution to the theory.

The authors also discuss limitations of Rogers' principles (*i.e.*, that they are too abstract and that terms have not been sufficiently operationalized).

For the reader unfamiliar with Rogers' *Theoretical basis of nursing*, this article presents a brief overview and summary. The examples of application to practice using the nursing process show the utility of the theory for practice, and this makes it more useful for the practitioner. In this way, the article contributes to our understanding and use of this theory and therefore to the science of nursing.

Katz, V. (1971) Auditory stimulation and developmental behavior of the premature infant. *Nursing Research*, 20(3), 196–201.

It has never been explicitly stated by the author; however, because she was a student in Martha Rogers' program and because this research was based on other research carried out at the same institution, it is assumed that Katz's study was developed based on assumptions of Rogers' theory. If this is correct, not presenting the theoretical framework would be a limitation.

If one were to try to guess which assumptions of Rogers underlie this study, the following might be included: (1) a human being and his environment are continuously exchanging matter and energy with one another, (2) the life process evolves irreversibly and unidirectionally along the space/time continuum, (3) pattern and organization identify a human being and reflect his innovative wholeness (Rogers, 1970).

"The focus of this study was to determine whether a variation in the environment of the low-birth-weight premature infant by the introduction of the maternal voice can influence behavior." (p. 196) The design of the study was quasi-experimental with a control group; it had a sample size of 62. The major statistical analysis was an analysis of variance, comparing those premature infants who received a regimen of auditory stimulation with those who did not. The behavioral outcomes measured were motor, tactile-adaptive, auditory, visual, muscle-tension, and irritability responses. All the tools used had reliability and validity data available.

The same two raters (not the investigator) who were used to test all infants were blind as to which groups the infants were in. Interscorer agreement between the raters and the investigator was obtained after the raters were trained. These and other measures are important safeguards that were used in this study to reduce the potential for bias in the data. In general, based on the write-up, it appears that the study was well-designed.

The study supported previous findings that had indicated that variations in behavioral development are evident after changes are made in sensory input in low-birth-weight premature infants. More important, and consistent with Rogers' belief that the purpose of nursing as an empirical science is to describe and explain the phenomena central to its concern (*i.e.*, person) and to predict about them, this study provides empirical data from which nursing intervention can then be planned. In Rogers' terms, "the identification of relationship between events provides for an ordering of knowledges and for the development of nursing's hypothetical generalizations and unifying principles (1980, pp. 84–85)."

For these reasons, this study supports Roger's theory and contributes both to empirical validation of it as well as to the science of nursing in general by the rigor of the research. An important omission in the write-up, however, was that the researcher did not indicate other potentially testable hypotheses generated by this research.

Porter, L.S. (1972) The impact of physical–physiological activity on infants' growth and development. *Nursing Research*, 21(3), 210–219.

This rigorous experimental study was explicitly based on two assumptions of Martha Rogers' theory: (1) the human organism is an open system in constant interaction with the environment, and (2) growth and developmental processes are unitary and integrative. The study was developed with the conceptualization that the human organism is an energy field in continuous motion. The researcher postulated a direct relationship between environmentally imposed motion and a speeding up of infant growth and development.

The research was built on earlier studies that also used Rogers' theory as a conceptual framework as well as the researcher's own earlier study of infants. Because the researcher believed that the results of her earlier study were not generalizable enough, this study was undertaken as a follow-up study to corroborate the earlier findings. (An earlier study by the author, Luz Sobong, tested Johnson's proposition of stimulation and growth.)

The study is methodically and systematically described, clearly enough so as to be reproducible. Background, hypotheses, methodology, data collection, and results are all described in detail. Tables showing the data are included as well as a summary of the analyses performed on the six measures of growth and development used in the study. The six measures of growth and development were gains in weight, length, motor, adaptive, language, and personal-social behavior. The design of the study was experimental, with random assignment of subjects who were then matched with a control group. One limitation in the data collection was that the investigator collected the data and was not blind to whether the subjects were in the experimental group or the control group (or so it appears from the write-up).

A question is raised here regarding the data analysis. For example, the subjects were pretested on the six measures. Results presented showed that the heaviest control subject initially weighed 325 ounces, while the corresponding experimental subject weighed 369 ounces. There is a difference between these two of 44 ounces. In the discussion, the author indicated that there was "no important initial difference" (p. 216) between the groups. The question is, Is this a significant difference between the two groups? A t-test would have provided this information and, although it may have been done by the investigator, the results were not reported here.

This research study has contributed to the science of nursing not only by contributing to knowledge about infants with implications for nursing intervention but also by providing support for the assumptions upon which it was based, namely those of Martha Rogers. This was a rigorous study and a scholarly report.

Rogers, M.E. (1970) *An introduction to the theoretical basis of nursing.* Philadelphia: F.A. Davis.

It is in this book that Martha Rogers first presents her ideas about the theoretical basis of nursing in a formal way. Some of the origins of her ideas, her earlier thinking, is seen in her 1963 article, which it is helpful to read either prior to or in conjunction with this book. (Rogers uses "man" to refer to the nursing client in this early writing.)

Essentially, the book is divided into three main sections. In the first section, "Book of modern nursing," she presents background material related to man's beginnings, the evolution of man's thinking, and theories of this century about how man and life originated. "The phenomenon of man: Nursing's concern" is the second section. Here Rogers states what it is she sees as the central concern of nursing: man in his entirety. Man as a whole, man as a system, is the prototypic theory used to present the underlying assumptions Rogers makes about man. The assumptions are explicitly numbered and labeled as such. Five assumptions upon which nursing science builds are identified.

In the third section, "Nursing's conceptual system," Rogers clearly points out the aims of nursing, nursing's conceptual model, the principle of nursing science, the principles of homeodynamics, evidence to support the concepts, ideas about formulating testable hypotheses, ways in which to translate the conception into practice and, finally, some ideas about the future. The essence of the theory is expressed in the first part of this section. The assumptions about man, the focus of nursing, were identified in the earlier section, but it is here that the concepts and principles are defined—the internal structure, aspects of the goals and consequences, and some dimensions of the theory are outlined.

An important chapter in this section relates to the potential of this theory for research. In fact, a whole body of research attempting to verify the principles of the real world (being carried out by doctoral students under Rogers' direction) is presented. The limitation in this chapter discussing the findings is that about 95% of it includes unpublished doctoral dissertations and is not generally available. Nevertheless, the important thing is that numerous studies, including cluster studies, have been and continue to be undertaken in attempts to accumulate evidence in support of the principles postulated by Rogers. This fact alone makes Rogers' formulations stand out from all of the other nursing theories and models, even to this day. Furthermore, implications of many of the studies give direction for practice as well as provide direction for additional research.

The major limitations of Rogers' formulations are well-known. These are that the principles of homeodynamics—reciprocity, synchrony, helicy, and resonance —are all quite abstract and have not been adequately operationalized. Some would say that because the principles are not easily understood, they are difficult to translate into practice. Also, because of the lack of operational definitions, the research carried out to verify the principles provides questionable results. The major counter argument, if one were to think along the lines of Rogers' theory and writing, is that research must focus on the range of human phenomena and that this will give substance to nursing's abstract system. There is, to a degree, an element of inductive reasoning, and an inductive approach is suggested; that is, the principles provide the framework, the direction for research, but the research results really provide the substance of the theory.

A chapter in the third section, in addition to discussing research, addresses the potential of the theory for practice. With the exception of citing four research studies suggesting direction for nursing practice, the discussion is more or less an abstract discussion of nursing interventions that purportedly are based on the different principles of homeodynamics. It does not indicate whether or not the theory is actually used in any practice settings.

In closing, we would recommend to anyone interested in Rogers' theory to read, at the minimum, the third section of the book; then for additional understanding of the assumptions about human beings, the second section, and for background in general, the first. The book is clearly and logically developed and very readable. In general, reading the whole book, elegant in its simplicity, sophisticated in its presentation, and erudite as its author, is highly recommended. Rogers stands out among the nursing theorists, and her work in theorizing, research, and education presents a major contribution to nursing as a science.

Rogers, M.E. (1975) Euphemisms in nursing's future. *Image*, 7(2), 3–9.

The focus of this paper is an argument against the many forms of nursing services parading under the guise of nice-sounding titles, when in fact they are cover-ups for physicians' assistants. This controversy was at its height in the early to mid-1970s, and Rogers was strongly opposed to the development of new roles or any new title, such as the family health practitioner, pediatric associate, and primary care nurse. She believed these were cover-ups for the physician's assistant, were "perpetrated to deny a future to nurses and nursing" (p. 3), and were coined to enhance the economic gains of the physicians.

This article bears little if any relevance to Rogers' theoretical basis of nursing per se. What comes through are her beliefs about roles and levels of education needed to prepare nurses and what the scope of nursing is. Her theme that a baccalaureate preparation for nursing is important is repeated here.

For those unfamiliar with the more personal side of the professional Martha Rogers, this article provides a touch of that side. It gives one a feel for the spontaneous way in which she makes her arguments and for the strength of her convictions. Her wit, sense of humor, and a touch of cynicism are well-demonstrated in this article. For this alone, this article is well worth reading.

Rogers, M.E. (1980) Nursing: A science of unitary man. In J.P. Riehl and C. Roy (Eds.), *Conceptual models for nursing practice* (2nd ed.). New York: Appleton-Century-Crofts.

In this chapter, Rogers brings us up to date on her thinking about nursing and a conceptual system in nursing. She in fact presents a few changes in the underlying assumptions and in the principles of homeodynamics, compared with her earlier book (1970). No explanation is set forth as to why the changes were made. In essence, no specific assumptions about man are identified. Rather, Rogers states that four building blocks are essential in the conceptual system presented in this paper. They are: (1) energy fields, (2) universe of open systems, (3) pattern and organization, and (4) four-dimensionality. Each is briefly discussed.

The principles of homeodynamics have been reduced from four to three, and one of the three is different from the original. The original four were the principles of reciprocity, synchrony, helicy, and resonance. The new three are the principles of helicy, resonance, and complementarity. The first two remain essentially the same in definition. The principles of complementarity have elements of the original principle of reciprocity with the added idea of interaction between man and environment.

There are some elements of the theory that appear to have been updated; for example, the title. Here the underlying assumptions are broadened to include more than those five assumptions about the human being. Here, they are also described as building blocks rather than assumptions. As already discussed, the principles of homeodynamics have changed somewhat.

Also updated are the theories deriving from the proposed conceptual system. Only a few of these are discussed. These include theory of accelerating evolution, explanations of paranormal events, and rhythmical correlates of change. The implications that advances in technology have for change are also taken into account by Rogers.

The last of these updates are in the discussion of implications for practice. Changes in nursing practice must result from changes in man, such as the evolutionary emergence of new behavior patterns (*e.g.*, hypertension and hyperactivity), new knowledge, and changes in values. This is an interesting point that Rogers makes and, indeed, one not commonly mentioned by most theorists.

It is recommended that this chapter be read in conjunction with Rogers' 1970 book.

Whelton, B.J. (1979) An operationalization of Martha Rogers' theory throughout the nursing process. *International Journal of Nursing Studies*, 16, 7–20.

This is the second of only two known articles referring to situations in which Rogers' theory is used throughout the nursing process. This whole article essentially focuses on that, whereas Falco and Lobo (1980) only present the nursing process in a section of their chapter.

The introduction clearly states the purpose of the paper and describes the content to be covered and then, clearly and precisely, the authors carry out their plan. This makes the paper very readable.

The version of Rogers' theory used here is the earlier (1970) version rather than the 1980 updates. In the presentation of the theory, the structural components are clearly spelled out; that is, basic assumptions about man, the five nursing concepts (stated more explicitly than Rogers really did), and the nursing principles of homeodynamics derived from the concepts. The five nursing concepts identified by this author are wholeness, openness, pattern and organization, unidirectionality, and sentience and thought.

The clinical population of interest identified to be the focus of the operationalization of Rogers' theory are those patients with decreased cardiac output and impaired neurological function. For example, the assessment of these patients would include data related to the five general concepts already mentioned. Tables are included that show what is assessed under each of these categories. For example, under wholeness, physical integrity and psychological integrity are listed. Then in a later table for a patient with impaired neurological functioning, the subitems are listed.

The general format is carried out in detail through each phase of the nursing process, here identified as assessment, nursing diagnosis, plan of care (including goal), and implementation and evaluation. Detailed tables present an actual nursing care plan showing diagnosis, plan, and goal. No examples are given for implementation and evaluation.

At least one example in this area would have complemented the other phases. In summarizing, Whelton indicates that assessment tools will vary with the patient population. However, it is not entirely reasonable to have an assessment tool for each and every different patient population. Therefore, the tool described here could be developed in more general terms and could thus be more generalizable to other patient populations.

This article has contributed significantly to the applicability of Rogers' theory to practice by making the somewhat abstract notions of the theory more concrete and by operationalizing the theory within the nursing process.

Sister Callista Roy

Brower, H.T. and Baker, B.J. (1976) Using the adaptation model in a practitioner curriculum. *Nursing Outlook*, 24(11), 686–689.

The practitioner curriculum described here is a geriatric nurse practitioner program that utilizes the adaptation model of Roy. The authors forthrightly state that Roy's model meets the following criteria: it outlines the features of the discipline and provides direction for practice, research, and education; it considers the values and goals of nursing, the client, and practitioner interventions; and, in essence, it is a theory at the prescriptive or situation-producing level. Because these criteria were met, the model was incorporated into this curriculum.

Another important aspect of the model identified was that it was helpful in differentiating between those aspects of care unique to nursing versus medical practice within the context of Roy's four modes of adaptation. Furthermore, in describing the application of the model, it appeared that examples used are the authors' interpretation of Roy's model. Although the potential of the model for practice is supported (*e.g.*, another area of practice is covered), the application offers neither refinement nor extension. On the other hand, some insights in the form of interventions for nursing are suggested. For example, in order to promote client adaptation, nursing interventions might include facilitation of adaptive tasks of aging through counseling, effective communication techniques, health education, active manipulation, providing support, and identifying resources. However, here the points of entry for the nursing intervention are not clearly spelled out. It is stated: "If inadequate adaptation is occurring, the practitioner can attempt to modify or manipulate focal stimuli, thereby making a positive response possible." (p. 687) This example simply is not specific enough; it suggests where to intervene but not when.

The third focus in this article is curriculum application. In this section, there is an elaboration of the content taught that provides information about what these authors draw on from other fields and other theoretical models for a knowledge base as it relates to this model. For example, crisis intervention theory, health anthropology, attitudes, life review, stage theory, and role theory are all included. This information may be interesting to those who want to plan a similar practitioner program.

Farkas, L. (1981) Adaptation problems with nursing home application for elderly persons: An application of the Roy adaptation nursing model. *Journal of Advanced Nursing*, 6(5), 363– 368.

The author suggested at the outset that the elderly are often dependent on significant others to provide care supplementary to home care in order for them to remain at home. The importance of this study, then, was to "assess the life circumstances surrounding nursing home applications for elderly people" (p. 364), and the Roy adaptation model was chosen as the framework to organize data collected about adaptation problems of elderly people and their significant others.

Three research questions were identified:

1. "In what way can a conceptual framework in nursing provide for the understanding of adaptation problems of elderly persons and significant others which contribute to nursing home applications?
2. If two groups of elderly persons are receiving at least one home care service, what similarities and differences exist in adaptation problems that allow one group to remain at home while the other group must apply for admission to a nursing home?
3. To what extent do the adaptation problems on the part of the elderly person of those persons closest to him contribute to the nursing home application for the elderly person?" (p. 364)

The discussion of the conceptual framework that followed those research questions briefly presented the underlying beliefs of the Roy adaptation model and identified the four adaptive modes and what was considered an "adaptive response." The nurse's role within the model was identified as promoting adaptation that involved two factors in the nursing process: assessment and intervention. Other than this brief overview, the author assumed that the reader was familiar with the model. Only one study was cited that documented characteristics or problems of elderly applicants to long-term care facilities, and no research, related to adaptation or to use of the adaptation model, was cited.

In the purpose statement, the general purpose to assess factors associated with nursing home application was repeated. A general statement that five hypotheses were formulated and tested was made, and a statement was made that they related to "overall adaptation problems, powerlessness, role reversal guilt, and knowledge and utilization of services, but the hypotheses were not explicitly stated. Furthermore, no theoretical connections between the hypotheses and the Roy model were explicated. It is not clear that all the hypotheses flowed from the research question. This led me to conclude that the conceptualization of this research within the Roy model was extremely limited; that is, it was conceptually inadequate.

The study group and the control group were described, but criteria for each subject group were not specific.

The method used in this study was described as an *ex post facto* design, appropriate to this population because admission to a nursing home is not a variable that can be controlled. Statistical analyses were completed using Chi-square. Both the elderly subjects and their significant others were interviewed in their homes.

The limitations of this research outweigh the contributions it might have made to the testing of the Roy adaptation model. What is more, in the conclusion, neither the limitations of the research nor the implications for future research are discussed.

Galligan, A.C. (1979) Using Roy's concept of adaptation to care for young children. *American Journal of Maternal Child Nursing*, 4(1), 24–28.

Given the psychosocial as well as the physical needs of children while they are hospitalized, this author has chosen Roy's concept of adaptation "as a means of guiding nurses in a more conscious effort to assist the child during hospitalization." Rationale for the choice of this model was not provided.

The author has divided the hospital stay into four different stages: prehospitalization, preoperative, postoperative, and discharge. The rationale for these divisions was that because "man" (child?) is in constant interaction with a changing environment, the nursing assessment and appropriate interventions must be revised periodically during the patient's stay. Each of the four stages are briefly discussed regarding their potential for assessment and intervention. Then, to illustrate how the Roy adaptation model might be used to assess and intervene with a young child, a hypothetical case was presented.

For three of the four stages of hospitalization, omitting discharge, each mode is discussed with examples of assessment—including focal, contextual, and residual stimuli—and intervention. In the second and third stages, the dimensions of diagnosis and evaluation were added. The discharge stage was discussed only very briefly, indicating that the child should be evaluated again in each of the four adaptive modes, and a discharge plan should be formulated.

For those interested in the applicability of the model for practice, especially with patients other than adults, this is an important contribution, demonstrating that the model is useful in the nursing care of children. On the whole, however, it does not increase our understanding of the Roy model itself.

Janelli, L.M. (1980) Utilizing Roy's adaptation model from a gerontological perspective. *Journal of Gerontological Nursing*, 6(3), 140–150.

The title of this article clearly indicates the focus, but more specifically, the author discusses two purposes. The first is general background about how the author came to use the theory and an overview of the model. Selye's stress theory was identified as the paradigmatic origin of the theory. The second purpose of the article is to present use of the model with specific clinical examples in gerontological nursing.

As far as contributions to the theory, the author presents her conception, in diagrammatic form, of a human being as a bio-psycho-social being interacting with the environment. Although the Roy adaptation model is basically a systems model, Roy does not use the word "tension" as it is used in this description. Other than the diagram, this article does not substantially add to our understanding of the model. It does, or at least did in this case, provide enough direction for practice with an elderly clientele.

This article is useful for those interested in gerontological nursing. Tables of needs and the schematic presentation of the human being–environment interactions are also useful.

Jones, P.S. (1978) An adaptation model for nursing practice. *American Journal of Nursing,* 78(11), 1900–1906.

The adaptation model described here is not related to the Roy adaptation model and, in fact, uses a different prototype theory as a basis for its development. The author suggested that having this second framework based on the idea of adaptation (in this case modeled after Selye) might be confusing, but she thought her model might have more to offer than other theories. She suggested that there were difficulties with other existing theories; however, the difficulties were not identified.

In addition to using Selye's theory as a prototype, Maslow's hierarchy of needs was also used "to provide structure and guidance for assessing all needs." Based on the hierarchy, the author developed an elaborate assessment tool.

In terms of the structural components of the model, assumptions and concepts were explicit. Eight underlying assumptions were listed. The major concepts used included wholeness, needs, adaptability, illness, and wellness. The author did not specifically develop propositional statements that described the relationship of the concepts.

On the whole, this article does not contribute to our understanding of Roy's adaptation model, although it may have contributed another perspective to the concept of the health/illness continuum (in this case, illness/wellness continuum), which is not terribly clear in Roy's model. Jones illustrates her model using a triangle to demonstrate the interaction of the three variables in an average person. This conceptualization helps to determine wellness when the person is physically ill but "well" in other areas, a problem in Roy's model.

Mastal, M.F. and Hammond, H. (1980) Analysis and expansion of the Roy adaptation model: A contribution to holistic nursing. *Advances in Nursing Science,* 2(4), 71–81.

Although believing that the Roy adaptation model has much to offer nursing by way of providing a framework to organize its body of nursing knowledge, these authors are highly critical of the model in its present form. Specifically, the criticisms focus on a lack of explicit theoretical components of assumptions and concepts, simple propositions, and relational propositions (criticisms noted in earlier critiques also).

The purpose, then, of this article is to make up for some of the above deficits. Assumptions underlying the mode, heretofore implicit, are explicitly stated. (Roy's 1980 edition of *Conceptual Models* was not yet published when this article was written because in that edition, the assumptions are outlined by Roy. Readers are encouraged to compare the two sets of assumptions.)

The five major concepts within the framework are identified, summarized, and discussed. These include: (1) person, (2) environment, (3) adaptation, (4) health/illness, and (5) nursing.

The authors focus on the lack of theoretical and operational definitions as well as on the narrow scope of health/illness. In attempting to elucidate this concept and to answer some questions, a continuum is defined, a new idea of transition is introduced, and nursing assessment along the continuum is clarified. This addition is justified on the basis that it expands the model's scope. However, based on this brief discussion, this is a critical addition to the concept of health/illness.

Two other major additions to the theory are a diagram depicting the relationships between the major concepts of the model and a set of propositional statements. The latter is a particularly important contribution because it is what the model was lacking at the time this article was published.

Overall, the article is clearly written and adds to our understanding of the theory. The contribution of propositional statements adds to the researchability of the theory, and ultimately to nursing as a science.

Mastal, M.F., Hammond, H., and Roberts, M.P. (1982) Theory into hospital practice: A pilot implementation. *Journal of Nursing Administration,* 12(6), 9–15.

This article describes both the process involved when the Roy Adaptation Model was implemented in one unit of a small community hospital, and how the process contributed to the validation of nursing theory. The description of the process is detailed enough to give guidance to clinicians or administrators who might choose to implement a theoretical model. Each step of the process is outlined and described.

Adequate review and understanding of any theoretical model to be used in a clinical setting is requisite. In this case, the review revealed that not all components (philosophical basis, assumptions, concepts, and propositions) had been specifically identified and defined. This led the authors to pursue this end directly with the theorist, Sister Callista Roy. From this, specific components were clarified, and what were perceived by the authors to be the model's components were depicted visually. This effort was later used to make the model understandable and usable for the hospital's nursing staff. (This process of clarification of the components of the model and the communications with Sister Roy would also make another significant contribution to the validation of the theory.) Once components of the model had been clarified, the administrative processes were initiated.

Planning and organizing were the major steps required administratively to start the pilot. Approval was sought, starting with the top levels of hospital and nursing administration. Congruence with the hospital philosophy, standards of patient care, and cost-effectiveness were all explored. One unit was selected for the pilot with justification for that choice outlined.

Organization was based on Di Vincenti's theoretical framework for change and required three major steps: (1) establishing the change structure, (2) developing appropriate procedures, and (3) determining requirements and allocating resources. Each of these steps was described and was discussed in some detail. In the change structure, shared power was the category of "how" to change. Group problem solving and group decision making, as part of shared power, was emphasized. Open communication and a method for addressing problems in an ongoing way was also important to the success of the project.

The development of procedures included review of existing forms and required revision of nursing assessment, although not of the nursing care plan. Procedures affecting unit function required guidelines for the following: "(1) using the assessment and planning tools, (2) nursing reports and rounds, (3) patient care conferences, (4) nursing documentation, (5) orientation of new personnel, (6) standards of performance and job descriptions for nurses involved in the project, and (7) audit criteria" (Mastal *et al.*, 1982, p. 13). Costs for these services and required materials were assumed by the hospital. The planning and organizational phase was reported to have taken five months.

Staff education required the next major block of time. One-hour sessions weekly for a period of 15 weeks were structured for all the staff—R.N.'s and L.V.N.'s—on the pilot unit. Cooperation of the head nurse and other departmental heads to cover staffing on the unit during this time period was critical to the success of the classes.

The authors believed that the overall components of success of the pilot implementation were authority, leadership, and communication. Clear lines of authority and administrative sanction for the implementation of the adaptation model were critical. Furthermore, open communication was fostered and facilitated through weekly group meetings, through frequent one-to-one talks between project directors and staff nurses, and through the use of an on-unit community log book for staff to express feelings.

Outcomes were measured indirectly both by improved patient care and by nurses' satisfaction with enhanced professional practice. Since then, patient satisfaction is being documented by conducting further research. There were more concrete measures of enhanced nursing practice. Namely, the development of a new tool to assess the bio-psycho-social status of patients (illustrated by Exhibit 1), more complete nursing care plans phrased in terms consistent with the model, and greater collegial sharing and rapport were reported.

This report was written clearly in a conversational style, without sacrificing scholarliness and thoroughness. It would be of interest to theorists, researchers, and clinicians alike who are interested in the Roy model because it clearly illustrates the helical nature of theory, research, and practice. What is more, it makes an important contribution to the science of nursing by demonstrating application to practice and by stimulating research.

Roy, C. (1970) Adaptation: A conceptual framework for nursing. *Nursing Outlook*, 18(3), 42–45.

The purpose of this article is to describe the framework of a conceptual model for nursing that was in the early stages of development by a nursing faculty group. Implications of the model for nursing science, practice, and education are suggested.

Implicit in the section, "Theoretical Model," are the functional components of assumptions and concepts. Examples of the underlying assumptions are: (1) man is a bio-psycho-social being, (2) man is constantly interacting with a changing environment, and (3) man has both innate and acquired coping mechanisms. The major concepts of the model are adaptation and coping, health and illness, and man and the environment. However, Roy, in this very first publication on her theory, does not yet explicitly identify either the assumptions or the concepts.

In the discussion of the concepts, the major concept of adaptation is described in terms of its origin in the physiological theory of Harry Helson. The definition is technical and somewhat tautological and does not answer the questions raised by the author, which are: "How does this adaptation take place?" and "What is behind the process?" These are difficult questions, and it was too early to answer them. Furthermore, when the author tries to answer the question about how the concept of adaptation applies to nursing, the answer is in terms of the function of nursing, which is "to support and promote patient adaptation."

Although the term "elements," as applied to conceptual models, was not used at the time this article was published, except in a course taught by Dorothy Johnson at the University of California, Los Angeles, where Roy was studying for her master's degree, this analysis reveals that the following elements are present: *goal of action*—to support and promote patient adaptation; *actor's role*—to assess and intervene and to promote adaptation. Less clear are the elements of *patiency*, which is when the nurse becomes involved with the patient on the health/illness continuum, and the *source of difficulty* (although it is similar to patiency). The recipient of nursing care is the human being. The *intervention focus* or *mode* is to promote adaptation by changing the person's response potential. Specific examples are given. Understanding man in health and illness is the essential focus of adaptation nursing.

That this developing theoretical model presents rudimentary outlines of a nursing science is an overstatement on the part of the author. However, considering that this is one of the earlier theoretical models developed in nursing, it is an important contribution to the growth of nursing as a science. This is a useful article to read for those interested in analyzing the development of theoretical thinking in nursing.

Roy, C. (1971) Adaptation: A basis for nursing practice. *Nursing Outlook*, 19(4), 254–257.
This article picks up where the earlier one (1970) left off; it is helpful to read both together. It offers a description of man as an adaptive system with four modes of coping. Assumptions underlying the model are offered; the four modes of adaptation and their components as well as examples are listed. The four modes—later called effector modes—are physiological needs, self-concept, role mastery (later, role function), and interdependence. All four modes were identified based on samples of behavior collected by nursing students of the author as well as on a synthesis of work done by other nurses. The other nursing sources included Abdellah and McCain. Ultimately, it appears that the categories are a synthesis of several sources, which may raise some questions about the validity of the categories. What data and what research supported these four choices? Are there other modes, such as the cognitive mode, which might be included?

A more rigorous approach that may have helped in the development of nursing knowledge would have been for the author to develop a research orientation and a scientific approach rather than a curricular one. Hindsight aside, the leap was immediately made to clinical application. Within the context of clinical application, new concepts then came up that had had insufficient elaboration. Examples of these included health/illness continuum, "positive" responses versus "negative" needs, and a diagram/figure describing the nursing process and first-level assessment.

The nursing goal, clearly stated, is "to bring about an adapted state in the patient, which frees him to respond to other stimuli which may be present." This remains a nursing goal of the theory in 1984 and continues to raise questions about what the nature of the adapted state is and the intended consequences (being (in 1984) the quality of life and the integrity of the individual).

To demonstrate the applicability of the model of adaptation to nursing, two case studies were presented. In each, the nurse used the model as a basis for assessment and intervention. Because it is clearly stated that the nurse establishes a nursing care plan and later evaluates it, and because the nursing process as it was known at the time encompasses four stages—assessment, planning, intervention, and evaluation—one wonders why Roy chose instead to use a nursing process including only two of the four—assessment and intervention. That question aside, the steps grew to six in 1984.

Although there is a discussion about planning, the "how to" of choosing nursing approaches is left to the process of nursing judgment outlined by McDonald and Harms. Additionally, the unintended consequences of the nursing intervention are not discussed.

Overall, this article continues to contribute to our understanding of processes, strategies, and phases of theory development in nursing.

Roy, C. (1976) The Roy adaptation model: Comment. *Nursing Outlook*, 24(11), 690–691.

Sister Callista Roy, who developed the Roy adaptation theory, herein presents her reactions to two articles by Brower and Baker (1976) and by Wolfer (1976). She thinks that the authors did a fine job in implementing ideas from her writings, considering that they used only her published material as a basis.

After more general reactions to Brower and Baker's article regarding the importance of a nursing model as a basis for role identification, Roy goes on to clarify her views, to identify what could be considered limitations, and to acknowledge difficulties with the model. Among these are the fact that the model "has not yet been submitted to the rigors of clinical research that will be necessary to establish its validity," and that the model is a deductive one and has not been developed by formal theory construction methods.

This interaction and feedback is an important process for the growth of nursing knowledge, and the thinking of scholars was evident later on in the development of Roy's theory.

Roy, C. (1979) Relating nursing theory to education: A new era. *Nurse Educator*, 4(2), 16–21.

This article examines the relationship between nursing theory and nursing education, from the meaning of theory to mechanisms of theory utilization, within a department of nursing.

Roy, C. (1980) The Roy adaptation model. In J.P. Riehl and C. Roy (Eds.), *Conceptual models for nursing practice* (2nd ed.). New York: Appleton-Century-Crofts.

Notably still missing in this updated version of the Roy model are data from research, a decade after the first publication appeared in *Nursing Outlook*.

Presented here is the more formal theory construction work that was promised in the earlier "Comment" (1976). Clearly presented and labeled as such are the basic assumptions underlying the model and the elements of the model; namely values, goal of action, patiency, source of difficulty, and intervention. What is still missing is an elaboration of the major concepts and the propositions, or those statements that show the relationship between the concepts. This important omission is not acknowledged by the author. More seriously at issue here is that the model is now 10 years old, is widely used as a curricular framework and in nursing practice settings, and yet research is still not being carried out.

There is a new diagram depicting the "source of difficulty," which is not clarified in the text. The source of difficulty is first "described as the originating point of deviations from the desired state or condition." However, the discussion continues in the vein of how the modes and coping mechanisms are called into play (*i.e.*, like a feedback system) rather than truly defining the source of difficulty. The discussion closes with this summary explanation: " "The source of difficulty," then, is coping activity that is inadequate to maintain integrity in the face of a need deficit or excess." This does not match the diagram that shows that there can exist either adaptive or maladaptive behaviors. The question unanswered by either the diagram or the text description is, When does a source of difficulty really exist? and, particularly and more important, When does the nurse intervene, at the originating point of deviation or at a later time, when the coping mechanisms called up are inadequate? The diagram is somewhat confusing in light of the discussion in the text.

In summarizing, the author points to areas in which "continuing development" is needed, such as validation of assumptions, explication of values, and clarification of elements.

Schmitz, M. (1980) The Roy adaptation model: Application in a community setting. In J.P. Riehl and C. Roy (Eds.), *Conceptual models of nursing practice* (2nd ed.) (pp. 193–206). New York: Appleton-Century-Crofts.

The Roy adaptation model was applied here in the home setting, which is quite different from the inpatient setting where it has heretofore exclusively been applied. This necessitated an expansion of the concept of client from individual with an identified need to include the "family of care." If this broadened definition of the client is accepted, and it seems appropriate to do so, this will be an important contribution to the model.

In the introduction, the author is careful to identify differences between the home and hospital, especially in terms of nursing goals and nursing interventions. Also identified in the home setting were variables influencing care. The introductory remarks laid the groundwork for a detailed case study, with a family requiring home nursing care, which was the major focus of the study.

The care presentation included six detailed tables describing the client behaviors with focal, contextual, and residual stimuli for each mode and an accompanying nursing care plan for each.

The author summarized how the Roy adaptation model was used to assess and intervene with a family. Application of the model was the focus of this article. A more theoretical discussion would also have been appropriate because an expansion of the concept of client resulted from the thinking and work of this author, which is an important theoretical contribution.

Starr, S.L. (1980) Adaptation applied to the dying client. In J.P. Riehl and C. Roy (Eds.), *Conceptual models for nursing practice* (2nd ed.). New York: Appleton-Century-Crofts.

In this very brief descriptive article, the author has elaborated on "elements of adaptive death" within four modes (Roy's): (1) physiologic mode, (2) self-concept mode, (3) role mode, and (4) interdependence mode. Within each mode, adaptive behaviors of the dying client are identified, stimuli affecting the behaviors are listed, and the nursing goal and interventions appropriate to each mode are presented.

Although this article is included in a set of three articles about the Roy adaptation model, there is no direct reference to Roy's work by the author. If one assumes that this is an application of the Roy model to practice, it is clear that it is timely, that the model can be applied to this group of patients, and that it is appropriate to nursing practice in this area. However, the article does not extend the Roy adaptation model.

Wagner, P. (1976) The Roy adaptation model: Testing the adaptation model in practice. *Nursing Outlook*, 24(11), 682–685.

The potential for practice in both episodic and distributive settings using the Roy adaptation model has been realized, according to this author. Graduate students who tested the feasibility of the model for practice concluded that "the model provided a good framework for ordering a variety of observations" and using the model for nursing enhanced assessment and intervention as well as the overall nursing process.

Before field-testing the model, the graduate students reviewed materials published about the model. They found discrepancies between sources and also, although not stated directly, they found limitations in the original assessment tools. They also identified limitations with a tool they subsequently developed even though their tool met the criterion that it was both theoretical and practical. These authors also expressed concern with overlap between the four modes as developed by Roy.

The author gives an indication that the model provides enough direction to affect practice in a variety of settings. Who is acted upon is not as clearly described as where or in what setting the person is acted upon. We are not any clearer as to the focus of the theory, nor are any definitions clarified such as health/illness, modes, positive and negative behavior, and adaptation.

Wagner added two dimensions—nursing diagnosis and evaluation—to Roy's nursing process of assessment and intervention. These later (1984) became an integral part of Roy's nursing process.

Overall, this article supports the notion that the conceptual model currently applies to practice and that it does have relevance for the way nursing is practiced today.

Joyce Travelbee

Travelbee, J. (1963) **What do we mean by rapport?** *American Journal of Nursing*, 63(2), 70–72.

This article provides an excellent example of an attempt to conceptualize a phenomenon. It could be used as an early exemplar in concept development. However, the lack of clinical referents limits its wide utility and curtails its research potential. The term "rapport" is commonly used in nursing but had previously been neither conceptualized, operationally defined, nor researched. Frequently, rapport is defined by what it is not rather than by what it is. The explicit assumption underlying this development is that a controlled type of emotional involvement with the patient is allowed to establish and maintain rapport. Implicit in this is the value judgment that rapport is good or positive and to be valued.

Rapport is described in a number of ways here. It is a process in the way people perceive and relate to each other. It is an entity with empathy, compassion, and sympathy as components. It is also an outcome, being the ability to communicate creatively and intelligently to others. To establish rapport, certain ingredients are essential. A patient has to feel a sense of trust in the nurse. The nurse's needs should have been met in the past to be able to give of herself, but a bit of previous "suffering" would help nurses in understanding others. Stages of rapport development begin with empathy, then sympathy (equated in 1964 with caring), and then rapport.

Travelbee's major concepts that later evolved into her theory were introduced in this article.

Chapter *19*

Metatheory and Theory Bibliography

The purpose of this chapter is to provide the reader with a comprehensive bibliography related to nursing theory and theorizing in nursing. The chapter is divided into 17 sections. Sections 1 through 12 include literature related to metatheory and theorizing in nursing. Section 13 includes the nursing theories organized alphabetically by theorist. Sections 14 through 24 include major paradigms that have influenced nursing or have been utilized in nursing. Section 25 includes video and audio tapes on theory. More specifically, the sections are the following:

There are several points to remember when using the bibliography.

1. Citations preceded by asterisks (*) refer to works that have been abstracted in Chapter 18, Section I. Citations preceded by daggers (†) refer to works that have been abstracted in Chapter 18, Section II.
2. Most of the abstracts in Chapter 18 are expansions of citations in Chapter 19, Sections 3, 6, 7, 8, 10, and 11. The emphasis was on providing a comprehensive view of literature cited in Sections 3 and 11.
3. There are many ways to use the bibliography, such as systematically reading within a section, reading within chronological themes, selecting readings according to years or decades of publication, and reading sections in conjunction with appropriate book chapters. Examples of the latter are Section 1 with Chapter 4, Sections 4 and 5 with Chapter 3, Section 10 with Chapter 11, Section 13 with Chapters 12, 13, 14, 15, and 16. Section 2 gives major books related to theory and metatheory and could be used concurrently with all other chapters and sections.

THEORY AND THEORIZING IN NURSING

1. Philosophy and Methods

Barber, B. and Hirsch, W. (Eds.) (1962) *The sociology of science.* New York: Free Press of Glencoe.

Bennis, W.G., Benne, K.D., and Chin, R. (1976) *The planning of change* (3rd ed.). New York: Holt, Rinehart & Winston.

Blake, R.M., Ducasse, C.J., and Madden, E.H. (1960) *Theories of scientific method: The Renaissance through the nineteenth century.* Seattle: University of Washington Press.

Blalock, H.M. (1969) *Theory construction.* Englewood Cliffs, NJ: Prentice-Hall.

Blumer, H. (1954) What is wrong with social theory? *American Sociological Review,* 19(1), 3–10.

Brodbeck, M. (1956) The philosophy of science and educational research. *Review of Educational Research,* 26(5), 427–441.

Brodbeck, M. (1959) Models, meanings, and theories. In L. Gross (Ed.), *Symposium on sociological theory* (pp. 373–403). Evanston, IL: Row, Peterson & Co.

Bruner, R.S. (1966) The social construction of social theory. In R.S. Rudner (Ed.), *Philosophy of social science.* Englewood Cliffs, NJ: Prentice-Hall.

*Burgess, G. (1978) The personal development of the nursing student as a conceptual framework. *Nursing Forum*, 17(1), 96–102.

Campbell, N. (1953) The structure of theories. In H. Feigl and M. Brodbeck (Eds.), *Readings in the philosophy of science* (pp. 288–308). New York: Appleton-Century-Crofts.

Carnap, R. (1966) *An introduction to the philosophy of science.* New York: Basic Books.

Chafetz, J.S. (1978) *A primer on the construction and testing of theories in sociology.* Itasca, IL: F.E. Peacock Publisher.

*Chapman, C.M. (1976) The use of sociological theories and models in nursing. *Journal of Advanced Nursing*, 1, 111–127.

Chinn, P.L. and Jacobs, M.K. (1987) *Theory and nursing: A systematic approach* (2nd ed.). St. Louis: C.V. Mosby.

Cohen, M.R. and Nagel, E. (1962) *An introduction to logic and the scientific method*, rev'd ed. New York: Harcourt Brace Jovanovich.

Copi, I.M. (1972) *Introduction to logic* (4th ed.). New York: Macmillan. (Note especially: Chapter 3, "Informal Fallacies," and Chapter 6, "Categorical Syllogisms.")

Copleston, F. (1963) *A history of philosophy* (Vol. 8). *Modern philosophy: Bentham to Russel, Part II, Idealism in America. The Pragmatic movement, The revolt against idealism.* Garden City, NJ: Image Books.

Costner, H. (1969) Theory, deduction, and rules of correspondence. *American Journal of Sociology*, 75, 245–263.

Costner, H. and Leik, R.K. (1964) Deductions from axiomatic theory. *American Sociological Review*, 29, 819–835.

Denisoff, R.S., Callahan, O., and Levine, M.H. (1974) *Theories and paradigms in contemporary sociology.* Itasca, IL: F.E. Peacock Publisher.

Dewey, J. (1958) *Experience and nature*, rev'd ed. New York: Dover Publications.

Dewey, J. (1964) *Reconstruction in philosophy*, rev'd ed. Boston: Beacon Press.

Dewey, J. (1980)*The quest for certainty*, rev'd ed. New York: Perigee Books.

Dubin, R. (1978) *Theory building.* New York: Free Press.

Durbin, P.R. (1968) *Philosophy of science: An introduction.* New York: McGraw-Hill.

*Ellis, R. (1968) Characteristics of significant theories. *Nursing Research*, 17(3), 217–222.

Gibbs, J. (1972) *Sociological theory construction.* Hinsdale, IL: Dryden Press.

Gibson, Q. (1960) *The logic of social inquiry.* New York: Humanities Press.

Goode, W.J. and Hatt, P.K. (1952) *Methods in social research.* New York: McGraw-Hill. (Note especially: Chapter 5, pp. 41–55, "Basic Elements of the Scientific Method: Concepts.")

Gouldner, A.W. (1961) Theoretical requirements of the applied social sciences. In H.J. Bennis, K.D. Benne, and R. Chin (Eds.), *The planning of change* (2nd ed.). New York: Holt, Rinehart & Winston.

Grinker, R.R. (Ed.). (1967) *Toward a unified theory of human behavior: An introduction to general systems theory* (2nd ed.). New York: Basic Books.

Hage, J. (1972) *Techniques and problem of theory construction in sociology.* New York: John Wiley & Sons.

Hardy, M.E. (1974) Theories: Components, development, evaluation. *Nursing Research*, 23(2), 100–107.

Harris, S. (1977) *What's so funny about science?*, rev'd ed. Los Altos, CA: William Kaufmann.

Hempel, C.G. (1952) *Fundamentals of concept formation in empirical science.* Chicago: University of Chicago Press.

Hempel, C.G. (1965) *Aspects of scientific exploration and other essays in the philosophy of science.* New York: Free Press.

Husserl, E. (1962) *Ideas: General introduction to pure phenomenology,* rev'd ed. (Trans. W.R. Boyce Gibson). New York: Collier Books.

Inkeles, A. (1964) *What is sociology?* Englewood Cliffs, NJ: Prentice-Hall. (Note especially: "Models of Society in Sociological Analysis," pp. 28–67.)

Kaplan, A. (1964) *The conduct of inquiry: Methodology for behavioral science.* San Francisco: Chandler.

*Kramer, S. (1969) Behavioral science and human biology in medicine. *The New Physician,* 18(11), 965–978.

Kuhn, T.S. (1970) The structure of scientific revolutions. In Neurath O. (Ed.), *International encyclopedia of unified science* (2nd ed.). (Vol. 2). Chicago: University of Chicago Press.

Kuhn, T.S. (1977) *The essential tension: Selected studies in scientific tradition and change.* Chicago: University of Chicago Press.

Lachman, R. (1963) The model in theory construction. In Melvin H. Marx (Ed.), *Theories in contemporary psychology.* New York: Macmillan.

Laudan, L. (1977) *Progress and its problems: Toward a theory of scientific growth.* Berkeley: University of California Press.

Lemaire, G., Macleod, R., Mulkay, M., and Weingart, P. (Eds.). (1976) *Perspectives on the emergence of scientific disciplines.* Chicago: Aldine.

Losee, J. (1980) *A historical introduction to the philosophy of science* (2nd ed.). Oxford: Oxford University Press.

MacKinnon, C.A. (1982) Feminism, Marxism, method, and the state: An agenda for theory. *Signs,* 7, 515–544.

Maris, R. (1970) The logical adequacy of Homan's social theory. *American Sociological Review,* 35, 1069–1081.

Marx, M.H. (1963) *Theories in contemporary psychology.* New York: Macmillan. (Note especially: "The General Nature of Theory Construction," pp. 4–46.)

McCall, R.J. (1963) *Basic logic: The fundamental principles of formal deductive reasoning* (2nd ed.). New York: Barnes & Noble.

*McKay, R. (1969) Theories, models and systems for nursing. *Nursing Research,* 18(5), 393–399.

Merton, R.K. (1973) *The sociology of science: Theoretical and empirical investigations* (edited with an introduction by N.W. Storer). Chicago: University of Chicago Press.

Merton, R.K. (1977) *The sociology of science: An episodic memoir.* Carbondale, IL: Southern Illinois University Press.

Miller, E.F. (1980) Epistemology and political inquiry: Comment on Kress' "Against epistemology." *Journal of Politics,* 42, 1160–1167.

Morgan, G. (1982) Cybernetics and organizational theory: Epistemology or technique? *Human Relations,* 35, 521–538.

Murphy, J.F. (Ed.). (1971) *Theoretical issues in professional nursing.* New York: Appleton-Century-Crofts. (Note especially Chapters 1, 2, and 3).

Northrup, F.S.C. (1965) *The logic of the sciences and the humanities,* rev'd ed. New York: The World Publishing Co.

Payne, G. (1973) Comparative sociology: Some problems of theory and method. *British Journal of Sociology,* 24(1), 13–29.

*Peterson, C.J. (1977) Questions frequently asked about the development of a conceptual framework. *Journal of Nursing Education*, 16(4), 22–32.

Popper, K.R. (1959) *The logic of scientific discovery*. New York: Basic Books.

Popper, K.R. (1971) *The open society and its enemies: The spell of Plato*, rev'd ed. Princeton: Princeton University Press.

Popper, K. (1976) *Unended quest: An intellectual autobiography*. La Salle, IL: Open Court.

Reynolds, P.D. (1971) *A primer in theory construction*. New York: Bobbs-Merrill.

Rudner, R.S. (1966) *Philosophy of social science*, Englewood Cliffs, NJ: Prentice-Hall. (Note especially: "The Construction of Social Theory.")

Russell, B. (1965) *On the philosophy of science*. New York: Bobbs-Merrill.

Sahakian, W.S. (1968) *History of philosophy from the earliest times to the present*. New York: Barnes & Noble.

Sarter, B. (1988) Philosophical sources of nursing theory. *Nursing Science Quarterly*, 1(2), 52–59.

Sheridan, A. (1980) *Michel Foucault: The will to truth*. New York: Tavistock.

Shils, E. (Ed.) (1968) *Criteria for scientific development, public policy, and national goals*. Cambridge, MA: M.I.T. Press.

Sidorsky, D. (Ed.) (1977) *John Dewey: The essential writings*. New York: Harper Torchbooks.

Simon, H.A. and Newell, A. (1963) The uses and limitations of models. In M.H. Marx (Ed.), *Theories in contemporary psychology* (pp. 89–104). New York: Macmillan.

Stinchcombe, A.L. (1968) *Constructing social theories*. New York: Harcourt Brace Jovanovich.

Suppe, F. and Jacox, A.K. (1989) Philosophy of science and the development of nursing theory. *Annual Review of Nursing Research*, 3, 241–267.

The search for knowledge. (1973) *Daedalus*, 102(2), 1–176.

Torres, G. and Yura, H. (1974) *Today's conceptual framework: Its relationship to the curriculum development process* (Publ. No. 15-1529). New York: National League for Nursing.

Toulmin, S. (1981) The tyranny of principles. *Hastings Center Report*, 11, 31–39.

Van Laer, P.H. (1956) *Philosophy of science: Part One—Science in general*. Pittsburgh, PA: Duquesne University Press.

Van Laer, P.H. (1962) *Philosophy of science: Part Two—A study of the division and nature of various groups of sciences*. Pittsburgh, PA: Duquesne University Press.

Wallace, W. (1971) Theories: Logical deduction, hypothesis, interpretation, instrumentation, scaling, and sampling. In *The logic of science in sociology* (pp. 63–74). New York: Aldine Atherton.

Weaver, W. (1970) *Science of change: A lifetime in American science*. New York: Charles Scribner's Sons.

Wolman, B.B. and Nagel, E. (Eds.). (1965) *Scientific psychology: Principles and approaches*. New York: Basic Books.

2. Nursing Theory: General

Barnum, B. (1990) *Nursing theory: Analysis, application and evaluation* (3rd ed.). Boston: Little, Brown & Co.

Chinn, P.L. (1983) *Advances in nursing theory development*. Rockville, MD: Aspen Systems.

Chinn, P.L. (Ed.) (1986) *Nursing research methodology issues and implementation*. Rockville, MD: Aspen Systems.

Chinn, P.L. and Jacobs, M. (1987) *Theory and nursing: A systematic approach* (2nd ed.). St. Louis: C.V. Mosby.

Cull-Wilby, B.L. and Pepin, J.I. (1987) Towards a coexistence of paradigms in nursing knowledge development. *Journal of Advanced Nursing*, 12(4), 515–521.

Fawcett, J. (1989) *Analysis and evaluation of conceptual models of nursing* (2nd ed.). Philadelphia: F.A. Davis.

Fitzpatrick, J. and Whall, A. (1989) *Conceptual models of nursing: Analysis and application* (2nd ed.). Norwalk, CT: Appleton & Lange.

Fitzpatrick, J., Whall, A., Johnston, R., and Floyd, J. (1982) *Nursing models and their psychiatric mental health applications.* Bowie, MD: Robert J. Brady Co.

Gebbie, K. (Ed.). (1976, March 4–7) *Summary of the second national conference: Classification of nursing diagnosis.* 1310 South Boulevard, St. Louis, MO 63104.

Kim, H.S. (1983) *The nature of theoretical thinking in nursing.* Norwalk, CT: Appleton-Century-Crofts.

Lundh, U., Soder, M., and Waerness, K. (1988) Nursing theories: A critical view. *Image: Journal of Nursing Scholarship*, 20, 36–40.

Marriner-Tomey, A. (1989) *Nursing theorists and their work* (2nd ed.). St. Louis: C.V. Mosby.

Newman, M. (1979) *Theory development in nursing.* Philadelphia: F.A. Davis.

Norris, C. (Ed.) (1969) Proceedings: Second Nursing Theory Conference, Kansas: University of Kansas Medical Center, Department of Nursing Education, Oct. 9–10, 1969.

Nursing Development Conference Group. (1977) *Concept formalization in nursing: Process and product.* Boston: Little, Brown & Co.

Parse, R.R. (1987) *Nursing science: Major paradigms, theories, and critiques.* Philadelphia: W.B. Saunders.

Riehl-Sisca, J.P. (1989) *Conceptual models for nursing practice* (3rd ed.). Norwalk, CT: Appleton & Lange.

Silva, M.C. (1987) Conceptual models of nursing. *Annual Review of Nursing Research*, 5, 229–246.

Torres, G. (1986) *Theoretical foundations of nursing.* Norwalk, CT: Appleton-Century-Crofts.

Walker, L.O. and Avant, K.C. (1989) *Strategies for theory construction in nursing.* Norwalk, CT: Appleton-Century-Crofts.

Winstead-Fry, P. (1986) *Case studies in nursing theory.* New York: National League for Nursing.

3. Metatheory and Theory Development in Nursing

Allen, D.G. (1987) The social policy statement: A reappraisal. *Advances in Nursing Science*, 10(1), 39–48.

Barnett, K. (1972) A theoretical construct of the concepts of touch as they relate to nursing. *Nursing Research*, 21(2), 102–110.

*Batey, M.V. (1977) Conceptualization: Knowledge and logic guiding empirical research. *Nursing Research*, 26(5), 324–329.

*Becker, C.H. (1983) A conceptualization of concept. *Nursing Papers: Perspectives in Nursing*, 15(2), 51–58.

*Beckstrand, J. (1978) The notion of a practice theory and the relationship of scientific and ethical knowledge to practice. *Research in Nursing and Health*, 1(3), 131–136.

*Beckstrand, J. (1978) The need for a practice theory as indicated by the knowledge used in conduct of practice. *Research in Nursing and Health*, 1(4), 175–179.

*Beckstrand, J. (1980) A critique of several conceptions of practice theory in nursing. *Research in Nursing and Health*, 3(2), 69–80.

Bergenson, B.S. (1971) Adaptation as a unifying theory. In J.F. Murphy (Ed.), *Theoretical issues in professional nursing*. New York: Appleton-Century-Crofts.

*Berthold, J.S. (1968) Prologue: Symposium on theory development in nursing. *Nursing Research*, 17(3), 196–197.

Bibace, R. and Walsh, M.E. (1982) Conflict of roles: On the difficulties of being both scientist and practitioner in one life. *Professional Psychology*, 13, 389–395.

Bohny, B.J. (1980) Theory development for a nursing science. *Nursing Forum*, 19(1), 50–67.

Botha, M.E. (1989) Theory development in perspective: The role of conceptual frameworks and models in theory development. *Journal of Advanced Nursing*, 14(1), 49–55.

*Brown, M.I. (1964) Research on the development of nursing theory: The importance of a theoretical framework in nursing research. *Nursing Research*, 13(2), 109–112.

*Brown, M.I. (1968) Theory development in nursing: Social theory in geriatric nursing research. *Nursing Research*, 17(3), 213–217.

*Brown, M.L. (1983) Research questions and answers: The use of theory and conceptual frameworks in nursing research and practice. *Oncology Nursing Forum*, 10(2), 111–112.

*Bush, H.A. (1979) Models for nursing. *Advances in Nursing Science*, 1(2), 13–21.

*Carper, B.A. (1978) Fundamental patterns of knowing in nursing. *Advances in Nursing Science*, 1(1), 13–23.

*Chapman, C.M. (1976) The use of sociological theories and models in nursing. *Journal of Advanced Nursing*, 1, 111–127.

*Chinn, P.L. and Jacobs, M.K. (1978) A model for theory development in nursing. *Advances in Nursing Science*, 1(1), 1–11.

*Clark, J. (1982) Development of models and theories on the concept of nursing. *Journal of Advanced Nursing*, 7(2), 129–134.

Cleary, F. (1971) A theoretical model: Its potential for adaptation to nursing. *Image*, 4(1), 14–20.

*Cleland, V.S. (1967) The use of existing theories. *Nursing Research*, 16(2), 118–121.

*Colaizzi, J. (1975) The proper object of nursing science. *International Journal of Nursing Studies*, 12(4), 197–200.

*Collins, R.J. and Fielder, J.H. (1981) Beckstrand's concept of practice theory: A critique. *Research in Nursing and Health*, 4(3), 317–321.

Conway, M.E. (1985) Toward greater specificity in defining nursing's metaparadigm. *Advances in Nursing Science*, 7(4), 73–81.

*Crawford, G., Dufault, S.K., and Rudy, E. (1979) Evolving issues in theory development. *Nursing Outlook*, 27(5), 346–351.

Crow, R. (1982) Frontiers of nursing in the 21st century: Development of models and theories on the concept of nursing. *Journal of Advanced Nursing*, 7, 111–116.

Cull-Wilby, B.L. and Pepin, J.I. (1987) Towards a coexistence of paradigms in nursing process. *Journal of Advanced Nursing*, 12, 515–521.

Derdiarian, A.K. (1979) Education: A way to theory construction in nursing. *Journal of Nursing Education*, 18(2), 36–47.

*Dickoff, J. and James, P. (1968) A theory of theories: A position paper. *Nursing Research*, 17(3), 197–203.

Dickoff, J. and James, P. (1971) Clarity to what end? *Nursing Research*, 20(6), 499–502.

*Dickoff, J., James, P., and Wiedenbach, E. (1968) Theory in practice discipline: Part I. Practice oriented theory. *Nursing Research*, 17(5), 415–435.

*Dickoff, J., James, P., and Wiedenbach, E. (1968) Theory in practice discipline: Part II. Practice oriented theory. *Nursing Research*, 17(6), 545–554.

*Donaldson, S.K. and Crowley, D. (1978) The discipline of nursing. *Nursing Outlook*, 26(2), 113–120.

Donnelly, G.F. (1986) Nursing theory: Evolution of a sacred cow. *Holistic Nursing Practice*, 1(1), 1–7.

Dubin, R. (1978) *Theory building*. New York: Free Press.

*Ellis, R. (1968) Characteristics of significant theories. *Nursing Research*, 17(3), 217–222. (See Section 2.)

Ellis, R. (1971) Commentary on Walker's "Toward a clearer understanding of the concept of nursing theory." *Nursing Research*, 20(6), 493–494.

Ellis, R. (1982, July–August) Conceptual issues in nursing. *Nursing Outlook*, 30(7), 406–410.

Flaskerud, J.H. and Halloran, E.I. (1980) Areas of agreement in nursing theory development. *Advances in Nursing Science*, 3(1), 1–7.

Flaskerud, J.H. and Halloran, E.J. (1981) Areas of agreement in nursing theory development. *Advances in Nursing Science*, 3(3), 31–42.

*Gebbie, K. and Lavin, M.A. (1974) Classifying nursing diagnoses. *American Journal of Nursing*, 74(2), 250–253.

Goode, W.J. and Hatt, P.K. (1952) Science: Theory and fact. In *Methods in social research* (pp. 7–17). New York: McGraw-Hill.

*Gortner, S.R. (1983) The history and philosophy of nursing science and research. *Advances in Nursing Science*, 5(2), 1–8.

Hadley, B.J. (1969) Evolution of a conception of nursing. *Nursing Research*, 18(5), 400–405.

*Hall, B.A. (1981) The change paradigm in nursing: Growth versus persistence. *Advances in Nursing Science*, 3(4), 1–6.

Hardy, L.K. (1986) Janforum: Identifying the place of theoretical frameworks in an evolving discipline, the nursing profession. *Journal of Advanced Nursing*, 11(1), 103–107.

Hardy, M.E. (1974) The nature of theories. In M.E. Hardy (Ed.), *Theoretical foundations for nursing* (pp. 10–22). New York: MSS Information Corp.

*Hardy, M.E. (1978) Perspectives on nursing theory. *Advances in Nursing Science*, 1(1), 37–48.

Harris, I.M. (1971) Theory building in nursing: A review of the literature. *Image*, 4(1), 6–10.

Hinshaw, A.S. (1987) Response to "Structuring the nursing knowledge system: A typology of four domains." *Scholarly Inquiry for Nursing Practice*, 1(2), 11–114.

Hurley, B.A. (1979) Why a theoretical framework in nursing research? *Western Journal of Nursing Research*, 1(1), 28–41.

Jacobs-Kramer, M.K. and Chinn, P.L. (1988) Perspectives on knowing: A model of nursing knowledge. *Scholarly Inquiry for Nursing Practice*, 2(2), 129–139.

Jacobson, M. (1971) Qualitative data: As a potential source of theory in nursing. *Image*, 4(1), 10–14.

*Jacox, A. (1974) Theory construction in nursing: An overview. *Nursing Research*, 23(1), 4–13.

Jennings, B.M. (1987) Nursing theory development: Successes and challenges. *Journal of Advanced Nursing*, 12(1), 63–69.

*Johnson, D.E. (1959) The nature of a science of nursing. *Nursing Outlook*, 7(5), 291–294.

*Johnson, D.E. (1968) Theory in nursing: Borrowed and unique. *Nursing Research*, 17(3), 206–209.

Johnson, D.E. (1974) Development of theory: A requisite for nursing as a primary health profession. *Nursing Research*, 23(5), 372–377.

*Johnson, D.E. (1978) Development of theory: A requisite for nursing as a primary health profession. In N. Chaska (Ed.), *The nursing profession: Views through the mist*. New York: McGraw-Hill.

Kaplan, A. (1964) *The conduct of inquiry: Methodology for behavioral science*. San Francisco, Chandler.

Ketefian, S. (1987) A case study of theory development: Moral behavior in nursing. *Advances in Nursing Science*, 9(2), 10–19.

Kidd, P. and Morrison, E.F. (1988) The progression of knowledge in nursing: A search for meaning. *Image: Journal of Nursing Scholarship*, 20(4), 222–224.

Kim, H.S. (1987) Structuring the nursing knowledge system: A typology of four domains. *Scholarly Inquiry for Nursing Practice*, 1(2), 111–114.

King, I.M. (1964) Nursing theory: Problems and prospect. *Nursing Science*, 10, 394–403.

King, I.M. (1971) *Toward a theory for nursing*. New York: John Wiley & Sons.

King, I.M. (1978) The "why" of theory development. In NLN, *Theory Development: What, why, and why*? (Publ. No. 15–1708). New York: National League for Nursing.

Klein, J.F. (1978) Theory development in nursing. In N.L. Chaska (Ed.), *The nursing profession: Views through the mist*. New York: McGraw-Hill.

Kristjanson, L.J., Tamblyn, R., and Kuypers, J.A. (1987) A model to guide development and application of multiple nursing theories. *Journal of Advanced Nursing*, 12, 523–529.

*Kritek, P.B. (1978) The generation and classification of nursing diagnoses: Toward a theory of nursing. *Image*, 10(3), 33–40.

Lancaster, W. and Lancaster, J. (1980) Models and model building in nursing. *Advances in Nursing Science*, 3(1), 1–7.

*Leininger, M.M. (1969) Introduction: Nature of science in nursing. *Nursing Research*, 18(5), 388–389.

Levine, M.E. (1988) Antecedent from adjunctive discipline: Creative of nursing theory. *Nursing Science Quarterly*, 1(1), 16–21.

Mathwig, G. (1971) Nursing science: The theoretical core of nursing knowledge. *Image*, 4(1), 20–23.

*McCarthy, R.T. (1972) A practice theory of nursing care. *Nursing Research*, 21(5), 406–410.

*McKay, R. (1969) Theories, models, and systems for nursing. *Nursing Research*, 18(5), 393–400.

McKay, R.P. (1977, May–June) Research question and answer: What is the relationship between the development and utilization of taxonomy and nursing theory? *Nursing Research*, 26(3), 222–223.

*McKay, R. (1977) What is the relationship between the development and utilization of a taxonomy and nursing theory? *Nursing Research*, 26(3), 222–224.

McMurry, P.H. (1982, Feb.–March) Toward a unique knowledge base in nursing. *Image*, 14(1), 12–15.

Meleis, A.I. (1985) International nursing for knowledge development. *Nursing Outlook*, 33(3), 144–147.

Meleis, A.I. (1987) ReVisions in knowledge development: A passion for substance. *Scholarly Inquiry: International Journal*, 1(1), 5–19.

Meleis, A.I. (1987) Theoretical nursing: Today's challenges, tomorrow's bridges. *Nursing papers: Perspectives in nursing. Canadian Journal of Nursing Research*, 19(1), 45–56.

*Menke, E.M. (1978) Theory development: A challenge for nursing. In N.L. Chaska (Ed.), *The nursing profession: Views through the mist*. New York: McGraw-Hill.

Moccia, P. (1986) *New approaches to theory development.* New York: National League of Nurses.

*Moore, M. (1968) Nursing: A scientific discipline. *Forum,* 7(4), 340–348.

Murphy, J.D. (1978) Toward a philosophy of nursing. In N.L. Chaska (Ed.), *The nursing profession: Views through the mist.* New York: McGraw-Hill.

Murphy, J.F. (Ed.). (1971) *Theoretical issues in professional nursing.* New York: Appleton-Century-Crofts. (Note especially Chapters 1, 2, and 3).

*Murphy, S.A. and Hoeffer, B. (1983) Role of the specialties in nursing science. *Advances in Nursing Science,* 5(4), 31–39.

National League for Nursing. (1978) *Theory development: What, why, how?* (Publ. No. 15-1708). New York: National League for Nursing.

*Newman, M. (1972) Nursing's theoretical evolution. *Nursing Outlook,* 20(7), 449–453.

Newman, M. (1977) *Theory development in nursing.* Philadelphia: F.A. Davis.

Nicoll, L. (1986) *Perspectives in nursing theory.* Boston: Little, Brown & Co.

Norris, C.M. (Ed.). (1969, 1970) *Proceedings, first, second, and third nursing theory conference.* Kansas City, KS: University of Kansas Medical Center, Department of Nursing Education.

Norris, C.M. (1982) *Concept classification in nursing.* Rockville, MD: Aspen Systems.

*Notter, L.E. (1975) The case for nursing research. *Nursing Outlook,* 23(12), 760–763.

Nursing Development Conference Group. (1979) *Concept formalization in nursing: Process and product.* Boston: Little, Brown & Co.

Ohashi, J.P. (1985) The contributions of Dickoff and James to theory development in nursing. *Image,* 17(1), 17–20.

Panel Discussion. (1968) Theory development in nursing. *Nursing Research,* 17(3), 223–227.

*Payne, L. (1983) Health: A basic concept in nursing theory. *Journal of Advanced Nursing,* 8(5), 393–395.

Perry, J. (1985) Has the discipline of nursing developed to the stage where nurses do "think nursing"? *Journal of Advanced Nursing,* 10(1), 31–37.

*Peterson, C.J. (1977) Questions frequently asked about the development of a conceptual framework. *Journal of Nursing Education,* 16(4), 22–23.

*Phillips, J.R. (1977) Nursing systems and nursing models. *Image,* 9(1), 4–7.

*Putnam, P. (1965) A conceptual approach to nursing theory. *Nursing Science,* 3, 430–442.

*Quint, J.C. (1967) The case for theories generated from empirical data. *Nursing Research,* 16(2), 109–114.

Ramos, M. (1987) Adopting an evolutionary lens: An optimistic approach in discovering strength in nursing. *Advances in Nursing Science,* 10(1), 19–26.

Reed, P.G. (1989) Nursing theorizing as an ethical endeavor. *Advances in Nursing Science,* 11(3), 1–9.

Rinehart, J.M. (1978) The "how" of theory development in nursing. In NLN, *Theory development: What, why, how?* (Publ. No. 15-1708, pp. 67–74). New York: National League for Nursing.

*Rogers, M. (1963) Some comments on the theoretical basis of nursing practice. *Nursing Science,* 1, 11–13, 60.

*Rubin, R. (1968) A theory of clinical nursing. *Nursing Research,* 17(3), 210–212.

Sasmor, J.L. (1968) Toward developing theory in nursing. *Nursing Forum,* 7(2), 191–200.

Schafer, P.J. (1987) Philosophic analysis of a theory of clinical nursing. *Maternal-Child Nursing Journal,* 16(4), 289–368.

Schlotfeldt, R.M. (1988) Structuring nursing knowledge: A priority for creating nursing's future. *Nursing Science Quarterly,* 1(1), 35–38.

Schultz, P. (1987) Toward holistic inquiry in nursing: A proposal for synthesis of patterns and methods. *Scholarly Inquiry for Nursing Practice*, 1(2), 135–146.

Schultz, P.R. (1987) When client means more than one: Extending the foundational concept of person. *Advances in Nursing Science*, 10(1), 71–80.

Schultz, P. and Meleis, A.I. (1988) Nursing epistemology: Traditions, insights, questions. *Image: Journal of Nursing Scholarship*, 20(4), 217–221.

*Silva, M.C. and Rothbart, D. (1984) An analysis of changing trends in philosophies of science on nursing theory development and testing. *Advances in Nursing Science*, 6(2), 1–13.

Simon, H. (1971) Logical, empirical approach to developing a body of knowledge. In J. Murphy (Ed.), *Theoretical issues in professional nursing*. New York: Appleton-Century-Crofts.

Smoyak, S.A. (1969) Toward understanding nursing situation: A transaction paradigm. *Nursing Research*, 18(5), 405–411.

Sorenson, G. (Ed.). (1986) *Setting the agenda for the year 2000: Knowledge development in nursing*. Kansas City, MO: American Academy of Nursing.

*Stainton, M.C. (1982) The birth of nursing science. *Canadian Nurse*, 78(10), 24–28.

Stember, M.L. (1986) Model building as a strategy for theory development. In P.L. Chinn (Ed.), *Nursing research methodology* (pp. 103–117). Rockville, MD: Aspen Systems.

Stevenson, J.S. and Woods, N.F. (1986) Nursing science and contemporary science: Emerging paradigms. In G. Sorenson (Ed.), *Setting the agenda for the year 2000: Knowledge development in nursing*. Kansas City, MO: American Academy of Nursing.

Suppe, F. and Jacox, A. (1985) Philosophy of science and the development of nursing theory. *Annual Review Nursing Research*, 3, 241–267.

*Tinkle, M.B. and Beaton, J.L. (1983) Toward a new view of science: Implications for nursing research. *Advances in Nursing Science*, 5(2), 27–36.

*Tucker, R.W. (1979) The value decisions we know as science. *Advances in Nursing Science*, 1(2), 1–12.

Visintainer, M.A. (1986) The nature of knowledge and theory in nursing. *Image: Journal of Nursing Scholarship*, 18(2), 32–38.

*Wald, F.S. and Leonard, R.C. (1964) Toward development of nursing practice theory. *Nursing Research*, 13(4), 309–313.

Walker, L.O. (1971) Toward a clearer understanding of the concept of nursing theory. *Nursing Research*, 20(5), 428–435.

Walker, L.O. (1972) Rejoinder to commentary: Toward a clearer understanding of the concept of nursing theory. *Nursing Research*, 21(1), 59–62.

Walker, L.O. and Avant, K.C. (1988) *Strategies for theory construction in nursing*. Norwalk, CT: Appleton & Lange.

*Weatherston, L. (1979) Theory of nursing: Creating effective care. *Journal of Advanced Nursing*, 4(7), 365–375.

4. Forces and Constraints in Theory Development: Women as Scientists

Abramson, J. (1975) *The invisible woman: Discrimination in the academic profession*. San Francisco: Jossey-Bass.

Andreoli, K. (1977) The status of nursing in academia. *Image*, 9(3), 52–58.

Arditti, R, Brennan, P., and Cavrak, S. (1980) *Science and liberation*. Boston: South End Press.

Armeger, B. (1974) Scholarship in nursing. *Nursing Outlook*, 22(3), 162–163.

Astin, H.S. (1967) Factors associated with the participation of women doctorates in the labor force. *Personnel and Guidance Journal*, 46(3), 24–246.

Bachtold, L.M. and Werner, E.E. (1972) Personality characteristics of women scientists. *Psychological Reports*, 31, 391–396.

Benoliel, J. (1975) Scholarship—A women's perspective. *Image*, 7(2), 22–27.

Bissel, M. (1978) Equality for women scientists. *Grants Magazine*, 4, 331–334.

Blankenship, V. (1973) The scientist as a "political man." *British Journal of Sociology*, 24(3), 269–287.

Briscoe, A.M. and Pfafflin, S.M. (Eds.). (1979) Expanding the role of women in the sciences. *Annals of New York Academy of Science*, 323.

Brown, C. (1975) Women workers in the health service industry. *International Journal of Health Services*, 5(2), 173–184.

Bullough, B. (1975) Barriers to the nurse practitioner movement: Problems of women in a woman's field. *International Journal of Health Services*, 5(2), 225–233.

Bullough, B. (1978) The struggle for women's rights in Denver: A personal account. *Nursing Outlook*, 26(9), 566–567.

Chafetz, J.S. (1978) *Masculine/feminine or human? An overview of the sociology of sex roles*. Itasca, IL, F.E. Peacock.

Cleland, V. (1974) To end sex discrimination. *Nursing Clinics of North America*, 9(3), 563–571.

Cole, J.R. (1979) *Fair science: Women in the scientific community*. New York: Free Press.

Cole, J.R. (1981, July–August) Women in Science. *American Scientist*, 69(4), 385–391.

Conant, L.H. (1968) On becoming a nurse researcher. *Nursing Research*, 17(1), 68–71.

Curran, L. (1980) Science education: Did she drop out or was she pushed? In L. Birke et al. (Eds.), *Alice through the microscope*. London: Virgo.

Epstein, C.F. (1973) Positive effects of the multiple negative: Explaining the success of black professional women. *American Journal of Sociology*, 78(4), 912–935.

Fausto-Sterling, A. (1981) Women in science. *Women Science International Forum*, 4, 41–50.

Feulner, P.A. (1979) *Women in the professions: A social psychological study*. Palo Alto, CA: R & E Research Association.

Fitzpatrick, M.L. (1977) Nursing: Review essay. *Signs*, 2(4), 818–833.

Grier, M.R. and Schnitzler, C.P. (1979) Nurses' propensity to risk. *Nursing Research*, 28(3), 186–191.

Grissum, M. and Spengler, C. (1976) *Woman power and health care*. Boston: Little, Brown & Co.

Humphreys, S.M. (1982) *Women and minorities in science: Strategies for increasing participation*. Boulder, CO: Westview Press.

Jaquette, J.S. (1976) Political science: Review essay. *Signs*, 2 (1), 147–176.

Keller, M.C. (1979) The effect of sexual stereotyping on the development of nursing theory. *American Journal of Nursing*, 79(9), 1584–1586.

Loomis, M.E. (1974, November) Collegiate nursing education: An ambivalent profession. *Journal of Nursing Education*, 39–48.

MacDonald, M.R. (1977) How do men and women students rate in empathy? *American Journal of Nursing*, 77(6), 998.

Martin, B.R. and Irvine, J. (1982) Women in science: The astronomical brain drain. *Women's Studies International Forum*, 5, 41–68.

May, K.M., Meleis, A.I. and Winstead-Fry, P. (1982) Mentorship for scholarliness: Opportunities and dilemmas. *Nursing Outlook*, 30, 22–28.

McCain, G. and Segal, E.M. (1977) *The game of science*. Monterey, CA: Brooks/Cole. (Note especially pp. 74–78).

Meleis, A.I. and Dagenais, F. (1981) Sex role identity and perception of professional self in graduates of three programs. *Nursing Research*, 30(3), 162–167.

Meleis, A.I. and May, K. (1981) Nursing theory and scholarliness in the doctoral program. *Advances in Nursing Science*, 4(2), 31–41.

Meleis, A.I. and May, K. (1982) Mentorship for scholarliness. *Proceedings for Doctoral Forum* (held in Seattle, Washington, 1981). University of Washington, Seattle.

Meleis, A.I., Wilson, H.S. and Chater, S. (1980) Toward the socialization of a scholar: A model. *Research in Nursing and Health*, 3, 115–124.

Merchant, C. (1980) *The death of nature: Women, ecology and the scientific revolution*. San Francisco: Harper & Row.

Moore, D., Decker, S., and Down, M.W. (1978) Baccalaureate nursing students' identification with the women's movement. *Nursing Research*, 27(5), 291–295.

Neusner, J. (1977, May 31) The scholars' apprentice. *The Chronicle of Higher Education Point of View*, p. 40.

Roe, A. (1951) A psychological study of eminent biologists. *Psychological Monographs*, 65, 1–67.

Roe, A. (1963) *The making of a scientist*. New York: Dodd Mead.

Roe, A. (1966) Women in science. *Personnel and Guidance Journal*, 54, 784–787.

Rossi, A. (1972) Women in science: Why so few? In C. Safilios-Rothchild (Ed.), *Toward a sociology of women* (pp. 141–153). New York: Xerox Corp.

Rossiter, M.W. (1982) *Women scientists in America: Struggles and strategies in 1940*. Baltimore: Johns Hopkins Press.

Seiden, A. (1976) Overview: Research on the psychology of women. I and II. Gender differences and sexual and reproductive life. *American Journal of Psychiatry*, 133(10), 1111–1118.

Speizer, J.J. (1981) Role models, mentors and sponsors: The elusive concepts. *Signs*, 6, 692–712.

Stroller, E.P. (1978) Perceptions of the nursing role: A case study of an entering class. *Journal of Nursing Education*, 17(6), 2–14.

Stromborg, M.F. (1976) Relationship of sex-role identity to occupational image of female nursing students. *Nursing Research*, 25(5), 363–369.

Vaughter, R. (1976, Autumn) Psychology: Review essay. *Signs*, 2(1), 120–146.

Wallsgrove, R. (1980) The masculine face of science. In L. Birke et al. (Eds.), *Alice through the microscope*. London: Virgo.

Watson, J.D. (1968) *The double helix*. New York: New American Library.

White, M.S. (1972) Psychological and social barriers to women in science. In C. Safilios-Rothchild (Ed.). *Toward a sociology of women*. New York: Xerox Corp.

5. Forces and Constraints in Theory Development: Nursing Profession

Ashley, J.A. (1980) Power in structured misogyny: Implications for the politics of care. *Advances in Nursing Science*, 2(3), 3–22.

Ashley, J. (1976) *Hospital paternalism and the role of the nurse*. New York: Teachers' College Press.

Aydelotte, M.K. (1968) Issues of professional nursing: The need for clinical excellence. *Nursing Forum*, 7(1), 72–86.

Babich, K.S. (1968) The perception of professionalism: Equality. *Nursing Forum*, 7(1), 14–20.

Barber, B. (1963, Fall) Some problems in the sociology of professions. *Daedalus*, 92(4), 669–688.

Bixler, G. and Bixler, R.W. (1959) The professional status of nursing. *American Journal of Nursing*, 59(8), 1142–1147.

Brown, E.L. (1948) *Nursing for the future*. New York: Russel Sage Foundation. (Especially note pp. 669–688).

Brown, M.I. (1964) Research in the development of nursing theory. *Nursing Research*, 13(2), 109–112.

Caplow, T. (1954) *The sociology of work*. Minneapolis, MN: University of Minnesota Press. (Especially note p. 139.)

Cogan, M.L. (1955, January) The problem of defining a profession. *Annals of the American Academy of Political and Social Sciences*, 297, 105–111.

Colodarci, A. (1963) What about the word "profession"? *American Journal of Nursing*, 63(10), 116–118.

Conant, L.H. (1968) On becoming a nurse researcher. *Nursing Research*, 17(1), 68–72.

Cox, C. (1979) Who cares? Nursing and sociology: The development of symbiotic relationship. *Journal of Advanced Nursing*, 4, 237–252.

Devereux, G. and Weiner, F. (1950, October) The occupational status of nurses. *American Sociological Review*, 15, 628–634.

Dilworth, A. (1963, May) Goals in nursing. *Nursing Outlook*, 11, 336–340.

Ellison, M., Diers, D., and Leonard, R. (1965) The use of the behavioral sciences in nursing: Further comment. *Nursing Research*, 14, 71–72.

Feldman, H.R. (1980) Nursing research in the 1980s: Issues and implications. *Advances in Nursing Science*, 3(1), 85–92.

Feldman, H.R. (1981, October) A science of nursing—to be or not to be? *Image*, 13, 63–66.

Fox, D. (1964, Winter) A proposed model for identifying research areas in nursing. *Nursing Research*, 13, 29–36.

Goode, W.J. (1959) Community within a community: The professions. *American Sociological Review*, 194–200. (Bobbs-Merrill Reprint S-99.)

Goode, W.J. (1960, December) Encroachment, charlatanism, and the emerging profession: Psychology, sociology, and medicine. *American Sociological Review*, 25, 902–914.

Gouldner, A. (1961) Theoretical requirements of the applied social sciences. In W.G. Bennis, K.D. Benne, and R. Chin (Eds.), *The planning of change*. New York: Holt, Rinehart & Winston.

Hughes, E.C. (1958) *Men and their work*. Glencoe, IL: Free Press. (Especially note p. 133.)

Hughes, E.C. (1963, Fall) Professions. *Daedalus*, 655–668.

Hurley, B.A. (1979) Why a theoretical framework in nursing research. *Western Journal of Nursing Research*, 1(1), 28–41.

Johnson, M. and Martin, H. (1958) A sociological analysis of the nurse role. *American Journal of Nursing*, 58(3), 373–377.

Lipton, N. (1968) Nursing education as a challenge to the professionalization of nursing. *Nursing Forum*, 7(2), 201–214.

Martin, H.W. (1958, October) The behavioral sciences and nursing education. *Social Forces*, 37, 61–67.

McGlothlin, W.J. (1960) *Patterns of professional education*. New York: G.P. Putnam Sons. (Especially note pp. 1–25.)

McGlothlin, W.J. (1961, April) The place of nursing among the professions. *Nursing Outlook*, 9, 216.

Mead, M. (1956) Nursing—primitive and civilized. *American Journal of Nursing*, 56(8), 948–950.

Meleis, A.I. and May, K. (1981) Nursing theory and scholarliness in the doctoral program. *Advances in Nursing Science*, 4(1), 31–41.

Montag, M. (1959) *Community college education for nursing.* New York: McGraw-Hill.

Parsons, T. (1939) The professions and social structure. *Social Forces* (S-219). The College Book Co. (Especially note pp. 457–467.)

Parsons, T. (1965) *Essays in sociological theory.* New York: Free Press.

Reissman, L. and Rorher, J.H. (Eds.). (1957) *Change and dilemma in the nursing profession.* New York: G.P. Putnam's Sons.

Rogers, M. (1975) Euphemisms in nursing's future. *Image*, 7(2), 3–9.

Tyler, R. (1952, April) Distinctive attributes of education for the professions. *Social Work Journal*, 33, 55–62.

Van Maanen, J.M.T. et al. (1979) Janforum: The nursing profession: Ritualized, routinized or research-based? *Journal of Advanced Nursing*, 1, 87–89.

Wolensky, R.P. (1981) The graduate student's double bind: A professional socialization problem in sociology. *Sociological Spectrum*, 1, 393–414.

6. Theory and Science

*Abdellah, F.G. (1969) The nature of nursing science. *Nursing Research*, 18(5), 390–393.

*Andreoli, K.G. and Thompson, C.E. (1977) The nature of science in nursing. *Image*, 9(2), 32–37.

Barber, B. and Hirsch, W. (Eds.). (1962) *The sociology of science.* New York: Free Press of Glencoe.

Bernstein, J. (1978) *Experiencing science.* New York: Basic Books. (Especially note p. 87.)

Bilitski, J.S. (1981) Nursing science and the laws of health: The test of substance as a step in the process of theory development. *Advances in Nursing Science*, 4(1), 15–29.

Blume, S. (Ed.) (1977) *Perspectives in the sociology of science.* New York: John Wiley & Sons.

Bohny, B. (1980) Theory development for a nursing science. *Nursing Forum*, 19(1), 50–67.

*Colaizzi, J. (1975) The proper object of nursing science. *International Journal of Nursing Studies*, 12(4), 197–200.

Crowley, D.M. (1968) Perspective of pure science. *Nursing Research*, 17(6), 497–501.

Danto, A. and Morgenbesser, S. (Eds.) (1966) Laws and theories. *Philosophy of Science.* New York: The World Publishing Co. (Especially note pp. 177–287.)

Gortner, S.R. (1980) Nursing science in transition. *Nursing Research*, 29(3), 180–183.

*Green, J.A. (1979) Science, nursing and nursing science: A conceptual analysis. *Advances in Nursing Science*, 2(1), 57–64.

*Johnson, D.E. (1959) The nature of a science of nursing. *Nursing Outlook*, 7(5), 291–294.

*Leininger, M.M. (1969) Introduction: Nature of science in nursing. *Nursing Research*, 18(5), 388–389.

Longino, H.E. (1981) Scientific objectivity and feminist theorizing. *Liberal Education*, 67, 187–195.

Mathwig, G. (1971) Nursing science: The theoretical core of nursing knowledge. *Image*, 4(1), 20–23.

Ravetz, J.R. (1971) *Scientific knowledge and its social problems.* New York: Oxford University Press. (Especially note pp. 152, 162.)

*Rogers, M.E. (1963) Some comments on the theoretical basis of nursing practice. *Nursing Science*, 1, 11–13, 60.

Schrag, C. (1968) Science and the helping professions. *Nursing Research*, 17(6), 486–496.

Schwab, J.J. (1966) The teaching of science as inquiry. In *The teaching of science*. Cambridge, MA: Harvard University Press. (Especially note pp. 12, 15, 17.)

Shermis, S.S. (1962, November) On becoming an intellectual discipline. *Phi Delta Kappa*, 84–86.

*Tucker, R.W. (1979) The value decisions we know as science. *Advances in Nursing Science*, 1(2), 1–12.

7. Theory and Research

Ader, R. (1980) Psychosomatic and psychoimmunologic research. *Psychosomatic Medicine*, 42(3), 307–321.

Allan, J.D. (1988) Knowing what to weigh: Women's self-care activities related to weight. *Advances in Nursing Science*, 11(1), 47–60.

*Batey, M. (1972) Values relative to research and to science in nursing as influenced by a sociological perspective. *Nursing Research*, 21(6), 504–508.

*Benoliel, J.Q. (1977) The interaction between theory and research. *Nursing Outlook*, 25(2), 108–113.

*Brown, M.I. (1964) Research in the development of nursing theory. *Nursing Research*, 13(2), 109–112.

Chinn, P. (1985) Debunking myths in nursing theory and research. *Image*, 17(2), 45–49.

Compton, P. (1989) Drug abuse. A self-care deficit. *Journal of Psychosocial Nursing and Mental Health Services*, 27(3), 22–26.

Cressler, D.L. and Tomlinson, P.S. (1988) Nursing research and the discipline of etiological science. *Western Journal of Nursing Research*, 10(6), 743–756.

Curtin, L.L. (1984) Who or why or which or what? . . . is nursing. *Nursing Management*, 15(11), 7–8.

*Dickoff, J. and James, P. (1968) Researching research's role in theory development. *Nursing Research*, 17(3), 204–205.

Fawcett, J. (1988) Conceptual models and theory development. *Journal of Obstetric, Gynecologic, and Neonatal Nursing*, 17(6), 400–403.

Fawcett, J. and Downs, F.S. (1986) *The relationship of theory and research*. Norwalk, CT: Appleton-Century-Crofts.

Fawcett, J. (1978) The relationship between theory and research: A double helix. *Advances in Nursing Science*, 1(1), 49–62.

Feldman, H.R. (1980) Nursing research in the 1980s: Issues and implications. *Advances in Nursing Science*, 3(1), 85–92.

Fitzpatrick, J.J. (1988) How can we enhance nursing knowledge and practice? *Nursing and Health Care*, 9(9), 517–521.

Gunter, L.J. (1962) Notes on a theoretical framework for nursing research. *Nursing Research*, 11(4), 219–222.

Haller, K.B. (1988) Beyond idle speculation. *American Journal of Maternal Child Nursing*, 13(5), 386.

Hardy, L.K. (1982) Nursing models and research: A restrictive view? *Journal of Advanced Nursing*, 7, 447–451.

Hurley, B.A. (1979) Why a theoretical framework in nursing research? *Western Journal of Nursing Research*, 1(1), 28–41.

Ingram, M.R. (1988) Origins of nursing knowledge. *Image: Journal of Nursing Scholarship*, 20(4), 233.

Johnson, M. (1983) Some aspects of the relation between theory and research in nursing. *Journal of Advanced Nursing*, 8, 21–28.

Kidd, P. and Morrison, E.F. (1988) Comment. The progression of knowledge in nursing: A search for meaning. *Image: Journal of Nursing Scholarship*, 20(4), 222–224.

Lindeman, C.A. (1984) Theory and research as basic to nursing practice. *ANA Publication* (Publ. No. NP-68C, pp. 1–19) (pamphlet).

Ludemann, R. (1979) Editorial comment: The paradoxical nature of nursing research. *Image*, 11(1), 2–8.

MacPherson, K.I. (1983) Feminist methods: A new paradigm for nursing research. *Advances in Nursing Science*, 5, 17–26.

McBride, A.B. (1986) Theory and research. *Journal of Psychological Nursing*, 24(9), 27–32.

McFarlane, J.K. (1976) Role of research in the development of nursing. *Journal of Advanced Nursing*, 1, 443–451.

Moody, L.E., Wilson, M.E., Smith, K., Schwartz, R., Tittle, M., and Van Cott, M.L. (1988) Analysis of a decade of nursing practice research: 1977–1986. *Nursing Research*, 37(6), 374–379.

Munhall, P.L. (1989) Philosophical pondering on qualitative research methods in nursing. *Nursing Science Quarterly*, 2(1), 20–28.

Murdaugh, C.L. (1989) Nursing research. The use of grounded theory methodology to study the process of life-style changes. *Journal of Cardiovascular Nursing*, 3(2), 56–58.

*Notter, L.E. (1975) The case for nursing research. *Nursing Outlook*, 23(12), 760–763.

Orcutt, J. (1972) Toward a sociological theory of drug effects: A comparison of marijuana and alcohol. *Sociology and Social Research*, 56(2), 243–253.

Parse, R.R. (1989) Qualitative research: Publishing and funding (editorial). *Nursing Science Quarterly*, 2(1), 1–2.

*Payne, G. (1973) Comparative sociology: Some problems of theory and method. *British Journal of Sociology*, 24(1), 13–29.

Phillips, J.R. (1989) Qualitative research: A process of discovery. *Nursing Science Quarterly*, 2(1), 5–6.

Phillips, J.R. (1989) Science of unitary human beings: Changing research perspectives. *Nursing Science Quarterly*, 2(2), 57–60.

*Quint, J.C. (1967) The case for theories generated from empirical data. *Nursing Research*, 16(2), 109–114.

Rubin, R. and Erickson, F. (1978) Research in clinical nursing. *Journal of Advanced Nursing*, 3(2), 131–144.

Salsberry, P.J., Smith, M.C., and Boyd, C.O. (1989) Phenomenological research in nursing: Commentary and responses. *Nursing Science Quarterly*, 2(1), 9–19.

Santopinto, M.D. (1989) The relentless drive to be ever thinner: A study using the phenomenological method. *Nursing Science Quarterly*, 2(1), 29–36.

Schlotfeldt, R.M. (1975) The conceptual framework of nursing research: The need for a conceptual framework. In P.J. Verhonick (Ed.), *Nursing Research*. Boston: Little, Brown & Co.

*Silva, M.C. (1977) Philosophy, science, theory: Interrelationships and implications for nursing research. *Image*, 9(3), 59–63.

Treece, E.W. and Treece, J.W. (1977) Theory and method. In *Elements of research in nursing* (2nd ed.). St. Louis: C.V. Mosby.

Zelauskas, B.A., Howes, D.G., Christmyer, C.S., and Dennis, K.E. (1988) Bridging the gap: Theory to practice–Part II, Research applications. *Nursing Management*, 19(9), 50–52.

8. Theory and Practice

Adam, E. (1983) Frontiers of nursing in the 21st century: Development of models and theories on the concept of nursing. *Journal of Advanced Nursing*, 8, 41–45.

Aggleton, P. and Chalmers, H. (1987) Models of nursing, nursing practice and nursing education. *Journal of Advanced Nursing*, 12(5), 573–581.

Arndt, C. and Huckabay, L.M.D. (1975) Administrative theory within a systems' frame of reference. In *Nursing Administration*. St. Louis: C.V. Mosby.

Baer, E.D. (1987) "A cooperative venture" in pursuit of professional status: A research journal for nursing. *Nursing Research*, 36(1), 18–25.

Barnard, K.E. (1980) Knowledge for practice: Directions for the future. *Nursing Research*, 29(4), 208–212.

*Beckstrand, J. (1978) The notion of a practice theory and the relationship of scientific and ethical knowledge to practice. *Research in Nursing and Health*, 1(3), 131–136.

*Beckstrand, J. (1978) The need for a practice theory as indicated by the knowledge used in the conduct of practice. *Research in Nursing and Health*, 1(4), 175–180.

*Beckstrand, J. (1980) A critique of several conceptions of practice theory in nursing. *Research in Nursing and Health*, 3, 69–79.

Buchanan, B.F. (1987) Conceptual models: An assessment framework. *Journal of Nursing Administration*, 17(10), 22–26.

Craig, S.L. (1980) Theory development and its relevance for nursing. *Journal of Advanced Nursing*, 5, 349–355.

Christmyer, C.S., Catanzariti, P.M., Langford, A.M., and Reitz, J.A. (1988) Bridging the gap: Theory to practice–Part I, Clinical applications. *Nursing Management*, 19(8), 42–43, 46–48, 50.

Curtin, L.L. (1988) Thought-full nursing practice (editorial). *Nursing Management*, 19(10), 7–8.

Davis, A.J. (1978) The phenomenological approach. In N.L. Chaska (Ed.), *The nursing profession: Views through the mist*. New York: McGraw-Hill.

DeGroot, H.A., Ferketich, S.L., and Larson, P.J. (1987) Theory development in a non-university setting unit. *Journal of Nursing Administration*, 17(4), 38–44.

Derstine, J.B. (1989) The development of theory-based practice by graduate students in rehabilitation nursing. *Rehabilitation Nursing*, 14(2), 88–89.

DeSocio, J. and Sebastian, L. (1988) Towards a theoretical model for clinical nursing practice at Menningers. *Kansas Nurse*, 63(12), 4–5.

*Dickoff, J., James, P., and Wiedenbach, E. (1968) Theory in a practice discipline: Part I. Practice oriented theory. *Nursing Research*, 17(5), 415–435.

*Dickoff, J., James, P, and Wiedenbach, E. (1968) Theory in a practice discipline: Part II. Practice oriented research. *Nursing Research*, 17(6), 545–554.

Fawcett, J. (1980) A declaration of nursing independence: The relation of theory and research to nursing practice. *Journal of Nursing Administration*, 10(6), 36–39.

Field, P.A. (1987) The impact of nursing theory on the clinical decision making process. *Journal of Advanced Nursing*, 12(5), 563–571.

Field, L. et al. (1985) Moving to a nursing model. *American Journal of Nursing*, 85(10), 1100–1101.

Fielding, R.G. and Llewelyn, S.P. (1987) Communication in nursing may damage your health and enthusiasm: Some warnings. *Journal of Advanced Nursing Science*, 12(3), 281–290.

Fitzpatrick, J.J. (1988) How can we enhance nursing knowledge and practice? *Nursing and Health Care*, 9(9), 517–521.

Friedmann, M.L. (1989) Closing the gap between grand theory and mental health practice with families. Part I: The framework of systemic organization for nursing of families and family members. *Archives of Psychiatric Nursing*, 3(1), 10–19.

Friedmann, M.L. (1989) The concept of family nursing. *Journal of Advanced Nursing*, 14(3), 211–216.

Frissell, S. (1988) So many models, so much confusion. *Nursing Administration Quarterly*, 12(2), 13–17.

Gottlieb, L. and Lowat, K. (1987) The McGill model of nursing: A practice-derived model. *Advances in Nursing Science*, 9(4), 51–61.

Greenwood, E. (1961) The practice of science and the science of practice. In W.G. Bennis, K.D. Benne, and R. Chin (Eds.), *The planning of change*. New York: Holt, Rinehart & Winston.

Gruending, D.L. (1986) Nursing theory: A vehicle of professionalization. *Journal of Advanced Nursing Science*, 10(6), 553–558.

Hanchett, E.S. and Clark, P.N. (1988) Nursing theory and public health science: Is synthesis possible? *Public Health Nursing*, 5(1), 2–6.

Harrell, J.S. (1986) Needed nurse engineers to link theory and practice. *Nursing Outlook*, 34(4), 196–198.

Harrison, J., Saunders, M.E., and Sims, A. (1977) Integrating theory and practice in modular schemes for basic nurse education. *Journal of Advanced Nursing*, 2, 503–519.

Hathaway, D. and Strong, M. (1988) Theory, practice, and research in transplant nursing. *ANNA Journal*, 15(1), 9–12.

Henderson, B. (1978) Nursing diagnosis: Theory and practice. *Advances in Nursing Science*, 1(1), 75–82.

Hinshaw, A.S. (1987) Response to "Structuring the nursing knowledge system: A typology of four domains." *Scholarly Inquiry for Nursing Practice*, 1(2), 111–114.

Huggins, E.A. and Scalzi, C.C. (1988) Limitations and alternatives: Ethical practice theory in nursing. *Advances in Nursing Science*, 10(4), 43–47.

*Jacobs, M.K. and Huether, S.E. (1978) Nursing science: The theory-practice linkage. *Advances in Nursing Science*, 1(1), 63–73.

Jameton, A. and Fowler, M.D. (1989) Ethical inquiry and concept of research. *Advanced Nursing Science*, 11(3), 11–24.

Jennings, B.M. and Meleis, A.I. (1988) Nursing theory and administrative practice: Agenda for the 1990s. *Advances in Nursing Science*, 10(3), 56–69.

Johnson, S.E. (1989) A picture is worth a thousand words: Helping students visualize a conceptual model. *Nurse Educator*, 14(3), 21–24.

Johnson, D. (1987) Evaluating conceptual models for use in critical care nursing practice. *Dimensions of Critical Care Nursing*, 6(4), 195–197.

Jones, S. (1989) Practice and theory. Is unity possible? *Nursing Standard*, 3(18), 22–23.

Kim, H.S. (1987) Response to "Structuring the nursing knowledge system: A typology of four domains." *Scholarly Inquiry for Nursing Practice*, 1(2), 111–114.

Ketefian, S. (1987) A case study of theory development: Moral behavior in nursing. *Advances in Nursing Science*, 9(2), 10–19.

Kristjanson, L.J., Tamblyn, R., and Kuypers, J.A. (1987) A model to guide development and application of multiple nursing theories. *Journal of Advanced Nursing*, 12(4), 523–529.

Lewis, T. (1988) Leaping the chasm between nursing theory and practice. *Journal of Advanced Nursing*, 13(3), 345–351.

Long, G.E. (1985) Professional advancement: Theory development through practice and research. *ANA Journal*, 12(1), 35–38.

Mathwig, G. (1971) Nursing science: The theoretical core of nursing knowledge. *Image*, 4(1), 20–23.

McBride, A.B. and McBride, W.L. (1981) Theoretical underpinnings for women's health. *Women and Health*, 6, 37–55.

*McCarthy, R.T. (1972) A practice theory of nursing care. *Nursing Research*, 21(5), 406–410.

McFarlane, J.K. (1977) Developing a theory of nursing: The relationship of theory to practice, education, and research. *Journal of Advanced Nursing*, 2(3), 261–270.

McIver, M. (1987) Putting theory into practice. *Canadian Nurse*, 83(10), 36–38.

Miller, S.R. (1978) Have we dichotomized theory and practice in nursing? *Nursing Leadership*, 1(1), 34–36.

Moody, L.E., Wilson, M.E., Smith, K., Schwartz, R., Tittle, M., and Van Cott, M.L. (1988) Analysis of a decade of nursing practice research: 1977–1986. *Nursing Research*, 37(6), 374–379.

Moore, M.A. (1968) Nursing: A scientific discipline? *Nursing Forum*, 7(4), 340–348.

Munhall, P.L. (1989) Philosophical pondering on qualitative research methods in nursing. *Nursing Science Quarterly*, 2(1), 20–28.

Rew, L., Stuppy, D., and Becker, H. (1988) Construct validity in instrument development: A vital link between nursing practice, research, and theory. *Advances in Nursing Science*, 10(4), 10–22.

Rodgers, J.A. (1976) Today's preparation for tomorrow's practice. The Lehman College nursing program. *Journal of Advanced Nursing*, 1(4), 311–322.

Roper, N. (1966) A model for nursing and nursology. *Journal of Advanced Nursing*, 1(2), 219–227.

Roy, C. and Obby, S.M. (1978) The practitioner movement: Toward a science of nursing. *American Journal of Nursing*, 78(10), 1698–1702.

Santopinto, M.D. (1989) The relentless drive to be ever thinner: A study using the phenomenological method. *Nursing Science Quarterly*, 2(1), 29–36.

Sarter, B. (1987) Evolutionary idealism: A philosophical foundation for holistic nursing theory. *Advances in Nursing Science*, 9(2), 1–9.

Schafer, P.J. (1987) Philosophic analysis of a theory of clinical nursing. *Maternal-Child Nursing Journal*, 16(4), 289–368.

Schultz, P.R. (1987) When client means more than one: Extending the foundational concept of person. *Advances in Nursing Science*, 10(1), 71–86.

Topham, D.L. and DeSilva, P. (1988) Evaluating congruency between steps in the research process. A critique guide for use in clinical nursing practice. *Clinical Nurse Specialist*, 2(2), 97–102.

Visintainer, M.A. (1986) The nature of nursing and theory in nursing. *Image: Journal of Nursing Scholarship*, 18(2), 32–38.

Wald, F.S. and Leonard, R.C. (1971) Toward development of nursing practice theory. *Nursing Research*, 20(5), 428–435.

Zelauskas, B.A., Howes, D.G., Christmyer, C.S., and Dennis, K.E. (1988) Bridging the gap: Theory to practice—Part II, Research applications. *Nursing Management*, 19(8), 42–43, 46–48, 50.

9. Theory and Nursing Diagnosis

Gordon, M. (1979) The concept of nursing diagnosis. *Nursing Clinics of North America*, 14(3), 487–496.

Gordon, M.D. (1985) Nursing diagnosis. *Annual Review of Nursing Research*, 3, 127–146.

Gordon, M. and Sweeny, M.A. (1979) Methodological problems and issues in identifying and standardizing nursing diagnosis. *Advances in Nursing Science*, 2(1), 1–15.

Guzzetta, C.E. and Dossey, B.M. (1983) Nursing diagnosis: Framework, process, and problems. *Heart and Lung*, 12(3), 281–291.

Henderson, B. (1978) Nursing diagnosis: Theory and practice. *Advances in Nursing Science*, 1(1), 75–83.

Kim, M.J. (1989) Nursing diagnosis. *Annual Review of Nursing Research*, 7, 117–142.

Kritek, P.B. (1978) The generation and classification of nursing diagnosis: Toward a theory of nursing. *Image: Journal of Nursing Scholarship*, 10(2), 33–40.

Kritek, P.B. (1985) Nursing diagnosis: Theoretical foundations. *Occupational Health Nursing*, 33(8), 393–396.

Kritek, P.B. (1985) Nursing diagnosis in perspective: Response to a critique. *Image: Journal of Nursing Scholarship*, 17(1), 3–8.

Porter, E.J. (1985) Validating a diagnostic label. *Nursing Clinics in North America*, 20(4), 641–655.

Porter, E.J. (1986) Critical analysis of NANDA nursing diagnosis taxonomy I. *Image: Journal of Nursing Scholarship*, 18(4), 136–139.

Shamansky, S.L. and Yanni, C.R. (1983) In opposition to nursing diagnosis: A minority opinion. *Image: Journal of Nursing Scholarship*, 19(4), 184–185.

Tilley, J.D., Gregor, F.M. and Thieson, V. (1987) The nurses' role in patient education: Incongruent perceptions among nurses and patients. *Journal of Advanced Nursing*, 12, 291–391.

Tribotti, S., Lyons, N., Blackburn, S., Stein, M., and Withers, J. (1988) Nursing diagnosis for the postpartum woman. *Journal of Obstetric, Gynecologic, and Neonatal Nursing*, 17, 410–416.

Turkoski, B. (1988) Nursing diagnosis in print, 1950–1985. *Nursing Outlook*, 36(3), 142–144.

10. Theory and Education

Aggleton, P. and Chalmers, H. (1987) Models of nursing, nursing practice and nursing education. *Journal of Advanced Nursing*, 12(5), 573–581.

Baer, E.D. (1987) "A cooperative venture" in pursuit of professional status: A research journal for nursing. *Nursing Research*, 36(1), 18–25.

Batra, C. (1987) Nursing theory for undergraduates. *Nursing Outlook*, 35(4), 189–192.

Bevis, E.O. (1989, February) Curriculum building in nursing: A process. *NLN Publications* (Publ. No. 15-227), i–xx, 1–282.

*Burgess, G. (1978) The personal development of the nursing student as a conceptual framework. *Nursing Forum*, 17(1), 96–102.

Cessario, L. (1987) Utilization of board gaming for conceptual models of nursing. *Journal of Nursing Education*, 26(4), 167–169.

Chick, N. and Paull, D. (1988) Collaboration between nurse educators in Australia and New Zealand extends educational opportunities for nurses. *International Journal of Nursing Studies*, 25(4), 279–286.

Chinn, P.L. (1988) Knowing and doing (editorial). *Advances in Nursing Science*, 10(3), vii–viii.

Christmyer, C.S., Catanzariti, P.M., Langford, A.M., and Reitz, J.A. (1988) Bridging the gap: Theory to practice—Part I, Clinical applications. *Nursing Management*, 19(8), 42–43, 46–48, 50.

Curtin, L.L. (1987) Education and licensure: Once more into the breach (editorial). *Nursing Management*, 18(5), 9–10.

DeGroot, H.A., Ferketich, S.L., and Larson, P.J. (1987) Theory development in a non-university service setting. *Journal of Nursing Administration,* 17(4), 38–44.

Derdiarian, A. (1979) Education: A way to theory construction in nursing. *Journal of Nursing Education,* 18(2), 36–47.

Derstine, J.B. (1989) The development of theory-based practice by graduate students in rehabilitative nursing. *Rehabilitation Nursing,* 14(2), 88–89.

Dickoff, J. and James, P. (1970) Beliefs and values: Bases for curriculum design. *Nursing Research,* 19(5), 415–427.

Diekelmann, N. (1988) Curriculum revolution: A theoretical and philosophical mandate for change. *NLN Publications* (Publ. No. 15-2224), 137–157.

Dowie, S. and Park, C. (1988) Relating nursing theory to students' life experiences. *Nurse Education Today,* 8(4), 191–196.

Downs, F.S. (1988) Doctoral education: Our claim to the future. *Nursing Outlook,* 36(1), 18–20.

Duff, V. (1989) Perspective transformation: The challenge for the RN in the baccalaureate program. *Journal of Nursing Education,* 28(1), 38–39.

Emden, C. and Young, W. (1987) Theory development in nursing: Australian nurses advance global debate. *Australian Journal of Advanced Nursing,* 4(3), 22–40.

Fawcett, J. (1985) Theory: Basis for the study and practice of nursing education. *Journal of Nursing Education,* 24(6), 226–229.

Fielding, R.G. and Llewelyn, S.P. (1987) Communication in nursing may damage your health and enthusiasm: Some warning. *Journal of Advanced Nursing Science,* 12(3), 281–290.

Fitzpatrick, J.J. (1987) Use of existing nursing models. *Journal of Gerontological Nursing,* 13(9), 8–9.

Graham, L. (1979) The development of a useful conceptual framework in curriculum design. *Nursing Papers Perspective in Nursing,* 9(3), 84–92.

Greenwood, J. (1988) More considerations concerning the application of nursing models to curricula: A reply to Lorraine Smith. *Nurse Education Today,* 8(4), 187–190.

Haggerty, L.A. (1987) An analysis of senior nursing students' immediate responses to distressed patients. *Journal of Advanced Nursing,* 12(4), 451–461.

Hall, K.V. (1979, April) Current trends in the use of conceptual frameworks in nursing education. *Journal of Nursing Education,* 18(4), 26–29.

Harrison, J., Saunders, M.E., and Sims, A. (1977) Integrating theory and practice in modular schemes for basic nursing education. *Journal of Advanced Nursing,* 2, 503–519.

Hartley, L.A. (1988) Congruence between teaching and learning self-care: A pilot study. *Nursing Science Quarterly,* 1(4), 161–167.

Heinrich, K. (1989) Growing pains: Faculty stages in adopting a nursing model. *Nurse Educator,* 14(1), 3–4, 29.

Jacobs-Kramer, M.K. and Huether, S.E. (1988) Curricular considerations for teaching nursing theory. *Journal of Professional Nursing,* 4(5), 373–380.

Jameton, A. and Fowler, M.D. (1989) Ethical inquiry and the concept of research. *Advances in Nursing Science,* 11(3), 11–24.

Johnson, S.E. (1989) A picture is worth a thousand words: Helping students visualize a conceptual model. *Nurse Educator,* 14(3), 21–24.

Kristjanson, L.J., Tamblyn, R., and Kuypers, J.A. (1987) A model to guide development and application of multiple nursing theories. *Journal of Advanced Nursing,* 12(4), 523–529.

Lawrence, S.A. and Lawrence, R.M. (1983) Curriculum development: Philosophy, objectives, and conceptual framework. *Nursing Outlook,* 31(3), 160–163.

Masters, M. (1988) Nursing theory: An electric approach in baccalaureate education. *Kansas Nurse,* 63(12), 1–2.

McMahon, R. (1988) The "24-hour reality orientation" type of approach to the confused elderly: A minimum standard for care. *Journal of Advanced Nursing*, 13(6), 693–700.

Meleis, A.I. and Price, M. (1988) Strategies and conditions for teaching theoretical nursing: An international perspective. *Journal of Advanced Nursing*, 13, 592–604.

Olsson, H.M. and Gullberg, M.T. (1987) Nursing education: A valuation of theoretical and practical sections of the education. Expectations and knowledge of the nurse role. *Vard i Norden*, 7(13), 412–416.

Pepler, C. (1977) The practical aspects of using a conceptual framework. *Nursing Papers*, 9(3), 93–101.

Punton, S. (1989) King's fund nursing development. The Oxford experience. *Nursing Standard*, 3(22), 27–28.

Rajabally, M. (1977) Frankly speaking. Nursing education: Another tower of Babel. *Canadian Nurse*, 73(9), 30–31.

Reid, B., Allen, A.F., Gauthier, T., and Campbell, H. (1989) Solving the Orem mystery: An educational strategy. *Journal of Continuing Education in Nursing*, 20(3), 108–110.

Rogers, M.E. (1989) Creating a climate for the implementation of a nursing conceptual framework. *Journal of Continuing Education in Nursing*, 20(3), 112–116.

Ross, M.M., Bourbonnais, F.F., and Carroll, G. (1987) Curricular design and the Betty Neuman systems model: A new approach to learning. *International Nursing Review*, 34(3), 75–79.

Roy, C. (1979) Relating nursing theory to education: A new era. *Nurse Educator*, 4(2), 16–21.

Sortet, J.P. (1989) Incongruence in the nursing profession. *Nursing Management*, 20(5), 64–66, 68.

Torres, G. and Yura, H. (1974) Today's conceptual framework: Its relationship to the curriculum development process (Publ. No. 15-1529). New York: National League for Nursing.

Walker, M.K. and Norby, R.B. (1987–1988) An essay on friendships of utility: Resolving the disalignment between nursing education and nursing service. *Nursing Forum*, 23(1), 30–35.

11. Theory and Administration

DeGroot, H.A., Ferketich, S.L., and Larson, P.J. (1987) Theory development in a non-university service setting. *Journal of Nursing Administration*, 17(4), 38–44.

Dorsey, K. and Purcell, S. (1987) Translating a nursing theory into a nursing system. *Geriatric Nursing*, 8(3), 136–137.

Fawcett, J., Botter, M., Burritt, J., Crossly, J., and Frink, B. (1989) Conceptual models of nursing and organization theories. In B. Henry, C. Arndt, M. DiVincenti, and A. Marriner-Tomey (Eds.), *Dimensions of Nursing Administration: Theory, Research, Education, Practice*. Boston: Blackwell Scientific Publications.

Fielding, R.G. and Llewelyn, S.P. (1987) Communication training in nursing may damage your health and enthusiasm: Some warnings. *Journal of Advanced Nursing*, 12(3), 281–290.

Henry, B., Arndt, C., DiVincenti, M., and Marriner-Tomey, A. (Eds.) (1989) *Dimensions of nursing administration: Theory, research, education, practice*. Boston: Blackwell Scientific Publications.

Jennings, B.M. and Meleis, A.I. (1988) Nursing theory and administrative practice: Agenda for the 1990s. *Advances in Nursing Science*, 10(3), 56–69.

Meleis, A.I. and Jennings, B.M. (1989) Theoretical nursing administration: Today's challenges, tomorrow's bridges. In B. Henry, C. Arndt, M. DiVincenti and A. Marriner-Tomey (Eds.), *Dimensions of nursing administration: Theory, research, education, practice*. Boston: Blackwell Scientific Publications.

Rogers, M.E. (1989) Creating a climate for the implementation of a nursing conceptual framework. *Journal of Continuing Education in Nursing*, 20(3), 112–116.

Scherer, P. (1988) Hospitals that attract (and keep) nurses. *American Journal of Nursing*, 88(1), 34–40.

Schmieding, N.J. (1988) Action process of nurse administrators to problematic situations based on Orlando's theory. *Journal of Advanced Nursing*, 13(1), 99–107.

Verran, J.A. and Reid, P.J. (1987) Replicated testing of the nursing technology model. *Nursing Research*, 36(3), 190–194.

Wewers, M.E. and Lenz, E.R. (1987) Relapse among ex-smokers: An example of theory derivation. *Advances in Nursing Science*, 9(2), 44–53.

12. Theory Analysis and Critique: Factors Affecting the Acceptance of Scientific Theories

Ashley, J.A. (1978) Foundations for scholarship: Historical research in nursing. *Advances in Nursing Science*, 1, 25–36.

Buchanan, B. (1987) Conceptual models: An assessment framework. *Journal of Nursing Administration*, 17(10), 22–26.

Chafetz, J.S. (1979) *A primer on the construction and testing of theories in sociology*. Itasca, IL: F.E. Peacock. (Especially note Chapter 8).

Chinn, P.L. and Jacobs, M.K. (1987) *Theory and nursing: A systematic approach*. St. Louis: C.V. Mosby.

Chinn, P.L. and Jacobs, M.K. (1983) The evaluation of theory. In *Theory and nursing: A systematic approach*. St. Louis: C.V. Mosby.

Dewey, J. (1958) *Experience and nature*, rev'd ed. New York: Dover Publications.

Dubos, R. (1963) *The cultural roots and social fruits of science*. Eugene: University of Oregon Books.

Duffey, M. and Muhlenkamp, A.F. (1974) A framework for theory analysis. *Nursing Outlook*, 22(9), 570–574.

Edwards, P. (Ed. in Chief). (1967) Pragmatic theory of truth: Pragmatism. *The encyclopedia of philosophy* (Vol. 6) New York: Macmillan and Free Press.

*Ellis, R. (1968) Characteristics of significant theories. *Nursing Research*, 17(3), 217–222.

*Fawcett, J. (1980) A framework for analysis and evaluation of conceptual models of nursing. *Nurse Educator*, 5(6), 10–14.

Fawcett, J. (1989) *Analysis and evaluation of conceptual models of nursing* (2nd ed.). Philadelphia: F.A. Davis.

Fitzpatrick, J. and Whall, A. (1989) *Conceptual models of nursing: Analysis and application* (2nd ed.). Bowie, MD: Robert J. Brady Co.

Frank, P.G. (1954) The variety of reasons for the acceptance of scientific theories. *The Scientific Monthly*, 79(3), 139–145.

Frank, P.G. (1956) The variety of reasons for the acceptance of scientific theories. In P.G. Frank (Ed.), *The validation of scientific theories*. Boston: Beacon Press.

Hunk, M. (1981, November 16) Taking it: The scandal that rocked science. *This World, San Francisco Chronicle*, 16–19, 21.

Jacobs, M.K. (1986) Can nursing theory be tested? In P.L. Chinn (Ed.), *Nursing research methodology: Issues and implementation* (Chapter 4, pp. 39–54). Rockville, MD: Aspen Systems.

Jacobson, S.F. (1987) Studying and using conceptual models of nursing. *Image: Journal of Nursing Scholarship*, 19(2), 78–82.

Kaplan, A. (1964) *The conduct of inquiry: Methodology of behavioral science.* San Francisco: Chandler.

Kuhn, T. (1977) *The essential tension: Selected studies in scientific tradition and change.* Chicago: University of Chicago Press. (Especially note Chapter 13).

Laudan, L. (1977) *Progress and its problems: Toward a theory of scientific growth.* Berkeley: University of California Press.

Meleis, A.I. (1983) A model for theory description, analysis, and critique. In N.L. Chaska (Ed.), *The nursing profession: A time to speak.* New York: McGraw-Hill.

Moore, B. (1954) Influence of political creeds on the acceptance of theories. *The Scientific Monthly*, 79(3), 146–148.

Parse, R.R. (1987) *Nursing science: Major paradigms, theories, and critiques.* Philadelphia: W.B. Saunders.

Reynolds, P.D. (1971) *A primer in theory construction.* Indianapolis: Bobbs-Merrill.

Riehl, Sisca, J.P. (1989) *Conceptual models for nursing practice* (3rd ed.). Norwalk, CT: Appleton & Lange.

Rudner, R. (1954) Remarks on value judgements in scientific validation. *The Scientific Monthly*, 79(3), 1951–1953.

Schrag, C. (1967) Elements of theoretical analysis in sociology. In L. Gross (Ed.), *Sociological theory: Inquiries and paradigms.* New York: Harper & Row.

Silva, M.C. (1986) Research testing nursing theory: State of the art. *Advances in Nursing Science*, 9(1), 1–11.

Silva, M.C. (in press). Testing of nursing theory: Four perspectives on meaning. *Proceedings of National League for Nursing's First National Conference on Measurement and Evaluation.* National League for Nursing.

Stevens, B.J. (1984) Criteria for evaluating theories. In *Nursing theory: Analysis, application, evaluation* (2nd ed.). Boston: Little, Brown & Co.

Torres, G. (1986) *Theoretical foundations of nursing.* Norwalk, CT: Appleton-Century-Crofts.

Watson, J. (1981, July) Nursing's scientific quest. *Nursing Outlook*, 29(7), 413–416.

Webster, G., Jacox, A., and Baldwin, B. (1981) Nursing theory and the ghost of the received view. In M. Grace and N. McCloskey (Eds.), *Current issues in nursing.* Scranton, PA: Blackwell Scientific Publications.

Winstead-Fry, P. (Ed.) (1986) *Case studies in nursing theory.* New York: National League for Nursing.

Zetterberg, H.L. (1965) *On theory verification in sociology* (3rd ed.). New York: Bedminister Press.

13. Nursing Theory and Theorists

Abdellah

Abdellah, F.G. (1969) The nature of nursing science. *Nursing Research*, 18, 390–393.

*Abdellah, F.G. (1970) Overview of nursing research 1955–1968, Part 1. *Nursing Research*, 19, 6–17.

Abdellah, F.G. (1970) Overview of nursing research 1955–1968, Part 2. *Nursing Research*, 19, 151–162.

Abdellah, F.G. (1970) Overview of nursing research 1955–1968, Part 3. *Nursing Research*, 19, 239–252.

Abdellah, F.G. (1971) Evolution of nursing as a profession: Perspective on manpower development. *International Nursing Review*, 19, 119–235.

Abdellah, F.G. (1972) The physician-nurse team approach to coronary care. *Nursing Clinics of North America*, 7, 423–430.

Abdellah, F.G. (1976) Nurse practitioners and nursing practice. *American Journal of Public Health*, 66, 245–246.

Abdellah, F.G. (1976) Nursing's role in future health care. *AORN Journal*, 24(2), 236–240.

Abdellah, F.G. (1978) Long term care policy issues. *Annals of the American Academy of Political and Social Science*, 438, 22.

Abdellah, F.G. (1981) Nursing care of the aged in the United States of America. *Journal of Gerontological Nursing*, 7(11), 657–663.

Abdellah, F.G. (1982) The nurse practitioner 17 years later: Present and emerging issues. *Inquiry*, 19, 105–116.

Abdellah, F.G., Beland, I.L., Martin, A., and Matheney, R.V. (1973) *New directions in patient centered nursing: Guidelines for systems of service, education and research.* New York: Macmillan.

Abdellah, F.G., Foerst, H.V., and Chow, R.K. (1979) PACE: An approach to improving care to the elderly. *American Journal of Nursing*, 79, 1109–1110.

Abdellah, F.G. and Levine, R. (1957) Developing a measure of patient and personnel satisfaction with nursing care. *Nursing Research*, 5, 100–108.

Abdellah, F.G. and Levine, R. (1965) Aims of nursing research. *Nursing Research*, 14, 31.

Abdellah, F.G. and Levine, R. (1965) *Better patient care through nursing research.* New York: Macmillan.

Abdellah, F.G. and Levine, R. (1979) *Better patient care through nursing research* (2nd ed.). New York: Macmillan.

Alward, R.R. (1983) Patient classification systems: The ideal vs. reality. *Journal of Nursing Administration*, 13(2), 14–19.

Bergman, R., Stockler, R.A., Shavit, N., Sharon, R., Feinberg, D., and Danon, A. (1981) Role, selection and preparation of head nurses—I. *International Journal of Nursing Studies*, 18(2), 123–152.

Bergman, R., Stockler, R.A., Shavit, N., Sharon, R., Feinberg, D., and Danon, A. (1981) Role, selection and preparation of head nurses—III. *International Journal of Nursing Studies*, 18(4), 237–250.

Chow, R. (1969) Postoperative cardiac nursing research: A method for identifying and categorizing nursing action. *Nursing Research*, 18(1), 4–13.

Copp, L.A. (1973) Professional change: Which trends do nurses endorse? *International Journal of Nursing Studies*, 10, 55–63.

Cornell, S.A. (1974) Development of an instrument for measuring quality of nursing care. *Nursing Research*, 23, 108–117.

Craig, S.L. (1980) Theory development and its relevance for nursing. *Journal of Advanced Nursing*, 5, 349–355.

Dickoff, J. and James, P. (1970) Beliefs and values: Bases for curriculum design. *Nursing Research*, 19, 415–427.

Downs, F.S. and Fitzpatrick, J.J. (1976) Preliminary investigation of the reliability and validity of a tool for the assessment of body position and motor activity. *Nursing Research*, 25, 404–408.

Dycus, D., Schmeiser, D., Taggart, F. and Yancey, R. (1989) Faye Glenn Abdellah: Twenty-one nursing problems. In A. Marriner-Tomey, *Nursing theorists and their work* (2nd ed.). St. Louis: C.V. Mosby.

Elms, R.R. (1972) Recovery room behavior and post-operative convalescence. *Nursing Research*, 21, 390–397.

Fortinsky, R.H., Granger, C.V. and Seltzer, G.B. (1981) The use of functional assessment in understanding home care needs. *Medical Care*, 19(5), 489–497.

Goodwin, J.O. and Edwards, B.S. (1975) Developing a computer program to assist the nursing process: Phase I—From systems analysis to an expandable program. *Nursing Research*, 24, 299–305.

Gordon, M. (1980) Determining study topics. *Nursing Research*, 29, 83–87.

Gordon, M. and Sweeney, M.A. (1979) Methodological problems and issues in identifying and standardizing nursing diagnosis. *Advances in Nursing Science*, 2(1), 1–15.

Greaves, F. (1980) Objectively toward curriculum improvement in nursing education in England and Wales. *Journal of Advanced Nursing*, 5, 591–599.

Green, J.A. (1979) Science, nursing, and nursing science: A conceptual analysis. *Advances in Nursing Science*, 2(1), 57–64.

Grier, M.R. and Schnitzler, C.P. (1979) Nurses' propensity to risk. *Nursing Research*, 28(3), 186–190.

Hardy, L.K. (1982) Nursing models and research—a restricting view? *Journal of Advanced Nursing*, 7, 447–451.

Jennings, C.P. and Jennings, T.F. (1977) Containing costs through prospective reimbursement. *American Journal of Nursing*, 77, 1155–1159.

Jones, P.E. (1979) A terminology for nursing diagnosis. *Advances in Nursing Science*, 2(1), 65–72.

King, I.M. (1968) A conceptual frame of reference for nursing. *Nursing Research*, 17, 27–31.

Lanara, V.A. (1976) Philosophy of nursing and current nursing problems. *International Nursing Review*, 23(2), 48–54.

Leke, J.T. (1978) Nigerian patients' perception of their nursing care needs. *Journal of Advanced Nursing*, 3, 181–187.

Majesky, S.J., Brester, M.H., and Nishio, K.T. (1978) Development of a research tool: Patient indicators of nursing care. *Nursing Research*, 27, 365–371.

McGilloway, F.A. (1980) The nursing process: A problem solving approach to patient care. *International Nursing Studies*, 17(2), 79–90.

McLane, A.M. (1978) Core competencies of masters-prepared nurses. *Nursing Research*, 27(1), 43–58.

Minckley, B.B. (1974) Physiological and psychological responses of elective surgical patients. *Nursing Research*, 23(5), 392–401.

Price, M.R. (1980) Nursing diagnosis: Making a concept come alive. *American Journal of Nursing*, 80(4), 668–671.

Rubenstein, L.Z. (1981) Specialized geriatric assessment units and their clinical implications. *Western Journal of Medicine*, 135(6), 497–502.

See, E.M. (1989) Abdellah's model for nursing: Twenty-one nursing problems. In J. Fitzpatrick and A. Whall, *Conceptual models of nursing: Analysis and application* (2nd ed.). Norwalk, CT: Appleton & Lange.

Stevens, B.J. (1971) Analysis of structural forms used in nursing curricula. *Nursing Research*, 20(5), 388–397.

Walker, C. and Deuble, H. (1968) A schema for analysis of accident prevention activities in public health nurses' records. *Nursing Research*, 17(5), 408–414.

Walker, L.O. (1971) Toward a clearer understanding of the concept of nursing theory. *Nursing Research*, 20(5), 428–435.

Hadley

Hadley, B.J. (1967, April) The dynamic interactionist concept of role. *Journal of Nursing Education*, 6(2), 5–10, 24–25.

Hadley, B.J. (1969) Evolution of a conception of nursing. *Nursing Research*, 18(5), 400–406.

Hall

Artinian, B.M. (1983) Implementation of the intersystem patient-care model in clinical practice. *Journal of Advanced Nursing*, 8, 117–124.

Hall, B.A. (1975) Mutual withdrawal: The nonparticipant in a therapeutic community. *Perspectives in Psychiatric Care*, 14(2), 75–77.

Hall, B.A. (1975) Socializing patients into the psychiatric sick role. *Perspectives in Psychiatric Care*, 13, 123–129.

Hall, B.A. (1977) The effect of interpersonal attraction on the therapeutic relationship: A review and suggestion for further study. *Journal of Psychiatric Nursing*, 15(9), 18–23.

Hall, B.A. (1977) Occupational values and family perspectives: A comparison of pre-nursing and pre-medical women. *Communicating Nursing Research*, 8, 124–132.

*Hall, B.A. (1981) The change paradigm in nursing: Growth versus persistence. *Advances in Nursing Science*, 3(4), 1–6.

Hall, B.A., McKay, R.P., and Mitsunaga, B.K. (1971) Dimensions of role commitment: Career patterns of deans of nursing. *Communicating Nursing Research*, 4, 84–98.

Hall, B.A. and Mitsunaga, B.K. (1979) Education of the nurse to promote interpersonal attraction. *Journal of Nursing Education*, 18(5), 16–21.

Hall, B.A., Mitsunaga, B.K., and DeTornyay, R. (1981) Deans of nursing: Changing socialization patterns. *Nursing Outlook*, 29, 92–95.

Hall, B.A., von Endt, B., and Parker, G. (1981) A framework for measuring satisfaction of nursing staff. *Nursing Leadership*, 4(4), 29–33.

Mitsunaga, B.K. and Hall, B.A. (1979) Interpersonal attraction and perceived quality of medical–surgical care. *Western Journal of Nursing Research*, 1(1), 5–26.

*Murphy, S.A. and Hoeffer, B. (1983) Role of the specialties in nursing science. *Advances in Nursing Science*, 5(4), 31–39.

Harms and McDonald

Bailey, J.T., McDonald, F.J., and Harms, M.T. (1966) A new approach to curriculum development. *Nursing Outlook*, 14(7), 33–36.

Harms, M.T. and McDonald, F.J. (1966) A new curriculum design, Part III. *Nursing Outlook*, 14(9), 50–53.

Harms, M.T. and McDonald, F.J. (1966) The teaching-learning process, Part IV. *Nursing Outlook*, 14(10), 54–58.

McDonald, F.J. and Harms, M.T. (1966) A theoretical model for an experimental curriculum, Part II. *Nursing Outlook*, 14(8), 48–51.

Henderson

DeMeester, D., Lauer, T., Neal, S., and Williams, S. (1989) Virginia Henderson: Definition of nursing. In A. Marriner-Tomey, *Nursing theorists and their work* (2nd ed.). St. Louis: C.V. Mosby.

Furukawa, C.Y. and Howe, J.K. (1980) Virginia Henderson. In the nursing theories conference group. *Nursing theories: The base for professional nursing practice*. Englewood Cliffs, NJ: Prentice-Hall.

Henderson, V. (1964) The nature of nursing. *American Journal of Nursing*, 64(8), 62–68.

Henderson, V. (1966) *The nature of nursing*. New York: Macmillan.

Henderson, V. (1969) Excellence in nursing. *American Journal of Nursing*, 69(9), 2133–2137.

Henderson, V. (1978) The concept of nursing. *Journal of Advanced Nursing*, 3, 113–130.

Henderson, V. (1980) Preserving the essence of nursing in a technological age. *Journal of Advanced Nursing*, 5, 245–260.

Runk, J.A. and Quillin, S.I.M. (1989) Henderson's definition of nursing. In J.J. Fitzpatrick and A.L. Whall, *Conceptual models of nursing: Analysis and application* (2nd ed.). Bowie, MD: Robert J. Brady Co.

Howland

Howland, D. (1963, Summer) Approaches to the systems problem, Part I. *Nursing Research*, 13, 172–174.

Howland, D. (1963, Fall) A hospital system model, Part II. *Nursing Research*, 12(4), 232–236.

Howland, D. (1966) Approach to nurse-monitor research. *American Journal of Nursing*, 66(3), 566–588.

Howland, D. and McDowell, W.E. (1964, Winter) The measurement of patient care: A conceptual framework. *Nursing Research*, 13(1), 4–7.

Johnson

Adam, E. (1987) Nursing theory: What it is and what it is not. *Nursing Papers/Perspectives on Nursing*, 19(1), 5–14.

†Auger, J.R. and Dee, V. (1983) A patient classification system based on the behavioral system model of nursing: Part 1. *Journal of Nursing Administration*, 13, 38–43.

Auger, J.R. (1976) *Behavioral systems and nursing*. Englewood Cliffs, NJ: Prentice-Hall.

Botha, M.E. (1989) Theory development in perspective: The role of conceptual frameworks and models in theory development. *Journal of Advanced Nursing*, 14(1), 49–55.

†Broncatello, K.F. (1980) Auger in action: Application of the model. *Advances in Nursing Science*, 2(2), 13–23.

Clough, D.H. and Derdiarian, A. (1980, Jan.–Feb.) A behavioral checklist to measure dependence and independence. *Nursing Research*, 29(1), 55–58.

Conner, S., Magers, J. and Watt, J. (1989) Dorothy E. Johnson: Behavioral system model. In A. Marriner-Tomey, *Nursing theorists and their work* (2nd ed.). St. Louis: C.V. Mosby.

Damus, K. (1980) An application of the Johnson behavioral system model for nursing practice. In J.P. Riehl and C. Roy (Eds.), *Conceptual models for nursing practice*. New York: Appleton-Century-Crofts.

†Dee, V. and Auger, J.R. (1983) A patient classification system based on the behavioral system model of nursing: Part 2. *Journal of Nursing Administration*, 13, 18–23.

Derdiarian, A.K. (1981) Nursing conceptual frameworks: Implications for education, practice, and research. In *Concepts of oncology nursing*. Englewood Cliffs, NJ: Prentice-Hall.

†Derdiarian, A.K. (1983) An instrument for theory and research development using the behavioral systems model for nursing: The cancer patient. Part I. *Nursing Research*, 32(4), 196–201.

Derdiarian, A.K. and Clough, D. (1980) A behavioral checklist to measure dependence and independence. *Nursing Research*, 28, 55–58.

†Derdiarian, A. and Forsythe, A.B. (1983) An instrument for theory and research development using the behavioral systems model for nursing: The cancer patient. Part II. *Nursing Research*, 32(4), 260–267.

Fawcett, J. (1989) Johnson's behavioral system model. In *Analysis and evaluation of conceptual models of nursing* (2nd ed.). Philadelphia: F.A. Davis.

Fruehwirth, S. (1989) An application of Johnson's behavioral model: A case study. *Journal of Community Health Nursing*, 6(2), 61–71.

†Grubbs, J. (1980) An interpretation of the Johnson behavioral system model for nursing practice. In J.P. Riehl and C. Roy (Eds.), *Conceptual models for nursing practice*. New York: Appleton-Century-Crofts.

Holaday, B. (1974) Achievement behavior in chronically ill children. *Nursing Research*, 23, 25–30.

†Holaday, B. (1980) Implementing the Johnson model for nursing practice. In J.P. Riehl and C. Roy (Eds.), *Conceptual models for nursing practice* (2nd ed.). New York: Appleton-Century-Crofts.

Holaday, B. (1981) The Johnson behavioral system model for nursing and the pursuit of quality health care. In G.E. Lasker (Ed.), *Applied systems and cybernetics* (Vol. 4) New York: Pergamon Press.

Holaday, B. (1981) Maternal response to their chronically ill infants' attachment behavior of crying. *Nursing Research*, 30(6), 343–347.

Holaday, B. (1982) Maternal conceptual set development: Identifying patterns of maternal response to chronically ill infant crying. *Maternal-Child Nursing Journal*, 11(1), 47–58.

Holaday, B. (1987) Patterns of interaction between mothers and their chronically ill infants. *Maternal-Child Nursing Journal*, 16, 29–45.

*Johnson, D.E. (1959) The nature of a science of nursing. *Nursing Outlook*, 7(5), 291–294.

†Johnson, D.E. (1959) A philosophy of nursing. *Nursing Outlook*, 7(4), 198–200.

†Johnson, D.E. (1961) The significance of nursing care. *Nursing Outlook*, 61(11), 63–66.

Johnson, D.E. (1964, June) Is there an identifiable body of knowledge essential to the development of a generic professional nursing program? Paper presented at First Interuniversity Faculty Work Conference Nursing Council, NEBHE, Stowe, VT.

Johnson, D.E. (1968, April) One conceptual model of nursing. Paper presented at Vanderbilt University, Nashville, TN.

*Johnson, D.E. (1968) Theory in nursing: Borrowed or unique. *Nursing Research*, 17(3), 206–209.

Johnson, D.E. (1974) Development of theory: A requisite for nursing as a primary health profession. *Nursing Research*, 23(5), 372–377.

†Johnson, D.E. (1980) The behavioral system model for nursing. In J.P. Riehl and C. Roy (Eds.), *Conceptual models for nursing practice* (2nd ed.). New York: Appleton-Century-Crofts.

Johnson, D.E. (1987) Evaluating conceptual models for use in critical care nursing practice. *Dimensions of Critical Care Nursing*, 6(4), 195–197.

Johnson, D.E. (1989) Some thoughts on nursing. *Clinical Nurse Specialist*, 3(1), 1–4.

†Lovejoy, N.C. (1983) The leukemic child's perceptions of family behaviors. *Oncology Nursing Forum*, 10(4), 20–25.

Lovejoy, N.C. (1983) The leukemic child's perceptions of family behaviors. *Oncology Nursing*. Presented at Vanderbilt University, Nashville, TN.

Loveland-Cherry, C. and Wilkerson, S.A. (1989) Dorothy Johnson's behavioral system model. In J.J. Fitzpatrick and A.L. Whall, *Conceptual methods of nursing: Analysis to application* (2nd ed.). Bowie, MD: Robert J. Brady Co.

Majesky, S.J., Brester, M.H., and Nishio, K.T. (1978) Development of a research tool: Patient indicators of nursing care. *Nursing Research*, 27, 365–371.

McCauley, K., Choromanski, J., and Liu, K. (1984) Learning to live with controlled ventricular tachycardia: Utilizing the Johnson model. *Heart and Lung*, 13(6), 633–638.

†Porter, L.S. (1972) The impact of physical-physiological activity on infants' growth and development. *Nursing Research*, 21(3), 210–219.

†Rawls, A.C. (1980) Evaluation of the Johnson behavioral model in clinical practice. Report of a test and evaluation of the Johnson theory. *Image*, 12, 13–16.

Roy, C. (1980) A case study viewed according to different models. In J.P. Riehl and C. Roy (Eds.), *Conceptual models for nursing practice*. New York: Appleton-Century-Crofts.

†Small, B. (1980) Nursing visually impaired children with Johnson's model as a conceptual framework. In J.P. Riehl and C. Roy (Eds.),*Conceptual models for nursing practice* (2nd ed.). New York: Appleton-Century-Crofts.

Wilkie, D.J., Lovejoy, N., Dodd, M., and Tesler, M. (1988) Cancer pain control behaviors: Description and correlation with pain intensity. *Oncology Nursing Forum*, 15(6), 723–731.

Wilkie, D.J., Lovejoy, N., Dodd, M., and Tesler, M. (1989) Pain control behaviors of patients with cancer. In S.G. Funk, E.M. Tornquist, M.T. Champagne, L.A. Copp, and R.A. Wiese (Eds.), *Key aspects of comfort: Management of pain, fatigue, and nausea*. New York: Springer-Verlag.

Wu, R. (1973) *Behavior and illness*. Englewood Cliffs, NJ: Prentice-Hall.

King

Ackermann, M., Brink, S., Clanton, J., Jones, C., Moody, S., Perlich, G., Price, D., and Prusinski, B. (1989) Imogene King: Theory of goal attainment. In A. Marriner-Tomey, *Nursing theorists and their work* (2nd ed.). St. Louis: C.V. Mosby.

Asay, M.K. and Osler, C.C. (Eds.) (1984) Conceptual models of nursing. Applications in community health nursing. Proceedings of the Eighth Annual Community Health Nursing Conference. Chapel Hill, NC: Department of Public Health Nursing, School of Public Health, University of North Carolina.

Austin, J.K. and Champion, V.L. (1983) King's theory for nursing: Explication and evaluation. In P. Chinn (Ed.), *Advances in nursing theory development* (pp. 49–61). Rockville, MD: Aspen Systems.

Brower, H.T. (1981) Social organization and nurses' attitudes toward older persons. *Journal of Gerontological Nursing*, 7, 293–298.

Brown, S.T. and Lee, B.T. (1980) Imogene King's conceptual framework: A proposed model for continuing nursing education. *Journal of Advanced Nursing*, 5(5), 467–473.

Bunting, S.M. (1988) The concept of perception in selected nursing theories. *Nursing Science Quarterly*, 1(4), 168–174.

Daubenmire, M.J. and King, I.M. (1973) Nursing process models: A systems approach. *Nursing Outlook*, 21(8), 512–517.

Daubenmire, M.J. (1989) A baccalaureate nursing curriculum based on King's conceptual framework. In J. Riehl-Sisca, *Conceptual models for nursing practice* (3rd ed.). Norwalk, CT: Appleton & Lange.

DiNardo, P.B. (1989) Evaluation of the nursing theory of Imogene M. King. In J. Riehl-Sisca, *Conceptual models for nursing practice* (3rd ed.). Norwalk, CT: Appleton & Lange.

Elberson, K. (1989) Applying King's model to nursing administration. In B. Henry, C. Arndt, M. DiVincenti, and A. Marriner-Tomey (Eds.), *Dimensions of nursing administration: Theory, research, education, practice*. Boston: Blackwell Scientific Publications.

Fawcett, J. (1989) King's interacting systems framework. In *Analysis and evaluation of conceptual models of nursing* (2nd ed.). Philadelphia: F.A. Davis.

Frey, M.A. (1989) Social support and health: A theoretical formulation derived from King's conceptual framework. *Nursing Science Quarterly*, 138–148.

Friedmann, M.L. (1989) The concept of family nursing. *Journal of Advanced Nursing*, 14, 211–216.

George, J.B. (1980) Imogene King. In The Nursing Theories Conference Group, *Nursing theories: The base for professional nursing practice*. Englewood Cliffs, NJ: Prentice-Hall.

Gonot, P.J. (1983) Imogene M. King: A theory for nursing. In J.J. Fitzpatrick and A.L. Whall (Eds.), *Conceptual models of nursing: Analysis and application*. Bowie, MD: Robert J. Brady Co.

Gonot, P.J. (1986) Family therapy as derived from King's conceptual model. In A.L. Whall, *Family therapy theory for nursing. Four approaches*. Norwalk, CT: Appleton-Century-Crofts.

Gonot, P.J. (1989) Imogene M. King's conceptual framework of nursing. In J.J. Fitzpatrick and A.L. Whall, *Conceptual models of nursing: Analysis and application* (2nd ed.). Bowie, MD: Robert J. Brady Co.

Gulitz, E.A. and King, I.M. (1988) King's general systems model: Application to curriculum development. *Nursing Science Quarterly*, 1(3), 128–132.

Hanucharurnkul, S. (1989) Comparative analysis of Orem's and King's theories. *Journal of Advanced Nursing*, 14, 365–372.

Husband, A. (1988) Application of King's theory of nursing to the care of the adult with diabetes. *Journal of Advanced Nursing*, 13(4), 484–488.

King, I.M. (1964, October) Nursing theory: Problems and prospects. *Nursing Science*, 2, 394–403.

King, I.M. (1968) A conceptual frame of reference for nursing. *Nursing Research*, 17(1), 27–31.

King, I.M. (1971) *Toward a theory for nursing: General concepts of human behavior*. New York: John Wiley & Sons.

King, I.M. (1975) A process for developing concepts for nursing through research. In P.J. Verhonick (Ed.), *Nursing Research* (Vol. 1). Boston: Little, Brown & Co.

King, I.M. (1976) The health care system: Nursing intervention subsystem. In W.H. Werley et al. (Eds.), *Health research: The systems approach*. New York: Springer-Verlag.

King, I.M. (1978) USA: Loyola University of Chicago School of Nursing. *Journal of Advanced Nursing*, 3, 390.

King, I.M. (1981) *A theory for nursing: Systems, concepts, process*. New York: John Wiley & Sons.

King, I.M. (1983) The family coping with a medical illness. Analysis and application of King's theory of goal attainment. In I.W. Clements and F.B. Roberts (Eds.), *Family health: A theoretical approach to nursing care*. New York: John Wiley & Sons.

King, I.M. (1983) King's theory of nursing. In I.W. Clements and F.B. Roberts (Eds.), *Family health: A theoretical approach to nursing*. New York: John Wiley & Sons.

King, I.M. (1984) Effectiveness of nursing care: Use of a goal oriented nursing record in end stage renal disease. *American Association of Nephrology Nurses and Technicians Journal*, 11(2), 11–17, 60.

King, I.M. (1984) Philosophy of nursing education: A national survey. *Western Journal of Nursing Research*, 6(4), 387–406.

King, I.M. (1986) King's theory of goal attainment. In P. Winstead-Fry (Ed.), *Case studies in nursing theory*. New York: National League for Nursing.

King, I.M. (1987) King's theory of goal attainment. In R.R. Parse, *Nursing science: Major paradigms, theories, and critiques*. Philadelphia: W.B. Saunders.

King, I.M. (1987) Translating research into practice. *Journal of Neuroscience Nursing*, 19(1), 44–48.

King, I.M. (1988) Concepts: Essential elements of theories. *Nursing Science Quarterly*, 1(1), 22–25.

King, I.M. (1989) King's systems framework and theory. In J. Riehl-Sisca, *Conceptual models for nursing practice* (3rd ed.). Norwalk, CT: Appleton & Lange.

King, I.M. (1989) King's systems framework for nursing administration. In B. Henry, C. Arndt, M. DiVincenti, and A. Marriner-Tomey (Eds.), *Dimensions of nursing administration: Theory, research, education, practice*. Boston: Blackwell Scientific Publications.

Magan, S. (1987) A critique of King's theory. In R.R. Parse, *Nursing science: Major paradigms, theories, and critiques*. Philadelphia: W.B. Saunders.

Rooke, L. and Norberg, A. (1988) Problematic and meaningful situations in nursing interpreted by concepts from King's nursing theory and four additional concepts. *Scandinavian Journal of Caring Sciences*, 2(2), 80–87.

Rosendahl, P.B. and Ross, V. (1982) Does your behavior affect your patient's response? *Journal of Gerontological Nursing*, 8, 572–575.

Smith, M. (1988) King's theory in practice. *Nursing Science Quarterly*, 1(4), 145–146.

Uys, L. (1987) Foundational studies in nursing. *Journal of Advanced Nursing*, 12(3), 275–280.

Levine

Bunting, S.M. (1988) The concept of perception in selected nursing theories. *Nursing Science Quarterly*, 1(4), 168–174.

†Esposito, C.H. and Leonard, M.K. (1980) Myra Estrin Levine. In The Nursing Theories Conference Group, *Nursing theories: The base for professional nursing practice* (pp. 150–163). Englewood Cliffs, NJ: Prentice-Hall.

Foli, K., Johnson, T., Marriner-Tomey, A., Poat, M., Poppa, L., Woeste, R., and Zoretich, S. (1989) Myra Estrin Levine: Four conservation principles. In A. Marriner-Tomey, *Nursing theorists and their work* (2nd ed.). St. Louis: C.V. Mosby.

Glass, J.L. (1989) Levine's theory of nursing: A critique. In J. Riehl-Sisca, *Conceptual models for nursing practice* (3rd ed.). Norwalk, CT: Appleton & Lange.

Fawcett, J. (1989) Levine's conservation model. In *Analysis and evaluation of conceptual models of nursing* (2nd ed.). Philadelphia: F.A. Davis.

†Hirschfeld, M.J. (1976) The cognitively impaired older adult. *American Journal of Nursing*, 76(12), 1981–1984.

†Levine, M. E. (1966) Adaptation and assessment: A rationale for nursing intervention. *American Journal of Nursing*, 66(11), 2450–2454.

Levine, M. (1966) Trophicognosis: An alternative to nursing diagnosis. In *Exploring progress in medical-surgical nursing practice* (pp. 55–70). New York: American Nurses' Association.

†Levine, M. (1967) The four conservation principles of nursing. *Nursing Forum*, 6(1), 45–59.

Levine, M. (1969) *Introduction to clinical nursing*. Philadelphia: F.A. Davis.

†Levine, M. (1969) The pursuit of wholeness. *American Journal of Nursing*, 69(1), 93–98.

†Levine, M.E. (1971) Holistic nursing. *Nursing Clinics of North America*, 6(2), 253–264.

†Levine, M.E. (1971, June) Time has come to speak of . . . health care. *AORN Journal*, 13, 37–43.

Levine, M.E. (1973) *Introduction to clinical nursing* (2nd ed.). Philadelphia: F.A. Davis.

Levine, M.E. (1977) Nursing ethics and the ethical nurse. *American Journal of Nursing*, 77(5), 845–849.

Levine, M.E. (1979) The science is spurious. *American Journal of Nursing*, 79(8), 1379–1383.

Levine, M.E. (1988) Antecedents from adjunctive disciplines: Creation of nursing theory. *Nursing Science Quarterly*, 1(1), 16–21.

Levine, M.E. (1988) Rationing health care (letter). *Nursing Outlook*, 36(6), 265.

Levine, M.E. (1989) Beyond dilemma. *Seminars in Oncology Nursing*, 5(2), 124–128.

Levine, M.E. (1989) The conservation principles: Twenty years later. In J. Riehl-Sisca, *Conceptual models for nursing practice* (3rd ed.). Norwalk, CT: Appleton & Lange.

Levine, M.E. (1989) The ethics of nursing rhetoric. *Image: Journal of Nursing Scholarship*, 21(1), 4–6.

Levine, M.E. (1989) Ethical issues in cancer care: Beyond dilemma. *Seminars in Oncology Nursing*, 5(2), 124–128.

Levine, M.E. (1989) The four conservation principles: Twenty years later. In J.P. Riehl-Sisca, *Conceptual models for nursing practice* (3rd ed.). Norwalk, CT: Appleton & Lange.

Levine, M.E. (1989) Ration or rescue: The elderly patient in critical care. *Critical Care Nursing Quarterly*, 12(1), 82–89.

Newport, M.A. (1984) Conserving thermal energy and social integrity in the newborn. *Western Journal of Nursing Research*, 6(2), 175–199.

Pieper, B.A. (1989) Levine's nursing model: The conservation principles. In J.J. Fitzpatrick and A.L. Whall, *Conceptual models of nursing: Analysis and application* (2nd ed.). Bowie, MD: Robert J. Brady Co.

Riehl, J.P. (1980) Nursing models in current use. In J.P. Riehl and C. Roy (Eds.), *Conceptual models for nursing practice* (2nd ed.). (pp. 393–398). New York: Appleton-Century-Crofts.

Taylor, J.W. (1974) Measuring the outcomes of nursing care. *Nursing Clinics of North America*, 9, 337–348.

Taylor, J.W. (1989) Levine's conservation principles: Using the model for nursing diagnosis in a neurological setting. In J. Riehl-Sisca, *Conceptual models for nursing practice* (3rd ed.). Norwalk, CT: Appleton & Lange.

Tompkins, E.S. (1980) Effect of restricted mobility and dominance on perceived duration. *Nursing Research*, 29(6), 333–338.

Meleis

Dagenais, F. and Meleis, A.I. (1982) Professionalism, work ethic, and empathy in nursing: The nurse self-description form. *Western Journal of Nursing Research*, 4(4), 407–422.

Dracup, K., Meleis, A.I., Baker, C., and Edlefsen, P. (1984) Family-focused cardiac rehabilitation: A role supplementation program for cardiac patients and spouses. *Nursing Clinics of North America*, 19, 112–124.

Mansell, D.M. and Porter-Chantemerle, K. (1979, March) Conceptualization and measurement of a role supplementation program: The effect of role supplementation on career success of neophyte nurses. *MINH undergraduate psychiatric nursing training and demonstration project*. Arizona State University, College of Nursing, Tempe, AZ.

Meleis, A.I. (1971) Self-concept and family planning. *Nursing Research*, 20, 229–236.

Meleis, A.I. (1974) Self-concept photographs: A research tool. *Videosociology*, 2(2), 46–62.

Meleis, A.I. (1975) Role insufficiency and role supplementation: A conceptual framework. *Nursing Research*, 24, 264–271.

Meleis, A.I. (1979) The graduate dilemma: The Kuwaiti experience. *International Journal of Nursing Studies*, 16, 337–343.

Meleis, A.I. and Burton, P. (1981) Educational innovations: A model. *International Journal of Nursing Studies*, 33–39.

Meleis, A.I. and Dagenais, F. (1981, May/June) Sex role identity and perception of professional self in graduates of three nursing programs. *Nursing Research*, 30, 162–167.

Meleis, A.I. and Swendsen, L. (1975) Role supplementation: An empirical test of nursing intervention. *Nursing Research*, 24, 264–271.

Meleis, A.I., Swendsen, L., and Jones, D. (1980) Preventive role supplementation: A grounded conceptual framework. In M.H. Miller and B. Flynn (Eds.), *Current perspectives in nursing: Social issues and trends* (Vol. 2). St. Louis: C.V. Mosby.

Swendsen, L., Meleis, A.I., and Jones, D. (1978) Role supplementation for new parents: A role mastery plan. *The American Journal of Maternal Child Nursing*, 3(2), 84–91.

Neuman

Beck, C.T. (1983) Parturients' temporal experiences during the phases of labor. *Western Journal of Nursing Research*, 5, 283–295.

Beddome, G. (1989) Application of the Neuman systems model to the assessment of community-as-client. In B. Neuman, *The Neuman systems model* (2nd ed.). Norwalk, CT: Appleton & Lange.

Beitler, B., Tkachuck, B., and Aamodt, D. (1980) The Neuman model applied to health, mental health and medical-surgical nursing. In J.P. Riehl and C. Roy (Eds.), *Conceptual models of nursing practice*. New York: Appleton-Century-Crofts.

Benedict, M.B. and Sproles, J.B. (1982) Application of the Neuman model to public health nursing practice. In B. Neuman, *The Neuman systems model. Application to nursing education and practice*. Norwalk, CT: Appleton-Century-Crofts.

Bertalanffy, L. (1968) *General system theory*. New York: George Braziller.

Bourbonnais, F.F. and Ross, M.M. (1985) The Neuman systems model in nursing. Course development and implementation. *Journal of Advanced Nursing*, 10(2), 117–123.

Breckenridge, D. (1989) Primary prevention as an intervention modality for the renal client. In B. Neuman, *The Neuman systems model* (2nd ed.). Norwalk, CT: Appleton & Lange.

Buchanan, B.F. (1987) Human environment interaction: A modification of the Neuman systems model for aggregates, families, and the community. *Public Health Nursing*, 4(1), 52–64.

Burke, M.E., Capers, C., O'Connell, R., Quinn, R., and Sinnott, M. (1989) Neuman-based nursing practice in a hospital setting. In B. Neuman, *The Neuman systems model* (2nd ed.). Norwalk, CT: Appleton & Lange.

Campbell, V. and Keller, K. (1989) The Betty Neuman health care systems model: An analysis. In J. Riehl-Sisca, *Conceptual models for nursing practice* (3rd ed.). Norwalk, CT: Appleton & Lange.

Capers, C.F. and Kelly, R. (1987) Neuman's nursing process: A model of holistic care. *Holistic Nursing Practice*, 1(3), 19–26.

Capers, C.F., O'Brien, C., Quinn, R., Kelly, R. and Fenerty, A. (1985) The Neuman systems model in practice. Planning phase. *Journal of Nursing Administration*, 15(5), 29–39.

Caplan, G. (1964) *Principles of preventive psychiatry*. New York: Basic Books.

Chardin, P.T. (1955) *The phenomena of man*. London: Collins.

Clark, J. (1982) Development of models and theories on the concept of nursing. *Journal of Advanced Nursing*, 7, 129–134.

Cornu, A. (1957) *The origins of Marxian thought*. Springfield, IL: Charles C. Thomas.

Craddock, R.B. and Stanhope, M.K. (1980) The Neuman health-care systems model: Recommended adaptation. In J.P. Riehl and C. Roy (Eds.), *Conceptual models of nursing practice*. New York: Appleton-Century-Crofts.

Deloughery, G.W., Gebbie, K.M., and Neuman, B.M. (1974) Teaching organizational concepts to nurses in community mental health. *Journal of Nursing Education*, 13, 8–14.

Deloughery, G.W., Neuman, B.M., and Gebbie, K.M. (1970) Change in problem-solving ability among nurses receiving mental health consultation. *Communicating Nursing Research*, 3(3), 41–53.

Drew, L., Craig, D., and Beynon, C. (1989) The Neuman systems model for community health administration and practice: Provinces of Manitoba and Ontario, Canada. In B. Neuman, *The Neuman systems model* (2nd ed.). Norwalk, CT: Appleton & Lange.

Dunn, S. and Trepanier, M. (1989) Application of the Neuman systems model to perinatal nursing. In B. Neuman, *The Neuman systems model* (2nd ed.). Norwalk, CT: Appleton & Lange.

Fawcett, J. (1984) Neuman's systems model. In *Analysis and evaluation of conceptual models of nursing*. Philadelphia: F.A. Davis.

Fawcett, J. (1989) Neuman's systems model. In J. Fawcett, *Analysis and evaluation of conceptual models of nursing* (2nd ed.). Philadelphia: F.A. Davis.

Field, P.A. (1987) The impact of nursing theory on the clinical decision making process. *Journal of Advanced Nursing*, 12(5), 563–571.

Flaskerud, J.H. and Halloran, E.J. (1980) Areas of agreement in nursing theory development. *Advances in Nursing Science*, 3(1), 1–7.

Gebbie, K.M., Deloughery, G.W., and Neuman, B.M. (1970) Levels of utilization: Nursing specialists in community mental health. *Journal of Psychiatric Nursing*, 8, 37–39.

Hamilton, P. (1983) Community nursing diagnosis. *Advances in Nursing Science*, 5(3), 21–36.

Harris, S., Hermiz, M., Meininger, M., and Steinkeler, S. (1989) Betty Neuman: Systems model. In A. Marriner-Tomey, *Nursing theorists and their work* (2nd ed.). St. Louis: C.V. Mosby.

Henderson, B. (1978) Nursing diagnosis: Theory and practice. *Advances in Nursing Science*, 1(1), 75–83.

Herrick, C.A. and Goodykoontz, L. (1989) Neuman's systems model for nursing practice as a conceptual framework for a family assessment. *Journal of Child and Adolescent Psychiatric and Mental Health*, 2(2), 61–67.

Hinton-Walker, P. and Raborn, M. (1989) Application of the Neuman model in nursing administration and practice. In B. Henry, C. Arndt, M. DiVincenti, and A. Marriner-Tomey (Eds.), *Dimensions of nursing administration: Theory, research, education, practice*. Boston: Blackwell Scientific Publications.

Johnson, M. (1983) Some aspects of the relation between theory and practice in nursing. *Journal of Advanced Nursing*, 8, 21–28.

Johnson, S.E. (1989) A picture is worth a thousand words: Helping students visualize a conceptual model. *Nurse Educator*, 14(3), 21–24.

Jones, P.S. (1978) An adaptation model for nursing practice. *American Journal of Nursing*, 78, 1900–1906.

Kelley, J., Sanders, N., and Pierce, J. (1989) A systems approach to the role of the nurse administrator. In B. Neuman, *The Neuman systems model* (2nd ed.). Norwalk, CT: Appleton & Lange.

Lancaster, D. and Whall, A. (1989) The Neuman systems model. In J.J. Fitzpatrick and A.L. Whall, *Conceptual models of nursing: Analysis and application* (2nd ed.). Norwalk, CT: Appleton & Lange.

Lebold, M. and Davis, L. (1980) A baccalaureate nursing curriculum based on the Neuman health-systems model. In J.P. Riehl and C. Roy (Eds.), *Conceptual models of nursing practice*. New York: Appleton-Century-Crofts.

Lillis, P. and Cora, V. (1989) A case study analysis using the Neuman nursing process format: An abstract. In B. Neuman, *The Neuman systems model* (2nd ed.). Norwalk, CT: Appleton & Lange.

Louis, M. (1989) An intervention to reduce anxiety levels for nurses working with long-term care clients using Neuman's model. In J. Riehl-Sisca, *Conceptual models for nursing practice* (3rd ed.). Norwalk, CT: Appleton & Lange.

Louis, M. and Koertvelyessy, A. (1989) The Neuman model in nursing research. In B. Neuman, *The Neuman systems model* (2nd ed.). Norwalk, CT: Appleton & Lange.

Lowry, L. and Jopp, M. (1989) An evaluation instrument for assessing an associate degree nursing curriculum based on the Neuman systems model. In J. Riehl-Sisca, *Conceptual models for nursing practice* (3rd ed.). Norwalk, CT: Appleton & Lange.

Mrkonich, D.E., Hessian, M., and Miller, M. (1989) A cooperative process in curriculum development using the Neuman health care systems model. In J. Riehl-Sisca, *Conceptual models for nursing practice* (3rd ed.). Norwalk, CT: Appleton & Lange.

Mrkonich, D., Miller, M., and Hessian, M. (1989) Cooperative baccalaureate education: The Minnesota intercollegiate nursing consortium. In B. Neuman, *The Neuman systems model* (2nd ed.). Norwalk, CT: Appleton & Lange.

Nelson, L., Hansen, M., and McCullagh, M. (1989) A new baccalaureate North Dakota-Minnesota nursing education consortium. In B. Neuman, *The Neuman systems model* (2nd ed.). Norwalk, CT: Appleton & Lange.

Neufeld, A. (1983) Curriculum revision: Making the process work. *Journal of Advanced Nursing*, 8, 213–220.

Neuman, B. (1974) The Betty Neuman health-care systems model: A total person approach to patient problems. In J.P. Riehl and C. Roy, *Conceptual models for nursing practice*. New York: Appleton-Century-Crofts.

Neuman, B.M. (1980) The Betty Neuman health care systems model: A total person approach to patient problems. In J.P. Riehl and C. Roy (Eds.), *Conceptual models of nursing practice*. New York: Appleton-Century-Crofts.

Neuman, B. (1982) *The Neuman systems model. Application to nursing education and practice*. Norwalk, CT: Appleton-Century-Crofts.

Neuman, B. (1989) In conclusion–in transition. In B. Neuman, *The Neuman systems model* (2nd ed.). Norwalk, CT: Appleton & Lange.

Neuman, B. (1989) The Neuman systems model. In B. Neuman, *The Neuman systems model* (2nd ed.). Norwalk, CT: Appleton & Lange.

Neuman, B. (1989) The Neuman nursing process format: Family case study. In J. Riehl-Sisca, *Conceptual models for nursing practice* (3rd ed.). Norwalk, CT: Appleton & Lange.

Neuman, B.M. and Wyatt, M. (1980) The Neuman stress/adaptation systems approach to education for nurse administrators. In J.P. Riehl and C. Roy (Eds.), *Conceptual models of nursing practice*. New York: Appleton-Century-Crofts.

Neuman, B.M. and Wyatt, M. (1981) Prospects for change: Some evaluative reflections from one articulated baccalaureate program. *Journal of Nursing Education*, 20(1), 40–46.

Neuman, B.M. and Young, R.J. (1972) A model for teaching a total person approach to patient problems. *Nursing Research*, 21, 264–269.

Putt, A. (1972) Entropy, evolution and equifinality in nursing. In J. Smith (Ed.), *Five years of cooperation to improve curricula in Western schools of nursing*. Boulder, CO: Western Interstate Commission for Higher Education.

Reed, K. (1989) Family theory related to the Neuman systems model. In B. Neuman, *The Neuman systems model* (2nd ed.). Norwalk, CT: Appleton & Lange.

Ross, M. and Bourbonnais, F. (1985) The Betty Neuman systems model in nursing practice: A nursing study approach. *Journal of Advanced Nursing*, 10(3), 199–207.

Ross, M., Bourbonnais, F., and Carroll, G. (1987) Curricular design and the Betty Neuman systems model: A new approach to learning. *International Nursing Review*, 34(3), 75–79.

Selye, H. (1950) *The physiology and pathology of exposure to stress.* Montreal: Acta.

Sipple, J. and Freese, B. (1989) Transition from technical to professional-level nursing education. In B. Neuman, *The Neuman systems model* (2nd ed.). Norwalk, CT: Appleton & Lange.

Smith, M.C. (1989) Neuman's model in practice. *Nursing Science Quarterly,* 2(3), 116–117.

Sohier, R. (1989) Nursing care for the people of a small planet: Culture and the Neuman systems model. In B. Neuman, *The Neuman systems model* (2nd ed.). Norwalk, CT: Appleton & Lange.

Stevens, B. (1984) *Nursing theory. Analysis, application, evaluation* (2nd ed.). Boston: Little, Brown & Co.

Story, E.L. and Ross, M.M. (1986) Family centered community health nursing and the Betty Neuman systems model. *Nursing Papers,* 18(2), 77–88.

Sullivan, J. (1986) Using Neuman's model in the acute phase of spinal cord injury. *Focus on Critical Care,* 13(5), 34–41.

Trepanier, M.J. (1989) Application of the Neuman systems model to perinatal nursing. In B. Neuman, *The Neuman systems model* (2nd ed.). Norwalk, CT: Appleton & Lange.

Venable, J.F. (1980) The Neuman health-care systems model: An analysis. In J.P. Riehl and C. Roy (Eds.), *Conceptual models of nursing practice.* New York: Appleton-Century-Crofts.

Whall, A.L. (1983) The Betty Neuman health care system model. In J.J. Fitzpatrick and A.L. Whall (Eds.), *Conceptual models of nursing: Analysis and application.* Bowie, MD: Robert J. Brady Co.

Ziemer, M.M. (1983) Effects of information on postsurgical coping. *Nursing Research,* 32, 282–287.

Newman

Engle, V. (1989) Newman's model of health. In J.J. Fitzpatrick and A.L. Whall, *Conceptual models of nursing: Analysis and application* (2nd ed.). Norwalk, CT: Appleton & Lange.

Field, L. and Newman, M. (1982) Clinical application of the unitary man framework: Case study analysis. In M.J. Kim and D.A. Moritz (Eds.), *Classification of nursing diagnosis* (pp. 249–263). New York: McGraw-Hill.

Hall, B. (1980, Sept.–Oct.) Book review of *Theory Development in Nursing* by Margaret Newman. *Nursing Research,* 29(5), 311.

Hensley, D., Keffer, M., Kilgore-Keever, K., Langfitt, J., and Peterson, L. (1989) Margaret A. Newman: Model of health. In A. Marriner-Tomey, *Nursing theorists and their work* (2nd ed.). St. Louis: C.V. Mosby.

Newman, M.A. (1972) Time estimation in relation to gait tempo. *Perceptual Motor Skills,* 34, 359–366.

Newman, M.A. (1972) Nursing's theoretical evolution. *Nursing Outlook,* 20, 449–453.

Newman, M.A. (1976) Movement tempo and the experience of time. *Nursing Research,* 25(4), 273–279.

Newman, M.A. (1979) *Theory development in nursing.* Philadelphia: F.A. Davis.

Newman, M.A. (1981) The meaning of health. In G.E. Lasker (Ed.), *Applied systems research and cybernetics: Vol. 4. Systems research in health care, biocybernetics and ecology* (pp. 1739–1743). New York: Pergamon.

Newman, M.A. (1982) Thoughts on Bohm's concept of implicate order and its meaning for nursing science. Presented at the Nursing Theory Think Tank, Dallas, TX.

Newman, M.A. (1982) Time as an index of consciousness with age. *Nursing Research,* 31, 290–293.

Newman, M.A. (1982) What differentiates clinical research? *Image*, 14(3), 86–88.

Newman, M.A. (1983) Health as expanding consciousness. *Proceedings of Seventh International Conference on Human Functioning*. Wichita, KS: Biomedical Synergistics Institute.

Newman, M.A. (1983) Newman's health theory. In I. Clements and F. Roberts (Eds.), *Family health: A theoretical approach to nursing care* (pp. 161–175). New York: John Wiley.

Newman, M. (1984) Nursing diagnosis. *American Journal of Nursing*, 84(12), 1496–1499.

Newman, M. (1986) *Health as expanding consciousness*. St. Louis: C.V. Mosby.

Newman, M. (1987) Aging as increasing complexity (Survey). *Journal of Gerontological Nursing*, 13(9), 16–18.

Newman, M. (1987) Perception of time among Japanese inpatients. *Western Journal of Nursing Research*, 9(20), 299–300.

Newman, M. (1989) The spirit of nursing. *Holistic Nursing Practice*, 3(3), 1–6.

Newman, M.A. and Gaudiano, J.K. (1984) Depression as an explanation for decreased subjective time in the elderly. *Nursing Research*, 33(3), 137–139.

Newman, M.A., Tompkins, E.S., Isenberg, M.A., Fitzpatrick, J.J., and Scott, D.W. (1980) Movement, time and consciousness: Parameters of health (Symposium). *Proceedings of Western Society for Research in Nursing Research*, 13, 45–49.

Nojima, Y., Oda, A., Nishii, H., Fukui, M., Seo, K., and Akiyoshi, H. (1987) Perception of time among Japanese inpatients. *Western Journal of Nursing Research*, 9(3), 288–300.

Roy, C., Rogers, M.E., Fitzpatrick, J.J., Newman, M., and Orem, D.E. (1982) Nursing diagnosis and nursing theory. In M.J. Kim and D.A. Moritz (Eds.), *Classification of nursing diagnosis* (pp. 215–231). New York: McGraw-Hill.

Sarter, B. (1988) Philosophical sources of nursing theory. *Nursing Science Quarterly*, 1(2), 52–59.

Nightingale

Armstrong, D. (1983) The fabrication of nurse-patient relationships. *Social Science and Medicine*, 17(8), 457–460.

Barnard, K. and Neal, M.U. (1977) Maternal-child nursing research: Review of the past and strategies for the future. *Nursing Research*, 26, 193–200.

Boland, L. (1988) Five Nightingale theories spell success. *Today's Nurse*, 10(12), 18–21.

Bourgeois, M.J. (1975) The special nurse research fellow: Characteristics and trends. *Nursing Research*, 24, 184–188.

Byrnes, M.A. (1982) Non-nursing functions: Nurses state their case. *American Journal of Nursing*, 82, 1089–1093.

Chinn, P.L. (1983) Editorial. *Advances in Nursing Science*, 6(1), ix–x.

Christoffel, T. (1976) Medical care evaluation: An old idea. *Journal of Medical Education*, 51(2), 83–88.

Cohen, I.B. (1984) Florence Nightingale. *Scientific America*, 250, 128–137.

Crow, R. (1982) How nursing and the community can benefit from nursing research. *International Journal of Nursing Studies*, 19(1), 37–45.

deGraaf, K., Marriner-Tomey, A., Mossman, C., and Slebodnik, M. (1989) Florence Nightingale: Modern nursing. In A. Marriner-Tomey, *Nursing theorists and their work* (2nd ed.). St. Louis: C.V. Mosby.

Dennis, K.E. and Prescott, P.A. (1985, January) Florence Nightingale: Yesterday, today and tomorrow. *Advances in Nursing Science*, 7(2), 66–81.

Francis, G. (1980) Gesellschaft and the hospital: Is total care a misnomer? *Advances in Nursing Science*, 2(4), 9–13.

Francis, H.W. (1982) On gossips, eavesdroppers and peeping toms. *Journal of Medical Ethics*, 8, 134–143.

Goldwater, M. (1987) Like Florence Nightingale, we use the political system. *The American Nurse*, 19(2), 15.

Grier, B. and Grier, M. (1978) Contributions of the passionate statistician. *Research in Nursing and Health*, 1(3), 103–109.

Hays, J.D. (1989) Florence Nightingale and the India sanitary reforms. *Public Health Nursing*, 6(3), 152–154.

Henderson, V.A. (1978) The concept of nursing. *Journal of Advanced Nursing*, 3, 113–130.

Henderson, V.A. (1980) Preserving the essence of nursing in a technological age. *Journal of Advanced Nursing*, 5, 245–260.

Heistand, W.C. (1982) Nursing, the family and the "new" social history. *Advances in Nursing Science*, 4(3), 1–12.

Hughes, L. (1980) The public image of the nurse. *Advances in Nursing Science*, 2, 55–72.

Johnson, D.E. (1974) Development of theory: A requisite for nursing as a primary health profession. *Nursing Research*, 23(5), 372–377.

Kalish, B.J. and Kalish, P.A. (1983) Heroine out of focus: Media images of Florence Nightingale. Part I: Popular biographies and stage productions. *Nursing and Health Care*, 4, 181–187.

Kalish, B.J. and Kalish, P.A. (1983) Heroine out of focus: Media images of Florence Nightingale. Part II: Film, radio, and television dramatizations. *Nursing and Health Care*, 4, 181–187.

Kalish, P.A. and Kalish, B.J. (1982) The image of nurses in novels. *American Journal of Nursing*, 82, 1220–1224.

Keith, J.M. (1988) Florence Nightingale: Statistician and consultant epidemiologist. *International Nursing Review*, 35(5), 147–151.

Kelly, L.Y. (1976) Our nursing heritage: Have we renounced it? *Image*, 8(3), 43–48.

Kopf, E.W. (1978) Florence Nightingale as statistician. *Research in Nursing and Health*, 1(3), 93–102.

Kovacs, A.R. (1978) The personality of Florence Nightingale. *International Nursing Review*, 20, 78–81.

Matthews, C.A. and Gaul, A.L. (1979) Nursing diagnosis from the perspective of concept attainment and critical thinking. *Advances in Nursing Science*, 2(1), 17–26.

Monteiro, L. (1972) Research into things past: Tracking down one of Miss Nightingale's correspondents. *Nursing Research*, 21(5), 526–529.

Novak, J.C. (1988) The social mandate and historical basis for nursing's role in health promotion. *Journal of Professional Nursing*, 4(2), 80–87.

Palmer, I.S. (1977) Florence Nightingale: Reformer, reactionary, researcher. *Nursing Research*, 26(2), 84–89.

Palmer, I.S. (1981) Florence Nightingale and international origins of modern nursing. *Image*, 13, 28–31.

Palmer, I.S. (1983, July–August) Nightingale revisited. *Nursing Outlook*, 31(4), 229–233.

Palmer, I.S. (1983) Origins of education for nurses. *Nursing Forum*, 22(3), 102–110.

Parker, P. (1977) Florence Nightingale: First lady of administrative nursing. *Supervisor Nurse*, 8(3), 24–25.

Reed, P.G. and Zurakowski, T.L. (1983) Nightingale: A visionary model for nursing. In J.J. Fitzpatrick and A.L. Whall (Eds.), *Conceptual models of nursing: Analysis and application*. Bowie, MD: Robert J. Brady Co.

Reed, P.G. and Zurakowski, T.L. (1989) Nightingale revisited: A visionary model for nursing. In J.J. Fitzpatrick and A.L. Whall, *Conceptual models of nursing: Analysis and application* (2nd ed.). Norwalk, CT: Appleton & Lange.

Rogers, P.S. (1972) Design for patient care. *International Nursing Review*, 19(3), 267–282.

Romano, C., McCormick, L.D., and NcNeely, L.D. (1982) Nursing documentation: A model for a computerized data base. *Advances in Nursing Science*, 1(2), 43–56.

Schlotfeldt, R.M. (1977) Nursing research: Reflection of values. *Nursing Research*, 26(1), 4–9.

Schrock, R.A. (1977) On political consciousness in nurses. *Journal of Advanced Nursing*, 2, 41–50.

Seelye, A. (1982) Hospital ward layout and nurse staffing. *Journal of Advanced Nursing*, 7, 195–201.

Seymer, L.R. (1960) One hundred years ago. *The American Journal of Nursing*, 60, 658–661.

Smith, F.T. (1981) Florence Nightingale: Early feminist. *American Journal of Nursing*, 81, 1021–1024.

Tebbe, S. (1988) Nightingale's environmental theory—A 20th century reality. *Today's Nurse*, 10(8), 8–15.

Thompson, J.D. (1980) The passionate humanist: From Nightingale to the new nurse. *Nursing Outlook*, 28(5), 290–295.

Torres, G. (1981) The nursing education administrator: Accountable, vulnerable and oppressed. *Advances in Nursing Science*, 3(3), 1–16.

Weiler, P.G. (1975) Health manpower dialectic: Physician, nurse, physician assistant. *American Journal of Public Health*, 65(8), 858–863.

Whittaker, E.W. and Olesen, V.L. (1967) Why Florence Nightingale? *American Journal of Nursing*, 67, 2338–2341.

Williams, B. (1965) Back to Florence Nightingale and Lawson Tait. *The Practitioner*, 194, 800–804.

Wolstenholme, G.E.W. (1970) Florence Nightingale: New lamps for old. *Proceedings of the Royal Society of Medicine*, 63, 1282–1288.

Orem

Aggleton, P. et al. (1985) Models and theories: Orem's self care model (Part 5). *Nursing Time*, 81(1), 36–39.

Allan, J. (1988) Knowing what to weigh: Women's self care activities related to weight. *Advances in Nursing Science*, 11(1), 47–60.

†Allison, S.E. (1973) A framework for nursing action in a nurse-conducted diabetic management clinic. *Journal of Nursing Administration*, 3(4), 53–60.

†Anna, D.J., Christensen, D.G., Hohn, S.A., Ord, L., and Wells, S.R. (1978) Implementing Orem's conceptual framework. *Journal of Nursing Administration*, 8(11), 8–11.

Backscheider, J. (1971) The use of self as the essence of clinical supervision in ambulatory patient care. *Nursing Clinics of North America*, 6(4), 785–794.

†Backscheider, J.E. (1974, December) Self-care requirements, self-care capabilities, and nursing systems in the diabetic nurse management clinic. *American Journal of Public Health*, 64(12), 1138–1146.

Behi, R. (1986, September) Look after yourself: Orem's self-care model. *Nursing Times*, 82(37), 35–37.

Bennett, J.G. (1980) Forward to the Symposium on the Self-care Concept in Nursing. *Nursing Clinics of North America*, 15(1), 129–130.

†Bromley, B. (1980) Applying Orem's self-care theory in enterostomal therapy. *American Journal of Nursing*, 80(2), 245–249.

†Buckwalter, K.C. and Kerfoot, K.M. (1982) Teaching patients self-care: A critical aspect of psychiatric discharge planning. *Journal of Psychiatric Nursing and Mental Health Services*, 20(5), 15–20.

†Caley, J.M., Dirkensen, M., Engally, M., and Hennrich, M.L. (1980) The Orem self-care model. In J.P. Riehl and C. Roy (Eds.),*Conceptual models for nursing practice* (2nd ed.). New York: Appleton-Century-Crofts.

Cammermeyer, M. (1983) Growth model of self-care for neurologically impaired people. *Journal of Neurosurgical Nursing*, 15, 299–305.

Campuzano, M. (1982, April–May) Self-care following coronary artery bypass surgery. *Focus on Critical Care*, 9(1), 55–56.

†Chang, B.L. (1980) Evaluation of health care professionals in facilitating self-care: Review of the literature and a conceptual model. *Advances in Nursing Science*, 3(1), 43–58.

Chapman, P. (1984) Specifics and generalities: A critical examination of two nursing models . . . Orem's and Preisner's. *Nurse Educator Today*, 4(6), 141–144.

Clark, M. (1986) Application of Orem's theory of self-care: A case study. *Journal of Community Health Nursing*, 3(3), 127–135.

Clinton, J.F., Denyes, M.J., Goodwin, J.O., and Koto, E.M. (1977) Developing criterion measures of nursing care: Case study of a process. *Journal of Nursing Administration*, 7(7), 41–45.

†Coleman, L.J. (1980) Orem's self-care concept of nursing. In J.P. Riehl and C. Roy (Eds.), *Conceptual models for nursing practice* (2nd ed.) (pp. 315–328). New York: Appleton-Century-Crofts.

Compton, P. (1989) Drug abuse, a self-care deficit. *Journal of Psychosocial Nursing*, 27(3), 22–26.

Dashiff, C. (1988) Theory development in psychiatric mental health nursing: An analysis of Orem's theory. *Archives of Psychiatric Nursing*, 2(6), 366–372.

Denyes, M.J. (1982) Measurement of self-care agency in adolescents (Abstract). *Nursing Research*, 31, 63.

Denyes, M.J. (1988) Orem's model used for health promotion: Directions from research. *Advances in Nursing Science*, 11(1), 13–21.

Denyes, M.J., O'Connor, N., Oakley, D., and Ferguson, S. (1989) Integrating nursing theory, practice and research through collaborative research. *Journal of Advanced Nursing*, 14, 141–145.

†Dickson, G.L. and Lee-Villasenor, H. (1982) Nursing theory and practice: A self-care approach. *Advances in Nursing Science*, 5, 29–40.

Dropkin, M.J. (1981, April) Development of a self-care teaching program for postoperative head and neck patients. *Cancer Nursing*, 103–106.

Eben, J., Gashti, N., Nation, M., Marriner-Tomey, A., and Nordmeyer, S. (1989) Dorothea E. Orem: Self-care deficit theory of nursing. In A. Marriner-Tomey, *Nursing theorists and their work* (2nd ed.). St. Louis: C.V. Mosby.

Ewing, G. (1989) The nursing preparation of stoma patients for self-care. *Journal of Advanced Nursing*, 14, 41–420.

Fawcett, J. (1984) Orem's self-care model. In *Analysis and evaluation of conceptual models of nursing*. Philadelphia: F.A. Davis.

Fawcett, J. (1989) Orem's self-care model. In *Analysis and evaluation of conceptual models of nursing* (2nd ed.). Philadelphia: F.A. Davis.

Feathers, R. (1989) Orem's self-care nursing theory. In J. Riehl-Sisca, *Conceptual models for nursing practice* (3rd ed.). Norwalk, CT: Appleton & Lange.

Fenner, K. (1979) Developing a conceptual framework. *Nursing Outlook*, 27, 122–126.

Field, P.A. (1987) The impact of nursing theory on the clinical decision making process. *Journal of Advanced Nursing*, 12(5), 653–571.

Fitzgerald, S. (1980) Utilizing Orem's self-care nursing model in designing an educational program for the diabetic. *Topics in Clinical Nursing*, 2(2), 57–65.

Foster, P.C. and Janssens, N.P. (1980) Dorothea E. Orem. In the Nursing Theories Conference Group, *Nursing theories: The base for professional nursing practice.* Englewood Cliffs, NJ: Prentice-Hall.

Geden, E. (1989) The relationship between self-care theory and empirical research. In J. Riehl-Sisca, *Conceptual models for nursing practice* (3rd ed.). Norwalk, CT: Appleton & Lange.

Green, L.W. et al. (1977) Research and demonstration issues in self-care: Measuring the decline of medicocentricism. *Health Education Monographs*, 5, 161–181.

Greenfield, E. and Pace, J. (1985) Orem's self-care theory of nursing: Practical application to the end stage renal disease (ESRD) patient. *Journal of Nephro Nursing*, 2(4), 187–193.

Harris, J.K. (1980) Self-care is possible after delivery. *Nursing Clinics of North America*, 15(1), 191–194.

Hartley, L. (1988) Congruence between teaching and learning self care: A pilot study. *Nursing Science Quarterly*, 1(4), 161–167.

Johnston, R.L. (1983) Orem self-care model of nursing. In J.J. Fitzpatrick and A.L. Whall (Eds.), *Conceptual models of nursing: Analysis and application.* Bowie, MD: Robert J. Brady Co.

Johnston, R.L. (1989) Orem's self care model for nursing. In J.J. Fitzpatrick and A.L. Whall, *Conceptual models of nursing: Analysis and application* (2nd ed.). Norwalk, CT: Appleton & Lange.

Joseph, L.S. (1980) Self-care and the nursing process. *Nursing Clinics of North America*, 15(1), 131–143.

†Karl, C.A. (1982) The effect of an exercise program on self-care activities for the institutionalized elderly. *Journal of Gerontological Nursing*, 8, 282–285.

Kearney, B.Y. and Fleischer, B.J. (1979) Development of an instrument to measure exercise of self-care agency. *Research in Nursing and Health*, 2(1), 25–34.

Kinlein, M.L. (1977) *Independent nursing practice with clients.* Philadelphia: J.B. Lippincott.

Kinlein, M.L. (1977) Self-care concept. *American Journal of Nursing*, 77, 598–601.

Kinlein, M.L. (1978) Point of view on the front: Nursing and family and community health. *Family and Community Health*, 1, 57–68.

King, C. (1980) The self-care, self-help concept. *Nurse Practitioner*, 5, 34–35.

Kuriansky, J., Gurland, B., Fleiss, J., and Cowan, D. (1976) The assessment of self-care capacity in geriatric psychiatric patients by objective and subjective methods. *Journal of Clinical Psychology*, 32, 95–102.

Lane, D.E. (1981) Self-medication of psychiatric patients. *Journal of Psychiatric Nursing and Mental Health Services*, 19, 27–28.

Levin, L.S. (1976) *Self-care: Lay initiatives in health.* New York: Neale Watson Academic Publications.

Levin, L.S. (1977) Forces and issues in the revival of interest in self-care: Impetus for redirection for health. *Health Education Monographs*, 5, 115–120.

Levin, L.S. (1978) Patient education and self-care: How do they differ? *Nursing Outlook*, 26(3), 170–175.

Lundh, U., Soder, M., and Waerness, K. (1987) Nursing theories: A critical review. *Image: Journal of Nursing Scholarship*, 20(1), 36–40.

McFarlane, E.A. (1980) Nursing theory: The comparison of four theoretical proposals. *Journal of Advanced Nursing*, 5, 3–9.

McIntyre, K. (1980) The Perry model as a framework for self-care. *Nurse Practitioner*, 5(6), 34–37.

Melnyk, K.A.M. (1983) The process of theory analysis: An examination of the nursing theory of Dorothea E. Orem. *Nursing Research*, 32(3), 170–174.

Michael, M.M. and Sewall, K.S. (1980) Use of the adolescent peer group to increase the self-care agency of adolescent alcohol abusers. *Nursing Clinics of North America*, 15, 157–176.

†Miller, J.F. (1980) The dynamic focus of nursing: A challenge to nursing administration. *Journal of Nursing Administration*, 10(1), 13–18.

†Miller, J.F. (1982) Categories of self-care needs of ambulatory patients with diabetes. *Journal of Advanced Nursing*, 7, 25–31.

Millio, N. (1977) Self-care in urban settings. *Health Education Monographs*, 5, 136–144.

Morse, W. and Werner, J. (1988) Individualization of patient care using Orem's theory. *Cancer Nursing*, 11(3), 195–202.

Mullin, V.I. (1980) Implementing the self-care concept in the acute care setting. *Nursing Clinics of North America*, 15(1), 177–190.

†Murphy, P.P. (1981) The hospice model and self-care theory. *Oncology Nursing Forum*, 8(2), 19–21.

Norris, C.M. (1979) Self-care. *American Journal of Nursing*, 79(3), 486–489.

Nowakowski, L. (1980) Health promotion/self-care programs for the community. *Topics in Clinical Nursing*, 2, 21–27.

Nursing Development Conference Group. (1973) *Concept formalization in nursing: Process and product*. Boston: Little, Brown & Co.

Nursing Development Conference Group. (1979) *Concept formulization in nursing: Process and product* (2nd ed.). Boston: Little, Brown & Co.

Orem, D.E. (1959) *Guides for developing curriculae for the education of practical nurses*. Washington, D.C.: U.S. Department of Health, Education, and Welfare; Office of Education.

Orem, D.E. (1971) *Nursing: Concepts of practice*. New York: McGraw-Hill.

Orem, D.E. (1980) *Nursing: Concepts of practice* (2nd ed.). New York: McGraw-Hill.

Orem, D.E. (1983) The self-care deficit theory of nursing: A general theory. In I.W. Clements and F.B. Roberts (Eds.), *Family health: A theoretical approach to nursing care* (pp. 205–217). New York: John Wiley & Sons.

Orem, D.E. (1985) *Nursing: Concepts of practice* (3rd ed.). New York: McGraw-Hill.

Orem, D.E. (1987) Orem's general theory of nursing. In R.R. Parse, *Nursing science: Major paradigms, theories, and critiques*. Philadelphia: W.B. Saunders.

Orem, D.E. (1988) The form of nursing science. *Nursing Science Quarterly*, 1(2), 75–79.

Orem, D.E. and Taylor, S.G. (1986) Orem's general theory of nursing. In P. Winstead-Fry (Ed.), *Case studies in nursing theory*. New York: National League for Nursing.

†Petrlik, J.C. (1976) Diabetic peripheral neuropathy. *American Journal of Nursing*, 76, 1794–1797.

†Porter, D. and Shamian, J. (1983) Self-care in theory and practice. *Canadian Nurse*, 79(8), 21–23.

Raven, M. (1988–1989) Application of Orem's self-care model to nursing practice in developmental disability. *Australian Journal of Advanced Nursing*, 6(2), 16–23.

Reid, B., Allan, A., Gauthier, T., and Campbell, H. (1989) Solving the Orem mystery: An educational strategy. *Journal of Continuing Education in Nursing*, 20(3), 108–110.

Riehl-Sisca, J. (1989) Orem's general theory of nursing: An interpretation. In J. Riehl-Sisca, *Conceptual models for nursing practice* (3rd ed.). Norwalk, CT: Appleton & Lange.

Roberts, C.S. (1982) Identifying the real patient problems. *Nursing Clinics of North America*, 17(3), 481–489.

Romine, S. (1986) Applying Orem's self-care to staff development. *Journal of Nursing Staff Development*, 2(2), 77–79.

Rosenbaum, J.N. (1986) Comparison of two theorists on care: Orem and Leininger. *Journal of Advanced Nursing*, 11, 409–419.

Roy, C. (1980) A case study viewed according to different models. In J.P. Riehl and C. Roy (Eds.), *Conceptual models for nursing practice* (2nd ed.). New York: Appleton-Century-Crofts.

†Smith, M.C. (1979) Proposed metaparadigm for nursing research and theory development: An analysis of Orem's self-care theory. *Image*, 11(3), 75–79.

Smith, M.C. (1987) A critique of Orem's theory. In R.R. Parse, *Nursing science: Major paradigms, theories, and critiques*. Philadelphia: W.B. Saunders.

Storm, D. and Baumgartner, R. (1987) Achieving self-care in the ventilator-dependent patient: A critical analysis of a case study. *International Journal of Nursing Studies*, 24(2), 95–106.

†Sullivan, T.J. (1980) Self-care model for nursing. In *New directions for nursing in the '80s*. Kansas City, MO: American Nurses' Association.

Taylor, S. (1988) Nursing theory and nursing process: Orem's theory in practice. *Nursing Science Quarterly*, 1(3), 111–119.

Titus, S. and Porter, P. (1989) Orem's theory applied to pediatric residential treatment. *Pediatric Nursing*, 15(5), 465–468.

Underwood, P.R. (1980) Facilitating self-care. In P. Pothier (Ed.), *Psychiatric nursing* (pp. 115–144). Boston: Little, Brown & Co.

Uys, L. (1987) Foundational studies in nursing. *Journal of Advanced Nursing*, 12(3), 275–280.

Walborn, K.A. (1980) A nursing model for hospice, primary and self-care. *Nursing Clinics of North America*, 15(1), 205–217.

Walton, J. (1985) An overview: Orem's self care deficit theory of nursing. *Focus Critical Care*, 12(1), 54–58.

Whelan, E. (1984) Analysis and application of Dorothea Orem's self-care practice model. *Journal of Nursing Education*, 24(6), 226–229.

Woods, N. (1989) Conceptualizations of self-care: Toward health-oriented models. *Advances in Nursing Science*, 12(1), 1–13.

Orlando

Anderson, B.J., Mertz, H., and Leonard, R.C. (1965) Two Experimental tests of a patient-centered admission process. *Nursing Research*, 14, 151–157.

Andrews, C.M. (1983) Ida Orlando's model of nursing. In J.J. Fitzpatrick and A.L. Whall (Eds.), *Conceptual models of nursing: Analysis and application*. Bowie, MD: Robert J. Brady Co.

Andrews, C.M. (1989) Ida Orlando's model of nursing practice. In J.J. Fitzpatrick and A.L. Whall, *Conceptual models of nursing: Analysis and application* (2nd ed.). Norwalk, CT: Appleton & Lange.

Barnard, K.E. (1980) Knowledge for practice: Directions for the future. *Nursing Research*, 29(4), 208.

Barron, M.A. (1966) The effects varied nursing approaches have on patients' complaints of pain (Abstract). *Nursing Research*, 15(1), 90–91.

Bochnak, M.A. (1963) The effect of an automatic and deliberative process of nursing activity on the relief of patients' pain: A clinical experiment. *Nursing Research*, 12, 191–192.

Burssen, B. and Diers, D.K. (1964) Pseudo-patient centered orientations. *Nursing Forum*, 3(2), 38–50.

Cameron, J. (1963) An exploratory study of the verbal responses of the nurse-patient interactions. *Nursing Research*, 12, 192.

Crane, M.D. (1980) Ida Jean Orlando. In The Nursing Theories Conference Group, *Nursing theories: The base for professional nursing practice.* Englewood Cliffs, NJ: Prentice-Hall.

Diers, D.K. (1966) The nurse orientation system: A method for analyzing the nurse-patient interactions (Abstract). *Nursing Research*, 15(1), 91.

Diers, D. (1970) Faculty research development at Yale. *Nursing Research*, 19(1), 64–71.

Dracup, K.A. and Breu, C.S. (1978) Using nursing research findings to meet the needs of grieving spouses. *Nursing Research*, 27(4), 212.

Dumas, R.G. (1963, August) Psychological preparation for surgery. *American Journal of Nursing*, 63(8), 52–55.

Dumas, R.G. and Leonard, R.C. (1963) The effect of nursing on the incidence of postoperative vomiting. *Nursing Research*, 12(1), 12–15.

Dye, M.C. (1963) A descriptive study of conditions conducive to an effective process of nursing activity. *Nursing Research*, 12, 194.

Dye, M.C. (1963, August) Clarifying patients' communication. *American Journal of Nursing*, 63(8), 56–59.

Dye, M., Orlando, I.J., and Dumas, R.G. (1963) Validating a theory of nursing practice. *American Journal of Nursing*, 63(8), 52–59.

Eisler, J., Wolfer, J., and Diers, D. (1972) Relationship between the need for social approval and postoperative recovery and welfare. *Nursing Research*, 21(5), 520–525.

Elder, R.G. (1963) What is the patient saying? *Nursing Forum*, 2(1), 25–37.

Elms, R.R. and Leonard, R.C. (1966) Effects of nursing approaches during admission. *Nursing Research*, 15(1), 39–48.

Fitzpatrick, J. and Whall, A. (1983) *Conceptual models of nursing: Analysis and application.* Bowie, MD: Robert J. Brady Co.

Gilliss, S.L. (1976) Sleeplessness—can you help? *Canadian Nurse*, 72(7), 32–34.

Gowan, N.I. and Morris, M. (1964) Nurses' responses to expressed patient needs. *Nursing Research*, 13, 68–71.

Haggerty, L.A. (1985) A theoretical model for developing students' communication skills. *Journal of Nursing Education*, 24(7), 296–298.

Haggerty, L.A. (1987) An analysis of senior nursing students' immediate response to distressed patients. *Journal of Advanced Nursing*, 12, 451–461.

Hampe, S.O. (1975) Needs of grieving spouses in a hospital setting. *Nursing Research*, 24(2), 113.

Johnson, D.E. (1974) Development of theory: A requisite for nursing as a primary health profession. *Nursing Research*, 23(5), 372.

Larson, P.A. (1977) Influence of patient status and health condition on nurse perceptions of patient characteristics. *Nursing Research*, 26(6), 416.

Leonard, R.C., Skipper, J.K., Jr., and Wodridge, P.J. (1967, Spring) Small sample field experiments for evaluating patient care. *Health Services Research* 2(1), 47–60.

Marriner-Tomey, A., Mills, D., and Sauter, M. (1989) Ida Jean Orlando (Pelletier): Nursing process theory. In A. Marriner-Tomey, *Nursing theorists and their work* (2nd ed.). St. Louis: C.V. Mosby.

Mertz, H. (1962) Nurse actions that reduce stress in patients. In *Emergency intervention by the nurse* (Monograph No. 1) (pp. 10–14). New York: American Nurses' Association.

New England Board of Higher Education. (1977) *Mental health continuing education for associate degree nursing faculties: Project report.* Wellesley, MA: New England Board of Higher Education. NIH Training Grant No. 715 MH13182.

Orlando, I. (1961) *The dynamic nurse-patient relationship.* New York: G.P. Putnam's Sons.

Orlando, I. (1972) *The discipline and teaching of nursing process.* New York: G.P. Putnam's Sons.

Orlando, I. (1987) Nursing in the 21st century . . . alternate paths. *Journal of Advanced Nursing,* 12(4), 405–412.

Orlando, I. and Dugan, A.B. (1989) Independent and dependent path: The fundamental issue for the nursing profession. *Nursing and Health Care,* 10(2), 76–80.

Peitchinis, J.A. (1972) Therapeutic effectiveness of counseling by nursing personnel. *Nursing Research,* 21(2), 138–148.

Pienschke, D. (1973) Guardedness or openness on the cancer unit. *Nursing Research,* 22(6), 484–490.

Rhymes, J. (1964) A description of nurse-patient interaction in effective nursing activity (Abstract). *Nursing Research,* 13(4), 365.

Schmieding, N.J. (1983) An analysis of Orlando's nursing theory based on Kuhn's theory of science. In P.L. Chinn (Ed.), *Advances in nursing theory development* (pp. 63–87). Rockville, MD: Aspen Systems.

Schmieding, N.J. (1984) Putting Orlando's theory into practice. *American Journal of Nursing,* 84(6), 759–761.

Schmieding, N.J. (1986) Orlando's theory. In P. Winstead-Fry (Ed.), *Case studies in nursing theory.* New York: National League for Nursing.

Schmieding, N.J. (1987) Face-to-face contacts: Exploring their meaning. *Nursing Management,* 18, 83–86.

Schmieding, N.J. (1987) Problematic situations in nursing: Analysis of Orlando's theory based on Dewey's theory of inquiry. *Journal of Advanced Nursing,* 12(4), 431–440.

Schmieding, N.J. (1988) Action process of nurse administrators to problematic situations based on Orlando's theory. *Journal of Advanced Nursing,* 13(1), 99–107.

Stevens, B.J. (1971) Analysis of structural forms used in nursing curricula. *Nursing Research,* 20(5), 388.

Theis, E.C. (1973) Book review of Ida J. Orlando's *The discipline and teaching of nursing process. Nursing Research,* 22(1), 73.

Tryon, P.A. (1962) The effect of patient participation in decision making on the outcome of a nursing procedure. In *Nursing and the patients' motivation* (Clinical Paper No. 19, pp. 14–18). New York: American Nurses' Association.

Tryon, P.A. (1963) An experiment of the effect of patients' participation in planning the administration of a nursing procedure. *Nursing Research,* 12, 262–265.

Tryon, P.A. and Leonard, R.C. (1964) The effect of patients' participation on the outcome of a nursing procedure. *Nursing Forum,* 3(2), 79–89.

Williamson, Y. (1978) Methodologic dilemmas in tapping the concept of patient needs. *Nursing Research,* 27(3), 172.

Wolfer, J. and Visintainer, M.A. (1975) Pediatric surgical patients' and parents' stress response and adjustment as a function of psychological preparation and stress-point nursing care. *Nursing Research,* 24(4), 244–255.

Parse

Banonis, B. (1989) The lived experience of recovering from addiction: A phenomenological study. *Nursing Science Quarterly,* 2(1), 37–43.

Butler, M. (1988) Family transformation: Parse's theory in practice. *Nursing Science Quarterly*, 1(2), 68–74.

Chrisman, M. and Riehl-Sisca, J. (1989) The systems-developmental-stress model. In J. Riehl-Sisca, *Conceptual models for nursing practice* (3rd ed.). Norwalk, CT: Appleton & Lange.

Cowling, W.R. (1989) Parse's theory of nursing. In J.J. Fitzpatrick and A.L. Whall, *Conceptual models of nursing: Analysis and application* (2nd ed.). Norwalk, CT: Appleton & Lange.

English, J. (1989) The systems-developmental-stress model in psychiatric nursing. In J. Riehl-Sisca, *Conceptual models for nursing practice* (3rd ed.). Norwalk, CT: Appleton & Lange.

Lee, R. and Schumacher, L. (1989) Rosemarie Rizzo Parse: Man-living-health. In A. Marriner-Tomey, *Nursing theorists and their work* (2nd ed.). St. Louis: C.V. Mosby.

Limandri, B.J. (1982) Review of "Man—living—health: A theory of nursing." *Western Journal of Nursing Research*, 4(1), 105–106.

Michell, G.J. (1988) Man-living-health: The theory in practice. *Nursing Science Quarterly*, 1(3), 120–127.

Parse, R.R. (1974) *Nursing fundamentals*. Flushing, NY: Medical Examination Publ.

Parse, R.R. (1981) *Man-living-health: A theory of nursing*. New York: John Wiley & Sons.

Parse, R.R. (1987) *Nursing science: Major paradigms, theories, and critiques*. Philadelphia: W.B. Saunders.

Parse, R.R. (1987) Paradigms and theories. In R.R. Parse, *Nursing science: Major paradigms, theories, and critiques*. Philadelphia: W.B. Saunders.

Parse, R.R. (1987) Parse's man-living-health theory of nursing. In R.R. Parse, *Nursing science: Major paradigms, theories, and critiques*. Philadelphia: W.B. Saunders.

Parse, R.R. (1987) The simultaneity paradigm. In R.R. Parse, *Nursing science: Major paradigms, theories, and critiques*. Philadelphia: W.B. Saunders.

Parse, R.R. (1989) Man-living-health: A theory of nursing. In J. Riehl-Sisca, *Conceptual models for nursing practice* (3rd ed.). Norwalk, CT: Appleton & Lange.

Parse, R.R. (1989) Parse's man-living-health model and administration of nursing service. In B. Henry, C. Arndt, M. DiVincenti, and A. Marriner-Tomey (Eds.), *Dimensions of nursing administration: Theory, research, education, practice*. Boston: Blackwell Scientific Publications.

Phillips, J.R. (1987) A critique of Parse's man-living-health theory. In R.R. Parse, *Nursing science: Major paradigms, theories, and critiques*. Philadelphia: W.B. Saunders.

Pugliese, L. (1989) The theory of man-living-health: An analysis. In J. Riehl-Sisca, *Conceptual models for nursing practice* (3rd ed.). Norwalk, CT: Appleton & Lange.

Reed, P.G. (1983) Implications of the life-span developmental framework for well-being in adulthood and aging. *Advances in Nursing Science*, 6(1), 18–25.

Sarter, B. (1988) Philosophy sources of nursing theory. *Nursing Science Quarterly*, 1(2), 52–59.

Smith, M.J. (1989) Research and practice application related to man-living-health. In J. Riehl-Sisca, *Conceptual models for nursing practice* (3rd ed.). Norwalk, CT: Appleton & Lange.

Winkler, S.J. (1983) Parse's theory of nursing. In J.J. Fitzpatrick and A.L. Whall (Eds.), *Conceptual models of nursing: Analysis and application*. Bowie, MD: Robert J. Brady Co.

Paterson and Zderad

Brouse, S.H. and Laffrey, S.C. (1989) Paterson and Zderad's humanistic nursing framework. In J.J. Fitzpatrick and A.L. Whall, *Conceptual models of nursing: Analysis and application* (2nd ed.). Norwalk, CT: Appleton & Lange.

Kleiman, S. (1986) Humanistic nursing: The phenomenological theory of Paterson and Zderad. In P. Winstead-Fry (Ed.), *Case studies in nursing theory.* New York: National League for Nursing.

McCance, C., Paterson, J.G., Nommo, A.W., and Hunter, D. (1987) Psychiatric geography: Where patients live and their use of services–A study of computerized mapping of case register data. *Health Bulletin,* 45(4), 197–210.

Paterson, J.G. (1971) From a philosophy of clinical nursing to a method of nursology. *Nursing Research,* 20(2), 143–146.

Paterson, J.G. (1978) The tortuous way toward nursing theory. In *Theory development: What, why, how?* (NLN Publ. No. 15-1708, pp. 49–65). New York: National League for Nursing.

Paterson, J.G. and Zderad L.T. (1970–1971) All together through complementary syntheses the worlds of the many. *Image,* 4(3), 13–16.

Paterson, J.G. and Zderad, L.T. (1976) *Humanistic nursing.* New York: John Wiley & Sons.

Paterson, J.G. and Zderad, L.T. (1988, March) Humanistic nursing. New York: *NLN Publications* (Publ. No. 41-2218, pp. i–iv, 1–129.)

Zderad, L.T. (1968) A concept of empathy. Unpublished doctoral dissertation, Georgetown University.

Zderad, L.T. (1969) Empathetic nursing: Realization of a human capacity. *Nursing Clinics of North America,* 4, 655–662.

Zderad, L.T. (1970) Empathy: From cliche to construct. *Proceedings of the Third Nursing Theory Conference* (pp. 46–75). University of Kansas Medical Center Department of Nursing.

Zderad, L.T. (1978) From here and now to theory: Reflections on "how." In J.G. Paterson (Eds.), *Theory development: What, why, how?* (NLN Publ. No. 15-1708, pp. 35–48). New York: National League for Nursing.

Peplau

Carey, E.T., Noll, J., Rasmussen, L., Searcy, B., and Stark, N. (1989) Hildegard E. Peplau: Psychodynamic nursing. In A. Marriner-Tomey, *Nursing theorists and their work* (2nd ed.). St. Louis: C.V. Mosby.

Forchuk, C. (1989) Establish a nurse-client relationship. *Journal of Psychosocial Nursing,* 27(2), 30–34.

Forchuk, C., Beaton, S., Crawford, L., Ide, L., Voorberg, N., and Bethune, J. (1989) Incorporating Peplau's theory and case management. *Journal of Psychosocial Nursing and Mental Health Services,* 27(2), 35–38.

Gregg, D.E. (1978) Hildegard E. Peplau: Her contributions. *Perspectives in Psychiatric Care,* 16(3), 118–121.

Peplau, H. (1952) *Interpersonal relations in nursing.* New York: G.P. Putnam's Sons.

Peplau, H. (1957, November) Interpersonal relations and the work of the industrial nurse. *American Association of Industrial Nurses,* 15, 74.

Peplau, H. (1962) Interpersonal techniques: The crux of psychiatric nursing. *The American Journal of Nursing,* 62(6), 50–54.

Peplau, H. (1963, Oct.–Nov.) Interpersonal relations and the process of adaptation. *Nursing Science,* 3, 272–279.

Peplau, H. (1964) *Basic principles of patient counseling.* Philadelphia: Smith Kline & French Laboratory.

Peplau, H. (1968) Operational definitions and nursing science. In L.T. Zderad and H.C. Belcher (Eds.), *Developing behavioral concepts in nursing*. Atlanta: Southern Regional Education Board.

Peplau, H. (1968) Psychotherapeutic strategies. *Perspectives in Psychiatric Care*, 6(6), 264–270.

Peplau, H. (1969) Professional closeness . . . as a special kind of involvement with a patient, client, or family group. *Nursing Forum*, 8(4), 342.

Peplau, H. (1970, Nov.–Dec.) Changed patterns of practice. *Washington Street Journal of Nursing*, 42, 4.

Peplau, H. (1971, Winter) Communication in crisis intervention. *Psychiatric Forum*, 2, 1–7.

Peplau, H. (1974) Biography. *Nursing '74*, 4(2), 13.

Peplau, H. (1978) Psychiatric nursing: Role of nurses and psychiatric nurses. *International Nursing Review*, 25(2), 41–47.

Peplau, H. (1986) Credentialing in nursing: Contemporary developments and trends: Internal and external regulation (pamphlet). *ANA Publication* (Publ. No. G-172B, pp. 1–10).

Peplau, H. (1987) Nursing science: A historical perspective. In R.R. Parse, *Nursing science: Major paradigms, theories, and critiques*. Philadelphia: W.B. Saunders.

Peplau, H. (1988) The art and science of nursing: Similarities, differences, and relations. *Nursing Science Quarterly*, 1(1), 8–15.

Peplau, H. (1988) Future directions in psychiatric nursing from the perspective of history. *Journal of Psychosocial Nursing and Mental Health Services*, 27(2), 18–21, 25–28.

Reed, P.G. and Johnston, R.L. (1983) Peplau's nursing model: The interpersonal process. In J.J. Fitzpatrick and A.L. Whall (Eds.), *Conceptual models of nursing: Analysis and application*. Bowie, MD: Robert J. Brady Co.

Reed, P.G. and Johnston, R.L. (1989) Peplau's nursing model: The interpersonal process. In J.J. Fitzpatrick and A.L. Whall, *Conceptual models of nursing: Analysis and application* (2nd ed.). Norwalk, CT: Appleton & Lange.

Roy, C. (1980) A case study viewed according to different models. In J.P. Riehl and C. Roy (Eds.), *Conceptual models for nursing practice* (2nd ed.). New York: Appleton-Century-Crofts.

Sills, G.M. (1978) Hildegard E. Peplau: Leader, practitioner, academician, scholar, theorist. *Perspectives in Psychiatric Care*, 16(3), 122–128.

Thompson, L. (1986) Peplau's theory: An application to short-term individual therapy. *Journal of Psychological Nursing and Mental Health Service*, 24(8), 26–31.

Rogers

Aggleton, P. and Chalmers, H. (1984, December) Rogers' unitary field model. *Nursing Times*, 80(50), 35–39.

Alligood, M. (1989) Rogers's theory and nursing administration: A perspective on health and environment. In B. Henry, C. Arndt, M. DiVincenti, and A. Marriner-Tomey (Eds.), *Dimensions of nursing administration: Theory, research, education, practice*. Boston: Blackwell Scientific Publications.

Banonis, B. (1989) The lived experience of recovering from addiction: A phenomenological study. *Nursing Science Quarterly*, 2(1), 37–43.

Barrett, E. (1989) A nursing theory of power for nursing practice: Derivation from Rogers' paradigm. In J. Riehl-Sisca, *Conceptual models for nursing practice* (3rd ed.). Norwalk, CT: Appleton & Lange.

Barrett, K. (1972, March–April) Theoretical construct of the concepts of touch as they relate to nursing. *Nursing Research*, 21, 102–110.

Blair, C. (1979) Hyperactivity in children: Viewed within the framework of synergistic man. *Nursing Forum*, 18, 293–303.

Botha, M.E. (1989) Theory development in perspective: The role of conceptual frameworks and models in theory development. *Journal of Advanced Nursing*, 14(1), 49–55.

Butcher, H. and Parker, N. (1988) Guided imagery within Rogers' science of unitary human beings: An experimental study. *Nursing Science Quarterly*, 1(3), 103–110.

Cerilli, K. and Burd, S. (1989) An analysis of Martha Rogers' nursing as a science of unitary human beings. In J. Riehl-Sisca, *Conceptual models for nursing practice* (3rd ed.). Norwalk, CT: Appleton & Lange.

Clarke, P.L. (1986) Theoretical and measurement issues in the study of field phenomena. The human field and self actualization in healthy women. *Advances in Nursing Science*, 9(1), 29–39.

Compton, M.A. (1989) A Rogerian view of drug abuse: Implications for nursing. *Nursing Science Quarterly*, 2(2), 98–105.

Dailey, J., Maupin, J., Satterly, M., Schnell, D., and Wallace, T. (1989) Martha E. Rogers: Unitary human beings. In A. Marriner-Tomey, *Nursing theorists and their work* (2nd ed.). St. Louis: C.V. Mosby.

Duffey, M. and Muhlenkamp, A.F. (1974) A framework for theory analysis. *Nursing Outlook*, 22(9), 570–574.

†Egbert, E. (1980, January) Concept of wellness. *JPN and Mental Health Services*, 18(1), 9–12.

†Falco, S.M. and Lobo, M.L. (1980) Martha E. Rogers. In The Nursing Theories Conference Group. *Nursing theories: The base for professional nursing practice*. Englewood Cliffs, NJ: Prentice-Hall.

Fawcett, J. (1977) The relationship between identification and patterns of change in spouses' body image during and after pregnancy. *International Journal of Nursing Studies*, 14, 199–213.

Fawcett, J. (1984) Rogers' life process model. In *Analysis and evaluation of conceptual models of nursing*. Philadelphia: F.A. Davis.

Ference, H. (1989) Comforting the dying: Nursing practice according to the Rogerian model. In J. Riehl-Sisca, *Conceptual models for nursing practice* (3rd ed.). Norwalk, CT: Appleton & Lange.

Ference, H. (1989) Nursing science theories and administration. In B. Henry, C. Arndt, M. DiVincenti, and A. Marriner-Tomey (Eds.), *Dimensions of nursing administration: Theory, research, education, practice*. Boston: Blackwell Scientific Publications.

Field, L. and Newman, M. (1982) Clinical application of the unitary man framework: Case study analysis (1980). In M.J. Kim and D.A. Moritz (Eds.), *Classification of nursing diagnosis: Proceedings of the third and fourth national conference*. New York: McGraw-Hill.

Fisher, L. and Reichenbach, M. (1987–1988) From Tinkerbell to Rogers (How a fairy tale facilitated an understanding of Rogers' theory of unitary being). *Nursing Forum*, 13(1), 5–9.

Fitzpatrick, J.J. (1980) Patient's perception of time: Current research. *International Nursing Review*, 27, 148–153, 160.

Fitzpatrick, J.J. (1988) Theory based on Rogers' conceptual model. *Journal of Gerontological Nursing*, 14(9), 14–16.

Floyd, J.A. (1983) Research using Rogers' conceptual system: Development of a testable theorem. *Advances in Nursing Science*, 5(2), 37–48.

Forker, J.E. and Billing, C.V. (1989) Nursing therapeutics in a group encounter. *Archives of Psychiatric Nursing*, 3(2), 108–112.

Gill, B.P. and Atwood, J.R. (1981) Reciprocity and helicy used to relate mEGF and wound healing. *Nursing Research*, 30(2), 68–72.

Gioiella, E. (1989) Professionalizing nursing: A Rogers legacy. *Nursing Science Quarterly*, 2(2), 61–62.

Goldberg, W.G. and Fitzpatrick, J.J. (1980) Movement therapy with the aged. *Nursing Research*, 29(6), 339–346.

Gueldner, S. (1989) Applying Rogers's model to nursing administration: Emphasis on client and nursing. In B. Henry, C. Arndt, M. DiVincenti, and A. Marriner-Tomey (Eds.), *Dimensions of nursing administration: Theory, research, education, practice.* Boston: Blackwell Scientific Publications.

Heggie, J., Schoenmehl, P., Chang, M., and Grieco, C. (1989) Selection and implementation of Dr. Martha Rogers' nursing conceptual model in an acute care setting. *Clinical Nurse Specialist*, 3(3), 143–147.

Heidt, P. (1981) Effect of therapeutic touch on anxiety level of hospitalized patients. *Nursing Research*, 30(1), 32–37.

Hektor, L.M. (1989) Martha E. Rogers: A life history. *Nursing Science Quarterly*, 2(2), 63–73.

Johnston, R.L., Fitzpatrick, J.J., and Donovan, M.J. (1982) Developmental stage: Relationship to temporal dimensions (Abstract). *Nursing Research*, 31, 120.

†Katz, V. (1971) Auditory stimulation and developmental behavior of the premature infant. *Nursing Research*, 20(3), 196–201.

Kim, H.S. (1983) Use of Rogers' conceptual system in research: Comments. *Nursing Research*, 32(2), 89–91.

Kim, M.J. and Moritz, D.A. (Eds.) (1982) *Classification of nursing diagnosis: Proceedings of the third and fourth national conference.* New York: McGraw-Hill.

Krieger, D. (1975) Therapeutic touch: The imprimatur of nursing. *American Journal of Nursing*, 75(5), 784–787.

Krieger, D. (1976) Healing by the laying on of hands as a facilitator of bioenergetic change: The response of in-vivo human hemoglobin. *International Journal of Psychoenergetic Systems*, 1, 121–129.

Krieger, D. (1979) *Therapeutic touch: How to use your hands to help and heal.* Englewood Cliffs, NJ: Prentice-Hall.

Krieger, D., Peper, E., and Ancoli, S. (1979) Therapeutic touch: Searching for evidence of physiological change. *American Journal of Nursing*, 79, 660–662.

Madrid, M. and Winstead-Fry, P. (1986) Rogers's conceptual model. In P. Winstead-Fry (Ed.), *Case studies in nursing theory.* New York: National League for Nursing.

Macrae, J. (1979) Therapeutic touch in practice. *American Journal of Nursing*, 79, 664–665.

Manhart, E.A. (1988) Using Rogers' science of unitary human beings in nursing practice. *Nursing Science Quarterly*, 50–51.

Moccia, P. (1985) A further investigation of "Dialectical thinking as a means of understanding systems in development: Relevance to Rogers's Principles" (Commentary). *Advances in Nursing Science*, 7(4), 33–38.

Newman, M. (1979) *Theory development in nursing.* Philadelphia: F.A. Davis.

Phillips, J.R. (1989) Science of unitary human being: Changing research perspective. *Nursing Science Quarterly*, 2(2), 57–60.

†Porter, L.S. (1972) The impact of physical-physiological activity on infant growth and development. *Nursing Research*, 21(3), 210–219.

Quillin, S.I.M. and Runk, J.A. (1983) Martha Rogers' model. In J.J. Fitzpatrick and A.L. Whall (Eds.), *Conceptual models of nursing: Analysis and application.* Bowie, MD: Robert J. Brady Co.

Quillin, S.I.M. and Runk, J.A. (1989) Martha Rogers' unitary person model. In J.J. Fitzpatrick and A.L. Whall, *Conceptual models of nursing: Analysis and application* (2nd ed.). Norwalk, CT: Appleton & Lange.

Quinn, J.F. (1979) One nurse's evolution as a healer. *American Journal of Nursing*, 79, 662–664.

Quinn, J.F. (1989) Therapeutic touch as energy exchange: Replication and extension. *Nursing Science Quarterly*, 2(2), 74–78.

Rogers, M.E. (1963) Building a strong educational foundation. *The American Journal of Nursing*, 63(6), 94–95.

Rogers, M.E. (1963) Some comments on the theoretical basis for nursing practice. *Nursing Science*, 63(1), 11–13, 60–61.

Rogers, M.E. (1964) *Reveille in nursing*. Philadelphia: F.A. Davis.

Rogers, M.E. (1969) Nursing research: Relevant to practice? *Fifth Annual Research Conference: ANA*, 352–359.

†Rogers, M.E. (1970) *An introduction to the theoretical basis of nursing*. Philadelphia: F.A. Davis.

†Rogers, M.E. (1975) Euphemisms in nursing's future. *Image*, 7(2), 3–9.

†Rogers, M.E. (1980) Nursing: A science of unitary man. In J.P. Riehl and C. Roy (Eds.), *Conceptual models for nursing practice* (2nd ed.). New York: Appleton-Century-Crofts.

Rogers, M.E. (1980) *The science of unitary man. Video-tapes.* New York: Media for Nursing.

Rogers, M.E. (1981) Beyond the horizon. In N. Chaska (Ed.), *The nursing profession: A time to speak.* New York: McGraw-Hill.

Rogers, M.E. (1981) Science of unitary man: A paradigm for nursing. In G.E. Lasker (Ed.), *Applied systems and cybernetics* (Vol. IV, pp. 219–228). New York: Pergamon Press.

Rogers, M.E. (1983, June). Nursing science: A science of unitary human beings. Paper presented at the First National Rogerian Conference, New York University.

Rogers, M.E. (1983) Science of unitary human being: A paradigm for nursing. In I.W. Clements and F.B. Roberts (Eds.), *Family health: A theoretical approach to nursing care.* New York: John Wiley & Sons.

Rogers, M.E. (1987, May) Nursing research in the future. *NLN Publications* (Publ. No. 14-2203, pp. 121–123).

Rogers, M.E. (1987) Rogers's science of unitary human beings. In R.R. Parse, *Nursing science: Major paradigms, theories, and critiques.* Philadelphia: W.B. Saunders.

Rogers, M.E. (1988) Nursing science and art: A prospective. *Nursing Science Quarterly*, 1(3), 99–102.

Rogers, M.E. (1989) Creating a climate for the implementation of a nursing conceptual framework. *Journal of Continuing Education in Nursing*, 20(3), 112–116.

Rogers, M.E. (1989) Nursing: A science of unitary human beings. In J. Riehl-Sisca, *Conceptual models for nursing practice* (3rd ed.). Norwalk, CT: Appleton & Lange.

Rossi, L. and Krekeler, K. (1982) Small-group reactions to the theoretical framework "Unitary Man" (1980). In M.J. Kim and D.A. Moritz (Eds.), *Classification of nursing diagnosis: Proceedings of the third and fourth national conference.* New York: McGraw-Hill.

Roy, C. (1980) Rogers' theoretical basis of nursing. In J.P. Riehl and C. Roy (Eds.), *Conceptual models for nursing practice* (2nd ed.). New York: Appleton-Century-Crofts.

Safier, G. (1977) *Contemporary American leaders: An oral history.* New York: McGraw-Hill.

Sanchez, R. (1989) Empathy, diversity, and telepathy in mother-daughter dyads: An empirical investigation utilizing Rogers' conceptual framework. *Scholarly Inquiry for Nursing Practice: An International Journal*, 3(1), 29–51.

Sarter, B. (1988) *The stream of becoming: A study of Martha Rogers' theory*. New York: National League for Nursing.

Sarter, B. (1989) Some critical philosophical issues in the science of unitary human being. *Nursing Science Quarterly*, 3, 74–78.

Schodt, C. (1989) Parental-fetal attachment and couvade: A study of patterns of human-environment integrality. *Nursing Science Quarterly*, 2(2), 88–97.

Smith, M.J. (1986) Human-environment process: A test of Rogers' principle of integrality. *Advances in Nursing Science*, 9(1), 21–28.

Smith, M.J. (1988) Testing propositions derived from Rogers' conceptual system. *Nursing Science Quarterly*, 60–67.

Whall, A. (1987) A critique of Rogers's framework. In R.R. Parse, *Nursing science: Major paradigms, theories, and critiques*. Philadelphia: W.B. Saunders.

†Whelton, B.J. (1979) An operationalization of Martha Rogers' theory throughout the nursing process. *International Journal of Nursing Studies*, 16, 7–20.

Uys, L.R. (1987) Foundational studies in nursing. *Journal of Advanced Nursing*, 12(3), 275–280.

In addition, the April 1979 volume of the *American Journal of Nursing* contains three articles on therapeutic touch based on Rogers' conceptual model.

Roy

Aggleton, P. and Chalmers, H. (1984) The Roy adaptation model. *Nursing Times*, 80(40), 45–48.

Andrews, H. (1989) Implementation of the Roy adaptation model: An application of educational change research. In J. Riehl-Sisca, *Conceptual models for nursing practice* (3rd ed.). Norwalk, CT: Appleton & Lange.

Andrews, H. and Roy, C. (1986) *Essentials of the Roy adaptation model*. Englewood Cliffs, NJ: Prentice-Hall.

Blue, C., Brubaker, K., Fine, J., Kirsch, M., Papazian, K., and Riester, C. (1989) Sister Callista Roy: Adaptation model. In A. Marriner-Tomey, *Nursing theorists and their work* (2nd ed.). St. Louis: C.V. Mosby.

†Brower, H.T. and Baker, D.J. (1976) Using the adaptation model in a practitioner curriculum. *Nursing Outlook*, 24(11), 686–689.

Bunting, S.B. (1988) The concept of perception in selected nursing theories. *Nursing Science Quarterly*, 1, 168–174.

Camooso, C., Green, M., and Reilly, P. (1981) Students' adaptation according to Roy. *Nursing Outlook*, 29, 108–109.

Clements, I.W. and Roberts, F.B. (Eds.) (1983) *Family health: A theoretical approach to nursing care*. New York: John Wiley & Sons.

Cottrell, B. and Shannahan, M. (1987) A comparison of fetal outcome in birth chair and delivery table births. *Nursing Research and Health*, 10, 239–243.

Dahlen, R. (1980) Analysis of selected factors related to the elderly person's ability to adapt to visual prostheses following senile cataract surgery. Doctoral dissertation, University of Maryland.

DiIorio, C. (1989) Application of the Roy model to nursing administration. In B. Henry, C. Arndt, M. DiVincenti, and A. Marriner-Tomey (Eds.), *Dimensions of nursing administration: Theory, research, education, practice*. Boston: Blackwell Scientific Publications.

Downey, C. (1974) Adaptation nursing applied to an obstetric patient. In J.P. Riehl and C. Roy (Eds.), *Conceptual models for nursing practice* (pp. 151–159). New York: Appleton-Century-Crofts.

†Farkas, L. (1981) Adaptation problems with nursing home application for elderly persons: An application of the Roy adaptation nursing model. *Journal of Advanced Nursing,* 6(5), 363–368.

Fawcett, J. (1981) Assessing and understanding the cesarean father. In C.F. Kehoe (Ed.), *The cesarean experience: Theoretical and clinical perspectives for nurses.* New York: Appleton-Century-Crofts.

Fawcett, J. (1981) Needs of cesarean birth parents. *Journal of Obstetric, Gynecologic, and Neonatal Nursing,* 10, 371–376.

Fawcett, J. (1984) Roy's adaptation model. In *Analysis and evaluation of conceptual models of nursing.* Philadelphia: F.A. Davis.

Field, P.A. (1987) The impact of nursing theory on the clinical decision making process. *Journal of Advanced Nursing,* 12(5), 563–571.

Galbreath, J.G. (1980) Sister Callista Roy. In The Nursing Theories Conference Group. *Nursing theories: The base for professional nursing practice.* Englewood Cliffs, NJ: Prentice-Hall.

†Galligan, A.C. (1979) Using Roy's concept of adaptation to care for young children. *The American Journal of Maternal Child Nursing,* 4(1), 24–28.

Goodwin, J.O. (1980) A cross-cultural approach to integrating nursing theory and practice. *Nurse Educator,* 5(6), 15–20.

Gordon, J. (1974) Nursing assessment and care plan for a cardiac patient. In J.P. Riehl and C. Roy (Eds.), *Conceptual models for nursing practice* (pp. 144–150). New York: Appleton-Century-Crofts.

Hallen, P. (1981) A holistic model of individual and family health based on a continuum of choice. *Advances in Nursing Science,* 3(4), 27–42.

Hoch, C. (1987) Assessing delivery of nursing care. *Journal of Gerontological Nursing,* 13(1), 10–17.

Huch, M.H. (1987) A critique of the Roy adaptation model. In R.R. Parse, *Nursing science: Major paradigms, theories, and critiques.* Philadelphia: W.B. Saunders.

Idle, B.A. (1978) SPAL: A tool for measuring self-perceived adaptation level appropriate for an elderly population. In E.E. Bauwens (Ed.), *Clinical nursing research: Its strategies and findings* (Monograph series No. 2). Indianapolis: Sigma Theta Tau.

†Janelli, L.M. (1980) Utilizing Roy's adaptation model from a gerontological perspective. *Journal of Gerontological Nursing,* 6(3), 140–150.

†Jones, P.S. (1978) An adaptation model for nursing practice. *American Journal of Nursing,* 78(11), 1900–1906.

Kasemwatana, S. (1982) An application of Roy's adaptation model. *Thai Journal of Nursing,* 31(1), 25–46.

Kehoe, C.F. (1981) Identifying the nursing needs of the postpartum cesarean mother. In C.F. Kehoe (Ed.), *The cesarean experience: Theoretical and clinical perspectives for nurses.* New York: Appleton-Century-Crofts.

Kehoe, C.F. and Fawcett, J. (1981) An overview of the Roy adaptation model. In C.F. Kehoe (Ed.), *The cesarean experience: Theoretical and clinical perspectives for nurses.* New York: Appleton-Century-Corfts.

Laros, J. (1977) Deriving outcome criteria from a conceptual model. *Nursing Outlook,* 25, 333–336.

Leuze, M., and McKenzie, J. (1987) Preoperative assessment: Using the Roy's adaptation model. *AORN Journal,* 46(6), 1126–1129, 1131–1134.

Levesque, L. (1980, October 22–24) Rehabilitation of the chronically ill elderly: A method of operationalizing a conceptual model for nursing. In R.C. MacKay and E.G. Zilm (Eds.), *Research for practice: Proceedings of the National Nursing Research Conference.* Halifax, Nova Scotia.

Lewis, F. et al. (1978) Measuring adaptation of chemotherapy patients. In J.C. Krueger, A.H. Nelson, and M. Opal (Eds.), *Nursing research: Development, collaboration, utilization*. Germantown, MD: Aspen Systems.

Lewis, F.M., Firsich, S.C., and Parsell, S. (1979) Clinical tool development for adult chemotherapy patients: Process and content. *Cancer Nursing*, 2(2), 99–108.

Limandri, B.J. (1986) Research and practice with abused women: Use of the Roy adaptation model as an explanatory framework. *Advances in Nursing Science*, 8(4), 52–61.

†Mastal, M.F. and Hammond, H. (1980) Analysis and expansion of the Roy adaptation model: A contribution to holistic nursing. *Advances in Nursing Science*, 2(4), 71–81.

†Mastal, M., Hammond, H., and Roberts, M. (1982, June) Theory into hospital practice: A pilot implementation. *Journal of Nursing Administration*, 12(6), 9–15.

Mengel, A., Sherman, S., Nahigian, E., and Coleman, I. (1989) Adaptation of the Roy model in an educational setting. In J. Riehl-Sisca, *Conceptual models for nursing practice* (3rd ed.). Norwalk, CT: Appleton & Lange.

Norris, S., Campbell, L., and Brenkert, S. (1982) Nursing procedures and alterations in transcutaneous oxygen tension in premature infants. *Nursing Research*, 31(6), 330–336.

Pioli, C. and Sandor, J. (1989) The Roy adaptation model: An analysis. In J. Riehl-Sisca, *Conceptual models for nursing practice* (3rd ed.). Norwalk, CT: Appleton & Lange.

Porth, C.M. (1977) Physiological coping: A model for teaching pathophysiology. *Nursing Outlook*, 25, 781–784.

Rambo, B. (1984) *Adaptation nursing: Assessment and intervention*. Philadelphia: W.B. Saunders.

Randell, B., Tedrow, M., and van Landingham, J. (1982) *Adaptation nursing: The Roy conceptual model applied*. St. Louis: C.V. Mosby.

Roy, C. (1967) Role cues and mothers of hospitalized children. *Nursing Research*, 16(2), 178–182.

†Roy, C. (1970) Adaptation: A conceptual framework for nursing. *Nursing Outlook*, 18(3), 42–45.

†Roy, C. (1971) Adaptation: A basis for nursing practice. *Nursing Outlook*, 19(4), 254–257.

Roy, C. (1973) Adaptation: Implications for curriculum change. *Nursing Outlook*, 21(3), 163–168.

Roy, C. (1975) Adaptation framework. In *Curriculum innovation through framework application*. Loma Linda, CA: Loma Linda University.

Roy, C. (1975) The impact of nursing diagnosis. *AORN Journal*, 21(6), 1023–1030.

Roy, C. (1976) *Introduction to nursing: An adaptational model*. Englewood Cliffs, NJ: Prentice-Hall.

†Roy, C. (1976) The Roy adaptation model: Comment. *Nursing Outlook*, 24(11), 690–691.

Roy, C. (1977) *Decision-making by the physically ill and adaptation during illness*. Doctoral dissertation, University of California, Los Angeles.

Roy, C. (1978) The stress of hospital events: Measuring changes in level of stress. In M.V. Batey (Ed.), *Symposium on stress: Conference on communicating nursing research*. Boulder, CO: Western Interstate Commission on Higher Education.

Roy, C. (1979, December) Nursing diagnosis from the perspective of a nursing model. *Nursing Diagnosis Newsletter* (Vol. 6) St. Louis: St. Louis School of Nursing.

†Roy, C. (1979) Relating nursing theory to education: A new era. *Nurse Educator*, 4(2), 16–21.

*Roy, C. (1980) The Roy adaptation model. In J.P. Riehl and C. Roy (Eds.), *Conceptual models for nursing practice* (2nd ed.). New York: Appleton-Century-Crofts.

Roy, C. (1981) *Introduction to nursing: An adaptation model*. Englewood Cliffs, NJ: Prentice-Hall.

Roy, C. (1981) A systems model of nursing care and its effect on the quality of human life. In *Proceedings of the International Congress on Applied Systems Research and Cybernetics*. London: Pergamon Press.

Roy, C. (1982) *Introduction to nursing: An adaptation model*. (Japanese translation by Yuriko Kanematsu.) Japan: UNI Agency.

Roy, C. (1983) The expectant family: Analysis and application of the Roy adaptation model. In I.W. Clements and F.B. Roberts (Eds.), *Family health: A theoretical approach to nursing care*. New York: John Wiley & Sons.

Roy, C. (1983) The family in primary care: Analysis and application of the Roy adaptation model. In I.W. Clements and F.B. Roy, C. (1987) Response to "Needs of spouses of surgical patients: A conceptualization within the Roy adaptation model." *Scholarly Inquiry for Nursing Practice*, 1(1), 45–50.

Roy, C. (1983) Roy adaptation model. In I.W. Clements and F.B. Roberts (Eds.), *Family health: A theoretical approach to nursing care*. New York: John Wiley & Sons.

Roy, C. (1983) Theory development in nursing: A proposal for direction. In N. Chaska (Ed.), *The nursing profession: A time to speak*. New York: McGraw-Hill.

Roy, C. (1984) *Introduction to nursing: An adaptation model* (2nd ed.). Englewood Cliffs, NJ: Prentice-Hall.

Roy, C. (1987) Response to "Needs of spouses of surgical patients: A conceptualization within the Roy adaptation model." *Scholarly Inquiry for Nursing Practice*, 1, 45–50.

Roy, C. (1987) Roy's adaptation model. In R.R. Parse, *Nursing science: Major paradigms, theories, and critiques*. Philadelphia: W.B. Saunders.

Roy, C. (1988) An explication of the philosophical assumptions of the Roy adaptation model. *Nursing Science Quarterly*, 1(1), 26–34.

Roy, C. (1988) Human information processing. *Annual Review of Nursing Research*, 6, 237–262.

Roy, C. (1989) The Roy adaptation model. In J. Riehl-Sisca, *Conceptual models for nursing practice* (3rd ed.). Norwalk, CT: Appleton & Lange.

Roy, C. and Anway, J. (1989) Roy's adaptation model: Theories for nursing administration. In B. Henry, C. Arndt, M. DiVincenti, and A. Marriner-Tomey (Eds.), *Dimensions of nursing administration: Theory, research, education, practice*. Boston: Blackwell Scientific Publications.

Roy, C. and McLeod, D. (1981) Theory of the person as an adaptive system. In C. Roy and S.L. Roberts, *Theory construction in nursing: An adaptation model* (pp. 49–69). Englewood Cliffs, NJ: Prentice-Hall.

Roy, C. and Obloy, M. (1978) The practitioner movement: Toward a science of nursing. *American Journal of Nursing*, 78, 1698–1701.

Roy, C. and Roberts, S. (1981) *Theory construction in nursing: An adaptation model*. Englewood Cliffs, NJ: Prentice-Hall.

Sato, M. (1986) The Roy adaptation model. In P. Winstead-Fry (Ed.), *Case studies in nursing theory*. New York: National League for Nursing.

†Schmitz, M. (1980) The Roy adaptation model: Application in a community setting. In J.P. Riehl and C. Roy (Eds.), *Conceptual models for nursing practice* (2nd ed.). (pp. 193–206). New York: Appleton-Century-Crofts.

Silva, M.C. (1987) Needs of spouses of surgical patients: A conceptualization within the Roy adaptation model. *Scholarly Inquiry for Nursing Practice*, 1, 29–44.

Smith, M. (1988) Roy adaptation model in practice. *Nursing Science Quarterly*, 1(2), 97–98.

†Starr, S.L. (1980) Adaptation applied to the dying patient. In J.P. Riehl and C. Roy (Eds.), *Conceptual models for nursing practice* (2nd ed.). New York: Appleton-Century-Crofts.

Tiedman, M.E. (1983) The Roy adaptation model. In J.J. Fitzpatrick and A.L. Whall, *Conceptual models of nursing: Analysis and application.* Bowie, MD: Robert J. Brady Co.

Tiedman, M.E. (1989) The Roy adaptation model. In J.J. Fitzpatrick and A.L. Whall, *Conceptual models of nursing: Analysis and application* (2nd ed.). Norwalk, CT: Appleton & Lange.

†Wagner, P. (1976) The Roy adaptation model: Testing the adaptation model in practice. *Nursing Outlook,* 24(11), 682–685.

Travelbee

Cook, L. (1989) Nurses in crisis: A support group based on Travelbee's nursing theory. *Nursing and Health Care,* 10(4), 203–205.

Doona, M.E. (1979) *Travelbee's intervention in psychiatric nursing* (2nd ed.). Philadelphia: F.A. Davis.

Frankel, V. (1963) *Man's search for meaning: An introduction to logotherapy.* New York: Washington Square Press.

Freihofer, P. and Felton, G. (1976) Nursing behaviors in bereavement: An exploratory study. *Nursing Research,* 25(5), 332–337.

Gadow, S. (1980) Introduction. In Spickor and S. Gadow (Eds.), *Nursing: Images and ideals—Opening dialogue with the humanities.* New York: Springer-Verlag.

Hobble, W., Lansinger, T., and Magers, J. (1989) Joyce Travelbee: Human-to-human relationship. In A. Marriner-Tomey, *Nursing theorists and their work* (2nd ed.). St. Louis: C.V. Mosby.

McBride, M.A. (1967) Nursing approach, pain, and relief: An exploratory experiment. *Nursing Research,* 16(4), 337–341.

Sloane, A. (1966) Review of "Interpersonal aspects of nursing" by J. Travelbee. *American Journal of Nursing,* 66(6), 77.

Stetler, C. (1977) Relationship of perceived empathy of nurses' communication. *Nursing Research,* 26(6), 432–438.

†Travelbee, J. (1963) What do we mean by "rapport"? *American Journal of Nursing,* 63(2), 70–72.

Travelbee, J. (1964) What's wrong with sympathy? *American Journal of Nursing,* 64(1), 68–71.

Travelbee, J. (1969) *Intervention in psychiatric nursing.* New York: Springer-Verlag.

Travelbee, J. (1971) *Interpersonal aspects of nursing* (2nd ed.). Philadelphia: F.A. Davis.

Travelbee, J. (1971) The nature of nursing. In J. Travelbee, *Interpersonal aspects of nursing* (2nd ed.). (pp. 7–21). Philadelphia: F.A. Davis.

Wolff, I.S. (1966, July) Review of "Interpersonal aspects of nursing" by J. Travelbee. *Nursing Outlook,* 1504–1506.

Watson

Bennet, P., Porter, B., and Sloan, R. (1989) Jean Watson: Philosophy and science of caring. In A. Marriner-Tomey, *Nursing theorists and their work* (2nd ed.). St. Louis: C.V. Mosby.

Boyd, C. and Mast, D. (1989) Watson's model of human care. In J.J. Fitzpatrick and A.L. Whall, *Conceptual models of nursing: Analysis and application* (2nd ed.). Norwalk, CT: Appleton & Lange.

Clayton, G. (1989) Research testing Watson's theory: The phenomena of caring in an elderly population. In J. Riehl-Sisca, *Conceptual models for nursing practice* (3rd ed.). Norwalk, CT: Appleton & Lange.

Jones, N., Kearins, J., and Watson, J. (1987) The human tongue show and observers willingness to interact: Replication and extensions. *Psychology Reports*, 60(3, Part 1), 759–764.

Krysl, M. and Watson, J. (1988) Existential moments of caring: Facets of nursing and social support. *Advances in Nursing Science*, 10(2), 12–17.

Ryan, L. (1989) A critique of nursing: Human science and human care. In J. Richl-Sisca, *Conceptual models for nursing practice* (3rd ed.). Norwalk, CT: Appleton & Lange.

Sithichoke-Rattan, N. (1989) A clinical application of Watson's theory. *Pediatric Nursing*, 15(5), 458–462.

Watson, J. (1979) *Nursing: The philosophy and science of caring.* Boston: Little, Brown & Co.

Watson, J. (1981) Conceptual systems of students, practitioners. *Western Journal of Nursing Research*, 3, 197–198.

Watson, J. (1981) The lost art of nursing. *Nursing Forum*, 20, 244–249.

Watson, J. (1981) Some issues related to a science of caring for nursing practice. In M. Leininger (Ed.), *Caring: An essential human need.* Thorofare, NJ: Charles Slack.

Watson, J. (1985) *Nursing: Human science and human care.* Norwalk, CT: Appleton-Century-Crofts.

Watson, J. (1987, May) The dream curriculum. *NLN Publications* (Publ. No. 15-2179, pp. 91–104).

Watson, J. (1987, December) The professional doctorate as an entry level into practice. *NLN Publications* (Publ. No. 41-2199, pp. 41–47).

Watson, J. (1987) Nursing on the caring edge: Metaphorical vignettes. *Advances in Nursing Science*, 10(1), 10–18.

Watson, J. (1988) New dimensions of human caring theory. *Nursing Science Quarterly*, 1(4), 175–181.

Watson, J. (1988, October) An ethic of caring/curing/nursing qua nursing: Introduction. *NLN Publications* (Publ. No. 15-2237, pp. 1–3).

Watson, J. (1988) Human caring as moral context for nursing education. *Nursing and Health Care*, 9(8), 422–425.

Watson, J. (1988, August) A case study: Curriculum in transition. *NLN Publications* (Publ. No. 15-2224, pp. 1–8).

Watson, J. (1988, May) Nursing: Human science and human care. A theory of nursing. *NLN Publications* (Publ. No. 15-2236, pp. 1–104).

Watson, J. (1989) Watson's philosophy and theory of human caring. In J. Riehl-Sisca, *Conceptual models for nursing practice* (3rd ed.). Norwalk, CT: Appleton & Lange.

Wiedenbach

Bennett, A.M. and Foster, P.C. (1980) Ernestine Wiedenbach. In the Nursing Theories Conference Group, *Nursing theories: The base for professional nursing practice.* Englewood Cliffs, NJ: Prentice-Hall.

Clausen, J. et al. (1977) *Maternity nursing today.* New York: McGraw-Hill.

Danko, M., Hunt, N., Marich, J., Marriner-Tomey, A., McCreary, C., and Stuart, M. (1989) Ernestine Wiedenbach: The helping art of clinical nursing. In A. Marriner-Tomey, *Nursing theorists and their work* (2nd ed.). St. Louis: C.V. Mosby.

Dickoff, J., James, P., and Wiedenbach, E. (1968) Theory in a practice discipline. *Nursing Research*, 19(5), 415–427.

Diers, D. (1966) The nurse orientation system: A method for analyzing nurse-patient interactions. *Nursing Research*, 15(1), 91.

Dracup, K. and Breu, C. (1978) Using nursing research findings to meet the needs of grieving spouses. *Nursing Research*, 27(4), 212–216.

Dumas, R. and Leonard, R. (1963) The effect of nursing on the incidence of postoperative vomiting. *Nursing Research*, 12(1), 12–15.

Eisler, J., Wolfer, J.A., and Diers, D. (1972) Relationship between the need for social approval and postoperative recovery welfare. *Nursing Research*, 21(5), 520–525.

Elms, R.R. and Leonard, R.C. (1966) Effects of nursing approaches during admission. *Nursing Research*, 15(1), 37–48.

Larson, P.A. (1977) Nurse perception of client illness. *Nursing Research*, 26(6), 416–421.

Leonard, R.C., Skipper, J.K., and Woolridge, P.J. (1967) Small sample field experiments for evaluating patient care. *Health Services Research*, 2(1), 46–50.

Raleigh, E. (1983) Wiedenbach's model. In J.J. Fitzpatrick and A.L. Whall (Eds.), *Conceptual models of nursing: Analysis and application*. Bowie, MD: Robert J. Brady Co.

Raleigh, E. (1989) Wiedenbach's model of nursing practice. In J.J. Fitzpatrick and A.L. Whall, *Conceptual models of nursing: Analysis and application* (2nd ed.). Norwalk, CT: Appleton & Lange.

Rickelman, B.L. (1971) Bio-psycho-social linguistics: A conceptual approach to nurse-patient interaction. *Nursing Research*, 20(5), 398–403.

Shields, D. (1978) Nursing care in labor and patient satisfaction. A descriptive study. *Journal of Advances in Nursing*, 3, 535–550.

Wiedenbach, E. (1962, June) A concept of dynamic nursing: Philosophy, purpose, practice, and process. A Conference on Maternal and Child Nursing, University of Pittsburg School of Nursing.

Wiedenbach, E. (1963) The helping art of nursing. *American Journal of Nursing*, 63(11), 54–57.

Wiedenbach, E. (1964) *Clinical nursing: A helping art*. New York: Springer-Verlag.

Wiedenbach, E. (1965, December) Family nurse practitioner for maternal and child care. *Nursing Outlook*, 13, 50–51.

Wiedenbach, E. (1968) Nurse's role in family planning: A conceptual base for practice. *Nursing Clinics of North America*, 3(2), 355–365.

Wiedenbach, E. (1969) *Meeting the realities in clinical teaching*. New York: Springer-Verlag.

Wiedenbach, E. (1970) Comment on beliefs and values: Basis for curriculum design. *Nursing Research*, 19(5), 427.

Wiedenbach, E. (1970) Nurses' wisdom in nursing theory. *American Journal of Nursing*, 70(5), 1057–1062.

Wiedenbach, E. (1973) The nursing process in maternity nursing. In J.P. Clausen et al., *Maternity nursing today*. New York: McGraw-Hill.

Wiedenbach, E. and Falls, C.E. (1978) *Communication: Key to effective nursing*. New York: Tiresias Press.

Wolfer, J. and Visintainer, M. (1975) Pediatric surgical patients' and parents' stress responses and adjustment. *Nursing Research*, 24(4), 244–255.

PARADIGMS THAT HAVE INFLUENCED NURSING

14. Psychoanalytic Theory

Alexander, F. (1958) Unexplored areas in psychoanalytic theory and treatment. *Behavioral Sciences*, 3, 293–316.

Brams, J. (1968) From Freud to Fromm. *Psychology Today*, 1, 32–35, 64–65.

Brenner, C. (1973) *An elementary textbook of psychoanalysis*. Garden City, NY: International Universities Press.

Brill, A.A. (1922) *Psychoanalysis, its theories and practical application* (3rd ed.). Philadelphia: W.B. Saunders.

Brill, A.A. (1969) Basic principles of psychoanalysis (1921). Garden City, NY: Doubleday & Co.

Burchard, E.M.L. (1960) Mystical and scientific aspects of the psychoanalytic theories of Freud, Adler, and Jung. *American Journal of Psychotherapy*, 15, 289–307.

Chertok, L. (1968) From Liebeault to Freud. *American Journal of Psychotherapy*, 22, 96–101.

Corsini, R. (1977) *Current personality theories*. Itasca IL: F.A. Peacock.

Desmonde, W.H., Mead, G.H., and Freud, S. (1957) American social psychology and psychoanalysis. *Psychoanalysis*, 4 & 5, 31–50.

Engel, G.L. (1980) The clinical application of the biopsychosocial model. *American Journal of Psychiatry*, 137(5), 535–544.

Engel, G.L. (1977, April) The need for a new medical model: A challenge for biomedicine. *Science*, 196, 129–135.

Fenichel, O. (1945) *The psychoanalytic theory of neurosis* (pp. 3–13). New York: W.W. Norton.

Fine, R. (1962) *Freud: A critical re-evaluation of his theories*. New York: McKay.

Fine, R. (1979) *A history of psychoanalysis*. New York: Columbia University Press.

Freedman, A., Kaplan, H., and Sadock, B. (1976) *Modern synopsis of comprehensive psychiatry* (2nd ed.). Baltimore: Williams & Wilkins.

Ford, D.H. and Urban, H.B. (1963) *Systems of psychotherapy: A comparative study*. New York: John Wiley & Sons.

Freud, S. (1924) *The complete introductory lectures on psychoanalysis*. New York: Pocket Books.

Freud, S. (1924) *A general introduction to psycho-analysis*. New York: Pocket Books.

Freud, S. (1925–1950) *Collected papers* (Vols. I–V). London: Hogarth.

Freud, S. (1938) The basic writings of Sigmund Freud, A.A. Brill (Ed.). New York: Random House.

Freud, S. (1946) An autobiographical study (1935), rev'd ed. London: Hogarth.

Freud, S. (1953–1955) *The standard edition of the complete psychological works* (24 Vols.). J. Strachey (Trans.). London: Hogarth.

Freud, S. (1954) *The origin of psychoanalysis: Letters to Wilhelm Fleiss*. E. Mosbacher and J. Strachey (Trans.), M. Bonaparte, A. Freud, and E. Dris (Eds.). New York: Basic Books.

Freud, S. (1957) *A general selection of the works of Sigmund Freud*. J. Rickman (Ed.). New York: Liveright.

Freud, S. (1959) *Beyond the pleasure principle*. J. Strachey, (Trans.). New York: Bantam Books.

Freud, S. (1959) *Collected papers*. New York: Basic Books.

Freud, S. (1962) *The ego and the id*. J. Riviere and J. Strachey (Trans.). New York: W.W. Norton.

Freud, S. (1963) *Dora: An analysis of a case of hysteria*. P. Reiff (Ed.). New York: Macmillan.

Freud, S. (1965) *The interpretation of dreams*. J. Strachey (Ed.). New York: Avon Books.

Freud, S. (1965) *The psychopathology of everyday life*. New York: W.W. Norton.

Freud, S. (1966) *On the history of the psychoanalytic movement*. New York: W.W. Norton.

Freud, S. (1969) *An outline of psycho-analysis*. New York: W.W. Norton.

Glover, E. (1959) *Freud or Jung*. New York: W.W. Norton.

Goshen, C.E. (1952) The original case material of psychoanalysis. *American Journal of Psychiatry*, 108, 829–832.

Hall, C. (1954) *A primer of Freudian psychology*. New York: New American Library.

Hall, C.S. and Lindzey, G. (1970) *Theories of personality*. New York: John Wiley & Sons.

Janger J. (1968) *Theories of development*. New York: Holt, Rinehart & Winston.

Johnstone, R.L. (1982) Individual psychotherapy: Relationship of theoretical approaches to nursing conceptual models. In J.J. Fitzpatrick, A.L. Whall, R.L. Johnstone, and J.S. Floyd (Eds.), *Nursing models and their psychiatric mental health applications*. Bowie, MD: Robert J. Brady.

Jones, E. (1953, 1955, 1957) *The life and work of Sigmund Freud* (3 Vols.). New York: Basic Books.

Kardinar, A., Karush, A., and Ovesey, L. (1966) A methodological study of Freudian theory. *International Journal of Psychiatry*, 2, 489–544.

Kolb, L.C. (1977) *Modern clinical psychiatry*. Philadelphia: W.B. Saunders.

Krech, D. and Klein, G.S. (1966) *Theoretical models and personality theory*. New York: Greenwood Press.

Mahler, M. et al. (1975) *The psychological birth of the human infant*. New York: Basic Books.

Mehrabian, A. (1968) *An analysis of personality theories*. Englewood Cliffs, NJ: Prentice-Hall.

Munroe, R.L. (1955) *Schools of psychoanalytic thought*. New York: Dryden Press.

Murphy, G. (1956) The current impact of Freud upon psychology. *American Psychologist*, 11, 663–672.

Pervin, L.A. (1975) *Personality: Theory, assessment, and research*. New York: John Wiley & Sons.

Reiser, M.F. (1979) Psychosomatic medicine: A meeting ground for oriental and occidental medical theory and practice. *Psychotherapy Psychosomatic*, 31, 315–323.

Schmid, F. (1952) Freud's sociological thinking. *Bulletin of the Menninger Clinic*, 16, 1–13.

Shakow, N. and Rapaport, D. (1964) The influence of Freud on American psychology. *Psychological Issues*, 4, 1–243.

Shaw, M.E. and Costanzo, P.R. (1982) *Theories of social psychology* (2nd ed.). New York: McGraw-Hill.

Sherman, M.H. (1966) *Psychoanalysis in America*. Springfield, IL: Charles C. Thomas.

Sherwood, M. (1969) *The logic of explanation in psychoanalysis*. New York: Academic Press.

Stafford-Clark, D. (1967) *What Freud really said*. New York: Schoken Books.

Stone, I. (1971) *The passions of the mind*. New York: Doubleday & Co.

Toman, W. (1960) *An introduction to psychoanalytic theory of motivation*. New York: Pergamon Press.

Turiell, E. (1967) An historical analysis of the Freudian conception of the superego. *Psychoanalytical Review*, 54, 118–140.

Waelder, R. (1960) *Basic theory of psychoanalysis*. New York: International Universities Press.

West, R. (1967) The social significance of the uncompleted father analysis of Sigmund Freud. *Psychotherapy Psychosomatic*, 15, 69.

Wolff, P.H. (1960) *The developmental psychologies of Jean Piaget and psychoanalysis*. New York: International University Press.

15. Symbolic Interaction

Allport, G.W. (1955) *Becoming: Basic considerations for a psychology of personality.* New Haven, CT: Yale University Press.

Banton, M. (1965) *Roles: An introduction to the study of social relations.* New York: Basic Books.

Biddle, B.J. and Thomas, E.J. (1966) *Role theory: Concepts and research.* New York, John Wiley & Sons.

Blasi, A. (1972) Symbolic interactions as theory. *Sociology and Social Research,* 56(4), 453–455.

Blumer, H. (1966) Sociological implications of the thought of George Herbert Mead, *American Journal of Sociology,* 71, 535–544.

Blumer, H. (1969) *Symbolic interactionism: Perspective and method.* Englewood Cliffs, NJ: Prentice-Hall.

Blumer, H. (1980) Mead and Blumer: The convergent methodological perspectives of social behaviorism and symbolic interactionism. *American Sociological Review,* 45, 409–419.

Bower, F. and Jacobson, M.J. (1979) Family theories: Frameworks for nursing practice. In S.E. Archer and R. Fleshman (Eds.), *Community health nursing: Patterns and practice* (2nd ed.). North Scituate, MA: Duxbury Press.

Burr, W.R., Leigh, G.K., Day, R.D., and Constantine, J. (1979) Symbolic interaction and the family. In W.R. Burr, R. Hill, F.I. Nye, and I.L. Reiss, (Eds.): *Contemporary theories about the family, Vol 2: General theories/theoretical orientations.* New York: Free Press.

Charon, J. (1979) *Symbolic interaction.* Englewood Cliffs, NJ: Prentice-Hall.

Coser, L.A. (1971) George Herbert Mead, 1863–1931. In *Masters of sociological thought* (pp. 333–355). New York: Harcourt Brace Jovanovich.

Cottrell, L.S., Jr. (1942) The adjustment of the individual to his age and sex roles. *American Sociological Review,* 7, 617–620.

Gordon, C. and Gerzen, K.J. (1968) *The self in social interaction, (Vol. I): Classic and contemporary perspectives.* New York: John Wiley & Sons.

Gordon, G. (1966) *Role theory and illness: A sociological perspective.* New Haven, CT: College and University Press.

Hammer, M.L. (1977) Symbols of aging as perceived by the young. *Journal of Gerontological Nursing,* 3(4), 17–18.

Hewitt, J. (1983) *Self and society: A symbolic interactionist social psychology* (3rd ed.) Boston: Allyn & Bacon.

Huber, J. (1973) Symbolic interaction as a pragmatic perspective: The bias of emergent theory. *American Sociological Review,* 38(2), 274–284.

Kuhn, M.H. (1964) Major trends in symbolic interaction theory in the past twenty-five years. *Sociological Quarterly,* 5, 61–84.

Laborde, J.M. (1979) Symbolism and gift-giving in family therapy. *Journal of Psychiatric Nursing,* 17(4), 32–35.

Linton, R. (1936) *The study of man.* New York: Appleton-Century-Crofts.

Manis, J.G. and Meltzer, B.N. (1972) *Symbolic interaction* (2nd ed.). Boston: Allyn & Bacon.

McPhail, C. and Rexroth, C. (1979) The divergent methodological perspectives of social behaviorism and symbolic interactionism. *American Sociological Review,* 44, 449–467.

Mead, G.H. (1937) *Mind, self and society.* Introduction by C.W. Morris. Chicago: University of Chicago Press.

Mead, G.H. (1956) *The Social Psychology of G.H. Mead.* Edited and with revised introduction by A. Strauss. Chicago: University of Chicago Press.

Meltzer, B.N. (1972) Mead's social psychology. In J.G. Manis and B.N. Meltzer (Eds.), *Symbolic interaction: A reader in social psychology* (2nd ed.). Boston: Allyn & Bacon.

Mowrer, O.H. (1960) *Learning theory and the symbolic process.* New York: John Wiley & Sons.

Porter, S.F. (1978) Interaction modeling: An educational strategy for new graduate leadership development. *Journal of Nursing Administration,* 8(4), 20–24.

Rickelman, B.L. (1971) Bio-psycho-social linguistics: A conceptual approach to nurse-patient interaction. *Nursing Research,* 20(5), 398–403.

Riehl, J.P. (1974) Application of interaction theory. In J.P. Riehl and C. Roy (Eds.), *Conceptual models for nursing practice.* New York: Appleton-Century-Crofts.

Rose, A. (1960) Incomplete socialization: Sociology and socialization. *Nursing Research,* 44, 244–250.

Rose, A. (Ed.). (1962) *Human behavior and social processes: An interactional approach.* Boston: Houghton-Mifflin.

Rose, A. (1974) A systematic summary of symbolic interaction theory. In J.P. Riehl and C. Roy (Eds.), *Conceptual models for nursing practice* (pp. 34–46). New York: Appleton-Century-Crofts.

Sarbin, T. (1954) Role theory. In G. Lindzey (Ed.), *Handbook of social psychology* (Vol. 1, pp. 223–258). Cambridge, MA: Addison-Wesley.

Sarbin, T. (1968) Role theory. In G. Lindzey and E. Aronson (Eds.), *Handbook of social psychology* (Vol. 1) (2nd ed.). (pp. 488–567). Cambridge, MA: Addison-Wesley.

Schroeder, K.A. (1981) Symbolic interactionism: A conceptual framework useful for nurses working with obese persons. *Image,* 13(3), 78–81.

Shibutani, T. (1961) *Society and personality.* Englewood Cliffs, NJ: Prentice-Hall.

Shott, S. (1979) Emotion and social life: A symbolic interactionist analysis. *American Journal of Sociology,* 84(2), 1317–1334.

Simmel, G. (1964) *The sociology of Geroge Simmel.* Translated and edited by K.H. Wolff. New York: Free Press.

Strauss, A. (Ed.). (1956) *The social psychology of George H. Mead.* Chicago: University of Chicago Press.

Strauss, A. (1977) Sociological theories of personality. In R. Corsini (Ed.), *Current personality theories* (pp. 277–281). Itasca, IL: F.E. Peacock Publisher.

Strauss, A. and Fisher, B.M. (1978) Interactionism (Working Paper), University of California San Francisco and New York University.

Stryker, S. (1959) Symbolic interaction as an approach to family research. *Marriage Family Living,* 21, 111–119.

Turner, R.H. (1956) Role taking, role standpoint, and reference group behavior. *American Journal of Sociology,* 61, 316–328.

Turner, R.H. (1962) Role taking: Process vs. conformity. In A. Rose (Ed.), *Human behavior and social processes* (pp. 20–40). Boston: Houghton-Mifflin.

Turner, R.H. (1968) The self-conception in social interaction. In C. Gordon and K.J. Gergen (Eds.), *Self in social interaction.* New York: John Wiley & Sons.

Turner, R.H. (1970) *Family interaction.* New York: John Wiley & Sons.

Turner, R.H. (1978) *The structure of sociological theory* (2nd ed.), Chapters 14–17. Homewood, IL: The Dorsey Press.

16. Holism

Abbot, E.A. (1984) *Flatland: A romance of many dimensions*. New York: Signet.

Agan, R.D. (1987) Intuitive knowing as a dimension of nursing. *Advances in Nursing Science,* 10(1), 63–70.

Duhl, L. (1986) Health and the inner and outer self. *Journal of Humanistic Psychology,* 26(3), 46–61.

Flynn, P. (1980) *Holistic health*. Bowie, MD: Robert J. Brady Co.

Fuller, G. (1978) Holistic man and the science and practice of nursing. *Nursing Outlook,* 26(11), 700–704.

Harmon, W. and Rheingold, H. (1984) *Higher creativity: Liberating the unconscious for breakthrough insights*. Los Angeles, CA: Jeremy P. Tarcher.

Mast, D. (1986) Effects of imagery. *Image,* 18(3), 118–120.

Schnect, K. (1985) Convergence, energy and optimal health. *Journal of Holistic Medicine,* 7(2), 178–193.

Smith, M. (1984) Transformation: The key to shaping nursing. *Image,* 16(1), 28–30.

Stevens, B. (1984) *Nursing theory: Analysis, application, evaluation* (2nd ed.). Boston: Little, Brown & Co.

17. Organizational Theory

Astley, W.G. (1985) Administrative science as socially constructed truth. *Administrative Science Quarterly,* 30, 497–513.

Daffe, R.L. (1986) *Organization theory and design* (2nd ed.). St. Paul: West.

Hegyvary, S., Duxbury, M., Hall, R., Krueger, J., Lindeman, C., Scott, J., and Scott, W. (1987) *The evolution of nursing professional organizations: Alternative models for the future*. Kansas City, MO: American Academy of Nursing.

Jennings, B.M. and Meleis, A.I. (1988) Nursing theory and administrative nursing practice: Agenda for the 1990s. *Advances in Nursing Science,* 10(3), 56–69.

Kast, F.E. and Rosenzweig, J.E. (1985) Chapter 1: The subject is organizations (pp. 3–22). In *Organization and management: A systems and contingency approach*. New York: McGraw-Hill.

Rakich, J., Longest, B., and Darr, K. (1985) *Managing health services organization* (2nd ed.). Philadelphia: W.B. Saunders.

Scott, W. (1987) Chapter 1: The subject is organizations (pp. 3–27). In *Organizations: Rational, natural and open systems*. Englewood Cliffs, NJ: Prentice-Hall.

18. Developmental Theory

Almy, M. (Ed.) (1967) *Young children's thinking*. New York: Teachers' College Press.

Baltes, P.B. (1987) Theoretical propositions of life-span developmental psychology: On the dynamics between growth and decline. *Developmental Psychology,* 23(5), 611–626.

Burnside, I.M., Ebersole, P., and Monea, H.E. (Eds.). (1979) *Psychosocial caring throughout the life span*. New York: McGraw-Hill.

Buhler, C. (1935) The curve of life as studied in biographies. *Journal of Applied Psychology,* 19, 405–409.

Buhler, C. (1959) Theoretical observations about life's tendencies. *American Journal of Psychotherapy,* 13(3), 561–581.

Buhler C. and Massarik, F. (1968) *The course of human life*. New York: Springer-Verlag.

Caldwell, B.M. and Richmond, J.B. (1962) The impact of theories of child development. *Children*, 9(2), 73–78.

Capps, D., Capps, W., and Bradford, M.G. (Eds.). (1977) *Encounter with Erikson*. Missoula, MT: Scholars Press.

Carroll E. (1977) *Human emotions*. New York: Plenum Press.

Chin, R. (1980) Developmental models. In J. Riehl and C. Roy (Eds.), *Conceptual models for nursing practice* (2nd ed.) (pp. 55–59). New York: Appleton-Century-Crofts.

Coles, R. (1970) *Erik H. Erikson*. Boston: Little, Brown & Co.

Davis, G. and Jones, A. (1980) Theories of personality development. In J. Lancaster (Ed.) *Adult psychiatric nursing: Current clinical nursing series*. Garden City, NY: Medical Examination Publishing Co.

Donabedian, A. (1966) Evaluating the quality of medical care. *Milbank Memorial Fund Quarterly*, 44(2), 174.

Erikson, E.H. (1953) Growth and crises of the healthy personality. In Kluckhohn and Murray (Eds.), *Personality in nature, society and culture*. New York: Alfred Knopf.

Erikson, E.H. (1964) Inner and outer space: Reflections on womanhood. *Daedalus*, 93(2).

Erikson, E.H. (1970) The quest for identity. *Newsweek*, December 21, 1976.

Erikson, E.H. (1978) Adulthood. New York: W.W. Norton.

Erikson, E.H. and Smelser, N. (Eds.). (1980) *Themes of work and love in adulthood*. Cambridge, MA: Harvard University Press.

Evans, R.I. (1967) *Dialogue with Erik Erikson* (pp. 11–58). New York: Harper & Row.

Flavel, J. (1963) *The developmental psychology of Jean Piaget*. Princeton, NJ: D. Nostrand Co.

Frenkel, E.B. (1968) Adjustments and reorientation in the course of the life span. In B.L. Neugarten (Ed.), *Middle age and aging* (pp. 77–84). Chicago: University of Chicago Press.

Furth, H.G. (1981) *Piaget and knowledge* (2nd ed.). Chicago: University of Chicago Press.

Goode, W. (1973) *Explorations in social theory*. London: Oxford University Press.

Gould, R.L. (1972) The phases of adult life: A study in developmental psychology. *American Journal of Psychiatry*, 129(5), 521.

Gruen, W. (1964) Adult personality: An empirical study of Erikson's theory of ego development. In B.L. Neugarten (Ed.), *Personality in middle and late life*. New York: Atherton Press.

Haan, N. (1976) Personality organizations of well-functioning younger people and older adults. *International Aging and Human Development*, 7(2), 117–127.

Handel, A. (1987) Personal theories about the life-span development of one's self in autobiographical self-presentations of adults. *Human Development*, 30, 83–98.

Harris, D.B. (Ed.). (1957) *The concept of development: An issue in the study of human behavior*. Minneapolis: University Press.

Harris, D.B. (1957) *Problems in formulating a scientific concept of development. The concept of development* (pp. 3—14). Minneapolis: University Press.

Janosik, E. (1982) Aspects of group development: Stages and levels. In E.H. Janosik and L.B. Phipps (Eds.), *Lifecycle group work in nursing*. Monterey, CA: Wadsworth.

Kimmel, D.C. (1980) *Adulthood and aging: An interdisciplinary developmental view* (2nd ed.). New York: John Wiley & Sons.

Kuhlen, R.G. (1968) Developmental changes in motivation during the adult years. In B.L. Neugarten (Ed.), *Middle age and aging*. Chicago: University of Chicago Press.

Lazarus, R.S. (1966) Psychological stress and the coping process. New York: McGraw-Hill.

LeFrancois, G.R. (1972) *Psychological theories and human learning: Kongor's report*. Monterey, CA: Brooks/Cole.

Levinson, D.J. (1978) *The seasons of a man's life*. New York: Ballantine Books.

Lidz, T. (1976) *The life cycle. The person* (2nd ed.). New York: Basic Books.

Loft, W.R. and Svoboda, C.P. (1975) Structuralism in cognitive developmental psychology: Past, contemporary and future perspective. In K.F. Riegel and G.C. Rosenwals (Eds.) *Structure and transformation*. New York: John Wiley & Sons.

Lowenthal, M.F., Thurnber, M., and Chiriboga, D. (1976) *Four stages of life*. San Francisco: Jossey-Bass.

Josselyn, I.M. (1948) *Psychosocial development of children*. New York: Family Service Association of America.

Maier, H.W. (1963) *Three theories of child development*. New York: Harper & Row.

Maier, H.W. (1978) The psychoanalytic theory of Erik H. Erikson. In *Three theories of child development*, rev'd ed. New York: Harper & Row.

Neugarten, B. (Ed.). (1968) *Middle age and aging*. Chicago: University of Chicago Press.

Papalia, D. and Wendkos Olds, S. (1981) The adolescent. In *Human development* (2nd ed.). New York: McGraw-Hill.

Peck, R.C. (1968) Psychological developments in the second half of life. In B.L. Neugarten, (Ed.), *Middle age and aging* (pp. 88–92). Chicago: University of Chicago Press.

Pulaski, M. (1971) *Understanding Piaget*. New York: Harper & Row.

Reed, P.G. (1983) Implications of the life-span developmental framework for well-being in adulthood and aging. *Advances in Nursing Science*, 6(1), 18–25.

Riegel, K.F. (1969) History as a nomothetic science: Some generalizations from theory and research in developmental psychology. *Journal of Social Issues*, 4, 99–127.

Riegel, K.F. (1972) Influence of economic and political ideologies on the development of developmental psychology. *Psychological Bulletin*, 78(2), 129–141.

Roazen, P. (1976) *Erik H. Erikson*. New York: Free Press.

Roberts, S. (1980) Piaget's theory reapplied to the critically ill. *Advances in Nursing Science*, 2(2), 61–79.

Rowe, G.P. (1966) The developmental conceptual framework to the study of the family. In F.I. Nye and F.M. Berardo (Eds.), *Emerging conceptual frameworks in family analysis*. New York: Praeger.

Sanford, N. (1966) *Self and society: Social change and individual development*. New York: Atherton Press.

Schaie, W.K. (1977–1978) Toward a stage theory of adult cognitive development. *International Journal of Aging and Human Development*, 8(2), 129–138.

Schuster, C. (1980) *The process of human development*. Boston: Little, Brown & Co.

Sheehy, G. (1976) *Passages: Predictable crises of adult life*. New York: E.P. Dutton & Co.

Sullivan, C., Grant, M.Q., and Grant, J.D. (1957) The development of interpersonal maturity: Application to delinquency. *Psychiatry*, 20, 373–385.

Sullivan, H.S. (1953) *Interpersonal theory of psychiatry*. New York: W.W. Norton.

Thibaut, J.W. and Kelley, H.H. (1967) *The social psychology of groups, Part I: Dyadic Relationships*. New York: John Wiley & Sons.

Thomas, H. (1970) Theory of aging and cognitive theory of personality. *Human Development*, 13(1), 1–16.

Thomas, A. (1981) Current trends in developmental theory. *American Journal of Orthopsychiatry*, 51(4), 580–609.

Toffler, A. (1971) *Future shock*. New York: Bantam/Random House.

Troll, L.E. (1975) *Early and middle adulthood: The best is yet to be—maybe*. Monterey, CA: Brooks/Cole.

Van Den Daele, L.D. (1975) Ego development and preferential judgment in life span perspective. In N. Datan and L.H. Ginsberg (Eds.), *Life-span developmental psychology*. New York: Academic Press.

Wadsworth, B.J. (1971) *Piaget's theory of cognitive development*. New York: David McKay Co.

Waechter, E.H. (1980) The developmental model. In M. Kalkman and A. Davis (Eds.) *New dimensions in mental health—psychiatric nursing* (2nd ed.). New York: McGraw-Hill.

Wahba, M. and Bridwell, L.G. (1976) Maslow reconsidered: A review of research on the need for hierarchy theory. *Organizational Behavior and Human Performance*, 15, 212–224.

Wolman, B.B. (Ed.) (1982) *Handbook of developmental psychology*. Englewood Cliffs, NJ: Prentice-Hall.

19. Systems Theory

Abbey, J.C. (1970) General system theory: A framework for nursing. In J. Smith (Ed.), *Improvement of curricula in schools of nursing through selection and application of care concepts of nursing: An interim report.* Boulder, CO: Western Interstate Commission for Higher Education.

Allport, G.W. (1960) The open system in personality theory. *Journal of Abnormal and Social Psychology*, 61, 310–21.

Altschul, A.T. (1978) A systems' approach to the nursing process. *Journal of Advanced Nursing*, 3(4), 333–340.

Battista, J.R. (1977) The holistic paradigm and general systems theory. *General Systems Yearbook*, 22, 65–71.

Beavers, W.R. (1977) Systems theory, family systems, and the self. In *Psychotherapy and growth: A family perspective* (pp. 19–41). New York: Brunner-Mazel.

Becht G. (1974, October) Systems theory, the key to holism and reductionism. *Bio Science*, 24(10), 569–578.

Bertalanffy, L. von. (1967) *Robots, men and minds*. Part 2. New York: George Braziller.

Bertalanffy, L. von. (1968) *General systems theory: Foundations, development application*, rev'd ed. New York: George Braziller.

Bertalanffy, L. von. (1969) General systems theory and psychiatry—an overview. In W. Gray et al. (Eds.) *General systems theory and psychiatry* (pp. 33–50). Boston: Little, Brown & Co.

Bertalanffy, L. von. (1975) *Perspectives on general systems theory*. New York: George Braziller.

Black, M. (1961) *The social theories of Talcott Parsons: A critical examination*. Englewood Cliffs, NJ: Prentice-Hall.

Boulding, K.E. (1956) General systems theory—the skeleton of science. *Management Science*, 2, 197–208.

Brody, H. and Sobel, D.S. (1980) A systems view of health and disease. *Holistic Health Review*, 3(3), 163–178.

Broderick, C. and Smith, J. (1979) The general systems approach to family. In W.R. Burr (Ed.), *Contemporary theories about the family* (pp. 112–129). New York: Free Press.

Buckley, W. (1967) *Sociology and modern systems theory*. Englewood Cliffs, NJ: Prentice-Hall.

Bunge, M. (1977) General systems and holism. *General Systems Yearbook*, 22, 87–90.

Bunge, M. (1979) A systems concept of society; beyond individualism and holism. *General Systems Yearbook*, 24, 27–44.

Chin, R. (1961) The utility of system models and developmental models for practitioners. In W.G. Bennis, K.D. Benne and R. Chin (Eds.), *The planning of change*. New York: Holt, Rinehart & Winston.

Chinn, P.L. (1979) Practice oriented theory: Part 2. *Advances in Nursing Science*, 1(2), 41–52.

Chrisman, M. and Riehl, J. (1980) The system-developmental stress model. In J.P. Riehl and C. Roy (Eds.), *Conceptual models for nursing practice* (2nd ed.). New York: Appleton-Century-Crofts.

Churchman, C.W. (1968) *The systems approach*. New York: Dell.

Cummings, T.G. (Ed.). (1981) *Systems theory for organizational development*. New York: John Wiley & Sons.

Demerath, N.J. and Peterson, R.A. (Eds.). (1967) *System, change and conflict*. New York: Free Press.

Emery, F.E. (Ed.). (1969) *Systems thinking*. Middlesex, UK: Penguin Books.

Ericson, R.F. (1979) Society for general systems research at twenty-five. What agenda for our second quarter century? *Behavioral Science*, 24(5), 225–237.

Gray, W. (1972) Bertalanffian principles as a basis for humanistic psychiatry. In E. Laszlo (Ed.), *The relevance of general systems theory*. New York: George Braziller.

Grinker, R.R. (Ed.). (1967) *Toward a unified theory of human behavior: An introduction to general systems theory*, rev'd ed. New York: Basic Books.

Hall, A.D. and Fagen, R.E. (1956) Definition of system. *General Systems Yearbook*, 1, 18–28.

Hamilton, G.A. (1979, January) Miller's living systems: A theory critique. *Advances in Nursing Science*, 1(2), 41–52.

Hazzard, M.E. (1971) An overview of systems theory. *Nursing Clinics of North America*, 6(3), 385–393.

Jantsch, E. (1970) Inter- and transdisciplinary university: A systems approach to education and innovation. *Policy Sciences*, 1, 403–428.

Kalmus, H. (Ed.). (1966) *Regulation and control in living systems*. New York: John Wiley & Sons.

Laszlo, E. (Ed.). (1972) *The relevance of general systems theory*. New York: George Braziller.

Laszlo, E. (1972) *The systems view of the world*. New York: George Braziller.

Laszlo, E. (1975) The meaning and significance of general systems theory. *Behavioral Science*, 20(1), 9–24.

Lilienfeld, R. (1978) *The rise of systems theory: An ideological analysis*. New York: John Wiley & Sons.

Maslow, A.H. (1970) *Motivation and personality* (2nd ed.). New York: Harper & Row.

Miller, J. (1965) Living systems: Basic concepts. *Behavioral Science*, 10, 193–237.

Parsons, T. (1951) *The social system*. London: Free Press of Glencoe.

Parsons. T. (1967) *Sociological theory and modern society*. New York: Free Press.

Pierce, L.M. (1972) Usefulness of a systems approach for problem conceptualization and investigation. *Nursing Research*, 21, 509–513.

Powers, P.S. and Girgenti, J.R. (1978) Analysis of a system. *JPN and Mental Health Services*, 17–22.

Prigogine, I. and Stengers, I. (1984) *Order out of chaos*. New York: Bantam Books.

Rapoport, A. (1970) Modern systems theory—an outlook for coping with change. *General Systems Yearbook*, 15, 15–25.

Ritterman, M.K. (1977) Paradigmatic classification of family therapy theories. *Family Process*, 16(1), 29–48.

Rudolph, E. (1980) Defining the parameters of general living systems theory. *The Family*, 7(2), 83–91.

Shrode, W.A. and Voich, D. (1974) *Organization and management: Basic systems concepts.* Homewood, IL: R.D. Irwin.

Sills, G.M. and Hall, J.E. (1977) A general systems perspective for nursing. In J.E. Hall and B.R. Weaver (Eds.), *Distributive nursing practice: A systems approach to community health* (pp. 19–28). Philadelphia: J.B. Lippincott.

Somers, J.B. (1977) Purpose and performance: A system analysis of nurse staffing. *Journal of Nursing Administration*, 7, 4–9.

Stephen W.R. (1978) Toward a redefinition of action theory: Paying the cognitive element its due. *American Journal of Sociology*, 83(6), 1317–1349.

Stevens, B.J. (1984) *Nursing theory, application, evaluation* (2nd ed.). Boston: Little, Brown & Co.

Sutherland, J.W. (1973) *A general systems philosophy for the social and behavioral sciences.* New York: George Braziller.

Tantsch, E. (1970) Inter- and transdisciplinary university: A systems approach to education and innovation. *Policy Sciences*, 1, 403–428.

Tashdjian, E. (1972) A systems approach to higher education with special reference to the core curriculum. *Policy Sciences*, 3, 219–33.

Wagner, P. (1977, Winter) Psychodynamic Formulation: General Systems Theory Model of a 19 Year-old Greek Paranoid Schizophrenic. UCSF, N 222B, Pat Underwood, Lecturer.

Weiner, N. (1948) *Cybernetics or control and communication in the animal and machine.* Paris: Herman and Cie.

Werley, H.H. et al. (Eds.). (1976) *Health research: The systems approach.* New York: Springer-Verlag.

20. Stress and Adaptation

Appley, M.H. (1971) *Adaptation—level theory: A symposium.* New York: Academic Press.

Auger, J.R. (1976) *Behavioral systems and nursing.* Englewood Cliffs, NJ: Prentice-Hall.

Bell, J.M. (1977) Stressful life events and coping methods in mental illness and wellness behaviors. *Nursing Research*, 26, 136–141.

Brower, H., Terri, F. and Baker, B.J. (1976) Using the adaptation model in a practitioner curriculum. *Nursing Outlook*, 24, 686–689.

Bruner, J. et al. (1966) *Studies in cognitive growth.* New York: John Wiley & Sons.

Coelho, G.V., Hamburg, D.A., and Adams, J.E. (1974) Introduction. In G.V. Coelho et al., *Coping and adaptation.* New York: Basic Books.

Cohen, F. and Lazarus, R. (1979) Coping with the stresses of illness. In G. Stine, F. Cohen, and N. Adler (Eds.), *Health psychology: A handbook.* San Francisco: Jossey-Bass.

Dobzhansky, T. (1962) *Mankind evolving.* New Haven, CT: Yale University Press.

Dobzhansky, T. (1967) Changing man. *Science*, 155, 409–415.

Dubos, R. (1965) Adaptation and its dangers. In *Man adapting* (pp. 254–280). New Haven, CT: Yale University Press.

Duffy, M.E. (1987) The concept of adaptation: Examining alternatives for the study of nursing phenomenon. *Scholarly Inquiry for Nursing Practice*, 3(1), 179–192.

Fagin, C. (1987) Stress: Implications for nursing research. *Image*, 19(1), 38–41.

Fielo, F.M.C. (1971) *Psychosocial nursing.* New York: Macmillan.

Folkman, S. and Lazarus, R. (1980) An analysis of coping in a middle-aged community sample. *Journal of Health and Social Behavior*, 21, 219–239.

Gossen, G. and Bush, H. (1979) Adaptation: A feedback process. *Advances in Nursing Science*, 1(4), 51–65.

Haan, N. (1969) A tripartite model of ego functioning values and clinical and research applications. *Journal of Nervous and Mental Disease*, 148, 14–30.

Hamburg, D.A., Coelho, G.V., and Adams, J.E. (1974) Coping and adaptation: Steps toward a synthesis of biological and social perspectives. In G.V. Coelho et al. (Eds.), *Coping and adaptation*. New York: Basic Books.

Harvey, O.J. (1966) *Experience, structure and adaptability*. New York: Springer-Verlag.

Helson, H. (1959) Adaptation level theory. In S. Koch (Ed.), *Psychology: A study of a science* (Vol. 1) (pp. 565–621). New York: McGraw-Hill.

Helson, H. (1964) *Adaptation level theory* (Chap. 2). New York: Harper & Row.

Mastal, M. and Hammond, H. (1980) Analysis and expansion of the Roy adaptation model: A contribution to holistic nursing. *Advances in Nursing Science*, 2(4), 71–81.

Minckley, B. et al. (1979) Myocardial infarct stress-of-transfer inventory: Development of a research tool. *Nursing Research*, 28(1), 4–10.

Murray, R. and Zentner, J. (1975) Application of adaptation theory to nursing. In R. Murray and J. Zentner (Eds.), *Nursing concepts for health promotion*. Englewood Cliffs, NJ: Prentice-Hall.

Murphy, J.F. (1971) *Adaptation as a unifying theory: Theoretical issues in professional nursing* (Chap. 4). New York: Appleton-Century-Crofts, Education Division.

Rabkin, J.G. and Struening, E.L. (1976) Life events, stress and illness. *Science*, 194, 1013–1020.

Redman, B.K. (1974) Why develop a conceptual framework? *Journal of Nursing Education*, 13, 2–10.

Riehl, J and Roy, C. (1974) *Conceptual models for nursing practice*. New York: Appleton-Century-Crofts.

Roy, C. (1971, April) Adaptation: A basis for nursing practice. *Nursing Outlook*, 21, 254–257.

Roy, C. (1973, March) Adaptation: Implications for curriculum change. *Nursing Outlook*, 21, 163–168.

Roy, C. (1974) The Roy adaptation model. In J. Riehl and C. Roy, *Conceptual models for nursing practice*. New York: Appleton-Century-Crofts.

Sander, L.W. (1969) The longitudinal course of early mother-child interaction-cross-case comparison in a sample of mother-child pairs. In B.M. Foss, (Ed.), *Determinants of infant behavior IV* (pp. 189–227). London: Methuen.

Scott, J. (1977, February) Stress and coping: A case for intervention. *Journal of Psychiatric Nursing and Mental Health Services*, 15, 14–17.

Scott, R. and Howard, A. (1970) Models of stress. In S. Levine and N. Scotch, (Eds.), *Social stress*. Chicago: Aldine.

Scott, D.W., Oberst, M., and Dropkin, M. (1980) A stress-coping model. *Advances in Nursing Science*, 3(1), 9–23.

Scott, D.W., Oberst, M. and Bookbinder, M. (1984) Stress-coping response to genitourinary carcinoma in men. *Nursing Research*, 32(6), 325–329.

Selye, H. (1950) *The physiology and pathology of exposure to stress*. Montreal: ACTA Medical Publishers.

Selye, H. (1950, June 17) Stress and the general adaptation syndrome. *British Medical Journal*, 1383–1392.

Selye, H. (1964) *From dream to discovery*. New York: McGraw-Hill.

Selye, H. (1965) The stress syndrome. *American Journal of Nursing*, 65(3), 97–99.

Selye, H. (1976) *The nature of adaptation. The stress of life* (Chap. 14). New York: McGraw-Hill.

Spielberger, C.D. (1972) Anxiety as an emotional state. In *Anxiety: Current trends in theory and research*. New York: Academic Press.

Stone, G., Cohen, F., and Adler, N. (1979) *Health psychology: A handbook*. San Francisco: Jossey-Bass.

Thetford, W.N. and Schucman, H. (1971) Motivational factors and adaptive behavior. In J.A. Downey and R.C. Darling (Eds.), *Physiological basis of rehabilitation medicine* (pp. 353–371). Philadelphia: W.B. Saunders.

Vailliant, G.E. (1977) *Adaptation to life*. Boston: Little, Brown & Co.

Wagner, P. (1976) Testing the adaptation model in practice. *Nursing Outlook*, 24, 682–685.

Wild, B.S. and Hanes, C. (1976) A dynamic conceptual framework of generalized adaptation to stressful stimuli. *Psychological Reports*, 37, 319–334.

21. Role Theory

Banton, M. (1965) *Roles: An introduction to the study of social relations*. New York: Basic Books.

Bem, S. (1975) Sex roles adaptability: One consequence of psychological androgeny. *Journal of Personality and Social Psychology*, 31(4), 634–43.

Berk, B.B. and Victor G. (1975) Selection vs. role occupancy as determinants of role-related attitudes among psychiatric aides. *Journal of Health and Social Behavior*, 16(2), 183–191.

Bertrand, A. (1972) *Social organization: A general systems of role theory perspective*. Philadelphia: F.A. Davis.

Biddle, B. and Thomas, E. (Eds.). (1966) *Role theory: Concepts and research*. New York: John Wiley & Sons.

Biddle, B.J. (1979) *Role theory: Expectations, identities, and behaviors*. New York: Academic Press Inc.

Blasi, A.J. (1971–1972) Symbolic interactionism as theory. *Sociology and Social Research*, 56, 453–465.

Blumer, H. (1969) *Symbolic interactionism: Perspective and method*. Englewood Cliffs, NJ: Prentice-Hall.

Brouse, S.H. (1985) Effect of gender role identity patterns on self concept scores from later pregnancy to early post-partum. *Advances in Nursing Science*, 7(3), 32–48.

Bunch, B. and Zahra, D. (1976) Dealing with death: The unlearned role. *American Journal of Nursing*, 76(9), 1486–1488.

Burke, P.J. and Tully, J.C. (1977) The measurement of role identity. *Social Forces*, 54, '881–897.

Burr, W.R. (1972) Role transitions: A reformulation of theory. *Journal of Marriage and the Family*, 34, 407–416.

Conway, M.E. (1978) Theoretical approaches to the study of roles. In M. Hardy and M. Conway (Eds.), *Role theory: Perspectives for the health professional*. Norwalk, CT: Appleton-Century-Crofts.

Goffman, E. (1969) *Stigma*. Englewood Cliffs, NJ: Prentice-Hall.

Gordon, G. (1966) *Role theory and illness: A sociological perspective*. New Haven, CT: College and University Press.

Gross, N.C., Mason, W.S., and McEachern, A.W. (1958) *Explorations in role analysis: Studies of the school superintendency role*. New York: John Wiley & Sons.

Habeeb, M. and McLaughlin, F. (1977) Health care professional's role expectation and patient needs. *Nursing Research*, 26, 288–298.

Hadley, B.J. (1964) Nursing a la Weber. *Nursing Science*, 4, 95–110.

Hadley, B.J. (1967) The dynamic interactionist concept of role. *Journal of Nursing Education*, 2, 5–10.

Hardy, M. and Conway, M.E. (1989) *Role theory: Perspectives for health professionals.* New York: Appleton-Century-Crofts.

Heiss, J. (1976) *Family roles and interaction: An anthology* (2nd ed.). Chicago: Rand McNally & Co.

Jones, S.L. (1976) Socialization vs. selection factors as sources of student definitions of the nurse role. *International Journal of Nursing Studies*, 13(3), 135–138.

Kassebaum, G. and Baumann, B. (1965) Dimension of the sick role in chronic illness. *Journal of Health and Human Behavior*, 6, 16–27.

Keller, N.S. (1973) The nurse's role: Is it expanding or shrinking? *Nursing Outlook*, 21, 236–240.

Levenstein, A. (1976) Role ambiguity in nursing. *Supervisor Nurse*, 7(6). 16–17.

Lewandowski, L.A. and Kramer, M. (1980) Role transformation of special care unit nurses: A comparative study. *Nursing Research*, 29(3), 170–179.

Lindersmith, A.R. and Strauss, A.L. (1968) Roles, role behavior and social structure. In A.R. Lindersmith, A.L. Strauss, and N.K. Denzin (Eds.), *Social Psychology* (3rd ed.). (pp. 276–298). New York: Holt, Rinehart & Winston.

Lindersmith, A.R., Strauss, A.L., and Denzin, N. (1975) *Social Psychology* (4th ed.). Hinsdale, Illinois: Dryden Press.

Meleis, A.I. (1975) Role insufficiency and role supplementation: A conceptual framework. *Nursing Research*, 24, 264–271.

Meleis, A.I. (1971) Self-concept and family planning. *Nursing Research*, 20, 299–236.

Meleis, A.I. and Swendsen, L.A. (1978) Role supplementation: An empirical test of a nursing intervention. *Nursing Research*, 27(1), 11–18.

Mercer, R.T. (1985) The process of role attainment over the first year. *Nursing Research*, 34, 198–204.

Miyamoto, F.S. (1963) The impact of research of different conceptions of role. *Sociological Inquiry*, 33, 144–123.

Miyamoto, F.S. and Dornbush, S. (1956) A test of the symbolic interactionist hypothesis of self-conception. *American Journal of Sociology*, 61, 399–403.

Morgan, W.R.B. (1975) Role theory: An attribution theory interpretation. *Sociometry*, 38, 429–444.

Morris, C.W. (Ed.) (1962) *Herbert Mead, 1863–1931. Mind, self and society from the standpoint of a social behaviorist.* Chicago: University of Chicago Press.

Murphy, J. (1968) Psychiatric nurses and their patients: A study of role perception of performance. *Communicating Nursing Research*, 1, 139–150.

Oda, D. (1977) Specialized role development, a three phase process. *Nursing Outlook*, 25(6), 374–377.

Plutchik, R., Conte, H.R., Wells, W., and Darasu, T.B. (1976) Role of the psychiatric nurse. *Journal of Psychiatric Nursing and Mental Health Services*, 14(9), 38–43.

Porter, S.F. (1978) Interaction modeling. *Journal of Nursing Administration*, 8, 2024.

Robischon, P. and Scott, D. (1969) Role theory and its application in family nursing. *Nursing Outlook*, 17, 52–57.

Sarbin, T.R. (1954) Role theory. In G. Lindzey (Ed.) *Handbook of social psychology, Vol. 1. Theory and method* (pp. 223–258). Cambridge, MA: Addison-Wesley.

Sarbin, T.R. and Jones, D.S. (1955, September) An experimental analysis of role behavior. *Journal of Abnormal Social Psychology*, 51, 236–241.

Swendsen, L.A., Meleis, A.I., and Jones, D. (1978) Role supplementation for new parents—a role mastery plan. *American Journal of Maternal Child Nursing*, 3, 84–91.

Thornton, R. and Nardi, P. (1975) The dynamics of role acquisition. *American Journal of Sociology*, 80, 870–885.

Turner, R.H. (1962) Role taking: Process vs. conformity. In A. Rose (Ed.), *Human behavior and social processes*. Boston: Houghton-Mifflin.

Turner, R.H. (1970) *Family interaction*. New York: John Wiley & Sons.

Turner, R.H. (1976) The real self from institution to impulse. *American Journal of Sociology*, 81(5), 989–1016.

Turner, R.H. (1978) The role and the person. *American Journal of Sociology*, 84, 1–23.

Turner, R.H. and Shosid, N. (1976) Ambiguity and interchangeability in role attribution: The effect of alter's response. *American Sociological Review*, 41, 993–1006.

Videbeck, R. and Bates, A. (1959) An experimental study of conformity to role expectations. *Sociometry*, 22(1).

Ward, C.R. (1986) The meaning of role strain. *Advances in Nursing Science*, 8(2), 39–49.

Weiss, S.J. (1983) Role differentiation between nurses and physician: Implications for nursing. *Nursing Research*, 32(3), 133–139.

22. Physiological Nursing Theory

Badgley, L.E. (1985) Therapeutic application of extra low frequency electromagnetic fields to living tissue. *Journal of Holistic Medicine*, 7(2), 135–144.

Carrieri, V.K., Lindsey, A.M., and West, C.M. (1986) *Physiological phenomena in nursing: Human responses to illness*. Philadelphia: W.B. Saunders.

Feldman, H.R. (1984) Psychological differentiation and the phenomenon of pain. *Advances in Nursing Science*, 6(2), 50–57.

Janson-Bjerklie, S., Broushey, H.D., Carrieri, V.K., and Lindsey, A.I. (1986) Emotionally triggered asthma as a predictor of airway response to suggestion. *Research in Nursing and Health*, 9, 43–59.

Janson-Bjerklie, S., Carrieri, V., and Hudes, M. (1986) The sensations of dyspnea. *Nursing Research*, 35(3), 154–159.

Longworth, J. (1982) Psychophysiological effects of slow stroke back massage in normotensive females. *Advances in Nursing Science*, 4(4), 44–61.

Ng, L. and McCormick, K. (1982) Position changes and their physiological consequences. *Advances in Nursing Science*, 4(4), 13–25.

23. Critical Theory and Hermeneutics

Bauman, Z. (1978) *Hermeneutics and society science*. New York: Columbia University Press.

Bubner, R. et al. (Eds.) (1975) Theory and practice in the light of the hermeneutic-criticist controversy. *Cultural Hermeneutics*, 2, 237–377.

Bubner R. et al. (1976) Is transcendental hermeneutics possible? In J. Manninen and R. Tuomela (Eds)., *Essays on explanation and understanding: Studies in the foundations of humanities and social sciences*. Boston: D. Reidel Publishing Co. (pp. 59–77).

Dallmayr, W. (1972) Critical theory criticized: Habermas' knowledge and human interests and its aftermath. *Philosophy of Social Sciences*, 2, 211–229.

Floistad, G. (1973) Understanding hermeneutics. *Inquiry*, 16, 445–465.

Fraser, N. (1987) What's critical about critical theory? In S. Benhabib and D. Cornell (Eds.), *Feminism as critique* (pp. 31–55). Cambridge, UK: Polity Press.

Frye, M. (1983) On being white: Thinking toward a feminist understanding of race and race supremacy. *The Politics of Reality: Essays in Feminist Theory*, 110–127. New York: The Crossing Press.

Gadamer, H.G. (1975) Hermeneutics and social science. *Cultural Hermeneutics*, 2, 307–336.

Gadamer, H.G. (1976) *Philosophical hermeneutics*. Translated and edited by David E. Linge. Berkeley/Los Angeles/London: University of California Press.

Habermas, J. (1970) On systematically distorted communication. *Inquiry*, 13, 205–218.

Habermas, J. (1970) Towards a theory of communicative competence. *Inquiry*, 13, 360–375.

Habermas, J. (1971) *Knowledge and human interests*. Boston: Beacon Press.

Habermas, J. (1976) Theory and practice in a scientific society. In P. Connerton (Ed.), *Critical sociology* (pp. 331–347). New York: Penguin Books.

Habermas, J. (1977). A review of Gadamer's *Truth and Method*. In Dallmayr and McCarthy, 1977, pp. 335–363.

Habermas, J. (1984) *The theory of communicative action*, Vol. 2. T. McCarthy (Trans.). Boston: Beacon Press.

Hegel, G.W.F. (1931) *The phenomenology of mind* (2nd ed.). Translated with an introduction and notes by J.B. Baillie. London/New York: Macmillan.

Heidegger, M. (1962) *Being and time*. MacQuarrie, J. and Robinson, E. (Trans.). London: SCM Press.

Held, D. (1980) *Introduction to critical theory*. Berkeley: University of California Press.

Holter, I.M. (1988) Critical theory: A foundation for the development of nursing theories. *Scholarly Inquiry for Nursing Practice*, 2, 223–232.

Horkheimer, M. (1976) Traditional and critical theory. In P. Connerton (Ed.), *Critical sociology* (pp. 206–224). New York: Penguin Books.

Howard, R.J. (1982) *Three faces of hermeneutics: An introduction to current theories of understanding*. Berkeley: University of California Press.

Marshall, B.L. (1988) Feminist theory and critical theory. *Canadian Review of Sociology and Anthropology*, 25(2), 208–230.

McLain, B.R. (1988) Collaborative practice: A critical theory perspective. *Research in Nursing Health*, 11, 391–398.

Ruane, J. and Tood, J. (1988) The application of critical theory. *Political Studies*, 36, 533–538.

Scott, J.P. (1978) Critical social theory: An introduction and critique. *British Journal of Sociology*, 29(1), 1–20.

Thompson, J.B. and Held, D. (Eds.) (1982) *Habermas: Critical debates*. Cambridge, MA: M.I.T. Press.

Thompson, J.L. (1987) Critical scholarship: The critique of domination in nursing. *Advances in Nursing Science*, 10(1), 27–38.

24. Feminist Perspectives

Bartky, S.L. (1979) Toward a phenomenology of feminist consciousness. In S. Bishop and M. Weinzweig (Eds.), *Philosophy and women* (pp. 252–258). Belmont, CA: Wadsworth.

Belenky, M.F., Clinchy, B.M., Goldberger, N.R., and Tarule, J.M. (1986) *Women's ways of knowing*. New York: Basic Books.

Breines, W. (1986) The 1950s: Gender and some social science. *Sociological Inquiry*, 6(1), 69–93.

Chinn, P.L. and Wheeler, C.E. (1985) Feminism and nursing: Can nursing afford to remain aloof from the women's movement? *Nursing Outlook*, 33(2), 74–77.

Chinn, P.L. (1986) Feminism, knowledge development, and client/environment interaction. *Doctoral Forum Proceedings, 1986*. San Francisco: University of California.

Chinn, P.L. (1986) Feminist nursing literature? *Cassandra*, 4, 9–11.

Chinn, P.L. (1988) From the editor: The politics of knowing. *Advances in Nursing Science*, 10(4), Editorial.

Connell, M.T. (1983) Feminine consciousness and the nature of nursing practice: A historical perspective. *Topics in Clinical Nursing*, 5(3), 1–10.

Cook, J.A. and Fonow, M. (1986) Knowledge and women's interests: Issues of epistemology and methodology in feminist sociological research. *Sociological Inquiry*, 6(1), 2–29.

Cooper, M.C. (1982) Gilligan's different voice: A perspective for nursing. *Journal of Professional Nursing*, 5(1), 10–16.

Davis, A.Y. (1989) *Women, culture and politics*. New York: Random House.

de Beauvoir, S. (1970) *The second sex*. New York: Bantam.

Donovan, J. (1985) *Feminist theory: The intellectual traditions of American feminism*. New York: Frederick Ungar.

DuBois, B. (1983) Passionate scholarship: Notes on values, knowing and method in feminist social science. In G. Bowles and R. Klein (Eds.), *Theories of women's studies*. London: Routledge & Kegan Paul.

Duffy, M.E. (1985) A critique of research: A feminist perspective. *Health Care for Women International*, 6(5-6), 341–352.

Duffy, M. and Hedin, B. (1988) New directives. In N. Woods and M. Catanzano (Eds.), *Research methods for nursing science* (pp. 530–539). St. Louis: C.V. Mosby.

Eisler, R. (1988) *The chalice and the blade: Our history, our future*. San Francisco: Harper & Row.

Eisenstein, Z. (1977) Developing a theory of capitalist patriarchy and socialist feminism. *The Insurgent Sociologist*, 7(3), 5–40.

Farganis, S. (1986) Social theory and feminist theory: The need for dialogue. *Sociological Inquiry*, 56(1), 50–68.

Flax, J. (1987) Postmodernism and gender relations in feminist theory. *Signs*, 12, 621–643.

Gilligan, C. (1982) *In a different voice: Psychological theory and women's development*. Cambridge, MA: Harvard University Press.

Grady, K. (1981) Sex bias in research design. *Psychology of Women Quarterly*, 5, 628–637.

Hagell, E.I. (1989) Nursing knowledge: Women's knowledge. A sociological perspective. *Journal of Advanced Nursing*, 14(3), 226–233.

Harding, S. (1983) Common causes: Toward a reflexive feminist theory. *Women and Politics*, 3(4), 27–42.

Harding, S. (1986) *The science question in feminism*. Ithaca, NY: Cornell University Press.

Harding, S. (Ed.). (1987) *Feminism and methodology*. Bloomington: Indiana University Press.

Harding, S. (1988) Feminism confronts the sciences: Reform and transformation. In C. Bridges and N. Wells (Eds.), *Proceedings of the fifth nursing science colloquium* (pp. 73–92). Boston: Boston University.

Hedin, B. (1986) Nursing, education, and emancipation: Applying the critical theoretical approach to nursing research. In P. Chinn (Ed.), *Nursing research methodology: Issues and implementation* (pp. 133–146). Rockville, MD: Aspen Systems.

Hedin, B. and Donovan, J. (1989) A feminist perspective on nursing education. *Nurse Educator*, 14(4), 8–13.

Jaggar, A. (1979) Political philosophies of women's liberation. In S. Bishop and M. Weinzweig (Eds.), *Philosophy and women*. Belmont, CA: Wadsworth.

Jaggar A. and Struhl, P.R. (1978) *Feminist frameworks: Alternative theoretical accounts of the relations between women and men*. New York: McGraw-Hill.

Jayaratne, T.E. (1983) The value of quantitative methodology for feminist research. In G. Bowles and R.D. Klein (Eds.), *Theories of Women's Studies* (pp. 140–161). Boston: Routledge & Kegan Paul.

Joseph, G.I. and Lewis, J. (1981) *Common differences: Conflicts in black and white feminist perspectives.* Boston: South End Press.

Karabenies, A., Miller, L., Nagel-Bamesberger, H., Rossiter, A., and Thompson, M. (1986) What makes a feminist social science? *Cassandra: Radical Feminist Nurses Newsjournal,* 4(1), 9–11.

Keller, E.F. (1982) Feminism and science. In N.O. Keohane, M.Z. Rosaldo, and B.C. Gelpi (Eds.), *Feminist theory: A critique of ideology* (pp. 113–126). Chicago: University of Chicago Press.

Keller, E.F. (1983) *A feeling for the organism. The life and work of Barbara McClintock.* New York: W.H. Freeman.

Keller, E.F. (1985) *Reflections on gender and science.* New Haven, CT: Yale University Press.

Keohane, N.O., Rosaldo, M.Z., and Gelpi, B.C. (1981) *Feminist theory: A critique of ideology.* Chicago: University of Chicago Press.

Klein, R.D. (1983) How to do what we want to do: Thoughts about feminist methodology. In G. Bowles and R.D. Klein (Eds.), *Theories of women's studies* (pp. 88–104). Boston: Routledge & Kegan Paul.

Lengermann, P.M. and Niegrugge-Brantley, J. (1988) Contemporary feminist theory. In G. Ritzer (Ed.), *Contemporary sociological theory* (2nd ed.). New York: Alfred A. Knopf.

Longino, H.E. (1986) Can there be a feminist science? *Hypatia: Journal of Feminist Science.*

MacKinnon, C. (1982) Feminism, Marxism, method and the state: An agenda for theory. *Signs: Journal of Women in Culture and Society,* 7(3), 515–544.

MacPherson, K.I. (1983) Feminist methods: A new paradigm for nursing research. *Advances in Nursing Science,* 5(2), 17–25.

MacPherson, K.I. (1988) The missing piece: Women as partners in feminist research. *Advances in Nursing Science,* 5(2), 17–26.

Marshall, B.L. (1988) Feminist theory and critical theory. *Canadian Review of Sociology and Anthropology,* 25(2), 208–230.

Mies, M. (1983) Towards a methodology for feminist research. In G. Bowles and R. Klein (Eds.), *Theories of women's studies* (pp. 117–139). London: Routledge & Kegan Paul.

Moccia, P. (1988) A critique of compromise: Beyond the methods debate. *Advances in Nursing Science,* 10(4), 1–9.

Moraga, C. (1986) From a long line of vendidas: Chicanas and feminism. In T. de Lauretis (Ed.), *Feminist studies/critical studies* (Chap. 11). Bloomington: Indiana University Press.

Oakley, A. (1981) Interviewing women: A contradiction in terms. In H. Roberts (Ed.), *Doing feminist research* (Chap. 2). New York: Routledge & Kegan Paul.

Reason, P. and Rowan, J. (1981) *Human inquiry: A sourcebook of new paradigm research.* New York: John Wiley & Sons.

Reinharz, S. (1983) Experimental analysis: A contribution to feminist research. In G. Bowles and R. Klein (Eds.), *Theories of women studies.* London: Routledge & Kegan Paul.

Roberts, H. (1981) *Doing feminist research.* London: Routledge & Kegan Paul.

Rose, H. (1983) Hand, brain, and heart: A feminist epistemology for the natural sciences. *Signs: Journal of Women in Culture and Society,* 9(1), 73–90.

Rose, H. (1986) Beyond masculinist realities: A feminist epistemology for the sciences. In R. Bleier (Ed.), *Feminist approaches to science.* New York: Pergamon Press.

Sherwin, S. (1987) Concluding remarks: A feminist perspective. *Health Care for Women International*, 8(4), 293–304.

Smith, D. (1974) Women's perspective as a radical critique of sociology. *Sociological Inquiry*, 44, 7–13.

Stacey, J. and Thorne, B. (1985) The missing feminist revolution in sociology. *Social Problems*, 32(4), 301–316.

Thompson, J.L. (1985) Practical discourse in nursing: Going beyond empiricism and historicism. *Advances in Nursing Science*, 7(4), 59–71.

Tronto, J. (1987) Beyond gender difference to a theory of care. *Signs: Journal of Women in Culture and Society*, 12(4), 644–663.

25. Video and Audio Tapes on Theory

Video Productions

A Conversation with Virginia Henderson.

Interview with Virginia Henderson about her life and work, conducted by Patricia Moccia.
Available from: National League for Nursing, Publication and Video Order Unit, 350 Hudson Street, New York, NY 10014, (212) 989-9393 or (800) 669-1656.

Care with a Concept.

A video by Mary Hale and Gates Rhodes that discusses the clinical application of Dorothea Orem's self-care model in a pediatric rehabilitation center.
Available from: Health Sciences Consortium, 201 Silver Cedar Court, Chapel Hill, NC 27514, (919) 942-8731.

Nursing in America: A History of Social Reform.

Video that examines nursing's history of social reform while chronicling social, political, and economic influences that shaped American nursing.
Available from: National League for Nursing, Publication and Video Order Unit, 350 Hudson Street, New York, NY 10014, (212) 989-9393 or (800) 669-1656.

Nursing Theory: A Circle of Knowledge.

Video hosted by Patricia Moccia that examines issues related to philosophy of nursing science, particularly the relevance of nursing theory to practice. Features discussions with Patricia Benner, Virginia Henderson, Dorothea Orem, Martha Rogers, Callista Roy, and Jean Watson.
Available from: National League for Nursing Publication and Video Order Unit, 350 Hudson Street, New York, NY 10014, (212) 989-9393 or (800 669-1656).

The Nurse Theorists: Portraits of Excellence.

Series of 14 videos about the lives and scholarly accomplishments of notable nurse theorists. Each video contains a biographical sketch of the theorist, an interview conducted by Jacqueline Fawcett, and a summary of the nursing theory. Video tapes include: (1) Virginia Henderson, "Definition of Nursing"; (2) Dorothy Johnson, "Behavioral Systems Model"; (3) Imogene King, "Interacting System Framework"; (4) Madeline Leininger, "Transcultural Nursing Care"; (5) Myra Levine, "The Conservative Model"; (6) Betty Neuman, "Neuman Systems Model"; (7) Florence Nightingale, "Special Edition"; (8) Dorothea Orem, "Self Care Framework"; (9) Ida Orlando Pelletier, "The Deliberative Nursing Process"; (10) Hildegard Peplau, "Interpersonal Relations in Nursing"; (11) Martha Rogers, "Science of Unitary Human Beings"; (12) Callista Roy, "The Adaptations Model of Nursing"; (13) Reva Rubin, "Theory of Maternal Identity"; and (14) Jean Watson, "A Theory of Caring."
Available from: Fuld Theorists Video Project, Samuel Merritt College, Studio Three, 370 Hawthorne Avenue, Oakland, CA 94609-9910, (415) 420-6193.

Theories at Work.

Video hosted by Patricia Moccia about innovative applications of nursing theory in nurse-managed health care systems. Moccia visits centers of nursing practice around the country and talks with Dorothy Powell, Bernadine Lacey, Jean Watson, and Janet Quinn about their theory-based nursing care.

Available from: National League for Nursing, Publication and Video Order Unit, 350 Hudson Street, New York, NY 10014, (212) 989-9393 or (800) 669-1656.

Conference Video Tapes
Nurse Theorist Conference 1985,

Pittsburgh, PA. Video taped presentations by Dorothea Orem and Hildegard Peplau as well as a video taped panel discussion featuring Dorothea Orem, Callista Roy, Imogene King, Martha Rogers, Rosemarie Parse, and Hildegard Peplau.

Available from: Meetings Internationale, Ltd., 1200 Delor Avenue, Louisville, KY 40217, (502) 634-8229.

Nurse Theorist Conference 1987,

Pittsburgh, PA. Video tapes include (1) Hildegard Peplau, "Art and Science of Nursing"; (2) Imogene King, "King's Theory"; (3) Rosemarie Parse, "Parse's Theory"; (4) Callista Roy, "Roy's Model"; (5) Martha Rogers, "Rogers' Framework"; (6) Jean Watson, "Watson's Model"; (7) Rozella Schlotfeldt, "Nursing Science in the 21st Century"; and (8) Panel Discussion with Theorists."

Available from: Meetings Internationale, Ltd., 1200 Delor Avenue, Louisville, KY 40217, (502) 634-8229.

Nurse Theorist Conference 1989,

Pittsburgh, PA. Video tapes include: (1) Afaf Meleis, "Being and Becoming Healthy: The Core of Nursing Knowledge"; (2) Betty Neuman, "Health as a Continuum in Neuman's Model"; (3) Rosemarie Parse, "Health as a Personal Commitment in Parse's Theory"; (4) Martha Rogers, "Evolutionary Emergence: Infinite Potential"; (5) Nola Pender, "Expressing Health Through Beliefs and Actions"; (6) Imogene King, "Health as the Goal of Nursing in King's Theory"; and (7) "Panel Discussion with Theorists."

Available from: Meetings Internationale, Ltd., 1200 Delor Avenue, Louisville, KY 40217, (502) 634-8229.

Conference Audio Tapes
Nursing Theory Congress 1986,

Toronto, Canada. Audio tapes of plenary sessions by Betty Neuman, Imogene King, Callista Roy, Rosemarie Parse, Martha Rogers, and Myra Levine. Other audio tapes include: (1) Moyra Allen, "A Developmental Health Model: Nursing as Continuous Inquiry"; (2) Patricia James and James Dickoff, "Overview of the Concept of Theoretical Pluralism"; (3) Bonnie Holaday, "Adaptation of Johnson's Framework"; (4) Susan Taylor, "Presenting Orem's Framework"; (5) Phyllis Kritek, "Impact of Nursing Theory on the Diagnostic Process"; and (6) Marian McGee, "Criteria for Selection and Use of a Nursing Model for Clinical Practice."

Available from: Audio Archives International, 100 West Beaver Creek, Unit 18, Richmond Hill, Ontario, Canada, L4B 1H4, (416) 889-6555.

Nursing Theory Congress 1988,

Toronto, Canada. Audio tapes include: (1) Carol Lindeman, "Nursing Theory: Elitism or Realism in 1988"; (2) Virginia Henderson, "Nursing Theory: A Historical Perspective"; (3) Jean Watson, "One Model or Many Models"; (4) Marjory Gordon, "Nursing Diagnosis: The Interface of Nursing Theory and Nursing Process"; (5) Rosemarie Parse, "Nursing Science as a Basis for Research"; (6) Phyllis Kritek and others, "Impact of Nursing Theory on the Profession"; and (7) Phyllis Kritek, "Agendas for the Future."

Available from: Audio Archives International, 100 West Beaver Creek, Unit 18, Richmond Hill, Ontario, Canada L4B 1H4, (416 888-6555). {*/ABIB*}

ACKNOWLEDGMENTS

The comprehensiveness of the bibliography in this chapter would not have been possible without the contributions of many doctoral students over the years. For the second edition, the assistance of Sirion Sindhu with the bibliography updating and of Patricia Stevens and Joanne Hall in compiling the list for audio and video tapes is particularly acknowledged and appreciated.

Index

The letter *t* after a page number indicates tabular material.

Author Index

Index

The letter *f* after a page number indicates a figure; *t* following a page number indicates tabular material.

Subject Index